S0-BXE-338

RECENT ADVANCES
IN CARDIOLOGY

JOHN HAMER

MD PhD FRCP
*Cardiologist, St Bartholomew's Hospital,
London.*

RECENT ADVANCES IN CARDIOLOGY

EDITED BY

JOHN HAMER

NUMBER SEVEN

RC681
E13
1977

CHURCHILL LIVINGSTONE
Edinburgh, London and New York
1977

338362

CHURCHILL LIVINGSTONE
Medical Division of Longman Group Limited

Distributed in the United States of America by
Longman Inc., 19 West 44th Street, New York,
N.Y. 10036, and by associated companies,
branches and representatives throughout the
world

© LONGMAN GROUP LIMITED 1977

All rights reserved. No part of this publication
may be reproduced, stored in a retrieval system,
or transmitted in any form or by any means,
electronic, mechanical, photocopying, recording
or otherwise, without the prior permission of
the publishers (Churchill Livingstone, 23 Ravelston
Terrace, Edinburgh EH4 3TL)

First published 1977

ISBN 0 443 01560 0
Library of Congress Cataloging in Publication Data
Main entry under title:
Recent advances in cardiology.
  Includes bibliographies and index.
  1. Cardiology.   I. Hamer, John.   [DNLM:
1. Cardiovascular diseases.   WG100 R293]
RC681.A25R43 1977   616.1′2   76–55787

Printed in Great Britain
by Adlard and Son, Dorking

PREFACE

The situation is still changing so fast in cardiology that we feel no need to apologise for a fresh edition of *Recent Advances in Cardiology* a few years after the previous one. While adhering to the previous policy of dealing with fundamental topics, major clinical problems and advances in therapeutics, the change in the contributors from the previous edition represents the new emphases of recent years. We return to presentation of new material on arrhythmias which have been neglected for several editions, although well covered years ago by East and Bain. Although once said to be the 'cardiological menopause' an interest in arrhythmias is no longer an old man's topic and the many new advances in our understanding of this subject produced by young workers in recent years are shown by Dr Krikler's descriptive chapter and Dr Spurrell's section on surgical treatment. The increased interest in coronary artery surgery has now been digested in Britain and is shown in Dr Rees' chapter on radiology and Mr Rees' section on the surgical aspects.

I have not thought it any part of my editorial duties to produce a uniformity of view among contributors, rather to encourage understanding by allowing overlap between chapters to show different points of view in controversial areas. You will find cardiac surgery in the neonate covered both by Dr Jordan from the physician's point of view and by Mr Rees speaking as a cardiac surgeon. The use of beta-adrenergic blocking agents in hypertension is discussed both by Dr Prichard, as an experienced user of these drugs and in my own chapter from a more theoretical point of view. Dr Aber's comments on arrhythmias in cardiac infarction add clinical flesh to the bones of Dr Krikler's largely diagnostic chapter on arrhythmias and Dr Kumana's contribution on anti-arrhythmic drugs. The appearance of two chapters on heart failure reflects the different research interests of Dr Taylor and myself, Dr Taylor being particularly interested in treatments aimed at reducing the load on the left ventricle and my own work being concerned with myocardial performance and the effects of digitalis and diuretic treatment.

London, 1977

JOHN HAMER

CONTRIBUTORS

CLIVE ABER MD FRCP
Cardiologist, Kingston-upon-Hull, North Humberside

PAUL V. L. CURRY MB MRCP
Honorary Senior Registrar, Hammersmith Hospital; Assistant Lecturer in Cardiovascular Diseases, Royal Postgraduate Medical School, London

C. R. W. EDWARDS MD MRCP
Senior Lecturer in Medicine and Honorary Consultant Physician, St Bartholomew's Hospital, London

D. G. GIBSON MB BChir FRCP
Cardiologist, Brompton Hospital, London

JOHN HAMER MD PhD FRCP
Cardiologist, St Bartholomew's Hospital, London

S. C. JORDAN MD FRCP
Cardiologist, Bristol General Hospital, Bristol

DENNIS M. KRIKLER MD FRCP
Cardiologist, Hammersmith Hospital; Lecturer in Cardiovascular Diseases, Royal Postgraduate Medical School, London

C. R. KUMANA MD MRCP
Lecturer in Clinical Pharmacology, Hamilton General Hospital, McMaster Clinical Unit, Hamilton, Ontario

J. R. MUIR DM FRCP
Professor of Cardiology, Welsh National School of Medicine, Cardiff

M. I. M. NOBLE PhD MD MRCP
Consultant Physician, King Edward VII Hospital, Midhurst, Charing Cross Hospital, and Midhurst Medical Research Institute, Midhurst, Sussex

FRANCIS O'GRADY MD MRCP FRCPath
Foundation Professor of Microbiology, University of Nottingham

E. G. J. OLSEN MD
Consultant Pathologist, National Heart Hospital; Honorary Lecturer, Cardiothoracic Institute, University of London

B. N. C. PRICHARD MB MSc MRCP
Consultant Physician, Hypertension Clinic, University College Hospital; Reader in Clinical Pharmacology, Medical Unit, University College Hospital Medical School, London

GARETH M. REES MS FRCS MRCP
Cardiothoracic Surgeon, St Bartholomew's Hospital, London

SIMON REES MA MB FRCP FRCR
Radiologist, St Bartholomew's Hospital and National Heart Hospital, London; Lecturer, Cardiothoracic Institute, University of London

LEON RESNEKOV MD(Cape Town) FRCP
Joint Director, Section of Cardiology, Professor of Medicine, University of Chicago, Illinois

T. R. D. SHAW BSc MB ChB MRCP
Senior Registrar in Cardiology, Western General Hospital, Edinburgh

R. A. J. SPURRELL MD BSc MRCP FACC
Cardiologist, St Bartholomew's Hospital, London

M. R. STEPHENS MD MRCP
Lecturer in Cardiology, Welsh National School of Medicine, Cardiff

S. H. TAYLOR MB ChB FRCP(Edin)
Senior Lecturer in Medicine, University of Leeds; Physician, Leeds General Hospital

J. TUCKMAN MD
Senior Research Fellow, Hypertension Clinic, University College Hospital and Department of Clinical Pharmacology, University College Hospital Medical School, London

CONTENTS

Preface   v

Contributors   vii

1. Paediatric Cardiology *S. C. Jordan*   1

2. Radioisotope Techniques in Cardiac Diagnosis *Leon Resnekov*   27

3. Radiology in Coronary Artery Disease *Simon Rees*   45

4. Coronary Care *Clive Aber*   63

5. Electrocardiographic Features of Cardiac Arrhythmias
   Dennis M. Krikler   Paul V. L. Curry   81

6. Drug Therapy in the Management of Cardiac Tachyarrhythmias
   C. R. Kumana   131

7. Therapeutic Uses of β-Adrenergic Blocking Drugs *John Hamer*   171

8. Aetiology of Hypertension *C. R. W. Edwards*   199

9. Treatment of Hypertension *B. N. C. Prichard   J. Tuckman*   227

10. Cardiac Metabolism *M. R. Stephens   J. R. Muir*   263

11. Myocardial Performance *M. I. M. Noble*   285

12. Clinical Assessment of Left Ventricular Function *D. G. Gibson*   315

13. Myocardial Biopsy *E. G. J. Olsen*   349

14. Heart Failure—I *S. H. Taylor*   369

15. Heart Failure—II *John Hamer*   399

16. Clinical Pharmacokinetics of Digitalis *T. R. D. Shaw*   425

17. Infective Endocarditis *John Hamer   Francis O'Grady*   447

18. Surgical Treatment *Gareth M. Rees   R. A. J. Spurrell*   473

Index   501

1

PAEDIATRIC CARDIOLOGY

S. C. Jordan

Today, paediatric cardiology in the Western World is almost exclusively concerned with the treatment of congenital heart disease, and brings physician and surgeon closer together than in almost any other branch of medicine. This cooperation has established firm principles for the treatment of individual lesions and the understanding of the abnormal anatomy and physiology on which advances in treatment of complex abnormalities can be planned.

SURGICAL TREATMENT

The Beginning

The successful resection of coarctation of the aorta and closure of patent ductus arteriosus in the 1930s and 1940s meant that about 12 per cent of congenital heart disease could be cured. In the 1950s the application of surface cooling ('conventional' hypothermia) with circulatory arrest for 5 to 7 min brought pulmonary stenosis and atrial septal defect within the curable category, making the total 'potentially correctable' group about 35 per cent, although, because of the benign nature of mild pulmonary stenosis and small or moderate sized atrial septal defects, the impact in terms of reducing mortality and morbidity was rather less than the figures imply.

Technical Developments

The end of the sixth and the early part of the seventh decade of the century brought the routine use of cardiopulmonary bypass and profound hypothermia for uncomplicated ventricular septal defect, severe aortic stenosis (with valvotomy or replacement), Fallot's tetralogy and a few less common lesions, notably total anomalous pulmonary venous connection. At this stage surgery was virtually limited to obstructive lesions and shunts, and to many it seemed fanciful to think that more complex lesions could be corrected. However, with Mustard's description of his operation for transposition of the great arteries in 1964 and its subsequent adoption on a large scale, all of the eight common forms of congenital heart disease, accounting for about 80 per cent of the total number of patients with congenital heart disease could now be cured. To this could be added a further 3 per cent consisting of the uncommon lesions of total anomalous pulmonary venous connection, atrioventricular canal of the less severe (ostium primum) type, left ventricular to right atrial shunt (Gerbode defect), subaortic stenosis, lone infundibular stenosis and cor triatriatum, so that in theory only about 15 per cent of children with congenital heart disease were unable to be cured. Subsequent progress in this group will be described later, but the difference between the potential and actual success rates of the 85 per cent of 'curable' patients needs to be considered.

Operations in the First Year of Life

Many of the poor results in this group of patients could be related to the early onset of symptoms and the need to carry out surgery within the first year of life. Miller (1974) reporting on the management of 111 infants presenting in the first week of life, found that the overall mortality was 69 per cent, although 50 per cent had curable lesions and only 11 per cent were unsuitable for any form of surgical treatment. There is therefore clearly a need for improvement in diagnosis, surgical techniques and pre- and postoperative care. The high incidence of pulmonary complications after the use of cardiopulmonary bypass in the first year of life and the technical difficulties of carrying out cannulation of right and left sides of the heart (quadruple cannulation) by Drew's technique in small infants have been responsible for the reluctance to advise early corrective surgery for such conditions as large ventricular septal defect, severe Fallot's tetralogy and transposition of the great arteries. This has led to the use of palliative rather than corrective operations in infancy.

Ventricular Septal Defect

Banding of the pulmonary artery was for many years the standard operation for infants with large ventricular septal defects. The operation proved to be simple and safe in experienced hands, but subsequent closure of the ventricular septal defect is made more hazardous. There are few reports of large series of patients, but Coleman et al (1972) had 4 deaths in 15 patients. The result of debanding may not be very satisfactory for Dobell et al (1973) in a study of 18 patients on average of four years after debanding and VSD closure found gradients of up to 72 mmHg (9.6 kPa) across the site of debanding and felt that these gradients would increase with further growth of the child. Girod et al (1974) had better results in 34 patients, all banded before the age of one year. There were four deaths from banding and one from debanding and closure of ventricular septal defect and the highest postoperative gradient across the repaired pulmonary artery was 25 mmHg (3.3 kPa).

Fallot's Tetralogy

Palliative operations for Fallot's tetralogy in the first two years of life have never been very satisfactory. Closed pulmonary valvotomy produces only temporary improvement, infundibular resection is technically difficult and also produces only temporary improvement. Blalock–Taussing shunts are difficult and rarely remain patent, Potts anastomosis is very difficult to close subsequently and the Waterston operation is difficult to judge and may lead to proximal obstruction of the right pulmonary artery and unilateral pulmonary oedema or pulmonary arterial hypertension in the right lung.

This led to something of a vicious circle with patients being operated on only when in extremis, with further worsening of the overall surgical mortality. The vicious circle was broken by the introduction of the technique of extended surface cooling, thus greatly reducing the period of bypass required. Good results were quickly reported for large ventricular septal defects, Fallot's tetralogy and transposition of the great arteries (Barratt Boyes, Simpson and Neutze, 1971; Venugopal et al, 1973). Encouraged by these results operation was extended to the less critically ill infant, and in this situation some surgeons found it possible to revert to conventional cardiopulmonary bypass or bypass-induced profound hypothermia with equally successful results, so avoiding the long period of time required for surface cooling (Stark, 1972). Many surgeons now operate routinely on infants in the first few months of life.

Another cause of high mortality, often linked with the necessity for early operation, was particularly unfavourable anatomy. This particularly applied to Fallot's tetralogy with a very under-developed right ventricular outflow tract and therefore a large right to left shunt. This problem is still largely unresolved, but the ability to use right ventricular outflow tract reconstruction at a later stage has made it more acceptable to carry out a palliative shunt in infancy, without the worry of being unable to correct the lesion later due to further atrophy of the outflow tract.

Total correction in infancy however has the advantage that muscular hypertrophy of the outflow tract of the right ventricle is less than in older patients. Rees and Starr (1973) reported nine patients aged 5 to 11 months with one death and virtually normal postoperative right ventricular pressures (30–40 mmHg, 3.8–5.0 kPa) and in a larger series of 25 patients corrected under two years of age Starr, Bonchek and Sunderland (1973) had only two deaths from total correction compared with five deaths in a similar group of 16 patients treated just with palliative shunts.

Adverse Factors in Infancy

Complicating factors, both physiological and anatomical, have also been a cause of poor surgical results.

Ventricular Muscle Disease

In severe obstructive lesions there may be hypoplastic ventricular cavities, gross ventricular hypertrophy or fibroelastosis. Freed et al (1973) found that of 19 patients presenting with cyanosis due to severe pulmonary stenosis in the neonatal period 13 had some degree of hypoplasia of the right ventricular cavity. However, all of the 12 who were treated by pulmonary valvotomy survived (although two required a further valvotomy subsequently). One patient was treated with a palliative shunt and died. Similarly Miller et al (1973) reported five patients with severe pulmonary stenosis treated by pulmonary valvotomy and all survived. However, of their 15 patients with pulmonary atresia, all of whom had small right ventricular cavities, seven died during or immediately following operation and five later, the only three survivors being those treated by systemic-pulmonary artery shunts. Until a few years ago pulmonary valvotomy was attempted in all cases of pulmonary atresia as it provided the only hope of ultimate correction. The development of the Fontan operation (see later), with its greater potential, now makes palliation by some form of shunt a better prospect when the right ventricular cavity is very small. In severe aortic stenosis presenting with symptoms in infancy the problems are even worse. Lakier et al (1974) found that of ten such patients only two had a small left ventricular cavity. Nevertheless three died prior to surgery and only one survived surgery. They attribute these poor results to a very hypertrophied, non-compliant left ventricle.

Hypertensive pulmonary vascular disease associated with intracardiac shunts, particularly ventricular septal defect, has been the most important physiological problem. It is likely that most patients with high pulmonary vascular resistance, including those who end up with the Einsemenger syndrome, have during early infancy gone through a stage when pulmonary blood flow is relatively high and hypertensive pulmonary vascular disease is reversible. Now that corrective surgery in infancy has an acceptable mortality, and provided these patients can be detected at the operable stage, the problem should be overcome.

Right Ventricular Outflow Reconstruction

Considerable progress has been made in treating the 15 per cent of patients with the more complex lesions. Right ventricular outflow tract reconstruction (Rastelli operation) has made curable pulmonary valve atresia with ventricular septal defect, persistent truncus arteriosus and transposition of the great arteries with ventricular septal defect and pulmonary or subpulmonary obstruction (the group having in common a discontinuity of pulmonary artery and right ventricle). In the least complicated of these lesions, pulmonary atresia with ventricular septal defect, the results of reconstruction have been good using a homograft aorta (with aortic valve in situ) and heterogenous valves sewn into a Dacron tube, but the use of fascia lata has proved unsatis-factory as there is shrinkage with recurrence of right ventricular outflow obstruction (Macartney, Scott and Ionescu, 1975). In the more complicated lesions problems have occurred in locating the graft so that kinking and obstruction do not occur. In order to ensure a free exit from the right ventricle into the conduit the latter must be angulated forwards and, particularly in small children, this has then become squashed when the sternum is closed over it. To avoid this some surgeons advise leaving a window in the sternum and McGoon, Wallace and Danielson (1973) suggest using a conduit directed more to the left and carefully measured for size. When the pulmonary artery lies behind the aorta, in transposition, greater care has also to be used to place the distal end of the conduit around the aorta without obstruction or tension. McGoon et al (1973) reported on their results in 111 operations, all using homografts of aorta, including the aortic valve. The overall mortality was 32 per cent and was similar in the three main lesions treated, persistent truncus arteriosus, transposition with ventricular septal defect and pulmonary stenosis and pulmonary atresia with ventricular septal defect. As might be expected the worst results were in patients under the age of two years with a mortality of 80 per cent and the best results (18 per cent mortality) were in the 5 to 12 year group. Over 12 years the mortality was again higher (32 per cent) mainly due to the presence of hypertensive pulmonary vascular disease and multiple previous operations.

The particular problems in the overall management of persistent truncus arteriosus (the lesion for which the Rastelli operation was originally designed) are highlighted by a report of Poirier, Berman and Stansel (1975). From the literature they estimated that in untreated patients the mean age at death was two and a half months. Twenty-two reports of banding of the pulmonary artery in 76 patients gave an overall mortality of 50 per cent, although in the most propitious, type I cases (where a common pulmonary trunk arises from the base of the truncus) it was 33 per cent. Against this must be set the known high mortality, untreated, in infancy and the virtual certainty of hypertensive pulmonary vascular disease in unbanded survivors. In eight reports of the Rastelli procedure, including the 58 in Rastelli's own group, mortality varied from 29 to 100 per cent.

Double Outlet Right Ventricle

On a slightly less dramatic note, progress has been made in dealing with varieties of malposition of the great arteries other than complete transposition. Much of the lack of success in the earliest attempts to cure these lesions resulted from a lack of definition of the exact anatomy. Both great arteries may arise from the right ventricle, with or without pulmonary stenosis. This may be associated with malposition of the aorta and pulmonary artery with respect to each other, as well as with respect to the two ventricles (Lincoln et al,

1975). When the ventricular septal defect is immediately below the aorta, repair is relatively straightforward as a patch can be inserted from the ventricular septal defect to the anterior margin of the aorta so that the left ventricular outflow through the ventricular septal defect is channelled exclusively into the aorta. Attempts to treat the other variety in which the ventricular septal defect lies below the pulmonary valve, by producing a much longer tunnel within the right ventricle from ventricular septal defect to aorta, have seldom been successful and a more promising approach is to direct left ventricular outflow into the pulmonary artery producing physiologically complete transposition and to make an intra-atrial baffle (Mustard procedure) to divert systemic venous return to the left ventricle and pulmonary venous return to the right.

Double Outlet Left Ventricle

Comparatively little has been written about the condition in which both great arteries arise from the left ventricle. Pacifico et al (1973) report on four cases (three with associated pulmonary stenosis). The same operation can be carried out irrespective of the relationship of the ventricular septal defect to the two great arteries, for the ventricular septal defect is closed, the outflow to the pulmonary artery from the left ventricle is also closed and a conduit containing a homograft or heterograft aortic vale is placed between the right ventricle and the pulmonary artery.

Since many operations on complex lesions, from severe Fallot's tetralogy to double outlet left ventricle, now require construction of a right ventricular outflow tract, the fate of this reconstruction is of considerable importance. Kaplan et al (1973) reviewed 150 patients, many with severe Fallot's tetralogy, treated by patching the outflow tract or by homograft reconstruction. They found that homografts continued to function very well (although the actual conduit may calcify) whereas patch reconstruction led to aneurysm formation and embolism into the lungs.

Single Ventricle

A significant advance in terms of lesions previously regarded as uncorrectable has occurred in the treatment of single or common ventricle. (The two terms are interchangeable in terms of physiology although their use is disputed on anatomic and embryologic grounds.) Previously the best that could be hoped for was to produce a circulation with adequate but not excessive pulmonary blood flow by either banding the pulmonary artery if there was no pulmonary stenosis or carrying out a Blalock shunt or Glenn operation for those with pulmonary stenosis and much reduced pulmonary blood flow. An optimal situation would be a pulmonary blood flow about twice normal, since this load is reasonably well tolerated, cyanosis is minimal and there is no significant elevation of pulmonary artery pressure. (Patients without pulmonary stenosis or pulmonary artery banding usually develop pulmonary hypertensive vascular disease which by the age of two to three years makes them inoperable.) Sporadic attempts have been made to divide the single ventricle in the past, and the use of the Fontan operation will be mentioned later but it is only recently that the principles on which successful septation of the single ventricle are based have been determined.

The first principle is to determine the *site of the conducting tissue* which, in single ventricle, is usually posteriorly situated (Anderson et al, 1974) but its position cannot always be predicted. Edie et al (1973) advocate the use of a probe to detect the His bundle activity. They reported four patients treated successfully by inserting a patch in the common ventricle, placing all sutures well away from areas in which His bundle activity was detected.

The second principle is to place the patch to give *the most direct pathway* between each AV valve and its nearest semilunar valve. This usually results functionally in the production of a situation of physiological transposition and it is then necessary to carry out an interatrial baffle procedure (Mustard operation) to provide physiological correlation (Edie et al, 1973). If there is an inadequate outflow to the pulmonary artery it may be necessary to reconstruct this in the same way as for pulmonary atresia or severe Fallot's tetralogy (Ionescu, Macartney and Wooler, 1973).

The third principle is to *correct associated abnormalities* which may include abnormalities of pulmonary venous drainage.

Clearly these complex operations still require considerable further experience before they can be regarded as standard procedures, but the results so far are promising, and although operation cannot usually be attempted before the age of 8 to 10 years, there is now a considerable stimulus to preserving infants with single ventricle by early palliative operations designed to produce a reasonable growth and exercise tolerance and to prevent the development of hypertensive pulmonary vascular disease. When there is no pulmonary stenosis this will usually entail banding of the pulmonary artery in infancy, and in the presence of severe pulmonary stenosis a palliative Blalock–Taussig shunt will be required to relieve cyanosis.

Tricuspid Atresia

Tricuspid atresia has until just recently been regarded by most surgeons with little enthusiasm. Although arterial to pulmonary artery shunt or Glenn (superior vena cava to right pulmonary artery) anastomosis provides palliation, the long-term outlook for affected children has been poor.

In the normal heart, and in cyanotic lesions with right heart obstruction and reduced pulmonary blood flow, it is known that the pulmonary artery pressure is only slightly higher than that in the right atrium. In the Glenn operation the additional pressure is provided by the hydrostatic pressure in the superior vena cava, especially when the patient is upright, but no similar way could be found to allow inferior vena caval blood to perfuse the lungs.

Fontan and Baudet (1971) realised that the right atrium could provide this small extra pressure (particularly when, as commonly occurs in tricuspid atresia, it is hypertrophied) provided that reflux down the inferior vena cava could be prevented during atrial contraction. The solution was to provide a conduit, from the right atrium to the pulmonary artery and place a homograft aortic valve at the junction of inferior vena cava and right atrium. In their first patient, aged 12, Fontan and Baudet carried out a Glenn procedure and then anastomosed the right atrial appendage to the proximal stump of the right pulmonary artery (Fig. 1.1A). In their second patient they used a conduit containing a homograft aortic valve from the right atrium to the main pulmon-

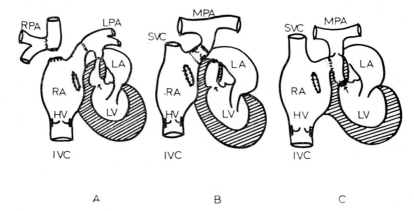

A   B   C

Figure 1.1   Fontan operation. (For description see text.) HV, homograft aortic valve; IVC, inferior vena cava; LA, left atrium; LV, left ventricle; LPA, left pulmonary artery; MPA, main pulmonary artery; RPA, right pulmonary artery; RA, right atrium. The arrow points to the ventricular septal defect, which is closed in C

ary artery (Fig. 1.1B) and used the right atrium to perfuse the whole pulmonary bed. Both these patients had a homograft inserted at the IVC–right atrial junction and both survived, although a third died. Kreutzer et al (1973) introduced a modification for patients in whom the pulmonary valve was normal, in which the conduit from the right atrium is inserted below the pulmonary valve into the rudimentary right ventricle and the ventricular septal defect closed, so avoiding the use of two homografts (Fig. 1.1C). Both their two patients survived.

Several groups have now reported their results with this operation (Stanford et al, 1973; Walker, Sbokos and Lennox, 1975) and it seems clear that dramatic improvement can be obtained. Most of the reports include patients who have previously had a Glenn operation and since in these the right atrium has only to handle a little over half the venous return these are a particularly favourable group. Most reports, though, are of only a few patients and it is equally clear that many problems need to be clarified. In most instances the immediate postoperative period is complicated by a considerable rise in right atrial pressure. One frequent consequence of this is that atrial fibrillation occurs and with the lack of atrial transport the right side of the heart acts only as a conduit. Long-term survival with atrial fibrillation has been reported but only at the price of a permanently raised venous pressure. In the few days following operation problems in fluid balance are almost invariable (Walker et al, 1975). Large amounts of intravenous fluids are required to maintain an adequate cardiac output and some of these problems are related to the effects of distension of the right atrium in stimulating stretch refluxes and producing both reflex cardiac acceleration and reflex suppression of antidiuretic hormone release.

The discovery that, even with the right atrium acting merely as a conduit, survival is possible has led some surgeons to perform the operation without the use of an IVC–RA homograft valve (Kreutzer et al, 1973). (The insertion of the valve is made difficult by the need to maintain cannulation of the IVC during cardiopulmonary bypass.) Although there have been some survivors using this simpler technique it has been necessary at times to insert the valve at a later stage in order to control severe right heart failure. Because of the need to insert a conduit and valve which will remain of adequate size into adult life the optimum age for operation is not before about seven to eight years although a few surgeons have reported success in younger children.

Since the success of the operation depends partly on the degree of the hypertrophy of the right atrium, the long-term possibility of the operation needs to be considered in the early palliative management of the condition. Formerly it was usual to perform balloon septostomy or surgical septectomy to ensure free drainage of blood from right atrium to left atrium, but now it may be better to leave the right atrium with a little obstruction to ensure adequate hypertrophy.

Fontan Operation in Other Lesions

Although the operation of right atrial to pulmonary artery conduit was originally designed for tricuspid atresia its potential use is more widespread. Because of the low pumping pressure possible it can only be applied where the pulmonary vascular resistance is normal. In pulmonary atresia with intact interventricular septum and hypoplastic right ventricle the haemodynamics are almost identical to those of tricuspid atresia. Although in some patients early pulmonary valvotomy may allow the right ventricle to grow this is not always the case and where the right ventricle retains its minute cavity and thick non-compliant walls, Fontan's operation represents a big improvement in prognosis. In single ventricle with pulmonary stenosis, or where the pulmonary artery has been banded early enough in life to prevent hypertensive pulmonary vascular disease, the operation is carried out as for tricuspid atresia, the tricuspid valve being closed over from the right atrium by a patch.

Stanley and Kolff (1973) made one interesting observation from their experience of this operation. It has been known that in severe cyanotic congenital heart disease there is a considerable collateral circulation to the lungs, but whether this joined the pulmonary circulation at the precapillary or capillary level was uncertain. However, during perfusion of two patients for Fontan operations for tricuspid atresia (both had had previous Glenn operation) they found that blood passed from the collaterals through the alveolar circulation to the pulmonary arteries, establishing the capillaries as the point of entry of the collateral vessels.

Valve Replacement in Children

One of the major disadvantages that confront the paediatric cardiac surgeon, which does not trouble his counterpart operating only on adults, is the impracticability of valve replacement during the years of rapid growth of the child. However, Klint et al (1972) have now reported their results in 14 children aged $4\frac{1}{2}$ to 15 years, all given prosthetic valves (including one triple valve replacement). There were five deaths and nine survivors. They also reviewed a total of 166 paediatric patients treated by valve replacement (176 valves in all). One hundred and eighteen of these patients were given anticoagulants, in general with no more problems than in adults and the overall rate of systemic embolism in the whole group was 5 per cent. In patients of 10 years and over requiring valve replacement it was generally found that the degree of cardiac enlargement was great enough to allow adult sized prostheses to be used. Cartmill et al (1974) also reported the use of tilting-disc prostheses in right ventricular outflow reconstruction. These results should certainly encourage wider use of valve replacement in life-threatening situations in children.

INVESTIGATION OF CONGENITAL HEART DISEASE

More complex operations call for more detailed and meticulous investigation and cardiac catheterisation and angiocardiography are still the mainstay of preoperative diagnosis. Advances have been mainly in the accurate and more detailed anatomical and physiological diagnosis of uncommon and complex lesions.

Blood supply in pulmonary atresia

In pulmonary atresia with ventricular septal defect it is necessary to know not only the anatomy of the blood vessels carrying blood to the lungs but also the pressures in the different parts of the pulmonary arterial tree. Macartney, Scott and Deverall (1974) demonstrated that the blood supply to the lungs may come from several sources but that only by catheterising individual vessels was it possible to detect those patients with a discrete pulmonary trunk with a low pressure which were suitable for operation. Similar findings were reported by Chestler, Matisonn and Beck (1974), although they found that the majority of patients had the least complicated system, that is central pulmonary arteries supplied by a single vessel, usually the ductus.

New Angiographic Studies

Although angiography has been employed routinely for well over 25 years in the diagnosis of congenital heart disease, new and specific patterns are still being demonstrated which have previously passed unrecognised. The classical example was the 'goose-neck' deformity of endocardial cushion defects (Baron et al, 1964). More recently at least three new angiographic patterns have been recognised and their surgical implications reported.

Aorto-left ventricular tunnel

Somerville, English and Ross (1974) reviewed their experience in diagnosing and treating patients with aorto-left ventricular tunnels. Although rare, the condition should be considered in any child with clinical signs of isolated, severe aortic regurgitation, because true aortic valve incompetence is itself rare in childhood. The lesion can readily be demonstrated by angiography because, unlike a sinus of Valsava aneurysm, the tunnel arises at right angles to the aorta before turning downwards to enter the left ventricle (Fig. 1.2). Early diagnosis and repair are indicated as distortion of the aortic valve ring with the production of valvar regurgitation resulted in their oldest patient.

Congenital mitral valve abnormalities

Mitral valve obstruction is uncommon as a congenital lesion, but when it is detected clinically or haemodynamically an accurate anatomical diagnosis is essential prior to surgery. Macartney et al (1974) reported on the angiographic features of two uncommon forms of mitral obstruction. Supravalvular rings were shown in two patients as discrete indentations within the left atrium, close to the valve ring. Four patients had evidence of parachute mitral valves. The single papillary muscle was demonstrated as a filling defect on left ventricular angiography (Fig. 1.3) almost dividing the left ventricular cavity into anterior and posterior portions (egg-timer deformity) and in one patient it was large enough to cause obstruction to left ventricular outflow. Treatment of supravalvar mitral rings is easily accomplished by excision. The parachute mitral valve cannot open or close properly because of its short chordae tendineae attached to the apex of the single papillary muscle. Although some success has been achieved by splitting the muscle, in many cases mitral valve replacement is required.

Tricuspid pouch

The specific angiographic features of endocardial cushion defect have already been mentioned. Kudo et al (1974) reported a previously unrecognised feature in 15 of 118 patients with endocardial cushion defects whom they investigated, namely the tricuspid pouch. This is best seen in the lateral view of a left ventricular angiogram and always occurs in the anterior third of the septal leaflet of the tricuspid valve, the posterior portion of this leaflet being hypoplastic. It does not cause obstruction to inflow or outflow in the right ventricle and its importance is that it always indicates a type II defect, that is

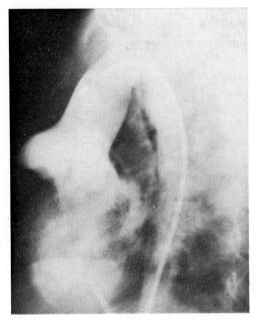

Figure 1.2   Aorta to left ventricular tunnel, filling from the back of the aorta. (Illustration supplied by Dr Jane Somerville.)

one with continuity of tricuspid and mitral valves across a depressed inter-ventricular septum.

Aneurysm of left ventricular septum

A lesion somewhat similar to tricuspid pouch is the aneurysm of the inter-ventricular septum. This was previously regarded as a rarity, but Lambert et al (1974) found 44 instances in a total of 250 left ventricular angiograms in patients with congenital heart disease, 34 of whom had small ventricular septal defects and Freedom et al (1974) found that of 56 children with small ventricular septal defects (pulmonary to systemic flow ratio of 2:1 or less) 20 had aneurysms of the membraneous septum at initial examination and a further 12 had developed by the time of repeat left ventricular angiography four years later. Seven of these 12 patients showed a reduction in the size of the shunt associated with the development of the aneurysm and it seems clear that the formation of the aneurysm is associated in some way with the process of closure in many children.

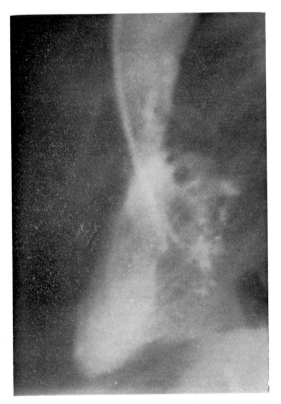

Figure 1.3 Parachute mitral valve. Left ventricular angiogram, left lateral view showing a large, single papillary muscle producing a filling defect (egg-timer defect)

Ultrasound Diagnosis

The use of diagnostic ultrasound in studying the heart is almost a quarter of a century old, yet it is only in the last five years that its potential in congenital heart disease has been realised. Undoubtedly the introduction of strip recorders and continuous M-mode presentation have made easier the recording and understanding of records from children with complex lesions. In principle there are several basic ways in which conventional ultrasound may give diagnostic information. The position and sizes of the two ventricles at end systole and end diastole allow an estimate of left ventricular stroke volume and cardiac output to be made. The extent and speed of movement of the mitral and tricuspid valves are an indication, amongst other things, of the volume of blood entering the left and right ventricles respectively and therefore are useful in assessing the size of intracardiac shunts. The relative positions of the aorta and pulmonary valve can be assessed and, particularly important in congenital heart disease, their continuity with structures inside the heart, particularly the anterior cusp of the mitral valve and the interventricular septum can be demonstrated. Abnormal structures (septa, aneurysms and tunnels) can also be shown. The movement of the aortic and (sometimes) pulmonary valve can be demonstrated. The thickness of the interventricular septum and the free wall of the left ventricle can also be measured and thickening of other structures, particularly the heart valves, often demonstrated.

Normal values

As is common with any new technique early reports were confined to recognition of specific qualitative abnormalities and it is only recently that normal values for the sizes of cardiac chambers and valve excursions have been made in children (Lunstrom, 1974; Meyer, Stockert and Kaplan, 1975) and neonates (Hagan et al, 1973; Solinger, Elbl and Minhas, 1973) and these validated against angiographic data (Lundstrom and Mortensson, 1974; Kaye, Tynan and Hunter, 1975). In addition Sahn et al (1974) have used ultrasound to study the changes in left ventricular function over the first few hours of life. They showed that left ventricular contractility, measured as mean velocity of circumferential left ventricular fibre shortening, increased to a maximum at the age of 1 h and then remained constant.

Septal defects

Atrial septal defect was the first congenital lesion to be systematically studied. The right ventricular dimension is increased and the excursion and speed of opening of the tricuspid valve are both increased (Diamond et al, 1971). A specific feature of the volume overload of the right ventricle in large defects is paradoxical movement of the interventricular septum, and this has been confirmed in children (Tajik et al, 1972). The septum normally moves posteriorly during ventricular systole, but in atrial septal defect this is reversed, so that it behaves more as part of the right ventricular wall than, as normally, part of the left ventricle. This paradoxical movement is restored to normal in most patients following operative closure of the defect.

Endocardial cushion defects show a variety of ultrasound abnormalities depending on the degree of the defect. In the mildest type, the 'ostium primum' defect, Williams and Rudd (1974) showed echoes from the anterior leaflet of the mitral valve anterior to the level of the posterior aortic wall, which they felt was the ultrasound counterpart of the 'goose-neck' deformity in the angiocardiogram. Pieroni, Homcy and Freedom (1975) described four abnormal patterns: prolonged mitral approximation to the septum in diastole with shortening of mitral–septal distance, a common atrioventricular leaflet traversing the interventricular septum, continuity of tricuspid valve with interventricular septum, 'capping' the mitral valve and a double mitral valve echo in systole.

Ventricular septal defects, when small, show no specific features, although when large it may be possible to demonstrate the actual defect as a disappearance of the septal echo as the probe scans up from apex to aortic root (Feigenbaum, 1973). In large defects, the left ventricular systolic and diastolic dimensions are increased, particularly the latter, reflecting the high left ventricular stroke output, and the mitral valve excursion and velocity of movement are increased indicating rapid left ventricular filling. When the defect is complicated by severe pulmonary hypertension and reversal of shunt, the ventricular dimensions return to normal and in some instances the septum may move paradoxically.

Patent ductus arteriosus is most difficult to assess when it occurs in the premature infant, often associated with pulmonary disease. A non-invasive way of assessing its haemodynamic effect is invaluable and Baylen et al (1975) have described the use of ultrasound in 37 such infants. A total of 129 studies were carried out to assess the size of the left atrium and the left ventricular end–diastolic dimension, since both are an indication of the size of the left-to-right shunt. When these dimensions were large surgical closure of the ductus was almost always required. Following surgical or spontaneous closure of the ductus the dimensions fell rapidly to normal.

Fallot's tetralogy shows variable features depending on the severity and exact anatomical situation. The overriding of the aorta which is found in about 60 per cent of patients can be demonstrated by a continuous recording as the transducer is 'swept' from the aorta downwards to the left ventricle. The anterior wall of the aorta then lies anterior to the plane of the septum and the two are referred to as discontinuous. The posterior aortic wall, however, retains its continuity with the anterior cusp of the mitral valve, an important point in distinguishing it from more complex abnormalities, such as double outlet right ventricle.

Left heart obstruction

Aortic stenosis shows changes which are usually readily detectable. The aortic valve cusps can almost always be demonstrated and these normally move apart almost to the aortic wall in systole and close in the centre of the aorta in diastole. In aortic stenosis the degree of movement is limited (Gramiak and Shah, 1970) and in diastole the point of closure may be eccentric, especially in patients with a bicuspid valve (Nanda et al, 1974). In subaortic stenosis the aortic valve cusps may also not open fully, but due to the impingement of the systolic jet from the subvalvar stenosis the cusps show a systolic vibration (Fig. 1.4) which is not found in other conditions (Davies et al, 1974) and may also demonstrate premature closure. In addition, Lundstrom and Edler (1971) were able to demonstrate echoes from the membrane below the aortic valve.

In supra-aortic stenosis Nasrallah and Nihil (1975) have demonstrated the narrowed segment by sweeping upwards over the ascending aorta (Fig. 1.5).

The echocardiographic features of *idiopathic hypertrophic subaortic stenosis* (IHSS, hypertrophic obstructive cardiomyopathy) have been extensively studied. The thickness of the left ventricular wall is increased, but the inter-ventricular septum is thickened to a greater degree so that the ratio of thickness of the septum to free wall exceeds 1.2. In addition the mitral valve behaves abnormally showing an abrupt forward movement towards the septum in the later half a systole (Fig. 1.6). (It has recently been suggested that the apparent systolic anterior movement of the mitral valve may actually be caused by the

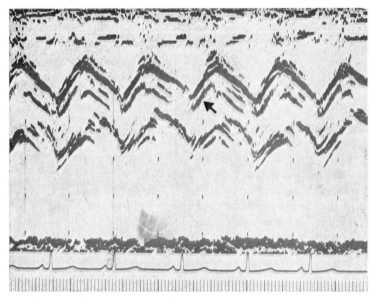

Figure 1.4   Discrete subaortic stenosis. The cusps of the aortic valve (arrowed) show fine vibrations during systole

hypertrophied papillary muscle which extends into the outflow tract of the left ventricle when the ventricle shortens in systole.) In addition, the aortic valve cusps may show early closure (Fig. 1.6) before the end of systole, in keeping with the fact that in hypertrophic obstructive cardiomyopathy (HOCM) almost all of left ventricular ejection takes place in the first half of systole. It is known that hypertrophic obstructive cardiomyopathy is some-what familial and Clark, Henry and Epstein (1973) used ultrasound to study relatives of patients with HOCM. They found an increased septal/free wall ratio in about 50 per cent of the first degree relatives, and always in one or other parent if they were both studied. They concluded that the disease was transmitted as an autosomal dominant but that many of the affected relatives did not show clinical or electrocardiographic abnormalities. Maron et al (1974)

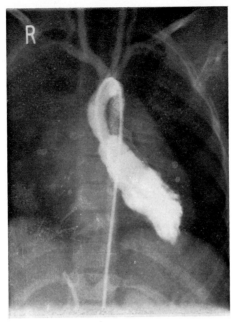

A.

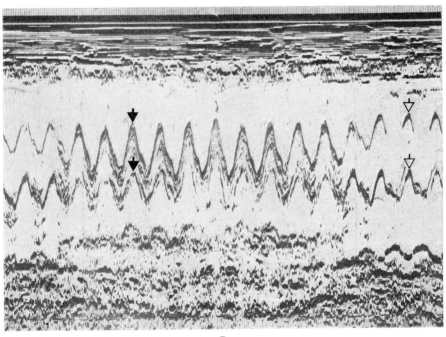

B.

Figure 1.5 Supra aortic stenosis. *A.* Angiogram. *B.* An ultrasound scan in which the transducer is angled from the aortic root upwards and then downwards again. The external diameter of the stenosed area (closed arrows) is reduced compared to the aortic root (open arrows) and the wall is thickened

studying relatives of infants with the condition also found at least one first-degree relative with echocardiogram or catheter evidence of thickening of the interventricular septum. These findings need to be confirmed but, if true, they raise important decisions regarding genetic counselling. More recently, however, Rossen et al (1974a) have found that in some patients with IHSS there is more generalised, concentric hypertrophy and stressed the import-ance of detecting systolic anterior movement of the mitral valve. The same authors in another report (Rossen et al, 1974b) found that in IHSS the thickened septum was functionally abnormal and showed less contractile

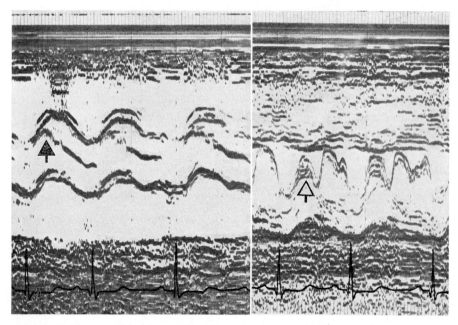

Figure 1.6   Hypertrophic obstructive cardiomyopathy. *A.* The aortic valve cusp (arrowed) shows premature closure and also systolic vibration. *B.* There is an echo (arrowed), apparent-ly continuous with the mitral valve, which moves forward in systole

movement so that the ratio of systolic thickness to diastolic thickness was less in IHSS than in normals.

Right heart lesions

The pulmonary valve is the most difficult of the heart valves to demonstrate by echocardiography and only a small portion of the valve can be demonstra-ted at any one time. In *pulmonary stenosis*, therefore, it is not possible to demonstrate the limited opening which is a feature of aortic stenosis. Weyman et al (1975) were able to demonstrate the presence of haemodynamically significant pulmonary stenosis in another way. When there is right ventricular hypertrophy the increased atrial contraction filling the right ventricle causes the pulmonary valve to make an opening movement prior to the onset of ventricular systole. This can be detected by ultrasound and the degree of movement is greater in severe stenosis. The same authors were able to distinguish valvular from infundibular stenosis for the latter condition produces a fluttering of the pulmonary valve in systole due to the turbulent jet from the infundibular obstruction.

Ebstein's anomaly of the tricuspid valve is usually easily diagnosed by a combination of clinical signs, radiology and electrocardiography, but the exact physiology of the valve function is still not well understood. Crews et al (1972) studied three patients and demonstrated that the most significant feature was greatly delayed tricuspid valve closure and Lundstrom (1973) confirmed these findings and also showed increased tricuspid excursion and a slow diastolic slope.

Miscellaneous lesions

The Gerbode defect (left ventricular to right atrial communication) is often difficult to distinguish clinically from ventricular septal defect. Nanda, Gramiak and Manning (1975) studied two patients and were able to demonstrate fluttering of the tricuspid valve during systole due to the jet of blood passing through the base of the valve. They were unable to find this in any other condition and regard it as specific for the Gerbode defect.

Cor triatriatum is a rare anomaly but its diagnosis often proves difficult. In particular, in children and adults with pulmonary hypertension it is one of the treatable causes which needs to be sought. Gibson, Honey and Lennox (1974) were able to demonstrate with echocardiograms a diaphragm behind the mitral valve. The pattern of movement was rather similar to that from the mitral valve ring. (The presence of a normal mitral valve movement is also useful in excluding mitral stenosis.) After operation the abnormal echo could no longer be demonstrated.

Complex congenital lesions, particularly those associated with a single ventricle, are difficult to diagnose accurately, even after angiography. It is important to differentiate single ventricle from tricuspid and mitral atresia, since the surgical treatment is different in each case, and in single ventricle the ultrasound cardiogram will show two valves (Chestler et al, 1970).

The more complicated forms of malposition of the great arteries are also difficult to diagnose angiographically, but echocardiography is helpful in establishing the presence or absence of continuity of one or other of the great arteries with the mitral valve. In double outlet right ventricle (origin of both great arteries from the right ventricle) neither pulmonary artery nor aorta are in continuity with the anterior cusp of the mitral valve and this can be demonstrated by the echocardiogram (Chestler et al, 1971) although it is important to demonstrate a sharp 'jump' between the anterior mitral valve leaflet and posterior aortic wall, as French and Popp (1975) have shown that an apparent, though more gradual, shift may be shown in other conditions, simply due to the differences in depth of the structures from the probe. In complete *transposition* the posterior aortic wall is continuous with the interventricular septum and the pulmonary valve and pulmonary artery can be demonstrated posteriorly, the posterior and anterior pulmonary artery echoes being continuous with those of the mitral valve and interventricular septum respectively (Gramaik et al, 1973). D-transposition is the only condition in which aortic and pulmonary valve echoes can be demonstrated at the same time (Dillon, Feigenbaum and Konecke, 1973).

Truncus arteriosus can also be diagnosed by ultrasound. The anterior and posterior truncal echoes are virtually continuous with anterior right ventricular wall and anterior mitral cusp echoes respectively, unlike pulmonary atresia with ventricular septal defect where the large aorta is continuous posteriorly with the mitral valve, but not anteriorly with the anterior right ventricular wall. However, it is important to search for echoes from the pulmonary valve since these features are not entirely specific (Chung et al, 1973).

In *total anomalous pulmonary venous connection* the right ventricle, tricuspid valve and interventricular septum show the same features of diastolic overload which are found in large atrial septal defects, but Paquet and Gutgesell (1975) found that the anomalous channel could also be demonstrated lying behind the left atrium.

Hypoplastic right and left heart syndromes are usually readily demonstrated by echocardiography, the small cavity of the hypoplastic ventricle contrasting with the large normal one (Meyer and Kaplan, 1972). Godman, Tham and Langford-Kidd (1974) reviewing their experience with 45 neonates with congenital heart disease found no false positives in the 12 patients they diagnosed with echocardiography as hypoplastic left heart syndrome. They suggested that the results in this lesion are sufficiently accurate to allow cardiac catheterisation to be dispensed with, particularly as this may be difficult to arrange in a rapidly deteriorating infant and as no surgical treatment is available.

Cardiac malposition

The congenital cardiac abnormalities associated with dextrocardia and isolated laevocardia are notoriously complex and difficult to establish, even by cardiac catheterisation. Meyer et al (1974) obtained useful information in 13 of 15 such patients, and in 11 a substantially correct diagnosis was established by echocardiography. Both they and Solinger, Elbl and Minhas (1975) recommend a similar approach to the problem. First the atrial situs is determined from chest radiographs, using the discovery of Van Meirop, Eisen and Schiebler (1970) that the longer of the two main bronchi is in relation to the anatomical 'left' atrium. The echocardiogram is then used to locate an atrioventricular valve in continuity with a semilunar valve and which must therefore be the mitral valve. The ventricular cavity in which this lies must be that of the anatomical 'left' ventricle. The other AV and semilunar valves are then detected and their relationship to the other chambers determined. Similarly the interventricular septum is located, if present.

Cardiac tumours

The use of ultrasound to detect atrial myxomas is well known. Farooki et al (1974) were also able to demonstrate two cases of ventricular rhabdomyoma. In one echoes were shown between the interventricular septum and mitral valve and in the other anterior to the ventricular septum in the right ventricle.

The measurement of left ventricular size and the calculation of stroke output and ejection fraction are important in the assessment of patients thought to have myocardial disease. Meyer et al (1975) studied 31 patients aged 2 to 15 years and found that left ventricular volumes could be determined by ultrasound as accurately as in adults. Sahn et al (1974) used a similar method for estimating left ventricular performance in the neonatal period and obtained consistent results. The electrocardiographic detection of left ventricular hypertrophy from measurement of QRS amplitude is often difficult in children since it is not uncommon to find values greater than the upper limits of normal in apparently healthy children. Morganroth et al (1975) studied 11 children in this group by echocardiography and were able to show that their measurement of interventricular septal and posterior left ventricular wall thickness were all within normal limits.

B-scan Techniques

The majority of echocardiography has been carried out using M-mode recording. Two-dimensional imaging of the heart, so useful in obstetrics and renal practice, is difficult to apply to the heart because of its rapid movement. However, using a scan triggered by the ECG so that all records are made at the same part in the cardiac cycle King (1973) has produced a technique which is useful in detecting the actual position of ventricular septal defects (King, Steeg and Ellis, 1973) and in determining the relative position of the great arteries (Henry et al, 1975).

Echocardiography has therefore shown its value in a wide range of paediatric problems from the sick neonate with complex congenital heart disease to the healthy child with a dubious electrocardiogram. Its great value in allowing repeated longitudinal studies is still to be exploited and doubtless many further advances will be made over the next few years.

REFERENCES

Anderson, R. H., Arnold, R., Thapar, M. I. C., Jones, R. S. & Hamilton, D. I. (1974) Cardiac specialised tissue in hearts with an apparently single ventricular chamber (double inlet left ventricle). *American Journal of Cardiology*, **33**, 95–106.

Baron, M. G., Wolf, B. S., Steinfeld, L. & Van Mierop, L. H. S. (1964) Endocardial cushion defects—specific diagnosis by angiocardiography. *American Journal of Cardiology*, **13**, 162–170.

Barratt Boyes, B. G., Simpson, M. & Neutze, J. M. (1971) Intracardiac surgery in neonates and infants using deep hypothermia with surface cooling and limited cardiopulmonary bypass. *Circulation*, **43** Suppl. 1, 25–30.

Baylen, B. G., Meyer, R. A., Kaplan, S., Ringenburg, W. E. & Korfhagen, J. (1975) The critically ill premature infant with patent ductus and pulmonary disease. An echocardiographic assessment. *Journal of Pediatrics*, **86**, 423–432.

Cartmill, T. B., Celermajer, D. S., Stuckey, D. S., Bowdler, J. D., Johnson, D. C. & Hawker, R. E. (1974) Use of Björk–Shiley tilting disc prosthesis in valved conduits for right ventricular outflow reconstruction. *British Heart Journal*, **36**, 1106–1114.

Chestler, E., Jaffe, H. S., Beck, W. & Schrire, V. (1970) Ultrasound cardiography in single ventricle and hypoplastic left and right heart syndromes. *Circulation*, **42**, 123–129.

Chestler, E., Jaffe, H. S., Beck, W. & Schrire, V. (1971) Echocardiographic recognition of mitral-semilunar valve discontinuity: an aid to the diagnosis of origin of both great vessels from the right ventricle. *Circulation*, **43**, 725–732.

Chestler, E., Matison,, R. & Beck, W. (1974) The assessment of the arterial supply to the lungs in pseudotruncus arteriosus and truncus arteriosus type IV in relation to surgical repair. *American Heart Journal*, **88**, 542–552.

Chung, K. J., Alexson, C. G., Manning, J. A. & Gramiak, R. (1973) Echocardiography in truncus arteriosus: the value of pulmonic valve detection. *Circulation*, **48**, 281–286.

Clark, C. E., Henry, W. L. & Epstein, S. E. (1973) Familial prevalence and genetic transmission of idiopathic hypertrophic subaortic stenosis. *New England Journal of Medicine*, **289**, 709–712.

Coleman, E. N., Reid, J. M., Barclay, R. S. & Stevenson, J. G. (1972) Ventricular septal defect repair after pulmonary artery banding. *British Heart Journal*, **34**, 134–138.

Crews, T. L., Pridie, R. B., Benham, R. & Leatham, A. (1972) Auscultatory and phonocardiographic findings in Ebstein's anomaly. Correlation of first heart sound with ultrasonic records of tricuspid valve movement. *British Heart Journal*, **34**, 681–693.

Davis, R. H., Feigenbaum, H., Chang, S., Konecke, L. L. & Dillon, J. C. (1974) Echocardiographic manifestations of discrete subaortic stenosis. *American Journal of Cardiology*, **33**, 277–280.

Diamond, M. A., Dillon, J. C., Haine, C. L., Chang, S. & Feigenbaum, H. (1971) Echocardiographic features of atrial septal defect. *Circulation*, **43**, 129–135.

Dillon, J. C., Feigenbaum, H. & Konecke, L. L. (1973) Echocardiographic manifestations of d-transposition of the great vessels. *American Journal of Cardiology*, **32**, 74–78.

Dobell, A. R. C., Murphy, D. A., Poirier, N. L. & Gibbons, J. E. (1973) The pulmonary artery after bebanding. *Journal of Thoracic and Cardiovascular Surgery*, **65**, 32–36.

Edie, R. N., Ellis, K., Gersony, W. M., Krongrad, E., Bowman, F. U. & Malm, J. R. (1973) Surgical repair of single ventricle. *Journal of Thoracic and Cardiovascular Surgery*, **66**, 350–360.

Farooki, Z. Q., Henry, J. G., Arciniegas, E. & Green, E. W. (1974) Ultrasonic pattern of ventricular rhabdomyoma in two infants. *American Journal of Cardiology*, **34**, 845–849.

Feigenbaum, H. (1973) Newer aspects of echocardiography. *Circulation*, **47**, 833–842.

Fontan, F. & Baudet, E. (1971) Surgical repair of tricuspid atresia. *Thorax*, **26**, 240–248.

Freed, M. D., Rosenthal, A., Bernhard, W. F., Litwin, S. B. & Nadas, A. S. (1973) Critical pulmonary stenosis with a diminutive right ventricle in neonates. *Circulation*, **48**, 875–882.

Freedom, R. M., White, R. D., Pieroni, D. R., Varghese, P. J., Krovetz, L. J. & Rower, R. D. (1974) The natural history of the so-called aneurysm of the membranous ventricular septum in childhood. *Circulation*, **49**, 375–384.

French, J. W. & Popp, R. (1975) Variability of echocardiographic discontinuity in double outlet right ventricle and truncus arteriosus. *Circulation*, **51**, 848–854.

Gibson, D. G., Honey, M. & Lennox, S. C. (1974) Cor triatriatum: diagnosis by echocardiography. *British Heart Journal*, **36**, 835–838.

Girod, D. A., Hurwitz, R. A., King, H. & Jolly, W. (1974) Recent results of two-stage surgical treatment of large ventricular septal defect. *Circulation*, **50**, Suppl. II, 9–12.

Godman, M. J., Tham, P. & Langford-Kidd, B. S. (1974) Echocardiography in the evaluation of the cyanotic newborn infant. *British Heart Journal*, **36**, 154–166.

Gramiak, R. & Shah, P. M. (1970) Echocardiography of the normal and diseased aortic valve. *Radiology*, **96**, 1–9.

Gramiak, R., Chung, K. J., Nanda, N. & Manning, J. (1973) Echocardiographic diagnosis of transposition of the great vessels. *Radiology*, **106**, 187–189.

Hagan, A. D., Deely, W. J., Sahn, D. & Friedman, W. F. (1973) Echocardiographic criteria for normal newborn infants. *Circulation*, **48**, 1221–1226.

Henry, W. L., Maron, B. J., Griffith, J. M., Redwood, D. R. and Esptein, S. E. (1975) Differential diagnosis of anomalies of the great arteries by real time, two-dimensional echocardiography. *Circulation*, **51**, 283–294.

Ionescu, M. I., Macartney, F. J. & Wooler, G. H. (1973) Intracardiac repair of single ventricle with pulmonary stenosis. *Journal of Thoracic and Cardiovascular Surgery*, **65**, 602–607.

Kaplan, S., Hemsworth, J. A., McKinivan, C. E., Benzing, G., Schwartz, D. C. & Schreiber, J. T. (1973) The fate of reconstruction of the right ventricular outflow tract. *Journal of Thoracic and Cardiovascular Surgery*, **66**, 361–369.

Kaye, H. H., Tynan, M. & Hunter, S. (1975) Validity of echocardiographic estimates of left ventricular size and performance in infants and children. *British Heart Journal*, **37**, 371–375.

King, D. L. (1973) Cardiac ultrasonography. Cross sectional imaging of the heart. *Circulation*, **47**, 843–847.

King, D. L., Steeg, C. N. & Ellis, K. (1973) Visualisation of ventricular septal defects by cardiac ultrasonography. *Circulation*, **48**, 1215–1220.

Kirklin, J. (1971) Pulmonary artery banding in babies with large ventricular septal defects. *Circulation*, **43**, 321–322.

Klint, R., Hernandez, A., Weldon, C., Hartmann, A. F. V. & Goldring, D. (1972) Replacement of cardiac valves in children. *Journal of Pediatrics*, **80**, 980–988.

Kreutzer, G., Galindez, E., Bond, H., dePalma, C. & Lavra, J. P. (1973) An operation for the correction of tricuspid atresia. *Journal of Thoracic and Cardiovascular Surgery*, **66**, 613–621.

Kudo, T., Yokoyama, M., Imai, Y., Konno, S. & Sakakibara, S. (1974) The tricuspid pouch in endocardial cushion defect. *American Heart Journal*, **87**, 544–549.

Lakier, J. B., Lewis, A. B., Heymann, M. A., Stanger, P., Hoffman, J. I. E. & Rudolph, A. M. (1974) Isolated aortic stenosis in the neonate. Natural history and haemodynamic considerations. *Circulation*, **50**, 801–808.

Lambert, M. E., Widlansky, Franken, E. A., Hurwitz, R. & Nasser, W. K. (1974) Natural history of ventricular septal defects associated with ventricular septal aneurysms. *American Heart Journal*, **88**, 566–569.

Lincoln, C., Anderson, R. H., Shinebourne, E. A., English, T. A. H. & Wilkinson, J. L. (1975) Double outlet right ventricle with 1-malposition of the aorta. *British Heart Journal*, **37**, 453–463.

Lundstrom, N. R. (1973) Echocardiography in the diagnosis of Ebstein's anomaly of the tricuspid valve. *Circulation*, **47**, 597–605.

Lundstrom, N. R. (1974) Clinical applications of echocardiography in infants and children. I. Investigation of infants and children without heart disease. *Acta pediatrica scandinavica*, **63**, 23–32.

Lundrom, N. R. & Edler, I. (1971) Ultrasound cardiography in infants and children. *Acta pediatrica scandinavica*, **60**, 117–123.

Lundstrom, N. R. & Mortensson, W. (1974) Clinical applications of echocardiography in infants and children. II. Estimation of aortic root diameter and left atrial size. A comparison between echocardiography and angiocardiography. *Acta pediatrica scandinavica*, **63**, 33–41.

Macartney, F. J., Scott, O. & Deverall, P. B. (1974) Haemodynamic and anatomical characteristics of pulmonary blood supply in pulmonary atresia with ventricular septal defect, including a case of persistent fifth aortic arch. *British Heart Journal*, **36**, 1049–1057.

Macartney, F. J., Scott, O. & Ionescu, M. I. (1975) Late haemodynamic results of fascia lata reconstruction of the right ventricular outlet. *American Heart Journal*, **89**, 195–199.

Macartney, F. J., Scott, O., Ionescu, M. I. & Deverall, P. B. (1974) Diagnosis and management of parachute mitral valve and supravalvar mitral ring. *British Heart Journal*, **36**, 641–652.

2

Maron, B. J., Edwards, J. E., Henry, W. L., Clark, C. E., Bingle, G. J. & Epstein, S. E. (1974) Asymmetric septal hypertrophy (ASH) in infancy. *Circulation*, **50**, 809–820.

McGoon, D. C., Wallace, R. B. & Danielson, G. K. (1973) The Rastelli operation. Its indications and results. *Journal of Thoracic and Cardiovascular Surgery*, **65**, 65–75.

Meyer, R. A. & Kaplan, S. (1972) Echocardiography in the diagnosis of hypoplasia of the left or right ventricle in the neonate. *Circulation*, **46**, 55–65.

Meyer, R. A., Schwartz, D. C., Covitz, W. & Kaplan, S. (1974) Echocardiographic assessment of cardiac malposition. *American Journal of Cardiology*, **33**, 897–903.

Meyer, R. A., Stockert, J. & Kaplan, S. (1975) Echographic determination of left ventricular volumes in pediatric patients. *Circulation*, **51**, 297–304.

Miller, G. A. H. (1974) Congenital heart disease in the first week of life. *British Heart Journal*, **36**, 1160–1166.

Miller, G. A. H., Restifo, M., Shinebourne, E. A., Paneth, M., Joseph, M. C., Lennox, S. C. & Kerr, I. H. (1973) Pulmonary atresia with intact ventricular septum and critical pulmonary stenosis presenting in first month of life. Investigation and surgical results. *British Heart Journal*, **35**, 9–15.

Morganroth, J., Maron, B. J., Krovetz, W., Henry, W. L. & Epstein, S. E. (1975) Electrocardiographic evidence of left ventricular hypertrophy in otherwise normal children. Clarification by echocardiography. *American Journal of Cardiology*, **35**, 278–285.

Nanda, N. C., Gramiak, R. & Manning, J. A. (1975) Echocardiography of the tricuspid valve in congenital left ventricular–right atrial communication. *Circulation*, **51**, 268–273.

Nanda, N. C., Gramiak, R., Manning, J. A., Mahoney, E. B., Lipchik, E. O. & Deweese, J. A. (1974) Echocardiographic recognition of the congenital bicuspid aortic valve. *Circulation*, **49**, 870–875.

Nasrallah, A. T. & Nihil, M. (1975) Supravalvular aortic stenosis: echocardiographic features. *British Heart Journal*, **37**, 662–667.

Pacifico, A. D., Kriklin, J. W., Bargeron, L. M. & Soto, B. (1973) Surgical treatment of double outlet left ventricle. Report of four cases. *Circulation*, **48**, Suppl. III, 19–23.

Paquet, M. & Gutgesell, H. (1975) Echocardiographic features of total anomalous pulmonary venous connection. *Circulation*, **51**, 599–605.

Pieroni, D. R., Homcy, E. & Freedom, R. M. (1975) Echocardiography in atrioventricular canal defect. A clinical spectrum. *American Journal of Cardiology*, **35**, 54–57.

Poirier, R. A., Berman, M. A. & Stansel, H. C. (1975) Current status of the surgical treatment of truncus arteriosus. *Journal of Thoracic and Cardiovascular Surgery*, **69**, 169–182.

Rees, G. M. & Starr, A. (1973) Total correction of Fallot's tetralogy in patients aged less than one year. *British Heart Journal*, **35**, 898–901.

Rossen, R. M., Goodman, D. J., Ingham, R. E. & Popp, R. L. (1974a) Ventricular septal thickening and excursion in idiopathic hypertrophic subaortic stenosis. *Circulation*, **50**, Suppl. III, 29.

Rossen, R. M., Goodman, D. J., Ingham, R. E. & Popp, R. L. (1974b) Echocardiographic criteria in the diagnosis of idiopathic hypertrophic subaortic stenosis. *Circulation*, **50**, 747–751.

Sahn, D. J., Deely, W. J., Hagan, A. D. & Friedman, W. F. (1974) Echocardiographic assessment of left ventricular performance in normal newborns. *Circulation*, **49**, 232–236.

Solinger, R., Elbl, F. & Minhas, K. (1973) Echocardiography in the normal neonate. *Circulation*, **47**, 108–118.

Solinger, R., Elbl, F. & Minhas, K. (1975) Deductive echocardiographic analysis in infants with congenital heart disease. *Circulation*, **50**, 1072–1096.

Somerville, J., English, T. & Ross, D. N. (1974) Aorto-left ventricular tunnel. Clinical features and surgical management. *British Heart Journal*, **36**, 321–328.

Stanford, W., Armstrong, R. G., Cline, R. E. & King, T. D. (1973) Right atrium-pulmonary artery allograft for correction of tricuspid atresia. *Journal of Thoracic and Cardiovascular Surgery*, **66**, 105–111.

Stanley, T. H. & Kolff, W. J. (1973) Reverse alveolar circulation in patients with cyanotic congenital heart disease. *Journal of Thoracic and Cardiovascular Surgery*, **66**, 16–21.

Stark, J. (1972) Cardiac surgery in early infancy. *Postgraduate Medical Journal*, **48**, 478–485.

Starr, A., Bonchek, L. I. & Sunderland, C. O. (1973) Total correction of tetralogy of Fallot in infancy. *Journal of Thoracic and Cardiovascular Surgery*, **65**, 45–57.

Tajik, A. J., Gau, G. T., Ritter, D. C. & Schattenberg, T. T. (1972) Echocardiographic pattern of right ventricular diastolic volume overload in children. *Circulation*, **46**, 36–43.

Van Mierop, L. H. S., Eisen, S. & Schiebler, E. S. (1970) The radiographic appearance of the tracheobronchial tree as an indication of visceral situs. *American Journal of Cardiology*, **26**, 432–438.

Venugopal, P., Olszowka, J., Wagner, H., Vlad, P., Lambert, E. & Subramanian, S. (1973) Early correction of congenital heart disease with surface induced deep hypothermia and circulatory arrest. *Journal of Thoracic and Cardiovascular Surgery*, **66**, 375–386.

Walker, D. R., Sbokos, C. G. & Lennox, S. G. (1975) Correction of tricuspid atresia. *British Heart Journal*, **37**, 282–389.

Weyman, A. E., Dillon, J. C., Feigenbaum, H. & Chang, S. (1975) Echocardiographic differentiation of infundibular from valvular pulmonary stenosis. *American Journal of Cardiology*, **36**, 21–26.

Williams, R. G. & Rudd, M. (1974) Echocardiographic features of endocardial cushion defect. *Circulation*, **49**, 418–422.

2
RADIOISOTOPE TECHNIQUES IN CARDIAC DIAGNOSIS

Leon Resnekov

The last decade has seen the emergence of a new subspecialty: cardiovascular nuclear medicine, as the parallel development of radiopharmaceuticals and detection devices, has permitted the unique properties of isotope tracers to be applied to the cardiovascular system for the detection of disease and for a more profound understanding of its physiology.

As long ago as 1927 a radioactive tracer was used to measure the velocity of blood in the arms. Between 1934 and 1946 the cyclotron became available, largely due to the pioneering efforts of Ernest Lawrence, who very early on foresaw its possible biomedical use. Up to this time, however, physiological tracer substances were very few and remained so until, during the war years (1939–1946), Enrico Fermi and others devised the reactor and some years later tracer production on a large scale followed. A cyclotron for medical use became available by 1960. Until 1963 iodine-131 was the nuclide of choice for medical use, but in that year the artificial compound technetium-99m became available due to the foresight of Harper and his colleagues of the University of Chicago.

Parallel with the development of nuclides suitable for biomedical use has been the development of detectors. Initially these were crude—photographic film exposed by x-rays or gamma rays. These early approaches soon gave way to using devices based on the piezoelectric phenomenon and later the cloud chamber was introduced. A great step forward was the detector invented in 1928 by Hans Geiger and perfected by him and Müller. Even so, the Geiger–Müller tube continued to have poor sensitivity and difficulty in differentiating gamma photon energies. The invention by Kallman in 1947 of the crystal scintillation detector was a major advance. A further important step forward was the development by Hal Anger towards the end of the 1950s of the scin-tillation camera, to permit measuring organ function by depicting the distri-bution in space of radioactivity over a selected period of time following the intravenous injection of a tracer substance.

As with other organs, investigation of the heart and cardiovascular system by radioactive tracers and appropriate detectors has continued apace.

Dr Resnekov is supported in part by USPHS Contract NO1-HV-81334 (Myocardial Infarction Research Unit) and NHLI Grant 1-P17-HL-17648 (Specialised Center of Research in Ischemic Heart Disease) and the Chicago Heart Association.

Printzmetal was one of the earliest workers to monitor the time course of a nuclide through the heart and measurements of cardiac output, shunt detection and valvar regurgitation followed. By 1963 lung scanning for the diagnosis of pulmonary emboli was introduced and with the development of specific nuclides and better detectors, nuclear techniques now available include measurement of total coronary flow, regional myocardial perfusion, localisation of myocardial infarction, systolic and diastolic volumes of the heart, ejection fractions, detection of akinetic and dyskinetic areas of the myocardium, the localisation and diagnosis of intracardiac tumours, shunt detection and quantitation as well as the diagnosis of pericardial effusions.

Principles of Radionuclide Diagnosis

Atomic nuclei consist of protons (charged particles) and neutrons (uncharged particles). When neutrons are insufficient or in excess, the nucleus becomes unstable and its spontaneous disintegration is accompanied by a loss of radiation energy, the phenomenon being known as radioactivity. An isotope of a particular element has the same number of protons but different numbers of neutrons and the total number of protons and neutrons in the nucleus is known as its mass number. This is used to designate a particular radioisotope, thus ^{131}I is the isotope of iodine with a total of 131 protons and neutrons in the nucleus.

Well over 1000 isotopes are known but only a few are stable and the majority are made artificially in reactors or cyclotrons. Some isotopes do not occur naturally, either in a stable or unstable form, and can be produced only by artificial methods of production. Such an isotope is technetium-99m. The m denotes a metastable form indicating that this radioactive atom will lose its energy by emitting gamma rays without changing the type or number of particles contained within its nucleus. Some artificially produced radioactive isotopes decay by emitting a positron from the nucleus which has the same mass as an electron but carries a positive charge. It combines with an electron giving rise to two photons which are given off in exact opposite directions and the detection of this form of annihilation radiation by coincidence counting has particular application in cardiac diagnosis.

Beta particles which are small and negatively charged (electrons) can be very damaging to biological tissues since their energy is given up in a very small region. Gamma radiation, on the other hand, is very penetrating and a great deal of lead shielding may be necessary to absorb its radiation completely. Although most isotopes emit both beta and gamma radiation, some are exclusive emitters of one or other type.

The curie is the unit of radioactivity. One curie is present if the rate of disintegration if $3.7 \times 10^{10}/s$. Disintegrations occur in a random manner until the atom will have changed its form or its energy state. After a certain period of time the number of the atoms will fall to half and this time is called the physical half-life of the radioisotope. The rate of disappearance of radioactivity from the body depends on the physical half-life of the nuclide and the rate at which its metabolism and elimination occur. Thus the time taken for the body radioactivity to fall to half is called the biological half-life. The combination of physical and biological half-lives is known as the effective half-life.

Usually a radioisotope is administered labelled or 'tagged' to some chemical substance which localises in a particular region or organ under consideration—thus chromium-51 which localises in the spleen is used extensively for haematological studies.

The amount of radiation absorbed depends on the given dose and on the energy of the radiation. This energy for beta and gamma rays is expressed as electron volts, more commonly as kiloelectron volts (keV). Gamma radiation energy of a few hundred keV can be usefully detected for clinical use.

Nuclides for Cardiac Use

For intravascular detection iodine-131 or 132 have been extensively used but, more recently, technetium-99m tagged to human red blood cells or to albumin has largely superseded earlier isotopes. For myocardial blood flow different techniques and isotopes are needed, thus rubidium-84 and coincidence counting introduced by Bing can give useful information despite its variable extraction ratio. More recently, potassium-43 and a gamma camera have been used to estimate myocardial blood flow. This isotope is not ideal since it emits a great deal of high energy gamma rays (619 keV) together with the clinically useful lower energy 379 keV rays. When energies are too high the gamma camera image is severely degraded necessitating complicated deconvolution procedures to correct for the resultant distortion. Others have used labelled oxygen-15 which results in a bolus of radioactive water being administered to the heart. This method, too, has its difficulties since correction factors have to be applied because of recirculation of the tracer. In addition, the very short half-life of ^{15}O imposes serious constraints on accuracy.

The monovalent cations potassium-43, caesium-129 and 131, nitrogen-13 attached to ammonia and thallium-201 have all been used with a variable measure of success. These isotopes are taken up in a relatively high concentration by cardiac muscle. Potassium has a better myocardial extraction ratio than caesium but its energies are not ideal for gamma camera detection. At present ^{13}N as ammonia or ^{201}Th seem advantageous for myocardial imaging although the short half-life of ^{13}N (9.96 min) restricts its use to institutions with their own cyclotron.

Scanners

Medical isotope scanners have been available since 1950. These devices consist of a moving scintillation detector attached to an electronic unit with noise rejecting circuits and counting devices. Multihole special purpose collimators are used to limit the field of view of the scintillation detector thus obtaining a high degree of sensitivity in a limited field for the particular region or organ of interest. At the end of its travel the detector moves from a preset position in a transverse direction.

Gamma Cameras

The gamma camera, introduced by Anger, produces a photographic image of the distribution of radioactivity without requiring the detector system to be moved. This is achieved by using a 30 cm sodium iodide crystal at the back of which is a bank of photomultiplier tubes. The pulse of light produced by the gamma ray striking the crystal is detected with different efficiencies by each of the photomultiplier tubes. The efficiency depends on the distance of each photomultiplier tube from the point at which light was produced in the crystal by the arrival of the gamma ray. The signals from all the photo-multiplier tubes are collected and processed electronically and the ultimate image can be in the form of a photographic print or recorded on an FM or digital tape for subsequent analysis. With suitable interfacing and program-ming the output can be analysed on line by a computer.

Image Display and Analysis

As important as the choice of nuclide and imaging device is the display and analysis of information obtained. A subjective interpretation can be obtained by critically inspecting a photographic print image, yet this method is hard to standardise, requires considerable training and even the most experienced is subject to observer variability. In consequence, a great deal of thought and effort is now being expended on analysis methods to provide reproducible and reliable quantitative information. As can be appreciated the radionuclide image information can easily be digitised and subjected to computer analysis. Algorithms are now available commercially based on small, dedicated, digital computers to provide not only quantification but also image enhancement and data reduction. When appropriate, the system can be modified so that images gated by the electrocardiogram can be analysed to provide information at specified points throughout the cardiac cycle, for example, during phases of systole or diastole. Gating the image in essence means that a considerable amount of available data is not analysed, and furthermore, sufficient counts have to be available during gating to permit meaningful analysis. To obviate some of these problems, programs are now being developed to permit collect-ing information throughout the cardiac cycle, at many discrete intervals during systole and diastole.

The descriptions which follow highlight some applications of radioisotope tracer techniques important in cardiac diagnosis. They do not include the detection of pericardial effusions (Wagner, McAfee and Mosley, 1960) or the diagnosis of pulmonary emboli (Wagner et al, 1964).

Radionuclide Angiogram

Folse and Braunwald (1962) recorded the time concentration curve following the selective injection of a nuclide into the left ventricle using a precordial detector and were also able to derive ventricular volumes and ejection fractions. Thereafter, attempts were made to obtain the same information following an

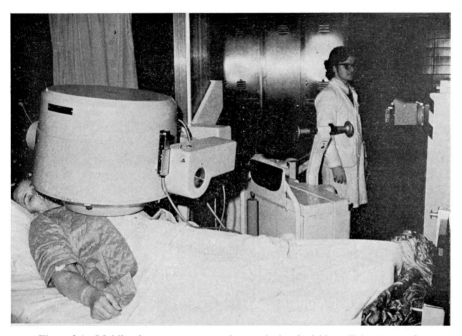

Figure 2.1   Mobile pho-gamma camera in use during bedside radioisotope study

intravenous injection of the radioactive tracer (Donato, 1962). Although the analysis of such precordial curves has had some practical appeal, the method continues to be limited, since each area of interest needs to be discretely monitored. More recently, such detailed analysis has now become available using a scintillation camera, data storage and computer analysis (Ishii and MacIntyre, 1971). Furthermore, useful information can be derived by analysing the beat-to-beat changes in the ventricular nuclide count rate to obtain ejection fractions. End diastolic volume can be calculated from area measurements of the scintigram (Sullivan et al, 1971; Weber, dos Remedios and Jasko, 1972) and using mobile equipment these techniques can be done at the bedside of the acutely ill patient (Fig. 2.1).

The preferred nuclide for isotope angiography is ^{99}Tc^m bound either to the patient's red cells or to human albumin to ensure that it remains an intravascular label. A rapid injection of 10 to 15 mCi is given and counting in the range of 25 to 50 thousand counts per second begun with the gamma camera routinely in the anteroposterior and left anterior oblique positions and positioned for left lateral and right anterior oblique views as needed. The image can be displayed on photographic film but it is highly advantageous to use data recording systems with instant replay. Using a computer and ECG gating, images corresponding to systole can be summed and compared to a composite image of diastole. This is useful in detecting left ventricular aneurysm and in demonstrating segmental contractility abnormalities (Hayden and Kriss, 1973; Strauss et al, 1972; Zaret et al, 1971). It is important to record in more

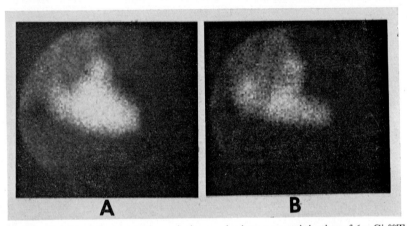

Figure 2.2 Bedside left ventricular scintigram. An intravenous injection of 6 mCi ^{99}Tc^m-labelled red blood cells has been made and ECG gated images obtained with the gamma camera in the left anterior oblique position. *A.* Diastole. *B.* Systole. Note the ventricular aneurysm shown in B

than one projection particularly when patients with coronary heart disease are being studied since non-uniform segmental abnormalities may not be apparent if only one plane is analysed. The whole study takes about 15 min to complete. Image quality is adequate for delineating the anatomical landmarks of the left ventricle including the planes of the aortic and mitral valves and the minor axis of the chamber. Cardiac output and left ventricular volume may then be calculated. Superimposition of end diastolic and end systolic frames permits abnormalities of wall motion to be determined (Kostuk et al, 1973).

The method, whilst capable of providing more sophisticated information if computer analysis of data is used, also serves as a useful photographic non-invasive screening method for excluding left ventricular aneurysm (Fig. 2.2) and for determining whether generalised hypokinesis is present rather than localised akinesis, to decide whether medical or surgical treatment is appropriate in an individual patient with coronary heart disease.

Intracardiac Shunts

In 1947 Printzmetal reported using sodium-24 and a Geiger counter, to determine the presence of an intracardiac shunt demonstrating the qualitative determination of shunts by precordial counting to be feasible. With a left-to-right shunt there is delay of entry of the tracer into the left ventricular field and greater delay in its clearance. A right-to-left shunt, on the other hand, shows an early peak which represents the shunted blood and a later peak representing major flow. Quantification of the volume of shunts remains a challenge (Swan, Zapata Diaz and Wood, 1953). In one method a detector is positioned over a remote arterial site, the presence and volume of the shunt being determined by deriving the cardiac output to that region (Strauss et al, 1969). For quantitating left-to-right shunts krypton-85 may be inhaled and samples of blood withdrawn from the right heart and analysed for radioactivity.

Regurgitant Volumes

Quantification of valvar regurgitant volumes has posed many problems. To a large extent reliance has traditionally been placed on selective angiography although faulty catheter placement and premature beats can cause spurious regurgitation. In addition, when both mitral and aortic regurgitation coexist, angiography is unreliable for assessing the severity of either lesion. In an attempt to solve some of the inherent problems indicator dilution techniques have been used but non-uniform mixing continues to give variable results (Frank et al, 1966). Morch, Klein and Richardson (1972) suggested a continuous infusion of xenon-133 which would obviate recirculation since it diffuses rapidly from the lungs. During left ventricular infusion of the tracer, sampling from the left atrium, aorta and brachial artery is done, permitting relative concentration measurements to be made in a steady state. The technique requires, however, many sampling catheters to be used which can limit its practical application in man.

A method of computerised radionuclide angiocardiography for the accurate computation of total forward and regurgitant fractions, based on a definition of the distribution of the tracer activity within the circulatory system during the wash-out phase following a bolus injection of the nuclide, has now been described (Kirch, Metz and Steele, 1974). It is applicable to both right and left sides of the heart and depends on the entry of the radionuclide bolus into the appropriate atrium. Thus selective injection of 8 to 10 mCi $^{99}Tc^{m}$-pertechnetate in a 1 ml volume is given into the superior vena cava for right heart studies or into the pulmonary arterial wedge position for left heart studies. Scintigraphic data is collected at 20 frames/s for 25 s after the injection. In the method described by Kirch the computer system consists of a PDP-12 computer interfaced to the pho-gamma camera. Differential equations solved by z-transformation permit an accurate definition of regurgitant volumes. The method has been validated in 12 patients with mitral or aortic regurgitation and there was good correlation with standard cineangiographic techniques.

Myocardial Imaging

Whereas blood pool agents such as $^{99}Tc^m$ provide information about segmental wall contractility, a promising, relatively new field is the use of nuclides which localise in normally functioning myocardial cells but which are poorly taken up by ischaemic or infarcted heart muscle thus providing a visual representation of the abnormal heart muscle ('cold spot scanning'). In contrast, some radioactive compounds seem to be taken up preferentially by damaged myocardial cells ('hot spot scanning'), thus offering the hope for the first time of being able to differentiate between infarcted tissue and ischaemic areas which could still be kept viable.

Among ions which are actively taken up by myocardial cells are rubidium-86 and 84, caesium-127, 129 and 131, potassium-42 and 43, and nitrogen-13 labelled ammonia. These compounds can be used to measure nutrient flow, the method depending on capillary surface area and flow rates, permeability of the capillary endothelium and myocardial cell membrane to the nuclide, and on the integrity of any specific transport system or metabolic processes of the tracer used (Bing, Rickart and Hellberg, 1972). The positron emitting rubidium-84 and coincidence counting have been extensively investigated by Bing et al (1964) as a non-invasive measurement of coronary flow. Others have used direct intracoronary infusion of solutions of radioactive inert gases, such as xenon-133, to obtain similar information (Ross et al, 1964; Bassingthwaite, Strandell and Donald, 1968).

Although useful for obtaining total coronary flow, these methods have been less widely used than originally predicted, probably due to the fact that the distribution of the total myocardial flow has been poorly defined. Total coronary flow provides little helpful information in the assessment of coronary heart disease where the information needed is the regional and segmental perfusion. Furthermore, wash-out curves of inert gases are in general unsatisfactory since local areas of decreased perfusion are obscured by the higher flows in adjacent areas and because of a non-exponential wash-out due to non-homogeneous perfusion (Cannon, Dell and Dwyer, 1972).

'Cold spot' myocardial scanning

Our own work has been largely centred around the use of the short-lived positron emitter nitrogen-13 (Harper et al, 1973). Its energies are advantageous for gamma camera detection and its half-life (9.96 min) permits sequential patient studies to be done in safety. Nitrogen-13 ammonia is prepared in our medical cyclotron as previously described (Harper et al, 1972; Monahan, Tilbury and Laughlin, 1972; Tilbury et al, 1971) by bombarding methane with 8 MeV deuterons; a 20-min run using an 8 to 10 μA beam provides sufficient energy for 20 to 30 mCi to be available after processing. Imaging is carried out using a pho-gamma camera and a specially designed collimator (Harper et al, 1973). More than 120 patients have now been studied, mainly in the early stages following acute myocardial infarction, the mobile equipment used permitting patient studies to be undertaken in the coronary care unit (Fig. 2.1). A dose of 10 to 30 mCi of the nuclide is administered intravenously and the total body radiation absorbed dose is estimated as 5 mrad/mCi, assuming uniform distribution, and 25 mrad/mCi to the liver, assuming 15 per cent of the injected dose to be in that organ on the basis of animal distribution studies (Harper et al, 1972, 1973). Myocardial images are usually of excellent quality and permit localisation of areas of infarction associated with poor perfusion to anterior, inferior or lateral surfaces of the ventricle (Fig. 2.3). Usually only the thick muscular wall of the left ventricle is visualised and there is, in addition, moderate uptake of activity in the lungs which washes out after 5 to 10 min. In patients who are heavy smokers, however, the pulmonary uptake of activity is frequently prolonged. Even so, satisfactory myocardial images are usually obtained in these individuals between 20 and 30 min after injection.

It is likely that there is an active transport in the myocardium for $^{13}NH_4^+$ which is similar to the transport of K^+. It is known that 90 per cent of the nuclide entering the coronary circulation is removed within a single pass (Harper et al, 1972). For rubidium or potassium ions this figure is between 50 and 60 per cent. For the radioactive ion to be taken up by the myocardial cell $^{13}NH_4^+$ is probably handled by the sodium-potassium activated transport mechanism of ATPase. There is therefore a relative passive barrier at the capillary wall and a concentrative transport process at the myocardial cell surface. This last is sensitive to ischaemia which limits substrate availability and ATP production. Once in the myocardial cell $^{13}NH_4^+$ enters the glutamine cycle and is metabolised.

More recently, thallium-201 has been investigated intensively for its cardiac applications and has been shown to provide myocardial images of superior quality, since its energies are even better than those of $^{13}NH_4^+$ for gamma camera detection. Furthermore, its longer physical half-life (78 h) means that its use is not restricted to institutions with their own cyclotron but, of course, it cannot be used for rapid sequential patient studies (Gehring and Hammond, 1967; Kawana et al, 1970).

'Hot spot' scanning

Although the nuclides discussed in the previous section give great diagnostic help by outlining poorly perfused tissue, they do not differentiate between acute infarction and ischaemia. Attempts at doing this were made initially by Dreyfuss, Ben-Porath and Menczel (1960) who undertook sequential precordial scanning over several days in patients with acute myocardial infarction using radioiodine. It was subsequently shown that the reported increased uptake was unlikely to have been myocardial and that it was almost certainly from the stomach.

Mercury-203 labelled with chlormerodrin was shown in experimental

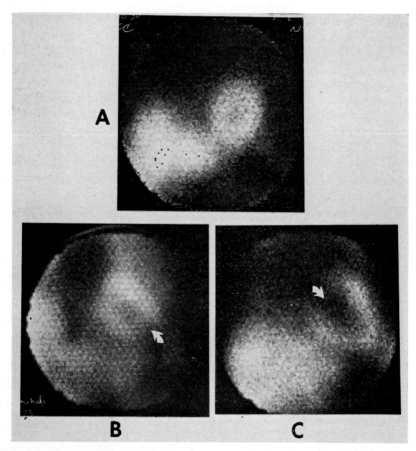

Figure 2.3   'Cold spot' bedside gamma camera myocardial imaging in three patients using the short half-life positron emitter ^{13}N as ammonia. Left anterior oblique views. *A*. Normal. *B*. Acute inferior myocardial infarction. *C*. Acute anteroseptal myocardial infarction. In *A*, note the uniform uptake of radioactivity by the myocardium whereas in *B* and *C* areas of underperfusion (arrowed) are related to the anatomical site of the infarction. Heavy uptake of radioactivity by the liver can be seen in all three images

animals to accumulate several-fold in infarcted myocardium (Carr et al, 1962). The clinical use of this substance has not been possible, however, since the quantity which has to be injected is far too high.

Malek, Kolc and Zastava (1963) demonstrated an accumulation of tetracycline in infarcted myocardium and ^{99}Tc^m-labelled tetracycline has been studied for detecting, localising and sizing infarction (Holman et al, 1973).

The mechanism by which tetracycline localises in infarcted tissue is as yet poorly understood but it may depend on the binding of a calcium tetracycline chelate to an anhydroxyapatite matrix (Riley, Paschall and Robinson, 1966). The method is still under investigation and has been used in man with some success (Holman et al, 1974).

A different approach has been suggested by Bonte (Bonte et al, 1974; Meyer et al, 1974), who has shown that $^{99}Tc^m$-pyrophosphate or diphosphonate accumulates in recently infarcted myocardium and can be imaged using a pho-gamma camera (Fig. 2.4). The nuclide is a bone-scanning compound and it has been suggested that the pyrophosphate or diphosphonate accumulates in the mitochondria of infarcted or ischaemic cells due to the increased presence of calcium ion from the damaged cells. Alternatively it may be that

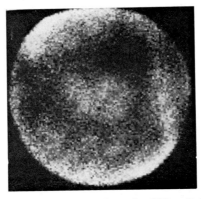

Figure 2.4 'Hot spot' bedside myocardial imaging using $^{99}Tc^m$-diphosphonate. Radioactivity has accumulated centrally in the region of acute myocardial infarction

the binding occurs to the damaged cell membranes, or that the compound binds to the organelles or even to leucocytes invading the infarcted area. The positive images obtained may be seen within a few hours of injection and repeated scanning may remain positive for about three weeks thereafter. It is as yet uncertain whether the $^{99}Tc^m$-polyphosphate is taken up by ischaemic tissue which is as yet not actually infarcted. Furthermore, Walsh et al (1975) have shown that following experimental myocardial infarction in animals there is an uneven uptake of the agent by infarcted tissues and that the nuclide localisation patterns in myocardial infarction appear to depend on the local collateral blood supply to the area of damage. They therefore suggest caution in using this technique for an accurate assessment of the size of infarcted regions of the myocardium.

Nevertheless, it is clear that a promising new investigative method has been opened which provides a positive image of damaged myocardial tissue. No doubt its clinical use will be extensively and carefully evaluated over the next few years.

Myocardial Blood Flow

The quantitation of coronary flow can be derived at present by one of four methods.

1. Diffusible gases. Nitrous oxide and a wash-out technique based on the original Kety–Schmidt method is used (Kety and Schmidt, 1948). This measures both nutrient and AV shunt flow and therefore cannot be used for inhomogeneous myocardial perfusion such as occurs in coronary heart disease.
2. Ions actively taken up by myocardial cells such as rubidium, xenon, caesium, potassium, nitrogen and thallium as previously described.
3. Indicator (dye) dilution (Nakamura et al, 1968) or thermodilution (Ganz and Swan, 1972) to measure coronary sinus flow.
4. Ultrasonic Doppler flowmeter (Franklin, Schleger and Watson, 1963; Benchimol and Desser, 1972). The position of the catheter tip flowmeter is critical.

In general, wash out techniques, even using nuclides, are not very satisfactory for obtaining quantitative data since areas of decreased perfusion may be obscured by adjacent areas with a larger or normal flow. Furthermore heterogeneous perfusion results in a non-exponential wash-out curve. Alternatively, microspheres (Domenech et al, 1969; Becker, Fortuin and Pitt, 1971) may be injected selectively into each coronary artery and will help in diagnosing dyskinetic segments, but will not differentiate viable from non-viable areas.

According to the Sapirstein principle (1958) the fraction of an injected indicator taken up by an organ equals the fraction of the cardiac output perfusing that organ for a finite time following the injection. Using this postulate a method for estimating myocardial blood flow can be formulated as follows:

$$\text{percentage myocardial uptake} = \frac{\text{myocardial blood flow}}{\text{cardiac output}}$$

and

$$\text{myocardial blood flow} = \frac{\text{myocardial uptake}}{\text{injected dose}} \times \text{cardiac output}$$

For this to be valid, however, it is essential that the extraction ratio of the myocardium for the nuclide equals that of the whole body and that the reduction of extraction ratio with an increased blood flow is identical for the myocardium and for the total body. It seems likely, however, that the extraction ratio of the monovalent cation nuclides used for estimating myocardial blood flow are different in ischaemic and normal areas of the myocardium and, if they move in the same way as potassium, it is probable that there will be a relative lack of uptake in ischaemic areas.

Whilst a great deal of work on fractionation methods for deriving myocardial blood flow based on the Sapirstein principle has been done (Glass, Buranapong and Doherty, 1975) others have preferred a static method which involves the selective injection into the coronary circulation of microspheres labelled with either ^{131}I or ^{99}Tc^m. This method provides a relative distribution of flow rather than absolute flow in millilitres per minute (Ashburn et al, 1970). Selective labelling of the microspheres injected into the right and left coronary arteries and multiple scintillation camera projections permit the distribution of radioactivity to be related to a particular anatomical lesion demonstrated by coronary arteriography (Jansen et al, 1973). These techniques may help therefore in assessing the functional importance of an obstructive coronary arterial lesion. In addition, they may be used to demonstrate hyperaemic changes in an attempt to delineate the need for revascularisation surgery (Ritchie et al, 1975).

Macroaggregates have been used clinically since 1964 with a mean particle size of 80 μm (Taplin et al, 1964). In 1969, Rhodes introduced human albumin microspheres for clinical use (Rhodes et al, 1969) and these range in size from 10 to 40 μm, the average being 30 μm and the number of particles per injected dose is 10 000 to 30 000. The theoretical basis and clinical validation of particle injection methods has been established (Wagner et al, 1969) and Schelbert et al (1971) have documented the feasibility of the intracoronary injection of these particles in man. Technetium-labelled particles may be injected into the left coronary artery and iodine-labelled particles into the right immediately following selective coronary arteriography (Jansen, Grames and Judkins, 1974). Images are obtained in multiple views using a high resolution collimator. Very few complications have been reported in over 1000 patients studied (Grames et al, 1974) and using this dual radionuclide technique the formulation and demonstration of myocardial perfusion anatomy and the collateral circulation has been possible.

The technique of microsphere scintigraphy provides, therefore, information about the integrity of the myocardial capillary bed beyond a stenosed coronary artery and such information cannot be obtained at present by any other technique in man. It permits a more careful selection of patients for revascularisation surgery and provides the surgeon help in the detailed planning of his operation.

Summary and Conclusion

A brief review is presented of the use of nuclear techniques in cardiovascular diagnosis—apart from the diagnosis of pericardial effusion and pulmonary embolism.

Newer developments in radiopharmaceuticals, scanning and detection devices and computer technology can provide not only a visual representation of lesions present but attempts are now being made to localise their position in the myocardium and to quantitate flow.

Using mobile equipment the seriously ill patient can be studied at the bedside following the intravenous injection of a suitable nuclide. Injecting blood-pool compounds and gating collecting counts to specific portions of the cardiac cycle provides a good visual representation of ventricular anatomy including the demonstration of ventricular aneurysm and dyskinetic myocardial segments. Cardiac output, ventricular volume and ejection fractions can all be derived.

Techniques are now available for the demonstration, localisation and quantification of intracardiac shunts and methods have been described for the measurement of valvar regurgitant volumes for both sides of the heart.

Short half-life monovalent cations have been extensively used for sequential studies in the coronary care unit following acute myocardial infarction for the diagnosis and localisation of regional areas of underperfusion. Technetium-pyrophosphate or diphosphonate localises to damaged myocardial cells providing help in differentiating infarcted from ischaemic areas.

Although total coronary flow can be measured without great difficulty it has proved less useful in man than originally predicted since the assessment of many disease states, particularly coronary heart disease, requires an estimation of regional perfusion. It is possible that nuclear techniques which depend on quantification of fractionation methods will not provide the accuracy needed for measuring segmental myocardial perfusion but the selective injection of suitably labelled microspheres into the coronary arteries at the time of coronary arteriography may give anatomical and functional assessments of the effects of coronary artery obstructive lesions and of collateral flow.

A combination of these techniques, therefore, will provide the clinician with a diagnostic precision which has previously been lacking and will enable therapeutic interventions, medical or surgical, to be planned more accurately and their effects to be determined more easily.

REFERENCES

Ashburn, W. L., Braunwald, E., Simon, A. L. & Gault, J. H. (1970) Myocardial perfusion imaging in man using 99m TcMAA. *Journal of Nuclear Medicine*, **11**, 618.

Bassingthwaite, J. B., Strandell, T. & Donald, D. S. (1968) Estimation of coronary blood flow by washout of diffusible indicators. *Circulation Research*, **23**, 259.

Becker, L. C., Fortuin, N. J. & Pitt, B. (1971) Effect of ischaemia and antiaginal drugs on the distribution of radioactive microspheres in the canine left ventricle. *Circulation Research*, **28**, 263.

Benchimol, A. & Desser, K. B. (1972) Clinical application of the Doppler ultrasonic flow-meter. *American Journal of Cardiology*, **29**, 540.

Bing, R. J., Bennish, A., Blümchen, G., Cohen, A., Gallagher, J. P. & Zaleski, E. J. (1964) The determination of coronary flow equivalent with coincidence counting technic. *Circulation*, **29**, 833.

Bing, R. J., Rickart, A. & Hellberg, K. (1972) Techniques to measure coronary blood flow in man. *American Journal of Cardiology*, **29**, 75.

Bonte, F. J., Parkey, R. W., Graham, K. D., Moore, R. T. & Stokeley, E. M. (1974) A new method for radionuclide imaging of myocardial infarcts. *Radiology*, **110**, 473.

Cannon, P. J., Dell, R. B. & Dwyer, E. M., Jr (1972) Measurement of regional myocardial perfusion in man with 133 xenon and a scintillation camera. *Journal of Clinical Investigation*, **51**, 964.

Carr, E. T., Bierwaltes, W. H., Patno, M. E., Bartlett, J. D. & Wegst, A. V. (1962) The detecting of experimental myocardial infarcts by photoscanning. *American Heart Journal*, **64**, 650.

Domenech, R. J., Hoffman, I. E., Noble, M. I. M., Saunders, K. B., Henson, J. R. & Subijanto, S. (1969) Total and regional coronary blood flow measured by radioactive microspheres in conscious and anesthetised dogs. *Circulation Research*, **25**, 581.

Donato, L. (1962) Selective quantitative radiography. *Progress in Cardiovascular Diseases*, **5**, 1.

Dreyfuss, F., Ben-Porath, M. & Menczel, J. (1960) Radioiodine uptake by the infarcted heart. *American Journal of Cardiology*, **6**, 237.

Folse, R. & Braunwald, E. (1962) Determination of fraction of left ventricular volume ejected per beat and of ventricular end-diastolic and residual volumes. *Circulation*, **25**, 674.

Frank, M. J., Casanegra, P., Nadimi, M., Megliori, A. J. & Levinson, G. E. (1966) Measurement of aortic regurgitation by upstream sampling with continuous infusion of indicators. *Circulation*, **33**, 545.

Franklin, D. L., Schleger, W. & Watson, N. W. (1963) Ultrasonic Doppler shift blood flowmeter: circuitry and practical application. *Biomedical Scientific Instrumentation*, **1**, 309.

Ganz, W. & Swan, J. H. C. (1972) Measurement of blood flow by thermodilution. *American Journal of Cardiology*, **29**, 241.

Gehring, P. J. & Hammond, P. B. (1967) The interrelationship between thallium and potassium in animals. *Journal of Pharmacology and Experimental Therapeutics*, **155**, 187.

Glass, H. I., Buranapong, P. & Doherty, P. (1975) Measurement of regional blood flow and distribution in myocardium using K-43. In *Nuklearmedezin*, ed. Pabst, H. W. & Hör, G. Stuttgart, New York: Schattaner FK.

Grames, G. M., Jansen, C., Gander, M. P., Wieland, H. C. & Judkins, M. P. (1974) The safety of the direct coronary injection of radiolabelled particles in 500 patients undergoing coronary angiography. *Journal of Nuclear Medicine*, **15**, 2.

Harper, P. V., Lathrop, K. A., Krizek, H., Lembares, N., Stark, V. & Hoffer, P. (1972) Clinical feasibility of myocardial imaging with [13]NH₃. *Journal of Nuclear Medicine*, **13**, 278.

Harper, P. V., Schwartz, J., Beck, R. N., Lathrop, K. A., Lembares, N., Krizek, H., Gloria, I., Dinwoodie, R., McLaughlin, A., Stark, V., Bekerman, C., Hoffer, P., Gottschalk, A., Resnekov, L., Al-Sadir, J., Mayorga, A. & Brooks, H. (1973) Clinical myocardial imaging with nitrogen-13 ammonia. *Radiology*, **108**, 613.

Hayden, W. G. & Kriss, J. P. (1973) Scintiphotographic studies of acquired cardiovascular disease. *Seminars of Nuclear Medicine*, **3**, 177.

Holman, B. L., Dewanjee, M. K., Iodine, J., Fliegel, C. P., Davis, M. A., Treves, S. & Eldh, P. (1973) Detection and localisation of experimental myocardial infarction with [99]Tc[m]-tetracycline. *Journal of Nuclear Medicine*, **14**, 595.

Holman, B. L., Lesch, M., Zweiman, E., Temte, J., Dewanjee, M. K., Lown, B. & Gorlin, R. (1974) Evaluation of acute myocardial infarction with technetium-99m tetracycline infarct imaging. *American Journal of Cardiology*, **33**, 144.

Ishii, Y. & MacIntyre, W. J. (1971) Measurement of heart chamber volumes by analysis of dye dilution curves simultaneously recorded by scintillation camera. *Circulation*, **44**, 37.

Jansen, C., Grames, G. M. & Judkins, M. P. (1974) Myocardial blood flow in man-albumin microsphere technique. In *Cardiovascular Nuclear Medicine*, ed. Strauss, H. W., Pitt, B. & James, A. E., Jr. St Louis: C. V. Mosby.

Jansen, C., Judkins, M. P., Grames, G. M., Gander, M. & Adams, R. (1973) Myocardial perfusion colour scintigraphy with MAA. *Radiology*, **109**, 369.

Kawana, M., Kuzek, H., Porter, J., Lathrop, K. A., Charleston, D. & Harper, P. V. (1970) Use of [199]Tl as a potassium analogy in scanning. *Journal of Nuclear Medicine*, **11**, 333.

Kety, S. S. & Schmidt, C. F. (1948) Nitrous oxide method for quantitative determinating cerebral blood flow in man: theory, procedure and normal values. *Journal of Clinical Investigation*, **27**, 476.

Kirch, D. L., Metz, C. E. & Steele, P. P. (1974) Quantitation of valvular insufficiency by computerised radionuclide angiocardiography. *American Journal of Cardiology*, **34**, 711.

Kostuk, W. J., Ehsani, A. A., Karliner, J. S., Ashburn, W. L., Peterson, K. L., Ross, J. & Sobel, B. E. (1973) Left ventricular performance after myocardial infarction assessed by radioisotope angiocardiography. *Circulation*, **47**, 242.

Malek, P., Kolc, J. & Zastava, V. L. (1963) Fluorescence of tetracycline analogues fixed in myocardial infarction. *Cardiology*, **42**, 303.

Meyer, S. L., Parkey, R. W., Bonte, F. J., Atkins, J. M., Curry, G. C. & Willerson, J. T. (1974) Technetium-99m stannous pyrophosphate myocardial scans in the diagnosis of acute myocardial infarction in patients. *Clinical Research*, **22**, 290A.

Monahan, W. G., Tilbury, R. S. & Laughlin, J. S. (1972) Uptake of ^{13}N labelled ammonia for medical use. *Journal of Nuclear Medicine*, **13**, 274.

Morch, J. E., Klein, S. W. & Richardson, P. (1972) Mitral regurgitation measured by continuous infusion of ^{133}xenon. *American Journal of Cardiology*, **29**, 812.

Nakamura, T., Katori, R., Miyazawa, K., Ishikawa, K., Yamaki, M., Tsuiki, K., Kobayashi, Y., Matsunga, A. & Haneda, T. H. (1968) Studies on dye-dilution method (XVI report): new method for measurement of coronary sinus blood flow in man. *Japanese Circulation Journal*, **32**, 1845.

Printzmetal, M., Corday, E., Spritzler, R. G. & Flieg, W. (1949) Radiocardiography and its clinical applications. *Journal of the American Medical Association*, **139**, 617.

Rhodes, B. A., Zolle, I., Buchanan, J. & Wagner, H. N., Jr (1969) Radioactive albumin microspheres for studies of the pulmonary circulation. *Radiology*, **92**, 1453.

Riley, L. H., Paschall, H. A. & Robinson, R. A. (1966) Intracellular calcification occurring in a transplanted human tumour. *Journal of Surgical Research*, **6**, 171.

Ritchie, J. L., Hamilton, G. W., Gould, K. L., Allen, D., Kennedy, J. W. & Hammermeister, K. E. (1975) Myocardial imaging with indium-113m macroaggregated albumin. *American Journal of Cardiology*, **35**, 380.

Ross, R. S., Veda, K., Lichtlen, P. R. & Rees, J. R. (1964) Measurement of myocardial blood flow in animals and man by selective injection of radioactive inert gas into the coronary arteries. *Circulation Research*, **15**, 28.

Sapirstein, L. A. (1958) Regional blood flow by fractional distribution of indicators. *American Journal of Physiology*, **193**, 161.

Schelbert, H., Ashburn, W., Covell, J., Simon, A. L., Braunwald, E. & Ross, J. (1971) Feasibility and hazards of the intracoronary injection of radioactive serum albumin macroaggregates for external myocardial perfusion imaging. *Investigative Radiology*, **6**, 379.

Strauss, H. W., Hurley, P. J., Rhodes, B. A. & Wagner, H. N., Jr (1969) Quantification of right to left transpulmonary shunts in man. *Journal of Laboratory Clinical Medicine*, **74**, 597.

Strauss, H. W., Zaret, B. L., Hurley, P. J., Natarajan, T. K. & Pitt, B. (1972) A scintiphotographic method for measuring left ventricular ejection in man without cardiac catheterisation. *American Journal of Cardiology*, **28**, 575.

Sullivan, R. W., Bergeron, D. A., Veller, W., Hyatt, K. H., Haughton, V. & Vogel, J. M. (1971) Peripheral venous scintillation angiocardiography in determination of left ventricular volume in man. *American Journal of Cardiology*, **28**, 563.

Swan, H. J. C., Zapata Diaz, J. & Wood, E. H. (1953) Dye dilution curves in cyanotic congenital heart disease. *Circulation*, **8**, 70.

Taplin, G. V., Johnson, D. E., Dore, E. J. & Kaplan, H. S. (1964) Lung photoscans with macroaggregates of human serum radioalbumin. Experimental basic and initial clinical trials. *Radiology*, **6**, 379.

Tilbury, R. S., Dahl, J. R., Monahan, W. G. & Laughlin, J. S. (1971) The production of 13-N labelled ammonia for medical use. *Radiochemical Radioanalytical Letters*, **8**, 317.

Wagner, H. N., Jr, McAfee, J. G. & Mosley, J. M. (1960) Medical radioisotope scanning. *Journal of the American Medical Association*, **174**, 162.

Wagner, H. N., Jr, Rhodes, B., Susaki, Y. & Ryan, J. (1969) Studies of the circulation with radioactive microspheres. *Investigative Radiology*, **4**, 374.

Wagner, H. N., Jr, Sabiston, D. C., McAfee, J. A., Tow, D. & Stern, H. S. (1964) Diagnosis of massive pulmonary embolism in man by radioisotope scanning. *New England Journal of Medicine*, **27**, 377.

Walsh, W., Schwartz, J., Bautovich, G., Booth, A., Harper, P. V., Al-Sadir, J. & Resnekov, L. (1975) Localisation patterns of ^{99} technetium^{m}-diphosphonate in experimental myocardial infarction. *Clinical Research*, **23**, 213A.

Weber, P. M., dos Remedios, L. V. & Jasko, I. A. (1972) Quantitative radioisotopic angiocardiography. *Journal of Nuclear Medicine*, **13**, 815.

Zaret, B. L., Strauss, H. W., Hurley, P. J., Natarajan, T. K. & Pitt, B. (1971) A non-invasive scintophotographic method for detecting regional ventricular dysfunction in man. *New England Journal of Medicine*, **284**, 1165.

3
RADIOLOGY IN CORONARY ARTERY DISEASE

Simon Rees

Clinical manifestations of myocardial ischaemia are nearly always due to coronary atherosclerosis, although other rare causes of coronary artery disease, such as congenital anomalies and syphilitic ostial stenosis are occasionally encountered. Angina pectoris may also occur with apparently normal coronary arteries, and although this is usually in association with other lesions, such as aortic or mitral valve disease, an important group of patients is also emerging in whom typical angina is associated with no demonstrable abnormality in the coronary arteries. This chapter is concerned with the current place of radiology in the investigation of patients with clinical manifestations of acute or chronic myocardial ischaemia.

PLAIN FILM CHANGES

Angina

Only a small proportion of patients presenting clinically with angina of effort show evidence of cardiac enlargement or pulmonary venous hypertension on the plain chest x-ray. Coronary artery calcification is, however, frequently encountered, and its presence is best confirmed by fluoroscopy. On the plain film, the calcification appears as a plaque, or more rarely as a double-line and is most frequently seen in the left main, proximal anterior descending or proximal circumflex coronary arteries on the penetrated anterior and lateral views. Fluoroscopy may be required to confirm that the calcification lies in the coronary arteries, as it may be difficult to distinguish it from costal cartilage or bronchial wall calcification. Calcification in the right coronary artery is much more difficult to see on plain films, as on the anterior view, the descending part overlies the spine, and on the lateral view, which is taken with a longer exposure time, the calcification is frequently obscured by motional blurr. Although calcification is much more likely to indicate significant coronary disease in the younger patient than in those over 50, areas of stenosis demonstrated on coronary arteriography do not necessarily correspond to sites of calcification (personal observation), and this particularly applies to the patient over 60 years.

Cardiac enlargement in patients with angina is an indication of previous infarction, left ventricular failure, dysrhythmia or other lesions such as hypertension or associated valve disease. Upper zone vessel dilatation is frequently present as well, and is a sensitive indicator of an elevated left ventricular end-diastolic pressure.

Infarction

Patients presenting with acute myocardial infarction usually also retain a normal chest x-ray throughout the course of their illness, and this applies to about three out of four patients passing through the coronary care unit. Using the pulmonary artery diastolic pressure as a parameter of left ventricular function, Bennett and Rees (1974) found a good correlation between radiological signs and left ventricular function. Absence of upper zone vessel dilatation on the chest radiograph always indicated that the pulmonary diastolic pressure was below 15 mmHg, unless elevated from another cause, such as pulmonary embolism. Radiological signs of pulmonary venous hypertension, including upper zone vessel dilatation and evidence of interstitial oedema, usually indicated a pressure over 15 mmHg. In most cases the discrepancies were due to a time lag between fall of pressure and radiological improvement, but occasionally oedema was found without any pressure rise— the reasons for this being obscure. They also found a good correlation between cardiac enlargement and the pulmonary venous pressure, and concluded that useful information can be obtained from a technically satisfactory portable film taken in the semi-erect position.

Pulmonary emboli are common after infarction and appear as small band-shadows at the bases, often with no clinical evidence of their presence. Larger infarcts are less common, and are associated with pleural effusion. Late pleural effusions, associated with cardiac enlargement, may be due to the postmyocardial infarction syndrome, which is probably a hypersensitivity reaction to necrotic cardiac muscle.

An acute rupture of the muscular ventricular septum is a rare complication, occurring within two weeks of infarction, and may follow occlusion of the anterior or posterior descending coronary arteries. The rupture may be associated with poor left ventricular function, aneurysm formation or mitral regurgitation. The shunt is frequently large and the pulmonary venous pressure is raised because of high pulmonary flow associated with poor left ventricular function. On the plain film there is cardiac enlargement with interstitial or alveolar oedema and pleural effusions. The pulmonary vessels are hidden by the oedema, so that the appearances of pulmonary plethora are not apparent in the acute stage. If the patient survives, evidence of pulmonary venous hypertension becomes less obvious and the picture may suggest a shunt, but the upper zone vessel dilatation remains.

Mitral regurgitation after infarction is often indistinguishable from rupture of the septum. It may be due to transient papillary muscle dysfunction

(Holloway, Whalen and McIntosh, 1965; Holmes and Logan, 1968), which later can become established (Burch, de Pasquale and Phillips, 1963; Burch, Phillips and de Pasquale, 1971; de Pasquale and Burch, 1971; Orlando et al, 1964) and is rarely the result of papillary muscle rupture (Cederquist and Söderström, 1964; Robinson, Stannard and Long, 1965). The posterior papillary muscle is most commonly affected and the syndrome is, therefore, seen with inferior infarction following occlusion of the dominant coronary artery supplying the posterior descending artery. Radiologically with acute regurgitation the heart may increase only slightly in size and the left atrium also rarely becomes more than slightly enlarged. It remains relatively incompliant, so that the systolic wave is transmitted to the lungs, giving striking changes of pulmonary venous hypertension. The pulmonary artery pressure also tends to be very high, with an elevated resistance. However, these florid changes of left-sided heart failure in the acute stage, are indistinguishable from rupture of the ventricular septum, and indeed clinical differentiation is also frequently difficult.

Another complication of infarction is left ventricular aneurysm (Baron, 1971; Dubnow, Burchell and Titus, 1965). Aneurysms vary in size and may be small and localised to the apex or anterior wall. On the plain film they may produce a characteristic bulge on the left border of the heart, although in most instances the contour remains normal and there is no evidence of pulmonary venous hypertension. Larger aneurysms which involve most of the anterior descending territory, classically present as a localised bulge on the left border of the heart, but in the majority of cases the enlarged heart has a non-specific shape which is indistinguishable from that seen in postinfarct left ventricular failure without localised aneurysm formation. Both have evidence of pulmonary venous hypertension on the plain film. Fluoroscopy in the diagnosis of left ventricular aneurysm has proved to be a disappointing technique and left ventricular angiography is necessary to make the diagnosis. In a series of aneurysms, proven by angiography, about 50 per cent showed a suggestive bulge on the left border of the heart.

LEFT VENTRICULAR ANGIOGRAPHY

Much valuable information is obtained about ventricular function from cine angiography. The ventricle is best studied by injecting 30 to 50 ml of contrast at 10 to 20 ml/s into the cavity with the patient in the right anterior oblique position and taking cine film at 50 frames/s. Difficulties in interpretation occur because of the frequent occurrence of ventricular ectopic beats during the contrast injection. This has partially been overcome by using a slow injection rate, although this does not necessarily guarantee a series of normal electrical beats during the injection. Ventricular contraction often has to be assessed by studying a postectopic beat, which is potentiated and occurs after a compensatory pause and is, therefore, not representative of normal sinus rhythm. However, the large ejection fraction of such a beat will generally make minor abnormalities of contraction more obvious. Left ventricular angiography is indicated in all patients undergoing coronary arteriography It is also the definitive diagnostic procedure in patients suspected of having ruptured ventricular septum, acute mitral regurgitation and left ventricular aneurysm; in these situations, biplane angiography is desirable.

Analysis of left ventricular angiograms obtained in ischaemic heart disease is the subject of much original work at the present time (Gibson and Brown, 1975; Harris et al, 1974; Rickards, Seabra-Gomez and Balcon, 1976). This is particularly being pursued by computer techniques in an attempt to define overall parameters of ventricular function and abnormalities of segmental wall motion (Harrison, 1965; Herman and Gorlin, 1969; Herman et al, 1967; Mourdjinis et al, 1968). Abnormal movement of the ventricular wall may occur in various forms and patterns:

1. *Localised dyskinesis*

May be defined as diminished or absent inward systolic movement and is synonomous with asynergy, hypokinesis, asyneresis and functional aneurysm. It typically involves a limited area of myocardium corresponding to the distribution of stenotic or occlusive coronary disease. It is seen most commonly at the apex, but also may occur on the anterolateral or posteroinferior surface, and in any combination of these three. Patients with normal ventricular angiograms at rest almost always exhibit dyskinesis in one or other part of the ventricle during angina induced by exercise or pacing, and such stress also increases the severity and extent of dyskinesis present at rest (Pasternac et al, Krayenbuehl et al, 1975; Sharma and Taylor, 1975). In some patients, dyskinetic areas may disappear following the administration of glyceryl trinitrate (Dumesnil et al, 1975). Revascularisation by aortocoronary saphenous vein grafting has frequently been shown to improve dyskinesis and some areas may return to normal contraction after operation. This is less likely to occur in patients with previous acute myocardial infarction (Chatterjee et al, 1973). Because dyskinetic areas contain ischaemic but potentially viable muscle, surgical resection would seem inappropriate.

2. *Generalised dyskinesis*

May be defined as uniform increase in ventricular systolic and diastolic volume with a reduced ejection fraction. It is indistinguishable angiographically from congestive cardiomyopathy. The patient usually has a history of heart failure, with or without angina, the end-diastolic pressure is raised and the prospects of improvement of ventricular function after revascularisation are, on the whole, poor.

3. *Left ventricular aneurysm*

The certain diagnosis of aneurysm on left ventricular angiography is frequently difficult and differentiation from an extensive area of dyskinesis may be impossible. The distinction is, however, important to make. An aneurysm suitable for resection may or may not have paradoxical outward systolic movement, but the endocardial surface is typically smooth because of the thrombus within it; the area involved is usually enlarged out of proportion to the rest of the ventricle and is therefore identifiable in diastole as well as systole. Only occasionally is a well-defined neck seen (Graber et al, 1972; Raphael et al, 1972). By far the most common site for aneurysm formation is the anterolateral and apical part of the ventricle, and this is due to a total occlusion of the left anterior descending coronary artery. In a typical case the subaortic area of the ventricle contracts vigorously, but may be dyskinetic in severely affected ventricles. Inferior aneurysms are rare and are not suitable for resection. Although the differentiation of aneurysm from extensive dyskinesis may be difficult angiographically, at surgery it is nearly always easy as a clear zone of demarcation is visible in an aneurysm (Cooley and Hallman, 1968).

Left ventricular angiography is also required to assess mitral regurgitation due to papillary muscle dysfunction which typically follows inferior infarction and is therefore associated with inferior dyskinesis (Sanders et al, 1971; Shelburne and Gorlin, 1972). Characteristically the regurgitant jet takes a circumferential course within the left atrial cavity, usually in a clockwise direction, an appearance similar to chordal rupture.

Left ventricular angiography is also necessary to diagnose and define the anatomy of a ruptured ventricular septum. The rupture may follow occlusion of the anterior or posterior descending coronary artery. With an anterior descending occlusion, an aneurysm may be present as well and with a posterior descending occlusion there may be additional mitral regurgitation from involvement of the posterior papillary muscle. Occasionally there is more than one defect. Perforation is commonest in first infarcts and in patients with hypertension. If the clinical situation allows, and if biplane cine angiography is not available, two ventriculograms—one in the left oblique and the other in the right oblique—are necessary for a total assessment of the situation. In the left anterior oblique the ventricular septum is in profile, and the exact site and size of the septal defect can be seen clearly. The right anterior oblique angiogram is necessary to assess ventricular function as a whole and also to confirm or exclude mitral regurgitation.

CORONARY ARTERIOGRAPHY

Technical Considerations

Coronary arteriography is rapidly becoming the most commonly performed invasive investigation on the heart. Over the years the technique has undergone much modification, and the developments have mainly been in the direction of easier, quicker and safer catheterisation, combined with the production of films of the highest quality compatible with a quick and safe examination. Suffice to say that at present the selective technique is exclusively employed, and the choice of brachial or femoral artery for insertion of the catheter depends partly on the preference and experience of the operator and partly on the clinical situation. For example, a patient suspected of having coronary heart disease with no other cardiac lesion can be investigated by either technique, whereas a patient with aortic valve disease, in whom pressure measurements across the aortic valve are required, is best investigated from the arm, as it is easier by this technique to pass the catheter through the valve into the ventricle. The x-ray equipment is of the greatest importance, but technical improvements have been so rapid and costs have escalated so fast, that few departments have been able to keep up to date with the latest and best installation. At the present time of writing, the requirements may be summarised as follows:

1. A high output, high mA generator, capable of producing rapid films with a low kV and short exposure time.
2. A fine focus high-speed anode tube with efficient heat dissipation.
3. An arrangement for taking various oblique views of the heart. This is best done with a rotating arm supporting the image intensifier and x-ray tube, with the patient lying still on a radiolucent moveable table top. An alternative is a cradle with fixed image intensifier and x-ray tube. It is also an advantage to be able to obtain a craniocaudal tilt to view the proximal left coronary artery, and various mechanical methods are now available to provide this facility.
4. A high resolution image intensifier with provision for filming on a small field with a magnified image.
5. A 35 mm cine camera with high quality lens capable of filming at 50 frames/s. Faster speeds for coronary arteriography seem to offer no particular advantage. The place of photofluorography using 70 or 100 mm film has yet to be established, but at the time of writing it seems unlikely to supplant cine, mainly because viewing a moving image eliminates most of the difficulties in interpretation caused by overlap of vessels.
6. Facilities for cine processing to produce a high contrast film with acceptable graininess.
7. A viewing system which is convenient to use, optically excellent, capable of allowing study of single frames as well as projection at slow and rapid speeds. Also, ideally, for larger audiences it should be possible to project on to a wide screen.
8. Contrast medium of the highest iodine content compatible with safety. At the present time the safety factor imposes a limit of about 40 per cent weight/volume.

Ideally, the end product should be a film of maximum contrast and resolution with minimal graininess, each of which is dependent on a number of factors. Contrast is enhanced by low kV and may be influenced by processing. Resolution is enhanced by short exposure time but reduced by excessive grain. Graininess, inherent in any image intensifier and film, is increased from quantum mottle as the radiation dose per frame on the intensifier face is reduced, but may be partly eliminated by processing.

Given an ideal developing and viewing system, the best results are probably achieved by keeping the dose per frame (and hence the kV and time) low, say about 10 μrad, so as to produce a reasonable balance between contrast, resolution and graininess. The correct degree of film blackening is then achieved by finding the appropriate aperture for the camera lens.

Projections for coronary arteriography

Numerous projections are necessary in order to demonstrate the coronary arterial tree completely. The following is widely used as the minimum standard routine:

1. Left coronary
    (a) Left anterior oblique
    (b) Anteroposterior
    (c) Shallow right anterior oblique
    (d) Steep right anterior oblique
    (e) Craniocaudal tilt (if possible), in left anterior oblique and right anterior oblique.
2. Right coronary
    (a) Left anterior oblique
    (b) Right anterior oblique

Complications of Coronary Arteriography

In skilled hands the investigation carries a very small risk, and this risk has been shown to be inversely proportional to the number of investigations carried out in any one unit. The conclusion of a recent survey was that arteriography should not be performed in units where the numbers are likely to be less than 100 per year, and it is also desirable that facilities for coronary arterial surgery should be available in the same unit. In such centres the mortality is of the order of 0.02 per cent (Royal College of Physicians of London and British Cardiac Society, 1975).

The most important non-fatal complication is myocardial infarction, due to dissection of the coronary artery by the catheter tip. This is fortunately rare.

Local arterial complications occur in approximately 5 per cent. In the brachial artery the commonest is loss of the radial pulse without clinical symptoms; ischaemic changes in the hand are fortunately very rare. In the femoral artery the commonest complications are haematoma, false aneurysm, thrombosis and dissection. Local surgical intervention may be necessary to treat these complications later.

Indications for Coronary Arteriography

The indications remain under constant review, but at the present time include:

1. Angina which has not responded to medical treatment, and where coronary artery surgery is being considered.
2. Crescendo or unstable angina, in which the pain has not settled with medical treatment.
3. An atypical history or electrocardiographic finding where the diagnosis of coronary heart disease cannot be established or refuted by other means.

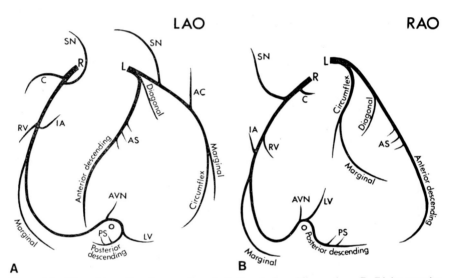

Figure 3.1   Disposition of major arteries. *A.* Left anterior oblique view. *B.* Right anterior oblique view. AC, left atrial circumflex branch; AS, anterior septal branches; AVN, atrioventricular node branch; C, conus branch; IA, right atrial circumflex artery (intermediate atrial); L, left coronary orifice; LV, posterior left ventricular branches; PS, posterior septal branches; R, right coronary orifice; RV, right ventricular branches; SN, sinoatrial node artery

4. Valve disease with angina as a symptom.
5. Heart failure of unknown cause.
6. Suspected congenital anomalies of the coronary arteries.

Coronary Artery Anatomy

The left coronary artery (Figs 3.1A, B, 3.2, 3.3A, B) arises from the left posterior aortic sinus (left coronary sinus). Its length is variable, but is rarely greater than 1 cm. In a small proportion of cases the artery has an immediate bifurcation, and occasionally there are two orifices in the left coronary sinus. In these circumstances, selective coronary arteriorgraphy and coronary perfusion at surgery are more difficult, in that one or other of the major branches only is likely to be entered, and this can lead to confusion in inter-pretation of arteriograms and errors of coronary perfusion. Beneath the left atrial appendix the main left coronary artery divides into the anterior descend-ing and the circumflex arteries.

The anterior descending artery passes to the left of the pulmonary trunk and turns forward to run downwards in the anterior interventricular groove. Its main trunk usually reaches the apex, but rarely runs beyond for any distance. It has two main groups of branches:

1. Septal branches which arise at right angles to the main trunk within a short distance of the origin, and pass vertically into the ventricular septum. The

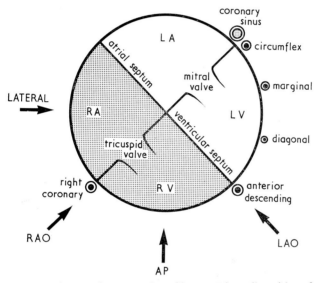

Figure 3.2 Diagrammatic central cross-section of heart to show disposition of major surface branches in various projections

first septal branch is generally the largest, and there are up to 10 other septal branches arising along the course of the main trunk. They supply the anterior two-thirds of the septum.
2. Surface branches which lie on the lateral aspect of the left ventricle and are called by convention diagonal branches. There may be more than one, and the origin of the first diagonal may be proximal or distal to the first septal.

The circumflex artery turns backwards shortly beyond its origin to run downwards in the left atrioventricular groove. Its size is extremely variable, and this is discussed below under the concept of coronary dominance. It too gives rise to a variable number of branches which lie on the lateral aspect of the left ventricle. They are termed by convention marginal branches of the circumflex; there may be up to four, and one or more of them is frequently larger than the main circumflex artery lying in the left atrioventricular groove.

The right coronary artery arises from the anterior aortic sinus (right coronary sinus), passes forward and then downward in the right atrioventricular groove, and continues around the margin of the heart towards the crux, a point inferiorly where the grooves of the heart meet. In the majority of individuals the right coronary continues forwards from the crux along the posterior interventricular groove to become the posterior descending artery, whence it approaches the apex of the heart. Important septal branches arise from the posterior descending artery, and ascend vertically in the septum. One of these is the artery to the atrioventricular node. Surface branches supplying the posteroinferior aspect of the left ventricle also arise from the posterior descending artery close to the crux, and these are normally referred to as posterior left ventricular branches.

In addition to the branches described, all of which supply the left ventricular myocardium, other smaller rather less constant branches may be present.

1. Sino-atrial node branch—usually from the proximal right coronary artery, occasionally from the circumflex.
2. Conus branch—from the proximal right coronary, to supply the outflow tract of the right ventricle. This vessel has a separate origin from the right aortic sinus in about one-third of patients.
3. Right atrial circumflex branch—from the right coronary artery.
4. Right ventricular branches—mostly from the descending portion of the right coronary but some from the anterior descending.
5. Left atrial circumflex branch—from the circumflex.

Coronary Dominance (Figs 3.3A, B)

The proportion of blood flow to the left ventricle derived from each artery is variable and is related to the size and number of distal branches arising from the right and left circumflex arteries. It presents a spectrum from extreme dominance of the right coronary, to extreme dominance of the left coronary. By convention, right coronary dominance is defined as origin of the posterior descending artery from the right coronary artery, and left dominance as origin of the posterior descending from the distal circumflex artery. Between these two situations all grades of variation occur, and some patients could reasonably be described as having balanced dominance, when the contribution to the inferior surface is about equal. In extreme right dominance the circumflex artery is small, its branch in the left AV groove may be completely absent, and the posteroinferior aspect of the left ventricle is supplied by large branches of the right coronary artery. Conversely, in extreme left dominance the right coronary artery is correspondingly small, and may contribute no branches at all to the left ventricular myocardium, terminating in the right atrioventricular groove about the margin of the heart. The circumflex artery will then not only give rise to the posterior descending but also supply the posterior left ventricular myocardium via large marginal

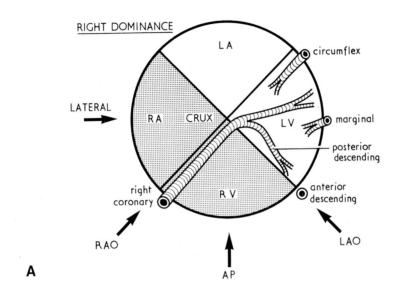

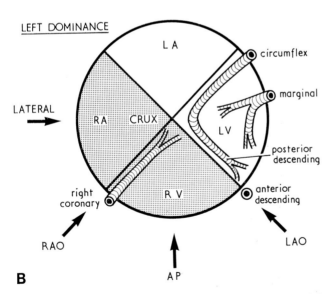

Figure 3.3   A, B. Diagram of arteries on inferior surface of heart viewed from above, to show difference between right and left coronary dominance

3

branches. If the dominant coronary artery is simply defined as the one giving rise to the posterior descending, then about 85 per cent of the population have a dominant right artery.

Patterns of Coronary Disease

The extent and distribution of narrowing of the coronary arteries by atherosclerosis is extremely variable, but some patterns are encountered more frequently than others.

Left main. Stenosis of this artery is not infrequent and, if significant, jeopardises the flow to the anterior descending and circumflex branches. Complete occlusion of the left coronary artery is rarely compatible with life, unless the onset is extremely gradual so that collaterals can develop from the right coronary artery.

Anterior descending. Block is common and may occur proximal or distal to the important first septal and diagonal branches. Stenotic lesions may be localised or diffuse, but are usually confined to the proximal part of the vessel. They frequently involve the origins of the proximal septal and diagonal branches. Localised stenoses in the distal part of the vessel are uncommon, unless the proximal part is also severely involved.

Circumflex. The circumflex artery, although commonly diseased, is involved by atheroma less often, and to a lesser extent than either the right or the anterior descending. Stenotic lesions may be localised or diffuse. If localised, they are usually proximal and may involve the main trunk, the proximal part of the AV branch and/or the marginal branches. Complete block of the circumflex is encountered less frequently than stenotic lesions, particularly complete block of the proximal circumflex. However, complete block of a marginal or the AV branch is occasionally encountered.

Right. Block is common and is more frequently found between the origin and the margin of the heart. Distal block is less frequent. Stenoses are also very common. They may be single or multiple, diffuse or localised and the patterns are extremely variable.

Collateral Pathways

Stenotic and occlusive lesions in the coronary arteries, providing they progress slowly over a period of months or years, stimulate the development of collateral pathways to the ischaemic area of myocardium (Paulin, 1967). Rapidly progressive disease which results in full thickness infarction is not followed by the development of collaterals. The common pathways encountered include:

1. To right coronary artery
   (a) To posterior descending from anterior descending via septal branches.

(b) To distal LV branches of right coronary and thence to posterior descending via marginal branches of circumflex.

(c) To posterior descending from anterior descending directly around apex.

(d) To proximal right coronary via atrial circumflex branches.

2. To anterior descending

(a) Via septals from posterior descending.

(b) To distal anterior descending from posterior descending around apex.

(c) To proximal anterior descending via conal branch of right coronary or atrial circumflex branches.

3. To circumflex

(a) To marginal or AV branch of circumflex via distal LV branches of right coronary.

(b) To AV branch from proximal right coronary via atrial circumflex branches.

In an artery with a proximal block, the distal lumen may opacify via collaterals arising from the same artery bypassing the block or, more often, from another artery pursuing one of the pathways mentioned above. In very severe proximal stenosis, filling of the distal lumen can sometimes be seen to occur both progradely and retrogradely via collaterals. In either case the true state of the distal lumen can be difficult to assess accurately, as incomplete filling is common. Surgical experience shows that the distal lumen of an artery filling retrogradely is often wider than would appear from the angiogram.

Interpretation of Coronary Arteriograms

It need hardly be said that the interpretation of coronary arteriograms is very greatly dependent on a technically adequate examination, and this includes proper opacification of the arteries with a film of high contrast and resolution. Each part of the coronary arterial tree is shown to best advantage when viewed exactly at right angles to the incident x-ray beam: each view therefore shows some parts better than others.

In the *left anterior oblique*, the main left and proximal parts of circumflex and anterior descending are greatly foreshortened. The distal anterior descending is well shown, but the circumflex and its branches are superimposed making accurate assessment difficult. The right coronary artery, in general, is well shown in this projection, except for foreshortening of the posterior descending.

The *anteroposterior view* is best for the main left coronary, and to a lesser extent the proximal part of the circumflex and anterior descending. The distal parts of both these vessels tend to be overlapped, although they can be separated on a cine film as they move in different directions during the cardiac cycle.

The *right anterior oblique* is a satisfactory view for the circumflex and its marginal branches. The proximal anterior descending is overlapped by its diagonal branch and may be difficult to see.

The distal anterior descending, may be blacked out at the edge of the heart, owing to the proximity of neighbouring lung.

The right coronary artery in its descending part is again well seen, and the posterior descending also is shown to best advantage. However, the portion of right coronary artery between margin and crux is greatly foreshortened, and overlaps the distal left ventricular branches. Figure 3.2 illustrates some of these points, and may be used by the beginner to help orientation in trying to identify the individual branches.

Pitfalls in Interpretation

Superselective catheterisation

Selective catherisation of either the anterior descending or the circumflex may be performed when the main left is short or absent and can result in complete failure to demonstrate a major portion of the coronary arterial tree. An erroneous conclusion of total block or congenital anomaly may be made. Similarly selective catheterisation of the conal artery may lead to an erroneous conclusion of right coronary block.

Incorrect identification of arteries

The anterior descending and cirumflex branches tend to overlap in the anteroposterior and right anterior oblique view, often leading to errors of identification. Although the different direction of movement of anterior descending and circumflex branches during the cardiac cycle may help, reference to the left anterior oblique view nearly always resolves the problem. The anterior descending always runs in the interventricular groove, and therefore is totally separated in position from any of the circumflex branches in this projection. It is, however, superimposed upon all the septal branches and must not be confused with them, particularly with the large first septal branch. The diagonal branch of the anterior descending bisects the angle between the anterior descending and proximal circumflex in the left anterior oblique. The circumflex and all its marginal branches are projected against the posterior wall of the heart, and their size and number can from this view be translated to the other views.

Extreme dominance

A very dominant system, either right or left, necessarily means that the opposite artery, be it the circumflex or right coronary, will be appropriately short and small and in the case of the AV branch of the circumflex, absent completely. Allowance must therefore be made for this before assuming that the small short vessel is diseased or blocked.

Method of Recording and Reporting on Coronary Arteriograms

A number of different methods of recording the findings on a coronary arteriogram have been suggested (Franklin, O'Reilly and Kranthamer, 1973). For practical purposes, when vein graft bypass surgery is being considered, only two basic pieces of information are necessary for a decision to be made:

1. The presence and site of a block and/or of stenoses and their severity.
2. The state of the distal artery into which the graft might be inserted.

A satisfactory method to record these is to indicate the lesions graphically on a diagram of a coronary arterial tree (Fig. 3.4), although by this method the

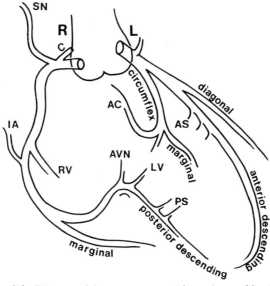

Figure 3.4   Diagram of the coronary arterial tree for marking lesions
(abbreviations as Fig. 3.1)

finer details cannot be adequately described. In the final analysis unless the film is lost it is obviously preferable to refer to the original angiogram.

Angiography of Saphenous Vein Grafts

Saphenous vein grafting is now a routine procedure in the surgical treatment of angina pectoris. Symptomatic relief is obtained in a high proportion of patients and large numbers have been investigated by selective contrast injections into the aortic end of the anastomosis (Morris et al, 1972 and Rosche et al, 1973). The incidence of patency of the vein grafts is roughly comparable to the incidence of symptomatic improvement, but will vary from one centre to another depending on the type of patient who is subjected to investigation. If done routinely on all patients, the incidence will be much higher than if done predominantly in those in whom there is an unsatisfactory clinical result. At the present time it would seem that the overall patency rate of grafts at one year is between 80 and 90 per cent (Flemma et al, 1972). Longer follow-ups with angiography performed at up to three years suggest that there is a small attrition rate of grafts at this stage and it would seem that the mechanism is intimal proliferation within the vein, rather than a recurrence of atheroma (Grondin et al, 1972). Grafting of an incompletely occluded coronary artery is frequently followed by an increase in the obstruction in the coronary vessel proximal to the anastomosis (Aldridge and Trimble, 1971; Malinow, et al, 1973), and it has been suggested that this occurs more quickly than would be expected without surgical treatment (Ben-Zui et al, 1974). It has also been suggested that the incidence of graft patency in those inserted into previously non-occluded but stenotic arteries, is greater than for those inserted into totally occluded arteries (Rees, 1976). The mechanism is possibly the creation of a watershed at the anastomosis where there may be phasic reversal of flow during the cardiac cycle which predisposes to thrombosis. If this is so, to achieve the highest patency rate it might be necessary to consider ligating the coronary artery at the time of surgery, preferably at its point of maximal narrowing. This would allow retrograde flow from the anastomotic site in to the branches distal to the stenosis and would also allow forward flow proximal to the stenosis into any important branches here.

REFERENCES

Aldridge, H. E. & Trimble, A. S. (1971) Progression of proximal coronary artery lesions to total occlusion after aortocoronary saphenous vein bypass grafting. *Journal of Thoracic and Cardiovascular Surgery*, **62**, 7.

Baron, M. G. (1971) Postinfarction aneurysm of the left ventricle. *Circulation*, **43**, 762.

Bennett, E. D. & Rees, S. (1974) The significance of radiological changes in the lungs in acute myocardial infarction. *British Journal of Radiology*, **47**, 879.

Ben-Zvi, K., Hildner, F. J., Javier, J. P., Fester, A. & Samet, P. (1974) Progression of coronary artery disease. Cinearteriographic and clinical observations in medically and surgically treated patients. *American Journal of Cardiology*, **34**, 295.

Burch, G. E., De Pasquale, N. P. & Phillips, J. H. (1963) Clinical manifestations of papillary muscle dysfunction. *Archives of Internal Medicine*, **112**, 158.

Burch, G. E., Phillips, J. H. & de Pasquale, N. P. (1971) Papillary muscle dysfunction. In *Coronary Heart Disease*, a symposium, ed. Russek, H. I. & Zohman, B. L. Philadelphia.

Cederquist, L. & Söderström, J. (1964) Papillary muscle rupture in myocardial infarction. *Acta medica scandinavica*, **176**, 287.

Chatterjee, K., Swan, H. J. C., Parmley, W., Sustaita, H., Marcus, H. & Matloff, J. (1973) Influence of direct myocardial revascularisation on left ventricular asynergy and function in patients with coronary heart disease: with and without previous myocardial infarction. *Circulation*, **47**, 276.

Cooley, D. A. & Hallman, G. L. (1968) Surgical treatment of left ventricular aneurysm: experience with excision of postinfarction lesions in 80 patients. *Progress in Cardiovascular Diseases*, **11**, 222.

de Pasquale, N. P. & Burch, G. E. (1971) Papillary muscle dysfunction in coronary (ischaemic) heart disease. *Annual Review of Medicine*, **22**, 327.

Dubnow, M. H., Burchell, H. B. & Titus, J. L. (1965) Post-infarction ventricular aneurysm. *American Heart Journal*, **70**, 753.

Dumesnil, J. G., Ritman, E. L., Davis, G. D., Gan, G. T., Rutherford, B. D. & Frye, R. L. (1975) Regional left ventricular wall dynamics before and after sublingual administration of nitroglycerin. *American Journal of Cardiology*, **36**, 419.

Flemma, R. J., Johnson, W. D., Lepley, D., Tector, A. J., Walker, J., Gale, H., Beddingfield, G. & Manley, J. C. (1972) Late results of saphenous vein bypass grafting for myocardial revascularisation. *Annals of Thoracic Surgery*, **14**, 232.

Franklin, M., O'Reilly, M. V. & Kranthamer, M. J. (1973) Standardised diagram for rapid tabulation of coronary arteriograms. *British Heart Journal*, **35**, 338.

Gibson, D. G. & Brown, D. J. (1975) Continuous assessment of left ventricular shape in man. *British Heart Journal*, **37**, 904.

Graber, J. D., Oakley, C. M., Pickering, B. N., Goodwin, J. F., Raphael, M. J. & Steiner, R. E. (1972) Ventricular aneurysm. An appraisal of diagnosis and surgical treatment. *British Heart Journal*, **34**, 830.

Grondin, C. M., Castonguay, Y. R., Lesperance, J., Bourassa, M. G., Campean, L. & Grondin, O. (1972) Attrition rate of aortocoronary saphenous vein grafts after one year. *Annals of Thoracic Surgery*, **14**, 223.

Harris, L. D., Clayton, P. D., Marshall, H. W. & Warner, H. R. (1974) A technique for the detection of asynergistic motion in the left ventricle. *Computers and Biomedical Research*, **7**, 380.

Harrison, T. R. (1965) Some unanswered questions concerning enlargement and failure of heart. *American Heart Journal*, **69**, 100.

Herman, M. V. & Gorlin, R. (1969) Implications of left ventricular asynergy. *American Journal of Cardiology*, **23**, 538.

Herman, M. V., Heinle, R. A., Klein, M. D. & Gorlin, R. (1967) Localised disorders in myocardial contraction. *New England Journal of Medicine*, **277**, 222.

Holloway, D. H., Whalen, R. E. & McIntosh, H. D. (1965) Systolic murmur developing after myocardial ischaemia or infarction. *Journal of the American Medical Association*, **191**, 888.

Holmes, A. M. & Logan, W. F. W. E. (1968) Transient systolic murmurs in angina pectoris. *American Heart Journal*, **76**, 680.

Krayenbuehl, H. P., Schoenbeck, M., Rutishauser, W. & Wirz, P. (1975) Abnormal segmental contraction velocity in coronary artery disease produced by isometric exercise and atrial pacing. *American Journal of Cardiology*, **35**, 785.

Malinow, M. R., Kremkau, E. L., Kloster, F. E., Bonchek, L. I. & Rosch, J. (1973) Occlusion of coronary arteries after vein bypass. *Circulation*, **47**, 1211.

Morris, G. C., Reul, G. J., Howell, J. F., Crawford, E. S., Chapman, D. W., Beazley, H. L., Winters, W. L., Peterson, P. K. & Lewis, J. M. (1972) Follow-up results of distal coronary artery bypass for ischaemic heart disease. *American Journal of Cardiology*, **29**, 180.

Mourdjinis, A., Olsen, E., Raphael, M. J. & Mounsey, J. P. D. (1968) Clinical diagnosis and prognosis of ventricular aneurysms. *British Heart Journal*, **30**, 497.

Orlando, M. D., Wooley, C. F., Scarpelli, D. & Ryan, J. M. (1964) Mitral regurgitation caused by infarcted papillary muscles: report of 15 cases (Abstract). *Circulation*, **30**, Suppl. 3, 36.

Pasternac, A., Gorlin, R., Sonnenblick, E. H., Haft, J. I. & Kemp, H. G. (1972) Abnormalities of ventricular motion induced by atrial pacing in coronary artery disease. *Circulation*, **45**, 1195.

Paulin, S. (1967) Interarterial coronary anastomoses in relation to arterial obstruction demonstrated in coronary arteriography. *Investigative Radiology*, **2**, 147.

Raphael, M. J., Steiner, R. E., Goodwin, J. F. & Oakley, C. M. (1972) Cine-angiography of left ventricular aneurysms. *Clinical Radiology*, **23**, 129.

Rees, S. (1976) The watershed: a factor in coronary vein graft occlusion. *British Heart Journal*, **38**, 197.

Rickards, A. F., Seabra-Gomes, R. & Balcon, R. (1976) A description of segmental wall motion abnormalities in patients with coronary disease (Abstract). *American Journal of Cardiology*, **37**, 165.

Robinson, J. S., Stannard, M. M. & Long, M. (1965) Ruptured papillary muscle after acute myocardial infarction. *American Heart Journal*, **70**, 233.

Rosch, J., Judkins, M. P., Green, G. S. & Kidd, H. (1972) Aortocoronary venous bypass grafts. Angiographic study of 84 cases. *Radiology*, **102**, 567.

Royal College of Physicians of London and British Cardiac Society (1975) The care of the patient with coronary heart disease. *Journal of the Royal College of Physicians of London*, **10**, 5.

Sanders, C. A., Armstrong, P. W., Willerson, J. T. & Dinsmore, R. E. (1971) Etiology and differential diagnosis of acute mitral regurgitation. *Progress in Cardiovascular Diseases*, **14**, 129.

Sharma, S. & Taylor, S. H. (1975) Localisation of left ventricular ischaemia in angina pectoris by cineangiography during exercise. *British Heart Journal*, **37**, 963.

Shelburne, J. C. & Gorlin, R. (1972) The diagnosis of papillary muscle dysfunction in coronary artery disease. *Geriatrics*, **27**, 116.

4
CORONARY CARE

Clive Aber

The routine management of acute myocardial infarction in coronary care units has assumed a fairly stable and comparatively uniform pattern over the past five to six years. The hospital mortality in efficient and experienced units varies between 10 and 15 per cent. This has been achieved mainly as a consequence of the immediate treatment of cardiac arrest and the prompt control of potentially lethal ventricular arrhythmias combined, perhaps, to some extent, with the prophylactic use of drugs in an attempt to prevent the development of such arrhythmias.

Having defined the principles of hospital management of postinfarction arrhythmias, more attention has been given to other possible means of reducing prehospital and hospital mortality and postinfarction morbidity. Areas of particular interest in this respect have been:

1. Prehospital coronary care—in an endeavour to stabilise myocardial irritability and to correct the autonomic disturbances that occur shortly after the onset of symptoms and/or in transit to hospital.
2. Regulation of infarct size—which would be expected to affect both the short- and the long-term prognosis.
3. The management of pump failure.
4. Physical and psychological rehabilitation.

PREHOSPITAL CORONARY CARE

Realisation that perhaps 60 per cent or more of the deaths that follow acute myocardial infarction occur outside hospital (Pantridge, 1974), within 1 h of the onset of acute symptoms (Bainton and Peterson, 1963; Gordon and Kannel, 1971), has promoted renewed interest and, in some countries, a greater endeavour to establish prehospital mobile coronary care facilities (Pantridge and Geddes, 1967; Grace and Chadbourn, 1970; Robinson and McLean, 1970; O'Rourke, 1972; Lund, 1973). Since more than 90 per cent of these early deaths take place either at home or en route to hospital from primary and potentially reversible ventricular fibrillation, often associated with relatively little ischaemic damage (Adgey et al, 1969), the need to reach these patients as soon as possible poses a continual challenge. None the less, often due to alleged concern about a limited budget and anticipated difficulties in staffing (medical, nursing, and paramedical), there remains a reluctance to establish mobile units of this type, even though it has been shown that the running and maintenance need not impose an undue financial burden and that where it has not been possible, or thought desirable, to provide medical cover an efficient service can be introduced with well-trained paramedical personnel (Binnion, Mandal and Makous, 1973; Cobb and Alvarex, 1973; White et al, 1973). Perhaps, to some extent, the inconclusive results of the south-western 'home and hospital treatment' study (Mather et al, 1971) in Great Britain have promoted this over-cautious attitude.

Collective international experience from mobile coronary care units has shown that by adopting a more aggressive therapuetic approach it has been possible to save lives (Adgey et al, 1969, 1971) and to collect additional information with regard to the nature, incidence, clinical significance and therapeutic implications of the early autonomic disturbances and arrhythmias that follow acute myocardial infarction (Geddes, Webb and Pantridge, 1972; Webb, Adgey and Pantridge, 1972; Epstein et al, 1973; Pantridge et al, 1974). For example, sinus bradycardia and major ventricular arrhythmias are common and often transient early events, although the relationship, if any, between these two arrhythmias remains debatable. The rationale for using atropine in the treatment of sinus bradycardia which occurs in about 30 per cent of patients within the first hour, often in association with a mild systolic hypotension, has been questioned (Epstein et al, 1973). Early AV block has also been shown to occur more frequently than previously recorded but, fortunately, rarely poses any major problem of management and usually responds to atropine therapy. The routine use of lignocaine in the management of early ventricular ectopic beats, whether unifocal, consecutive, multifocal, or of the R on T variety, has also been challenged. It now appears likely that when these arrhythmias occur early they are less responsive to this form of therapy than when similar arrhythmias develop later (Chopra et al, 1971; Lie, Wellens and Durrer, 1974; British Medical Journal, 1975).

The combined intravenous administration of atropine (0.6 mg) and a beta blocking agent (sotalol 10 mg) to prevent undue bradycardia or sinus tachycardia has been reported by Mulholland and Pantridge (1974), but the effectiveness of this routine as a means of preventing the development of major arrhythmias and reducing the amount of ischaemic myocardial damage has not been thoroughly established.

If we acknowledge that efficient, more 'aggressive', early intensive care, by controlling heart rate, hypotension or hypertension, heart failure, and arrhythmias, may also limit ultimate infarct size, additional benefit could be envisaged from the introduction of mobile units since the incidence of major postinfarction complications, particularly pump failure, would be expected to be reduced and this in turn might effect a shorter mean hospital stay.

REGULATION OF INFARCT SIZE

Identification of the major determinants of myocardial oxygen consumption in the normal and ischaemic heart (Table 4.1) (Sarnoff et al, 1958; Ross et al, 1965; Boerth, Covell and Pool, 1969; Braunwald, 1971; Karliner and Ross, 1971, Burns and Covell, 1972; Watanabe et al, 1972), combined with results of experiments which show that in the first few hours following coronary occlusion there is no clear-cut demarcation between normal myocardium and tissue which has been irreversibly damaged by ischaemia, indicate that the fate of a substantial quantity of myocardium would seem to be delicately poised after acute myocardial infarction—'jeopardised myocardium' (Cox et al, 1968; Becker, Ferreira and Thomas, 1973; Lubbe et al, 1974). This has promoted the examination of potential means of limiting the extent of myocardial necrosis which succeeds acute coronary occlusion. Animal experiments (Maroko et al, 1971, 1972a, b; Ginks et al, 1972; Redwood, Smith and

Table 4.1   Major determinants of myocardial oxygen consumption

1. Ventricular wall tension (Sarnoff et al, 1958)
2. Contractile state of the myocardium (myocardial contractility) (Ross et al, 1965; Braunwald, 1971)
3. Heart rate (Boerth et al, 1969)
4. Shortening against a load—Fenn effect (Coleman et al, 1969; Burns and Covell, 1972)
5. External cardiac work (Braunwald et al, 1958)

Epstein, 1972; Maroko and Braunwald, 1973) and exploratory clinical studies have now been completed which demonstrate that the amount of irreversibly damaged myocardium can be favourably modified during the early evolution of infarction by manipulating the balance between myocardial oxygen supply and demand, bearing in mind that the amount of jeopardised myocardium available for salvage is determined by (1) the duration of ischaemia prior to commencing therapy, (2) the size of the vessel occluded, (3) the completeness of the occlusive lesion, (4) the adequacy and availability of collateral blood flow and (5) appreciation that the microvasculature in an area of severe ischaemic myocardium 'collapses' irreversibly if the period of ischaemia is prolonged—'the no-flow phenomenon' (Leaf, 1973).

In an attempt to limit infarct size the potential therapeutic value of a wide range of pharmacological agents (Redwood, Kent and Smith, 1973; Chatterjee and Swan, 1974), metabolic adjustments (Maroko et al, 1972a, c; Mjos, Kjekshus and Lekven, 1974), mechanical circulatory support, and surgical revascularisation procedures (Sanders et al, 1972; Resnekov, 1974; O'Rourke et al, 1975) have been evaluated and continue to deserve consideration (Table 4.2).

β-Adrenergic Blockade

Since myocardial oxygen consumption is a direct function of heart rate and left ventricular pre- and afterload, the use of β-adrenergic blockade in an attempt to limit infarct size demanded evaluation. Preliminary experimental 'animal' and clinical studies using epicardial and precordial electrocardiographic mapping (Maroko et al, 1972a) or serial CPK measurements (Shell, Kjekshus and Sobel, 1971) as indices of the extent of myocardial necrosis appear to show that propranolol and practolol diminish or delay ischaemic myocardial injury if administered during acute ischaemic myocardial syndromes. Mueller et al (1974) reported the effects of intravenous propranolol (0.1 mg/kg in three divided doses at 5 min intervals) given to 20 patients with

Table 4.2 Potential methods of reducing ischaemic myocardial injury

A. Decreasing myocardial oxygen demand
　　1. β-Adrenergic blockade[a]
　　2. (i) Vasodilators[a]
　　　 (ii) Hypotensives[a]
　　　 (iii) Nitroglycerin[a]
　　3. External or intra-aortic balloon counterpulsation[a]
　　4. Digitalis (in heart failure)

B. Increasing myocardial oxygen supply by
　　1. Elevating arterial oxygen tension
　　2. Elevation of cornary perfusion pressure (drugs[a]; counterpulsation[a])
　　3. Thrombolytic agents[a]
　　4. Coronary artery revascularisation[a]
　　5. Increasing plasma osmolarity (mannitol; hypertonic glucose)

C. Augmentation of anaerobic glycolysis—glucose–inculin–potassium[a]; hyptertonic glucose

D. Improved diffusion of oxygen and substrate to the ischaemic zone—hyaluronidase[a]

E. Stabilisation of the autolytic and heterolytic processes—hydrocortisone

[a] Already under clinical investigation—see text

acute myocardial infarction of at least 6 to 8 h duration. Having excluded patients with previous or current heart failure, hypotension (blood pressure less than 100 mmHg), bradycardia (pulse less than 65 beats/min), atrioventricular and intraventricular conduction delay, or a history of chronic obstructive lung disease, they observed an approximate 20 per cent reduction in mean arterial pressure, heart rate, heart work, coronary blood flow, and myocardial oxygen uptake. By contrast, there was a definite increase in lactate extraction by the heart during this study which, in the absence of any significant changes in the arterial free fatty acid concentrations or free fatty acid uptake, almost certainly reflected a reduction in myocardial ischaemia. Pelides et al (1972), using precordial ST segment shift as an indirect index of the severity of myocardial necrosis, administered practolol intravenously (20 mg over a period of 5 min) to nine patients within 72 h of the onset of acute symptoms of myocardial infarction and observed that there was a significant reduction in ST segment elevation subsequent to giving this preparation. The observations of Fox et al (1975a) also suggest that the severity of ischaemic myocardial injury associated with prolonged ischaemic myocardial pain in patients with established coronary heart disease who enter coronary care units with likely acute myocardial infarction is less if they had been receiving long-term β-adrenergic blocking drugs.

Recognising that the reduction in heart rate was relatively mild in some of these studies and that Mueller et al (1974) found a reduction in coronary flow as a consequence of propranolol therapy, the overall benefits of β-adrenergic blockade in acute myocardial infarction may well be multifactoral, reflecting not only a reduction in heart work but also a possible redistribution of coronary blood flow without decreasing the flow to the jeopardised zones— subendocardial perfusion being maintained. There may also be effects on cell metabolism—reduction in cell membrane sodium and calcium transport and decreased glycolysis and lypolysis.

Vasodilator and Hypotensive Therapy

Awareness that transient or sustained systemic hypertension and all grades of heart failure are common after acute myocardial infarction, coupled with theoretical considerations which suggest that left ventricular pump efficiency can be altered profoundly by changes in systemic vascular resistance (SVR), promoted the study of vasodilator and hypotensive agents in acute myocardial infarction. These drugs are known to lower SVR and increase stroke volume and cardiac output thereby effecting an improvement of pump function, as well as possibly limiting infarct size. However, a prerequisite of this form of therapy is that the resultant fall in blood pressure and subsequent anticipated reflex tachycardia should not be severe enough to either significantly impair coronary flow or augment myocardial oxygen consumption.

Redwood et al (1972), using ST segment recordings from intramyocardial electrodes as an index of ischaemic myocardial injury during the evolution of acute myocardial infarction in dogs found that nitroglycerin diminished ischaemic myocardial injury and, to some extent, also prevented the lowering of the ventricular fibrillation threshold that occurs after coronary occlusion. Moreover, these effects occurred despite an associated fall in arterial blood pressure and an increase in heart rate. Paradoxically, they then observed (Smith et al, 1973) that when the reduction in blood pressure caused by nitroglycerin was abolished by the simultaneous administration of methoxamine or phenylephrine the degree of ischaemic injury due to coronary occlusion diminished to an even greater extent, suggesting that not all the apparent benefits of nitroglycerin were the direct consequences of the observed haemodynamic changes. Similar observations have been made by Hirshfield et al (1974).

In 1973 Chatterjee et al reported their haemodynamic evaluation of nitroprusside and phentolamine therapy in 38 patients following acute myocardial infarction. Using infusion rate of 16 to 200 μg/min of nitroprusside or 0.1 to 2.0 mg/min of phentolamine, they achieved either a reduction of mean arterial blood pressure of not more than 30 mmHg or a 'significant decrease' in capillary wedge or pulmonary end-diastolic blood pressures. This resulted in a decrease in SVR, pulmonary vascular resistance, pulmonary arterial pressure, right and left ventricular filling pressures, together with a slight to moderate fall in systemic arterial pressures in most patients, whether or not there had been evidence of heart failure prior to commencing vasodilator therapy. A consistent rise in cardiac index only occurred in patients with initially high left ventricular filling pressures (greater than 15 mmHg) who, in most instances, also displayed both clinical and radiographic features of left ventricular failure. Some of these patients were appreciably hypotensive and/or in cardiogenic shock before treatment was commenced. The authors comment that despite a fall in systemic arterial pressure their metabolic studies failed to reveal any deleterious effect on overall myocardial oxygen metabolism. Kelly et al (1973) likewise were able to show that the short-term (10–20 min) administration of intravenous phentolamine in hypertensive patients in left ventricular failure following acute myocardial infarction promoted an increase in cardiac index and reduction in left ventricular filling pressure. Their results suggest that the greatest benefit was afforded to those patients with acute hypertension and it is noteworthy that treatment had to be discontinued in two patients with established hypertension due to the development of chest pain and tachycardia. Similarly, Gould et al (1973) have examined the value of phentolamine (0.4 mg/min for 30 min) in the treatment of 10 normotensive patients within 24 h of the onset of symptoms of acute myocardial infarction. This promoted a rise in cardiac index from 2.44 to 3.58 litres/min/m^2 and an increase in stroke volume from 26 to 34 ml/beat/m^2. The left ventricular filling pressure fell in every patient from a mean of 21 to 13 mmHg during phentolamine infusion and the mean arterial pressure fell from 86 to 72 mmHg with a corresponding lowering of SVR from 1627 to 952 dyn s cm^5. More recently Shell and Sobel (1974) demonstrated that by reducing left ventricular afterload in a group of 38 hypertensive and normotensive patients with acute myocardial infarction with intravenous trimethaphan (Arfonad) (100–700 μg/min) it was possible to promote a significant diminution in infarct size in the hypertensive group, as measured by serial enzyme studies. The trimethaphan infusion was adjusted to decrease arterial pressure and maintain either systolic blood pressure values of 115 to 130 mmHg or to effect a reduction of 30 to 40 mmHg below the control pretreatment values. Therapy was commenced on average at 11 h after the onset of acute chest pain and intravenous methyldopa (1 g daily in divided doses) was administered 10 h afterwards to maintain a suitable reduction in blood pressure. It was also noted that the overall mortality in treated patients at one month was less than the untreated group.

Whereas it is essential to remain aware that most of these observations were made on animal models with an otherwise intact coronary circulation and that to date the clinical investigations have been carried out on small and not always well-matched groups of patients, there would appear to be reasonable optimism that vasodilator and/or hypotensive drugs may prove valuable therapeutic additions to the routine management of acute myocardial infarction, particularly in the presence of acute hypertension where the studies of Fox et al (1975b) have shown that the immediate and late prognoses are worse than in normotensive patients.

Counterpulsation

Failure of drug therapy significantly to influence the mortality from cardiogenic shock following acute myocardial infarction has encouraged the use of mechanical procedures that afford temporary circulatory support (Sanders et al, 1972; Soroff et al, 1972; Al-Sidir et al, 1973; Dilley, Ross and Bernstein, 1973; Gold et al, 1973). Reduction of left ventricular pre- and afterload effects a decrease in myocardial oxygen consumption by lowering the cardiac work level, whilst enhancement of arterial diastolic coronary filling pressure should allow augmentation of coronary perfusion along with limitation of ischaemic myocardial injury and subsequent improvement of left ventricular function and tissue perfusion. Although it has also been suggested that brief periods of counterpulsation open up intercoronary collaterals in the acutely ischaemic heart (Jacobey et al, 1968), to date clinical experience has not substantiated this concept and experimental studies have shown that weeks or even months are required for the development of intercoronary collaterals in response to an ischaemic stimulus (Baird and Manktelow, 1969).

Currently mechanical ventricular support with intra-aortic balloon counterpulsation (IABP) represents the most promising therapeutic approach to postinfarction cardiogenic shock where at least 40 to 50 per cent of the left ventricular myocardium has usually been damaged (Caulfield, Dunkman and Leinbach, 1972). The immediate clinical status can be improved substantially within 24 to 48 h in about 90 per cent of patients when this diagnosis has been based on the following criteria (Scheidt et al, 1973):

1. arterial blood pressure of less than 90 mmHg for 1 to 2 h which has failed to respond to drug therapy,
2. oliguria with urinary output of less than 20 ml/h, combined with
3. clinical features of shock—peripheral vasoconstriction, mental confusion, and drowsiness with a prepump (counterpulse) cardiac index of less than 2 litres/min/m^2 and/or with a pulmonary capillary pressure greater than 20 mmHg.

However, before accepting a complex method of patient care which demands a team of highly trained and skilled medical, nursing, and technical staff, we must know whether it will effect sufficient recovery of cardiac function to present reasonable optimism with regard to the long-term prognosis. So far information on this point is inconclusive, but preliminary studies suggest that perhaps 30 to 35 per cent of patients who have been offered mechanical circulatory support for 'cardiogenic shock' after acute myocardial infarction survive to leave hospital (Mundth et al, 1971; Leinbach et al, 1973). In some of these studies, however, the diagnostic criteria of cardiogenic shock has been imprecise and O'Rourke et al (1975) now suggest that better results would be obtained if counterpulsation were offered earlier and on a more flexible haemodynamic basis after acute ischaemic myocardial injury.

After establishing intra-aortic balloon counterpulsation features which appear to favour successful revascularisation as the treatment of choice in acute myocardial infarction complicated by cardiogenic shock are:

(a) beneficial response to IABP with objective haemodynamic improvement—indicative of potential myocardial functional reserve
(b) haemodynamic dependence on IABP persisting 24 to 48 h—a stable but suboptimal haemodynamic status with a cardiac index of about 2 litres/min/m^2, PC wedge of approximately 20 mmHg or mean aortic pressure of about 60 mmHg with IABP temporarily discontinued
(c) relatively short duration of shock (12–24 h)
(d) relatively short time interval (five days) from onset of myocardial infarction or extension of myocardial infarction.

The use of temporary circulatory support to cover preoperative cardiac catheterisation and coronary angiography when postinfarction surgery is under consideration has undoubtedly made it possible to salvage patients who otherwise would have died, either as a consequence of rupture of the ventricular septum or papillary muscle or where the development of either a left ventricular aneurysm or extreme left ventricular wall dyskinesia frequently combined with recurrent ventricular arrhythmias severely jeopardised their clinical progress (Mundth et al, 1972; Sanders et al, 1972; Scheidt et al, 1973; Miller et al, 1974).

Factors mitigating against surgical survival under such circumstances would appear to be (i) rapidly deteriorating clinical progress, (ii) a poor response to inotropic agents, (iii) severe hypokinesia or akinesia involving more than 60 per cent of the left ventricular wall, (iv) inadequate distal coronary arteries for satisfactory bypass, and (v) avascularity of hypokinetic areas of the left ventricular wall adjacent to the infarct.

Thrombolytic Therapy

The therapeutic value of thrombolytic agents in the early management of acute myocardial infarction has been examined in recent years but clear-cut beneficial results have not emerged (Praetorius et al, 1970; Dioguardi et al,

1971; European Working Party, 1971; Bett et al, 1973). Likewise, the results of a multicentred trial of streptokinase in the United Kingdom has failed to reveal any worthwhile value of this form of treatment which, if adopted as routine, would impose a further load on already overworked medical, nursing, and laboratory staff (Aber et al, 1976).

Preliminary observations of the effectiveness of this form of therapy in the intermediate coronary syndrome appear more optimistic.

INTERMEDIATE CORONARY SYNDROME

Crescendo angina, acute coronary insufficiency without myocardial infarction, variant angina, and intermediate coronary syndrome describe ischaemic myocardial syndromes intermediate in severity between angina pectoris and myocardial infarction (Graybiel, 1955; Vakil, 1961). Between 10 and 20 per cent of all admissions to coronary care units fall into this category, where the immediate and short-term prognosis is relatively good with an acute mortality of approximately 6 per cent (Vakil, 1961; Murnaghan and Hickey, 1970; Krauss, Hutter and DeSanctis, 1972). Rapid progression to infarction occurs in about 14 per cent. In contrast, the long-term outlook in this often ill-defined ischaemic myocardial syndrome would appear to be less favourable (Vakil, 1961; Murnaghan and Hickey, 1970; Gazes, Mobley and Faris, 1972; Krauss et al, 1972).

Both acute intensive β-adrenergic blockade (Fischl, Herman and Gorlin, 1973) and aortic coronary bypass surgery (Anagnostopoulos and Kittle, 1971; Hill et al, 1971; Lambert et al, 1971; Scanlon et al, 1971) have been used with varying success in attempts to control this unstable coronary circulatory syndrome. Linhart, Beller and Talley (1972) and Fischl et al (1973) reported their observations with respect to the clinical behaviour and angiographic findings in this condition. The Boston group described the effectiveness of β-adrenergic blockade in a clearly defined group of 23 patients. An increase in systolic blood pressure and heart rate during pain were common features and left ventricular failure developed in about one-third of this group. Definite ST segment changes (elevation and depression) and/or T-wave inversion was invariable and subsequent coronary angiography revealed significant arterial wall lesions in all but one patient. It was noted, however, that collateral vessels were less frequent than in patients with long-standing stable coronary heart disease (with or without previous infarction). Left ventricular dysfunction was usually only mild or absent. Seventeen out of the 20 patients treated with propranolol (20 mg orally every 4 h with rapid dosage increments until either pain was alleviated or the heart rate remained persistently below 60 beats/min during pain) gained prompt symptomatic relief and a corresponding reduction in blood pressure and heart rate with resolution of left ventricular failure when it had been evident before treatment.

A dosage of 40 to 400 mg of propranolol daily was required to achieve this effect. Elective revascularisation was then performed in 14 patients.

Coronary artery surgery

Successful saphenous vein bypass surgery for unstable angina pictures after detailed evaluation by coronary angiography has been described over the past three or four years (Anagnostopoulos and Kittle, 1971; Lambert et al, 1971). Conti et al (1971) reported marked symtomatic relief in 18 of 21 survivors of surgery. Although the initial surgical mortality appeared to be high when contrasted with the relatively low death rate following the establishment of beta blockade in this group of patients, the results of two recent prospective studies which compared medically and surgically treated patients failed to substantiate this difference (Bertolasi et al, 1974; Seldon et al, 1975). None the less, it must be borne in mind that the performance of acute coronary angiography in this high risk group of patients has a significant and relatively high mortality level.

Surgical Management of Acute Myocardial Infarction

Improvement in surgical and diagnostic techniques, combined with the introduction of mechanical circulatory support procedures, has encouraged acute surgery in the management of acute myocardial infarction. Infarctectomy, ventricular septal closure, mitral valve repair/or replacement, and revascularisation deserve consideration, since left ventricular wall rupture occurs in approximately 10 per cent of patients and a further 1 per cent develop either ventricular septal defect or papillary muscle rupture. Early diagnosis of these complications, which are frequently accompanied by recurrent ventricular arrhythmias, heart failure, and/or cardiogenic shock demands constant clinical awareness during the initial stages of the illness. It is also highly desirable that facilities should be available nearby to effect immediate mechanical circulatory support and diagnostic help. Indications for this type of surgery after clinical, haemodynamic, and angiographic confirmation of the diagnosis would seem to be:

(a) *Infarctectomy*—when there is progressive or persistent shock, sometimes associated with recurrent ventricular arrhythmias, and where the left ventricular angiogram reveals a dyskinetic or clear-cut paradoxical segment of the left ventricular wall.

(b) *Closure of a ventricular septal defect*—when there is intractable shock, heart failure, or recurrent ventricular (or sometimes supraventricular) arrhythmias or when a previously stable clinical and haemodynamic status suddenly deteriorates.

(c) *Early mitral valve replacement/repair*—when the valve incompetence has promoted the development of acute severe and drug resistant pulmonary oedema or when lesser grades of heart failure prove refractory to medical therapy.

(d) *Revascularisation*—is rarely indicated as the elective treatment for an established infarct per se in the absence of cardiogenic shock. It may, however, be carried out as a supportive procedure with the above forms of surgery. When acute coronary occlusion follows coronary angiography or in some cases of the intermediate coronary artery syndrome it can offer worthwhile benefit.

REHABILITATION

Economic, domestic, psychological, and social factors dictate that patients who survive acute myocardial infarction should return to as normal a life-style as possible as soon as practicable. Sixty to seventy per cent of patients in the working age group resume work within four months (Sharland, 1964; Kushnir et al, 1975a) although initial job modification may be required. Ninety per cent are working again within 10 months of their heart attack, usually without the assistance of specialised rehabilitation centres (Kushnir et al, 1975a). Fear of sudden death or recurrence of ill-health, ill-conceived ideas of the cause of their heart condition, combined with a lack of satisfactory professional guidance, may delay optimal rehabilitation and can lead to chronic invalidism (Wynn, 1967).

Mobilisation

Early mobilisation and discharge from hospital after uncomplicated acute myocardial infarction appears to have no detrimental effects (Harpur et al, 1971; Royal Infirmary, Glasgow, Study, 1973; Hutter et al, 1973; Lamers et al, 1973; Chaturvedi et al, 1974). Indeed, it may well promote psychological benefit and allow a more positive approach to subsequent rehabilitation. On the other hand, the value of a predischarge consultation in achieving a rapid return to normal living is in doubt (Kushnir et al, 1976). In contrast, hospital review within 8 to 10 weeks appears to offer the patient and sometimes the general practitioner considerable help with respect to the speed with which the 'normal' level of activity is attained (Kushnir et al, 1975a).

Physical training

Whilst involvement in an active training programme is sometimes adopted where appropriate facilities and staff are available (Clausen, Larsen, Trap-Jensen, 1969; Carson et al, 1973), there is as yet no conclusive data which shows that such formalised training either prolongs life or prevents reinfarction. None the less, angina of effort can be improved or relieved as a consequence of reducing the heart rate and systolic blood pressure response to exercise in the trained patient (Clausen et al, 1969; Detry and Bruce, 1971; Detry et al, 1971). This again must effect considerable psychological benefit in some instances (Kellerman et al, 1968; Nagle, Gangola and Picton-Robinson, 1971). Whether or not patients with established coronary heart disease who are otherwise in good physical condition tolerate further infarction better than those who are less 'fit' is speculative but remains a possibility.

Return to normal life

Patients frequently express concern about the resumption of sexual activity or the development of impotence following acute myocardial infarction. Unfortunately, these problems are often handled with restraint and uncertainty by many physicians. Attempts to evaluate the cardiovascular cost of conjugal sexual intercourse have been made (Hellerstein and Friedman, 1970) but the very personal nature of this aspect of a patient's life means that advice must be individualised. Impotence following acute myocardial infarction is relatively common and occasions sympathetic counselling, recognising that there is usually no obvious physical cause and that sometimes it is the result of fear and anxiety or is the side effect of drug therapy.

Interestingly, but perhaps not surprisingly, patients who have survived cardiac arrest due to primary ventricular fibrillation after their first myocardial infarction are slower to resume a 'normal' life-style as judged by resumption of work, sexual activity, and driving of motor vehicles (Kushnir et al, 1975b). Even so, their long-term prognosis is otherwise known to be similar to that of patients who had not developed this complication.

The recent report of the Joint Working Party of the Royal College of Physicians (London) and the British Cardiac Society (1975) and previously that of the International Society of Cardiology (1973) presents a more informed approach to rehabilitation after acute myoardial infarction. Many recommendations are made in general terms, although emphasis is placed on the avoidance of isometric exercise training with its known high cardiovascular demands and caution is also expressed with respect to the awarding of licences to pilots or patients previously holding public service or heavy goods vehicle licences in the United Kingdom. It is stressed that few patients in the working age group show persisting severe physical incapacity as a consequence of heart failure, breathlessness, or angina following acute myocardial infarction, hence a wide variety of jobs could and should be pursued after recovery from the acute illness.

REFERENCES

Aber, C. P., Bass, N. M., Berry, C. L., Carson, P. H. M., Dobbs, R. J., Fox, K. M., Hamblin, J. J., Haydu, S. P., Howitt, G., MacIver, J. E., Portal, R. W., Raftery, E. B., Rousell, R. H. & Stock, J. P. P. (1976) Streptokinase in acute myocardial infarction: a controlled multicentre study in the United Kingdom. *British Medical Journal*, 2, 1100–1104.

Adgey, A. A. J., Nelson, P. G., Scott, M. E., Geddes, J. S., Allen, J. D., Zaidi, S. A. & Pantridge, J. F. (1969) Management of ventricular fibrillation outside hospital. *Lancet*, 1, 1169–1171.

Adgey, A. A. J., Allen, J. D., Geddes, J. S., James, R. G. G., Webb, S. W., Zaidi, S. A. & Pantridge, J. F. (1971) Acute phase of myocardial infarction. *Lancet*, 2, 501–504.

Al-Sidir, J., Zimmet, L., Brooks, H., King, S. & Resnekov, L. (1973) Haemodynamic evaluation of external counterpulsation in acute myocardial infarction. *Clinical Research*, **21**, 396 (abstract).

Anagnostopoulos, C. E. & Kittle, C. F. (1971) Surgical aspects of acute myocardial infarction: current status of infarctectomy, ventricular septal defect closure, mitral valve replacement and revascularisation. *Surgical Clinics of North America*, **51**, 69–84.

Bainton, C. R. & Peterson, D. R. (1963) Deaths from coronary heart disease in persons fifty years of age and younger (a community-wide study). *New England Journal of Medicine*, **268**, 569–575.

Baird, R. J. & Manktelow, R. T. (1969) Systolic pressure in the tunnelled portion of a myocardial vascular implant. *Journal of Thoracic and Cardiovascular Surgery*, **57**, 714–720.

Becker, L. C., Ferreira, R. & Thomas, M. (1973) Mapping of left ventricular blood flow with radioactive microspheres in experimental coronary artery occlusion. *Cardiovascular Research*, **7**, 391–400.

Bertolasi, C. A., Trongé, J. E., Carreno, C. A., Jalon, J. & Vega, M. R. (1974). Unstable angina—Prospective and a randomised study of its evolution with and without surgery. Preliminary report *American Journal of Cardiology*, **33**, 201–208.

Bett, J. H. N., Biggs, J. C., Castaldi, P. A., Chestermann, C. N., Hale, G. S., Hirsh, J., Isbister, J. P., McDonald, I. G., McLean, K. H., Morgan, J. J., O'Sullivan, E. F. & Rosenbaum, M. (1973) Australian multicentre trial of streptokinase in acute myocardial infarction. *Lancet*, **1**, 57–60.

Binnion, P. F., Mandal, S. & Makous, N. (1973) The mobile coronary care unit. *Journal of the American Medical Association*, **223**, 923.

Boerth, R. C., Covell, J. W. & Pool, P. E. (1969) Increased myocardial oxygen consumption and contractile state associated with increased heart rate in dogs. *Circulation Research*, **24**, 725–734.

Braunwald, E., Sarnoff, S. J., Case, R. B., Stainsby, W. N. & Welch, G. H., Jr (1958) Haemodynamic determinants of coronary flow: effect of changes in aortic pressure and cardiac output on the relationship between myocardial oxygen consumption and coronary flow. *American Journal of Physiology*, **192**, 157–163.

Braunwald, E. (1971) Control of myocardial oxygen consumption (physiologic and clinical considerations). *American Journal of Cardiology*, **27**, 416–432.

British Medical Journal (1975) Doubts about lignocaine, **1**, 473–474.

Burns, J. W. & Covell, J. W. (1972) Myocardial oxygen consumption during isotonic and isovolumic contractions in the intact heart. *American Journal of Physiology*, **223**, 1491–1497.

Carson, P., Neophytou, M., Tucker, H. & Simpson, T. (1973) Exercise programme after myocardial infarction. *British Medical Journal*, **4**, 213–216.

Caulfield, J. B., Dunkman, W. B. & Leinbach, R. C. (1972) Cardiogenic shock: myocardial morphology with and without artificial left ventricular counterpulsation. *Archives of Pathology*, **93**, 532–536.

Chatterjee, K., Parmley, W. W., Ganz, W., Forrester, J., Walinsky, P., Crexells, C. & Swan, H. J. C. (1973) Hemodynamic and metabolic responses to vasodilator therapy in acute myocardial infarction. *Circulation*, **48**, 1183–1193.

Chatterjee, K. & Swan, H. J. E. (1974) Vasodilator therapy in acute myocardial infarction. *Modern Concepts of Cardiovascular Disease*, **63**, 119–124.

Chaturvedi, N. C., Walsh, M. J., Evans, A., Munro, D., Boyle, D. McC. & Barber, J. M. (1974) Selection of patients for early discharge after acute myocardial infarction. *British Heart Journal*, **36**, 533–535.

Chopra, M. P., Thadani, U., Portal, R. W. & Aber, C. P. (1971) Lignocaine therapy for ventricular ectopic activity after acute myocardial infarction: a double-blind trial. *British Medical Journal*, **3**, 668–670.

Clausen, J. P., Larsen, O. A. & Trap-Jensen, J. (1969) Physical training in the management of coronary artery disease. *Circulation*, **40**, 143–154.

Cobb, L. A. & Alvarez, H. E. (1973) Medic I. The Seattle system for management of out-of-hospital emergencies. *National Conference on Emergency Cardiac Care*, National Research Council and National Academy of Sciences, Washington, DC.

Conti, C. R., Green, B., Pitt, B., Griffith, L., Brawley, R., Taylor, D., Bender, H., Gott, V. & Ross, R. S. (1971) Coronary artery surgery in unstable angina pectoris. *Circulation*, **44**, Suppl. 2, 154.

Cox, J. L., McLaughlin, V. W., Flowers, N. C. & Horan, L. G. (1968) The ischaemic zone surrounding acute myocardial infarction. Its morphology as detected by dehydrogenase staining. *American Heart Journal*, **76**, 650–659.

Detry, J. M. & Bruce, R. A. (1971) Effects of physical training on exertional ST segment depression in coronary heart disease. *Circulation*, **44**, 390–396.

Detry, J. M., Rousseau, M., Vanden Brouke, G., Kusumi, F., Brasseur, L. & Bruce, R. A. (1971) Increased arteriovenous oxygen difference after physical training in coronary heart disease. *Circulation*, **44**, 109–118.

Dilley, R. B., Ross, J. J. & Bernstein, E. F. (1973) Serial haemodynamics during intra-aortic balloon counterpulsation for cardiogenic shock. *Circulation*, **47**, Suppl. 3, 99–104.

Dioguardi, N., Mannucci, P. M., Lotto, A., Rossi, P., Levi, G. F., Lomento, B., Rota, M., Mattei, G., Proto, C. & Fiorelli, C. (1971) Controlled trial of streptokinase and heparin in acute myocardial infarction. *Lancet*, **2**, 891–895.

Epstein, S. E., Goldstein, R. E., Redwood, D. R., Kent, K. M. & Smith, E. R. (1973) The early phase of acute myocardial infarction: pharmacological aspects of therapy. *Annals of Internal Medicine*, **78**, 918–936.

European Working Party (1971) Streptokinase in recent myocardial infarction—a controlled multicentre trial. *British Medical Journal*, **3**, 325–331.

Fischl, S. J., Herman, V. & Gorlin, R. (1973) The intermediate coronary syndrome. *New England Journal of Medicine*, **288**, 1193–1198.

Fox, K. M., Chopra, M. P., Portal, R. W. & Aber, C. P. (1975a) Long-term beta blockade: possible protection from myocardial infarction. *British Medical Journal*, **1**, 117–119.

Fox, K. M., Tomlinson, I. W., Portal, R. W. & Aber, C. P. (1975b) Prognostic significance of acute systolic hypertension after myocardial infarction. *British Medical Journal*, **3**, 128–130.

Gazes, P. C., Mobley, E. M. & Faris, H. M. (1972) Pre-infarction angina—prospective study —ten-year follow-up. *Circulation*, **46**, Suppl. 2, 23.

Geddes, J. S., Webb, S. & Pantridge, J. F. (1972) Limitations of lignocaine in control of early ventricular dysrhythmias complicating the acute myocardial infarction. *British Heart Journal*, **34**, 964–965.

Ginks, W. R., Sybers, H. D., Maroko, P. R., Covell, J. W., Sobel, B. E. & Ross, J., Jr (1972) Coronary artery reperfusion—reduction of myocardial infarct size at 1 week after coronary occlusion. *Journal of Clinical Investigation*, **51**, 2717–2723.

Gold, H. K., Leinbach, R. C., Sanders, C. A., Buckley, M. J., Mundth, E. D. & Austen, W. G. (1973) Intra-aortic balloon pumping for ventricular septal defect or mitral regurgitation complicating acute myocardial infarction. *Circulation*, **42**, 1191–1196.

Gordon, T. & Kannel, W. B. (1971) Premature mortality from coronary heart disease. The Framingham study. *Journal of the American Medical Association*, **215**, 1617–1625.

Gould, L., Reddy, C. V. R., Kalanithi, P., Espina, L. & Gomprecht, R. F. (1973) Use of phentolamine in acute myocardial infarction. *American Heart Journal*, **88**, 144–148.

Grace, W. J. & Chadbourn, J. A. (1970) The first hours in acute myocardial infarction (AMI): observations on 50 patients. *Circulation*, **41**, Suppl. 3 (abstract), 160.

Graybiel, A. (1955) The intermediate coronary syndrome. *U.S. Armed Forces Medical Journal*, **6**, 1–7.

Harpur, J. E., Conner, W. T., Hamilton, M., Kellett, R. J., Galbraith, H. J. B., Murray, J. J., Swallow, J. H. & Rose, G. A. (1971) Controlled trial of early mobilisation and discharge from hospital in uncomplicated myocardial infarction. *Lancet*, **2**, 1331–1334.

Hellerstein, H. K. & Friedman, E. H. (1970) Sexual activity and the postcoronary patient. *Archives of Internal Medicine*, **125**, 987–999.

Hill, J. D., Kerth, W. J., Kelly, J. J., Selzer, A., Armstrong, W., Popper, R. W., Langston, M. F. & Cohn, K. E. (1971) Emergency acute coronary bypass for impending or extending myocardial infarction. *Circulation*, **43**, Suppl. 1, 105–110.

Hirshfield, J. W., Jr, Borer, J. S., Goldstein, R. E., Barrett, M. J. & Epstein, S. E. (1974) Reduction in severity and extent of myocardial infarction when nitroglycerin and methoxamine are administered during coronary occlusion. *Circulation*, **49**, 291–297.

Hutter, A. M., Sidell, V. W., Shine, K. I. & DeSanctis, R. W. (1973) Early hospital discharge after myocardial infarction. *New England Journal of Medicine*, **288**, 1141–1144.

International Society of Cardiology, Council on Rehabilitation (1973) *Myocardial Infarction— How to Prevent, How to Rehabilitate.* International Society of Cardiology.

Jacobey, J. A., Chaddock, L. D., Wolf, P. S. & Beckwitt, H. G. (1968) Clinical experience with counterpulsation in coronary artery disease. *Journal of Thoracic and Cardiovascular Surgery*, **56**, 816–819.

Joint Working Party of the Royal College of Physicians of London and the British Cardiac Society (1975) Report on rehabilitation after cardiac illness. *Journal of the Royal College of Physicians of London*, **9**, 281.

Karliner, J. S. & Ross, J., Jr (1971) Left ventricular performance after acute myocardial infarction. *Progress in Cardiovascular Diseases*, **13**, 374–391.

Kellerman, J. J., Modan, B., Levy, M., Feldman, S. & Kariv, I. (1968) Return to work after myocardial infarction. Comparative study of rehabilitated and non-rehabilitated patients. *Geriatrics*, **23**, 151–156.

Kelly, D. T., Delgado, C. E., Taylor, D. R., Pitt, B. & Ross, R. S. (1973) Use of phentolamine in acute myocardial infarction associated with hypertension and left ventricular failure. *Circulation*, **47**, 729–735.

Krauss, K. R., Hutter, A. M. & DeSanctis, R. W. (1972) Acute coronary insufficiency: course and follow-up. *Circulation*, **45**, Suppl. 1, 66–71.

Kushnir, B., Fox, K. M., Tomlinson, I. W., Portal, R. W. & Aber, C. P. (1975a) The influence of psychological factors on early hospital follow-up on return to work after first myocardial infarction. *Scandinavian Journal of Rehabilitation Medicine*, **7**, 158–162.

Kushnir, B., Fox, K. M., Tomlinson, I. W., Portal, R. W. & Aber, C. P. (1975b) Primary ventricular fibrillation and resumption of work, sexual activity, and driving after first acute myocardial infarction. *British Medical Journal*, **4**, 609–611.

Kushnir, B., Fox, K. M., Tomlinson, I. W. & Aber, C. P. (1976) The effect of a pre-discharge consultation on the resumption of work, sexual activity, and driving following acute myocardial infarction. *Scandinavian Journal of Rehabilitation Medicine* **8**, 155–159.

Lambert, C. J., Adam, M., Geisler, G. F., Verzosa, E., Nazarian, M. & Mitchell, B. F. (1971) Surgical myocardial revascularisation for impending infarction and arrhythmias. *Journal of Thoracic and Cardiovascular Surgery*, **62**, 522–528.

Lamers, H. J., Drost, W. S. J., Kroon, B. J. M., Van Es, L. A., Melink-Hoedwaker, L. J. & Birkenhager, W. H. (1973) Early mobilisation after myocardial infarction: a controlled study. *British Medical Journal*, **1**, 257–259.

Leaf, A. (1973) Cell swelling: a factor in ischaemic tissue injury. *Circulation*, **48**, 455–458.

Leinbach, R. E., Gold, R. K., Buckely, M. J., Austen, W. G. & Sanders, C. A. (1973) Reduction of myocardial injury during acute infarction by early application of intra-aortic balloon pumping and propranolol. *Circulation*, **48**, Suppl. 4, 100.

Lie, K. I., Wellens, H. J. & Durrer, D. (1974) Characteristics and predictability of primary ventricular fibrillation. *European Journal of Cardiology*, **1**, (4), 379–384.

Linhart, J. W., Beller, B. M. & Talley, R. C. (1972) Pre-infarction angina: clinical haemodynamic and angiographic evaluation. *Chest*, **61**, 312–316.

Lubbe, W. F., Peisach, M., Praetorius, R., Bruyneel, K. J. J. & Ofie, L. H. (1974) Distribution of myocardial blood flow before and after coronary artery ligation in the baboon. Relation to early ventricular fibrillation. *Cardiovascular Research*, **8**, 478–487.

Lund, I. (1973) Resuscitation of cardiac arrest by doctor-manned ambulance services in Oslo. National Conference on Emergency Cardiac Care, National Research Council and National Academy of Sciences, Washington, DC.

Maroko, P. R., Kjekshus, J. K., Sobel, B. E., Watanabe, T., Covell, J. W., Ross, J., Jr & Braunwald, E. (1971) Factors influencing infarct size following experimental coronary artery occlusions. *Circulation*, **43**, 67–82.

Maroko, P. R., Libby, P. & Covell, J. W. (1972a) Precordial ST segment elevation mapping: an intra-aortic method for assessing alterations in the extent of myocardial ischaemic injury. The effects of pharmacologic and haemodynamic interventions. *American Journal of Cardiology*, **29**, 223–230.

Maroko, P. R., Libby, P., Sobel, B. E., Bloor, C. M., Sybers, H. D., Shell, W. E., Covell, J. W. & Braunwald, E. (1972b) Effect of glucose–insulin–potassium infusion on myocardial infarction following experimental coronary occlusion. *Circulation*, **45**, 1160–1175.

Maroko, P. R., Libby, P., Ginks, W. R., Bloor, C. M., Shell, W. E., Sobel, B. E. & Ross, J., Jr (1972c) Coronary artery reperfusion. 1. Early effects on local myocardial function and the extent of myocardial necrosis. *Journal of Clinical Investigation*, **51**, 2710–2715.

Maroko, P. R. & Braunwald, E. (1973) Modification of myocardial infarction size after coronary occlusion. *Archives of Internal Medicine*, **79**, 720–733.

Mather, H. G., Pearson, N. G., Read, K. L. Q., Shaw, D. B., Steed, G. R., Thorne, M. G., Jones, S., Guerrier, C. J., Eraut, C. D., McHugh, P. M., Chowdhury, N. R., Jafary, M. A. & Wallace, T. J. (1971) Acute myocardial infarction: home and hospital treatment. *British Medical Journal*, **3**, 334–338.

Miller, M. G., Weintraub, R. M., Hedley-Whyte, J., Restall, D. S. & Alexander, M. (1974) Surgery for cardiogenic shock. *Lancet*, **2**, 1342–1345.

Mjos, O. D., Kjekshus, J. K. & Lekven, J. (1974) Importance of free fatty acids as a determinant of myocardial oxygen consumption and myocardial ischaemic injury during norepinephrine infusion in dogs. *Journal of Clinical Investigation*, **53**, 1290–1299.

Mueller, H. S., Ayres, S. M., Religa, A. & Evans, R. G. (1974) Propranolol in the treatment of acute myocardial infarction: effect on myocardial oxygenation and haemodynamics. *Circulation*, **49**, 1078–1087.

Mulholland, H. C. & Pantridge, J. F. (1974) Heart rate changes during movement of patients with acute myocardial infarction. *Lancet*, **1**, 1244–1247.

Mundth, E. D., Buckley, M. J., Leinbach, R. C., Sanders, C. A., Kantrowitz, A. & Austen, W. G. (1971) Myocardial revascularisation for the treatment of cardiogenic shock complicating acute myocardial infarction. *Surgery*, **70**, 73–87.

Mundth, E. D., Buckley, M. J., Daggett, W. M., Sanders, C. A. & Austen, W. G. (1972) Surgery for complications of acute myocardial infarction. *Circulation*, **45**, 1279–1291.

Murnaghan, D. & Hickey, N. (1970) Immediate and long-term experience of acute coronary insufficiency. *British Heart Journal*, **32**, 555.

Nagle, R., Gangola, R. & Picton-Robinson, I. (1971) Factors influencing return to work after myocardial infarction. *Lancet*, **2**, 454–456.

O'Rourke, M. (1972) Modified coronary ambulance. *Medical Journal of Australia*, **1**, 875–878.

O'Rourke, M. F., Chang, V. P., Windsor, H. M., Shanahan, M. X., Hickie, J. B., Morgan, J. J., Gunning, J. F., Seldon, A., Hall, G. V., Michell, G., Goldfarb, D. & Harrison, D. G. (1975) Acute severe cardiac failure complicating myocardial infarction—experience with 100 patients referred for consideration of mechanical left ventricular assistance. *British Heart Journal*, **37**, 169–181.

Pantridge, J. F. & Geddes, J. S. (1967) A mobile intensive care unit in the management of myocardial infarction. *Lancet*, **2**, 271–273.

Pantridge, J. F. (1974) Pre-hospital coronary care. *British Heart Journal*, **36**, 233–237.

Pantridge, J. F., Webb, S. W., Adgey, A. A. J. & Geddes, J. S. (1974) The first hour after the onset of acute myocardial infarction. In *Progress in Cardiology*, ed. Yu, P. V. & Goodwin, J. F., Vol. 3, Ch. 5. Philadelphia: Lea & Febinger.

Pelides, L. J., Reid, D. S., Thomas, M. & Shillingford, J. P. (1972) Inhibition by β-blockade of the ST segment elevation after acute myocardial infarction in man. *Cardiovascular Research*, **6**, 295–301.

Praetorius, F., Gillman, H., Gebauer, D., Kortge, P., Schmutzler, R., Van de Loo, J. & Zekorn, D. (1970) Plenary Session Papers. *Sixth World Congress of Cardiology*, London.

Redwood, D. R., Smith, E. R. & Epstein, S. E. (1972) Coronary artery occlusion in the conscious dog. Effects of alteration in heart rate and arterial pressure on the degree of myocardial ischaemia. *Circulation*, **46**, 323–332.

Redwood, D. R., Kent, K. M. & Smith, E. R. (1973) The early phase of acute myocardial infarction: pharmacologic aspects of therapy. *Archives of Internal Medicine*, **78**, 918–936.

Resnekov, L. (1974) Mechanical assistance for the failing ventricle. *Modern Concepts of Cardiovascular Disease*, **63**, 81–86.

Robinson, J. S. & McLean, A. C. J. (1970) Mobile coronary care. *Medical Journal of Australia*, **2**, 439–442.

Ross, J., Jr, Sonnenblick, E. H., Kaiser, G. A., Frommer, P. L. & Braunwald, E. (1965) Electro-augmentation of ventricular performance and oxygen consumption by repetitive application of pained electrical stimuli. *Circulation Research*, **16**, 332–342.

Royal Infirmary, Glasgow, Medical Division (multiple participating physicians) (1973) Early mobilisation after uncomplicated myocardial infarction—prospective study of 538 patients. *Lancet*, **2**, 346–349.

Sanders, C. A., Buckley, M. J., Leinbach, R. C., Mundth, E. D. & Austen, W. G. (1972) Mechanical circulatory assistance: current status and experience with combining circulatory assistance, emergency coronary angiography and acute myocardial revascularisation. *Circulation*, **45**, 1292–1313.

Sarnoff, S. J., Braunwald, E., Welch, G. H., Jr, Case, R. B., Stainsby, W. N. & Macruz, R. (1958) Haemodynamic determinants of oxygen consumption of the heart with special reference to the tension time index. *American Journal of Physiology*, **192**, 148–156.

Scanlon, P. J., Nemickas, R., Tobin, J. R., Jr, Anderson, W., Montoya, A. & Pifarre, R. (1971) Myocardial revascularisation during acute phase of myocardial infarction. *Journal of the American Medical Association*, **218**, 207–212.

Scheidt, S., Wilner, G., Mueller, H., Summers, D., Lesch, M., Wolfe, G., Krakauer, J., Rubenfire, M., Fleming, P., Noon, G., Oldham, N., Killip, T. & Kantrowitz, A. (1973) Intra-aortic balloon counterpulsation in cardiogenic shock. Report of a co-operative clinical trial. *New England Journal of Medicine*, **288**, 979–984.

Seldon, R., Neill, W. A., Ritzmann, L. W., Okies, J. E. & Anderson, R. P. (1975) Medical versus surgical therapy for acute coronary insufficiency. *New England Journal of Medicine*, **293**, 1329–1333.

Sharland, D. E. (1964) Ability of men to return to work after cardiac infarction. *British Medical Journal*, **2**, 718–720.

Shell, W. E., Kjekshus, J. K. & Sobel, B. E. (1971) Qualitative assessment of the extent of myocardial infarction in the conscious dog by means of analysis of serial changes in serum creatinine phosphokinase (CPK) activity. *Journal of Clinical Investigation*, **50**, 2614–2625.

Shell, W. E. & Sobel, B. E. (1974) Protection of jeopardised ischaemic myocardium by reduction of ventricular afterload. *New England Journal of Medicine*, **291**, 481–486.

Smith, E. R., Redwood, D. R., McCarson, W. E. & Epstein, S. E. (1973) Coronary artery occlusion in the conscious dog. Effects of alterations in arterial pressure produced by nitroglycerin hemorrhage and alpha-adrenergic agonists on the degree of myocardial ischaemia. *Circulation*, **47**, 51–57.

Soroff, H. S., Cloutier, C. T., Birkwell, W. C., Banas, J. S., Brilla, A. H., Begley, L. A. & Messer, J. V. (1972) Clinical evaluation of external counterpulsation in cardiogenic shock. *Circulation*, **45**, Suppl. 2, 75.

Vakil, R. J. (1961) Intermediate coronary syndrome. *Circulation*, **24**, 557–571.

Watanabe, I., Covell, J. W., Maroko, P. R., Braunwald, E. & Ross, J., Jr (1972) Effects of increased arterial pressure and positive inotropic agents on the severity of myocardial ischaemia in the acutely depressed heart. *American Journal of Cardiology*, **30**, 371–377.

Webb, S. W., Adgey, A. A. J. & Pantridge, J. F. (1972) Autonomic disturbance at onset of acute myocardial infarction. *British Medical Journal*, **3**, 89–92.

White, N. M., Parker, W. S., Binning, R. A., Kimber, E. R., Ead, H. W. & Chamberlain, D. A. (1973) Mobile coronary care provided by ambulance personnel. *British Medical Journal*, **3**, 618–622.

Wynn, A. (1967) Unwarranted emotional distress in man with ischaemic heart disease (IHD). *Medical Journal of Australia*, **2**, 847–851.

5
ELECTROCARDIOGRAPHIC FEATURES OF CARDIAC ARRHYTHMIAS

Dennis M. Krikler   Paul V. L. Curry

The cardiac arrhythmias—disturbances of the rate and/or rhythm of cardiac impulse formation and/or conduction—cover a wide range of possibilities. From the clinical point of view it is convenient to divide them into brady-arrhythmias and tachyarrhythmias, reflecting the mode of presentation in terms of the ventricular response. There is however a certain amount of overlap, especially where mechanisms are concerned, and, in addition, one must pay attention to disturbances of conduction that may arise from the rhythm problems themselves, e.g. atrioventricular (AV) block secondary to atrial tachycardia.

There are many reasons for the increased interest in this topic that is now being seen. The basic electrophysiologic features are now better understood (Krikler, 1974), and improved diagnostic techniques have facilitated the analysis of arrhythmias and have developed simultaneously with a number of therapeutic advances in the fields of pharmacology, cardiac pacing and surgery. In this chapter the diagnostic aspects will be considered with especial attention to those arrhythmias in which there are highly characteristic features and in particular where knowledge has recently been advanced.

DIAGNOSTIC METHODS

The truism that clinical examination yields much useful information bears repetition. Careful history-taking is often of the utmost value especially when trying to analyse paroxysmal events. This applies as much to the brady-arrhythmias as to the tachyarrhythmias, and one should extract all the information contained within the history as well as the physical examination. Many have attested to the value of careful clinical examination in the analysis of attacks of tachyarrhythmia, but it is important to remember the basis on which the premises are founded. Fluctuations in the intensity of heart sounds due to changes in the P–R interval, while of great academic interest, are extremely difficult to observe in practice, and various abnormalities in the jugular pulse, e.g. giant 'a' waves, attributable to atrial contraction against closed atrioventricular valves are useful pointers, but by no means as valuable as have been claimed.

Conventional electrocardiography

Objective recordings of cardiac activity or of changes in peripheral pulses (MacKenzie, 1892) were clearly a great step forward, but it was not long before the advent of the electrocardiograph provided a most direct, non-invasive, method of rhythm analysis. Indeed, within the first decade of clinical electrocardiography, many of the basic rhythm disturbances were categorised (Lewis, 1910), often to be rediscovered some years later. In the vast bulk of cases, a properly executed electrocardiographic tracing taken during an attack of rhythm disturbance will yield the answer, but there are many cases in which the diagnosis has nevertheless to be deduced rather than directly observed. Proper attention to proper electrocardiographic principles is essential but often forgotten (Krikler and Macfarlane, 1974). The use of machines with adequate high and low frequency responses and the ability to

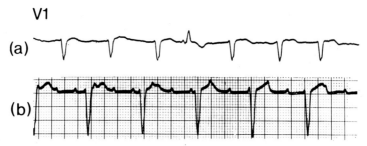

Figure 5.1   ECGs from a patient with paroxysmal atrial tachycardia. In the recording made with a machine showing poor high and low frequency responses (a), the abnormal P waves can only be discerned with great difficulty (note right bundle branch block pattern in fourth beat); with a machine meeting the American Heart Association standards (b) the arrhythmia is apparent

select different sensitivities and various paper speeds (American Heart Association, 1967) is of great practical importance. Machines with poor frequency responses may fail to show genuine abnormalities: Figure 5.1 reveals paroxysmal atrial tachycardia with well marked pathological and unduly frequent P waves, seen with a unit meeting the American Heart Association standards, but not in one that failed to do so. The ability to show fine notches or to measure the intervals between complexes to see whether they are regular or not demands the availability of rapid paper speeds as well as the selection of higher sensitivities (Fig. 5.2). Indeed, when intracardiac electrograms are recorded as in His bundle electrography, it is conventional to use a paper speed of 100 mm/s for this purpose, instead of the usual clinical speed of 25 mm/s; and there are many electrocardiographers, especially on the Continent, who regularly use a paper speed of 50 mm/s for routine ECGs with this in mind. This is not always wise; occasionally it is easier to recognise abnormal P waves at normal than at slow paper speeds (Fig. 5.3).

Intracardiac electrography

More sophisticated techniques have been developed in recent years, involving intracardiac electrography. It is not proposed to discuss the technicalities of these methods here, but some knowledge of their performance is

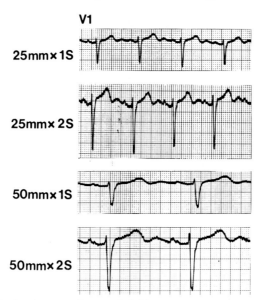

Figure 5.2   ECGs showing poor P wave definition at normal standardisation (1S) at paper speeds of 25 and 50 mm/s, clarified when the sensitivity was doubled (2S)

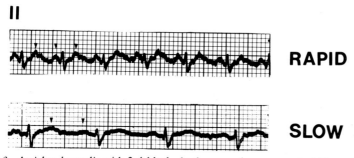

Figure 5.3   Atrial tachycardia with 2:1 block. At the normal paper speed of 25 mm/s (rapid), abnormal P wave activity is better seen than at the slow paper speed of 50 mm/s. Selected P waves are indicated by arrows

essential, if only to recognise patients in whom they are needed. Although there have been many attempts to record intracardiac electrograms beforehand, the method was effectively introduced into clinical practice by Latour and Puech (1957), and further refined and made practical by Scherlag et al (1969). The technique is carried out under local anaesthesia, with full aseptic precautions, in an appropriately equipped catheter laboratory. Catheters tipped with suitable electrodes are inserted percutaneously into one or more peripheral veins, usually the femoral, occasionally the brachial vein, and advanced, under fluoroscopic control, into the heart (Fig. 5.4). The key recording position is adjacent to the septal leaflet of the tricuspid valve, where, with manipulation, it is usually possible to obtain clear evidence of deflections produced from the low right atrium, bundle of His, and right ventricle: this tracing is called a His bundle electrogram. In order to show its relevance, it

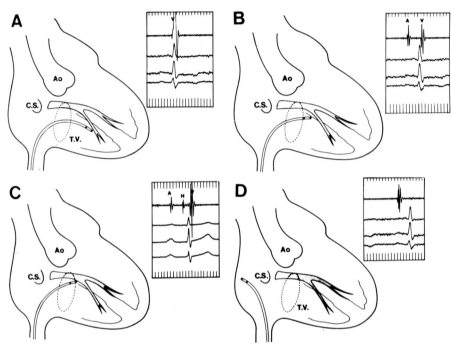

Figure 5.4 Diagrams showing lead placement during intracardiac electrography. CS = coronary sinus; Ao = aorta; T.V. = tricuspid valve; A = atrial, H = His, V = ventricular deflections. Insets show intracardiac electrogram from each position together with three simultaneous surface leads. (A) right ventricular electrogram; (B) ventriculogram recorded from right ventricle just distal to tricuspid valve, showing atrial as well as ventricular activation. (C) His bundle electrogram, showing A, H and V deflections. (D) high right atrial electrogram, showing atrial activation only

is analysed in conjunction with one or more simultaneously recorded surface ECG leads. Conventionally, leads I and III and chest leads V1 and V6 are used; these enable the patterns of frontal plane axis changes and the presence or absence of bundle branch block to be seen at the same time. Further recordings can be obtained from other electrodes which can be positioned high in the right atrium, in various parts of the right ventricle, or in the left atrium. The left atrium may be reached indirectly by passing the catheter into the coronary sinus or directly by passing it through the interatrial septum, either through a patent foramen ovale if one is present, or by transseptal puncture. In tachycardia, the direction of activation of the chambers is often revealed in this way; and one realises that the relative quietness, electrically speaking, of the P–R interval in the surface ECG, hides many important deflections recordable using intracardiac tracings.

Intracardiac electrography, especially His bundle electrograms, can be of particular importance in the diagnosis of the location of atrioventricular block; tracings taken during tachycardia can, as indicated above, reveal the direction of the travel of the cardiac impulse, and the possibility of initiating and terminating tachycardia and the study of pharmacological behaviour, using pacing or programmed electric stimulation, adds a considerable dimension to the analysis of arrhythmias. Detailed exposition is beyond the scope of this survey, but the relevance of these techniques will be mentioned as appropriate under the headings of the various rhythm disturbances; more detailed information can be obtained from Damato, Schnitzler and Lau (1973), Puech and Grolleau (1972) and Curry (1975).

Thus, the electrocardiograph remains the key tool for the arrhythmia analyst and further discussion will be based on its use. Between attacks of rhythm disturbance, there may be evidence to suggest a possible explanation for the symptoms; during an attack, specific features might be present. Often enough, however, there is more than one explanation and the ECG provides the basis for a deductive diagnosis rather than a firm committed interpretation. Intelligent use of the ECG thus requires much forethought. Casual glances lead to guesses, more often wrong than right; complicated tabulations of points to seek are impractical for they are rarely appropriate to the problem under consideration. Decision trees can be constructed as one analyses tracings, and adapted to the approach of the individual; in our experience they are more useful in the tachyarrhythmias than in the brady-arrhythmias.

BRADYARRHYTHMIAS

A general definition for bradyarrhythmia that defines the situation as a heart rate sufficiently slow to impede cardiac or cerebral function is inadequate, for bradycardia is often surprisingly well tolerated. There is a wide range of physiological variations from individual to individual and, as is well known, athletes, especially long distance runners, tends to have inherently slow heart rates. The various possibilities and their electrocardiographic identification (supplemented where necessary by intracardiac recordings) can be considered in the conventional anatomical terms.

Sinus Bradycardia

Here the heart rate is unduly slow but the site and direction of impulse formation and propagation is normal. A firm definition of a rate below which this is diagnosed is difficult, but rates below 50 beats/min, in adults, merit consideration as reflecting sinus bradycardia. With sinus bradycardia, the degree of fluctuation in the discharge rate under the influence of autonomic factors, e.g. sinus arrhythmia, is often exaggerated. The identification of sinus bradycardia on an ECG does not necessarily point to a pathological cause. For this, one must turn to other aspects, and look at the clinical context. Certain infections, particularly those of virus origin, or those due to salmonellae (e.g. enteric fever), are often associated with sinus bradycardia, but this may be a relative bradycardia, i.e. the sinus discharge rate is slower than might be expected from the degree of fever from which a patient may be suffering. An important cause of sinus bradycardia that must always be remembered today is iatrogenic: many drugs, especially the β-adrenergic blockers, tend to cause sinus bradycardia, and this possibility should always be borne in mind, often being the explanation for unexpected sinus bradycardia found in hypertensive subjects. In acute situations, ischaemia of the sinus node, during acute myocardial infarction (usually inferior but sometimes located elsewhere) may be the cause. In the absence of acute disease, and especially at more advanced ages, sinus bradycardia may reflect the presence of sinoatrial disease, and this possibility should be very much in mind if there is a history of syncope. It may be impossible to distinguish, on the surface ECG, between sinus bradycardia and 2:1 sinoatrial block, where every second sinoatrial beat is blocked or not initiated within the sinoatrial node; it may be possible to recognise its presence if it is intermittent and the sinoatrial rate is suddenly doubled or halved.

Sinoatrial Block

Under this heading lie a host of possible clinical expressions, often seen in various diagnostic labels which can justifiably be attached, and which do not at once suggest a common origin. With advancing age, progressive fibrosis may develop in the sinoatrial node, due perhaps to ischaemia as blood flow decreases in the artery to the SA node, or more likely to pathological changes, the precise nature of which remain poorly understood. Sinoatrial block may be seen as the dropping of occasional beats. It maybe impossible to recognise first-degree block in the sinoatrial node, for this has no influence on the P–R interval, or on the intervals between successive P waves. It may take a long time for impulses to generate, or an unduly long time for them to be conducted from the sinoatrial node into the atrium, but if this is unaccompanied by dropped beats, there is no way of diagnosing its absence or presence. Second-degree sinoatrial block is of course diagnosible, because cardiac impulses are dropped. This may take the form either of type I (Wenckebach, Möbitz type I) or type II (Möbitz type II) block (see p. 94 for explanation of these terms in relation to AV block). In type I block, most P–P intervals are equal, actually tending to shorten but occasional beats are dropped; the interval between the P waves surrounding the dropped beat is less than that of two cycles (Fig. 5.5); one can calculate the sinus node rate of discharge and confirm a Wenckebach (type I) block (Schamroth, 1971). In Figure 5.6, on the other hand, the interval between successive P waves separated by a gap is equal to double that of the normal cycle length, i.e. one beat is completely dropped without prior warning; this is quite analogous to the situation in Möbitz type II block seen in the His–Purkinje system. However, information as to whether or not the risk of complete sinoatrial block is greater in Möbitz type II than in type I is lacking, and patients with type I SA block have been known to develop complete sinoatrial arrest.

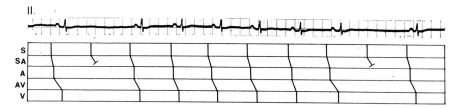

Figure 5.5   AV block (type I), the Wenckebach phenomenon, affecting the sinoatrial node. P waves are omitted after the first and seventh QRS complexes, and the R–R intervals encompassing these cycles are less than twice normal. Failure of impulse generation or propagation from the sinoatrial node is inferred as indicated in the ladder diagram (S = sinoatrial node; SA = junction between sinoatrial node and atrium; A = atrium; AV = atrioventricular node; V = ventricle)

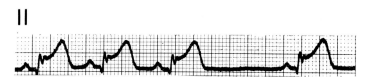

Figure 5.6   Sinoatrial block, Möbitz type II. The cycle length between the last two beats is equal to that between the first and third beats, indicating complete omission of a sinus cycle

In complete sinoatrial block, there will be failure of impulse formation in the sinoatrial node, or, if the impulse is formed, it is not conducted beyond the confines of the node into the atrium so as to initiate atrial depolarisation. This may well be interrupted by junctional pacemaker activation, a life-saving escape beat (Fig. 5.7), unless of course there is more widespread disease of the conducting system. Transient complete sinoatrial block may be induced in those with latent sinoatrial disease by carotid sinus massage (Fig. 5.8), though the precise significance of undue sensitivity of the carotid sinus is not clearly established. Thus this is an inadequate tool to decide whether or not sinoatrial block is present. At the moment, the clinical history and electrocardiographic evidence are particularly important as the precise role of tests of sinoatrial nodal function remain to be clarified.

4

Tests for sinoatrial nodal function fall into two categories; the pharmacological and the electrophysiological. Good correlation between either of these and the presence of pathologically confirmed sinoatrial disease is not always obtained, and at present the electrophysiological techniques show the greatest promise, though admittedly imperfect. There are two types of electrophysiological tests that can be used: the response of the sinoatrial node after the cessation of rapid right atrial pacing, and its behaviour after the injection

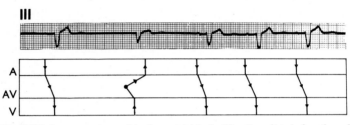

Figure 5.7   ECG from a patient with sinoatrial block. The first, third, fourth and fifth are sinus beats; the sinoatrial node fails to discharge at the proper time after the first beat and the second beat is due to junctional escape, with the same QRS configuration and a retrograde P′ wave in the subsequent T

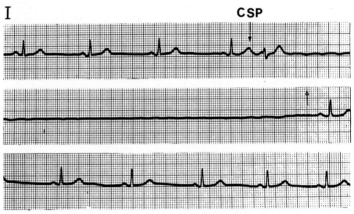

Figure 5.8   ECG from a patient with intermittent sinoatrial block and syncope. Immediately after carotid sinus pressure was applied, an extrasystole occurred (? junctional with aberrant conduction), and was followed by prolonged asystole (7 s)

of premature atrial stimuli using a special external pacemaker. There is no firm agreement on the duration of atrial pacing or the speed at which it should be carried out, to enable a firm diagnosis to be made (Mandel et al, 1972; Medvedowsky et al, 1975). The test depends on the inherent properties of the sinoatrial node and its ability to recover spontaneously after having been subjected to rapid over-drive suppression. Pacing at the rate of 120 beats/min for 1 min is recommended by some (Medvedowsky et al, 1975) as being satisfactory, though as the pacing rate is increased, we sometimes find a paradoxical improvement in sinoatrial nodal function. The sinoatrial node is considered to be diseased when it fails to recover spontaneous firing within 1.5 s after cessation of such pacing, and to be normal when it does so within 1.2 s, there being an intermediate grey zone where diagnostic confidence is lacking. Alternatively, recovery times greater than 125 per cent of the basic cycle length are considered pathological (Mandel et al, 1972). We have not found correction for basic cycle length of additional help. Narula, Samet and Javier (1972) subtract the basic cycle length from the recovery time and consider values over 525 ms suggestive of disease. This is clearly not a universally applicable test of sinoatrial nodal function.

Others have attempted to apply a technique of injecting premature atrial stimuli at different parts of the cardiac cycle to find the stage at which the sinoatrial node can be invaded and reset, and to see whether there is conduction block (Strauss et al, 1973). Many have attempted to apply this test, and publications continue to appear; a detailed analysis will not be made in view of the many conflicting reports, and the uncertainties as to whether the chosen indices reflect in any meaningful fashion the liability of the sinoatrial node to function normally or not. The spontaneous tendency to sinus arrhythmia, or the occurrence of extrasystoles, tends to complicate analysis.

Should complete sinoatrial nodal block occur, syncope, exactly analogous to Adams–Stokes attacks complicating atrioventricular block, may occur (Cohn and Lewis, 1912), though, as indicated, junctional pacemakers may well adequately take over cardiac function unless the conducting system is widely diseased. Sometimes it is possible to improve sinoatrial nodal function by blocking vagal tone following the administration of atropine by intravenous injection, but sometimes when the SA node is diseased, it fails to respond to this, and the function of a junctional pacemaker may be enhanced paradoxically, as illustrated in Figure 5.9.

The sinoatrial node normally, in discharging, suppresses all distal pacemakers. One problem thus, if it fails to discharge, that might occur is the functioning of subsidiary pacemakers, in the atrium or AV junction, or in the ventricles if there is AV conducting system disease. Thus, paradoxically, sinoatrial disease may present as a syndrome with alternating bradycardia and tachycardia (Short, 1954; Slama et al, 1969). The tachycardias that may thus occur can take various forms. Atrial fibrillation is a common expression of sinoatrial nodal disease which may well explain atrial fibrillation for which there is no other cause, especially in the elderly (Fig. 5.10). However, ectopic atrial tachycardias and reciprocating tachycardias involving the atrial musculature or the AV junction are other possible factors. This is of some importance as drugs that may be given to suppress such ectopic pacemakers or abnormal tachycardias may further depress an already diseased sinoatrial node and actually aggravate the tendency to tachycardias (Krikler et al, 1977). Thus, when a syndrome of alternating bradycardia and tachycardia is identified, the choice of therapeutic agent must be very careful, aided where possible by intracardiac recordings during pharmacological assessment. It is for this reason that it may be necessary to implant a ventricular demand pacemaker, which will fire off if the sinoatrial node discharge rate falls, at a rate sufficiently high to suppress proximal subsidiary foci that might otherwise initiate a paroxysmal tachyarrhythmia. Should the patient develop

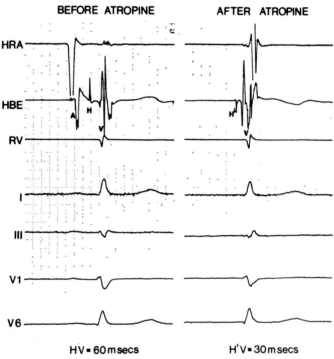

Figure 5.9   Intracardiac and surface electrograms in a patient with sinoatrial disease. HRA = high right atrial electrogram; HBE = His bundle electrogram; RV = right ventricular electrogram. A = atrial deflection, H = His bundle deflection, V = ventricular deflection. The left hand panel shows sinus rhythm, with an HV interval of 60 ms, just above the upper limit of normal. The right hand panel, after intravenous atropine: the complex indicates a junctional rhythm on the surface ECG, and there is no preceding atrial activation. The H deflection is now of different configuration and the H′V interval is shortened, suggesting retrograde His bundle activation from a slightly more distal focus, within the distal common bundle of His

established atrial fibrillation, he is often more comfortable, for then the ventricular response can be controlled with the use of drugs acting on the AV node in the conventional fashion.

Incomplete degrees of SA block can be closely mimicked by concealed extrasystoles that do not manifest themselves in the surface ECG but that re-enter the sinoatrial node and reset it, delaying its next discharge (Fig. 5.11). This is a difficult concept, convincingly argued by deductive electrocardiographers; a similar example is perhaps more appropriate as an introduction

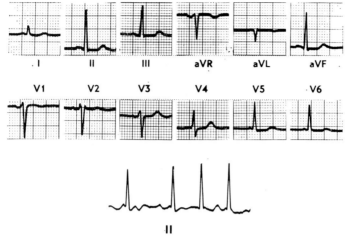

Figure 5.10 ECG from patient with alternating bradycardia and tachyarrhythmia. The 12 lead ECG is normal; the sinus rate was however 40/min. The strip of lead II below indicates that the arrhythmia was atrial fibrillation

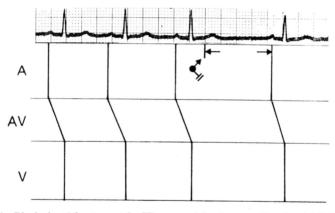

Figure 5.11 Blocked atrial extrasystole. The unexplained pause after the third sinus beat is consistent with an atrial extrasystole blocked in the antegrade direction, and conducted retrogradely so as to reset the SA node; the differential diagnosis is from sinoatrial block

to this possibility. If an atrial extrasystole occurs sufficiently early in the cycle, very soon after the preceding sinus beat, it may well find the AV node refractory and there will be no anterograde conduction to the ventricles and thus no QRS complex; but an isolated P wave will be seen. It can easily be visualised how this beat, arising close to the sinoatrial node, may re-enter and reset it (Childers et al, 1973) or, as in this case suppress it (Fig. 5.12). In V1, the ectopic P waves are clearly seen; but if lead II is scrutinised, it is only with great care that ectopic P waves can be seen to fall within the T waves that precede gaps; it is very easy to make the erroneous diagnosis of second-degree sinoatrial block under these circumstances. A concealed atrial or junctional extrasystole (Brat, 1975) can now be visualised as an extension of this state of affairs, which manifests itself exclusively by the resetting of the sinoatrial node, analogous to other forms of concealed conduction (Langendorf and Pick, 1956).

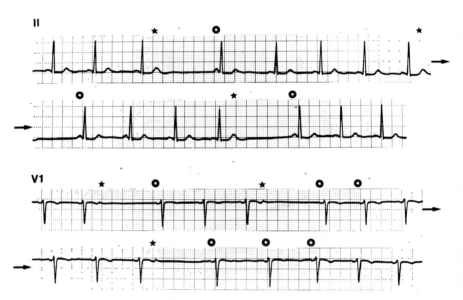

Figure 5.12   ECG showing blocked atrial extrasystoles (solid stars); the subsequent beats are different from sinus beats, and suggest simultaneous atrial and junctional escapes (open circles)

Atrioventricular Block

It is particularly in this field that clearer definition of mechanisms has resulted from judicious application of the technique of His bundle electro-graphy (Puech, 1975; Puech and Grolleau, 1972). Oversimplified classifica-tions based on the rather coarse discrimination that can be obtained judging whether blocks are above or below the level of the bundle of His, are to be avoided. The activation of the bundle of His provides an important landmark (Fig. 5.4, p. 84), blocks proximal to it tending to occur within the atrio-ventricular node, though blocks within the atria themselves may also occur on rare occasions. Where blocks are distal to the His bundle deflection, they have different implications in that complete heart block can only result if all the major fascicles of the His–Purkinje system are implicated. Such simplistic classifications do however fall down on a number of aspects. Firstly, blocks may well occur within the bundle of His itself, and these may be more frequent than are realised (Puech, 1975); very careful and perhaps even tedious technical aspects need to be explored before a block of the main trunk can be diagnosed or eliminated (Schuilenburg and Durrer, 1975). Perhaps more important, blocks may occur at multiple levels. This is of particular importance in infranodal blocks, for the disease process here is very often an obscure and progressive fibrosis. The definition of block at one particular level should not lead the investigator to forget that more distal blocks may occur. This is of importance in that more proximal blocks tend to have a more benign prognosis, for reasons that will be discussed below.

In practice, it is a useful rule that blocks within the AV node or proximal portion of the bundle of His will, as expected, result in QRS complexes that are narrow and that are of the same configuration as might previously have been seen during sinus rhythm. Correspondingly, with involvement of the major fascicles of the conduction system resulting in complete heart block, broad bizarre QRS complexes, perhaps resembling the pattern seen in bundle branch block, are the rule. Exceptions however abound and, while careful consideration of the surface ECG may enable these to be identified, a substantial proportion of cases can only be properly clarified using intracardiac electrography.

As with sinoatrial block—and even better recognised in practice—there are various degrees of incomplete atrioventricular blocks under the headings of 'nodal' and 'distal' but it must always be recognised that these statements involve many generalisations, providing no more than a working framework for clarification of individual cases.

Proximal AV block

By this is meant block in the atrium just proximal to the AV node, within the AV node itself, or within the trunk of the bundle of His. Congenital lesions are of particular importance in this location (Lev et al, 1971) and usually reflect anatomical discontinuity between the AV node and the origin of the bundle of His. Other possible causes include inflammatory diseases, including diphtheria and rheumatic fever, myocardial ischaemia, in particular inferior infarction, and surgical trauma (Slama, Motté and Coumel, 1971).

First-degree block is defined as prolongation of conduction from the low right atrium through the AV node to the bundle of His, beyond the usual physiological limits which, in an adult, is 0.22 s. Where this is seen in, for example, patients with mitral stenosis with left atrial enlargement, delay in conduction through the atrial musculature may be the explanation; in His bundle electrography, prolongation of the time from the start of the P wave to the onset of the atrial A deflection in the intracardiac electrogram, which should not exceed 25 to 40 ms, will indicate that this is so or not. First degree block within the AV node itself is more commonly seen transiently during the first few days of acute inferior myocardial infarction, and if intracardiac studies are carried out, the A–H interval, reflecting conduction time within the AV node, will be seen to be prolonged. In both cases the P–R interval will be prolonged; intracardiac electrography will show at which level this has occurred. Figure 5.13 shows chronic first-degree AV block at the nodal level in a subject also displaying right bundle branch block.

Second-degree block is defined as a situation where some beats but not others are normally conducted and can take two forms:

(a) *Wenckebach phenomenon:* Wenckebach AV block (*Möbitz type I block*) consists in the occurrence of progressive prolongation of AV nodal conduction until one beat is dropped; then the series restarts. Classically, the greatest

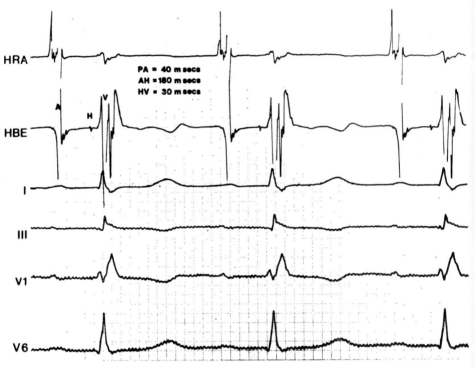

Figure 5.13 Intracardiac and surface ECGs showing first degree AV block (right bundle branch block also present). The A–H interval is 180 ms (upper limit of normal = 120)

increment in the degree of block occurs between the first and second conducted beats, which are closest to each other; the amount of the increment then decreases (Schamroth, 1971), but this typical pattern is not always seen. It usually occurs at the AV node, and when this occurs we see the typical appearances that make the Wenckebach phenomenon recognisable to most observers. However, it may occur anywhere within the condition system, and has been described in the infranodal His–Purkinje fascicles. When located in the AV node, the QRS complex has a normal morphology and is narrow, provided there was no pre-existing bundle branch block. Under these circumstances, His bundle electrograms show that the blocked beat is dropped

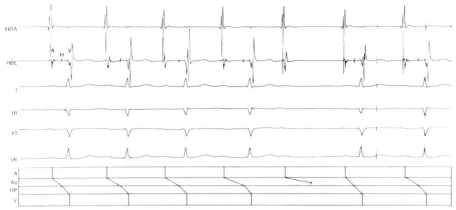

Figure 5.14 AV nodal block (type I) with the Wenckebach phenomenon. Note progressive increase in the P–R and A–H intervals from the first to fourth beats, with block after the P (and, in HBE, A waves) of the fifth sinus complex. The cycle restarts with the sixth sinus complex (stimulus artefact can be seen in T wave) with normal A–H and P–R intervals; final beat already shows prolongation of AV nodal conduction times

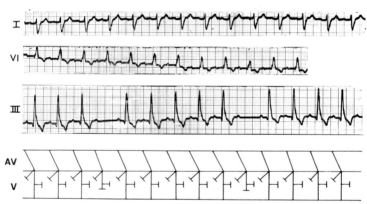

Figure 5.15 Second degree AV block, Möbitz type II. The tracings are not simultaneous: leads I and V1 indicate the presence of marked right axis deviation and right bundle branch block. In lead III, the QRS complex is dropped without antecedent P–R lengthening after the fourth and tenth P waves, due to failure of conduction in the residual portion of the left bundle branch

in the AV node and fails to reach the bundle of His, as evidenced by lack of an H potential (Fig. 5.14).

(b) *Möbitz type II block* characteristically occurs infranodally (Puech, 1975), and in this disorder beats are dropped suddenly, without prior lengthening of anterograde conduction times, i.e. the P–R interval remains unchanged in the beats preceding and following the blocked impulse. As the location is almost invariably infranodal, the QRS complexes are widened by bundle branch block, perhaps with evidence of bilateral involvement (Fig. 5.15).

A difficult point arises when 2:1 AV block is seen. This may either be an extreme form of the Wenckebach phenomenon with 2:1 AV block (Fig. 5.16) (Krikler, 1971), or it may reflect the Möbitz type II phenomenon. Many workers automatically describe 2:1 block as being Möbitz type II, but it is impossible to deduce this unless two consecutive normally conducted impulses can be seen with normal P–R intervals; the problems are well discussed by Barold and Friedberg (1974). It is still useful, at least clinically, to distinguish between Möbitz type I and II block, for the former is less often followed by complete heart block and, even if it is, the proximal location of the lesion usually permits the functioning of a high subsidiary escape focus,

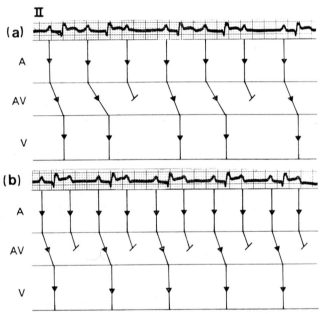

Figure 5.16   ECG of a patient with recent inferior myocardial infarction. (a) 3:2 Wenckebach block in the AV junctional area; (b) 2:1 block

able to drive the ventricles at a sufficiently rapid rate to prevent syncope. Because Möbitz type II block is so regularly due to widespread His–Purkinje disease, it is an important harbinger of distal complete heart block, with the possibilities of Adams–Stokes attacks and indeed death. However, having said this, information derived from intracardiac studies is often needed to define the situation more precisely.

Complete (third-degree) AV block indicates total interruption of the passage of the supraventricular impulse to the ventricles, which are depolarised from a subsidiary focus. Where the block is proximal, e.g. in the AV node or bundle of His, the escape focus will produce a narrow QRS complex (Fig. 5.17) unless there is pre-existing bundle branch or unless the slow rate of

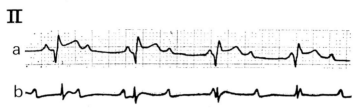

Figure 5.17 ECG (lead II) showing complete heart block in the AV node or bundle of His: note narrow QRS complexes and relatively rapid ventricular rates, 65 in each case. (a) Inferior myocardial infarction; (b) congenital

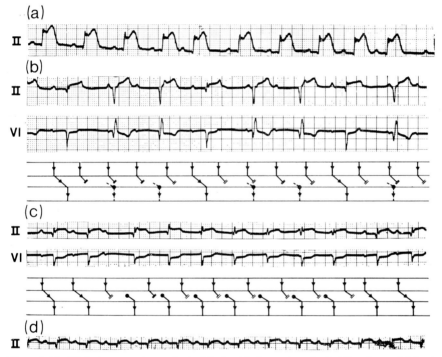

Figure 5.18 High degree atrioventricular block with aberration of subsidiary focus. (a) Acute inferior myocardial infarction. (b) Two days later, high degree atrioventricular block, conducted beats showing normal QRS complexes, with P–R prolongation; escape beats show appearances of right bundle branch block. (c) Following day, both conducted and escape beats show normal intraventricular conduction; (d) fifth day, sinus rhythm with first degree AV block only

discharge is accompanied by bradycardia-dependent bundle branch block (Fig. 5.18) (Rosenbaum et al, 1973); this usually permits an adequate ventricular escape rate.

That blocks may be of high grade and yet not quite complete has already been seen (Fig. 5.18). Provided the supraventricular beat reaches the blocked area at a critical time in the cycle, it may be conducted—because of so-called supernormal conduction at the end of the refractory period (Krikler, 1974) or the *Wedensky phenomena* (Schamroth and Friedberg, 1969). The *Wedensky effect* occurs when a preceding strong stimulus enables an otherwise insufficient one to reach the threshold and produce a response; *Wedensky facilitation* is defined as the enhancement of conduction across a blocked zone by the occurrence of a previous impulse reaching but not traversing it. Thus P waves that fall on the T wave of escape beats may initiate a beat that can be conducted to the ventricles (Fig. 5.19).

His bundle block
   During His bundle electrography, with careful right atrial pacing, conduction disturbance in the bundle of His has been defined in 18 per cent of

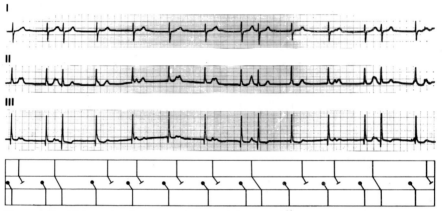

Figure 5.19   High grade, almost complete, block in the proximal conducting system. Where a sinus P wave falls critically on the T wave of a preceding junctional escape beat, it is conducted to the ventricles (third, ninth and thirteenth QRS complexes)

his cases by Puech (1975); roughly two-thirds of these were isolated and one-third associated with intraventricular conduction disturbance. Widening or duplication of the His potential, with the usual expressions of first, second and third degree block, have been carefully defined by this worker. The more carefully this lesion is sought the more frequently it will be found, as is exemplified in Figures 5.20 and 5.21 taken from a child who had undergone repair of tetralogy of Fallot, but who thereafter developed syncopal episodes. As can be seen in Figure 5.20a, complete heart block was evident with narrow QRS complexes. Intracardiac electrography (Fig. 5.20b) showed abnormally wide separation of two potentials recorded from the bundle of His (Ha and Hb) by 65 ms; with rapid right atrial pacing Ha and Hb were further separated, leading to 2:1 and then complete block in the bundle of His with complete ventricular standstill (Fig. 5.21). The patient immediately underwent implantation of a permanent ventricular demand pacemaker. That intrahisian block might be important under these circumstances is proposed by Steeg et al (1975). The tendency for block to occur within the bundle of His itself is still inadequately recognised even in otherwise thorough studies of intraventricular conduction disturbances in patients in whom cardiac pacing was considered justified (Cohen et al, 1975). This may be due to the fact that it can be difficult to record both components simultaneously on the same tracing using a single bipolar catheter, and one may have to be content with seeing the split potentials on separate tracings, making sure that the

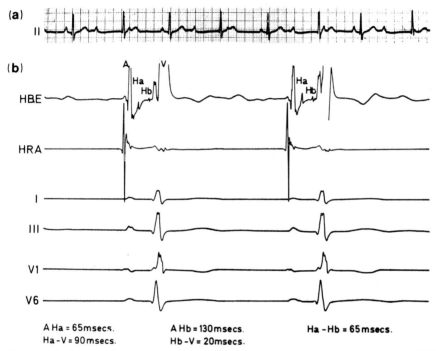

AHa = 65msecs.   AHb = 130msecs.   Ha -Hb = 65msecs.
Ha -V = 90msecs.   Hb -V = 20msecs.

Figure 5.20 Patient with repaired tetralogy of Fallot and syncopal attacks. (a) Surface ECG showing complete heart block with narrow QRS complexes. Atrial rate 79 beats/min, ventricular rate, 47. (b) His bundle electrogram (HBE), high right atrial electrogram (HRA) and four surface leads from the same case, showing split His potential (Ha–Hb = 65 ms)

first H complex is not obscured by the atrial complex (Schuilenburg and Durrer, 1975).

Distal AV or intraventricular block
    More distal AV block, now often called trifascicular block, is due to interruption of function of the major intraventricular conducting tissue. Prior tracings in sinus rhythm often show pre-existing bundle branch block patterns; when block supervenes, these may alter depending on the site of the subsidiary pacemaker, but the QRS complexes remain wide and often bizarre. Because the impulses arise distally in His–Purkinje tissue that has a slow response rate of spontaneous diastolic depolarisation, the heart rate tends

to be much slower than in more proximal complete AV block (Fig. 5.22), and a reduced response to neurogenic influences means that there is less possibility for the heart rate to increase in response to any demands on the circulation. This is the type of block that is characteristically complicated by Adams–Stokes attacks, and there is an appreciable incidence of death, unless a pacemaker is implanted.

Discussion of the anatomy of the intraventricular conduction system (Kulbertus and Demoulin, 1975), or of the patterns of QRS complexes that

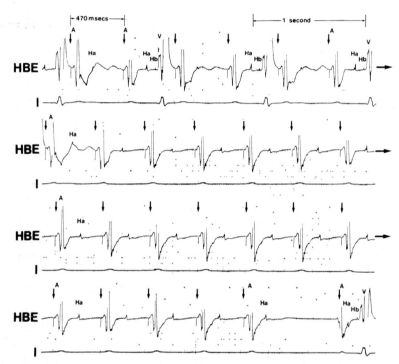

Figure 5.21   The same case as Figure 5.20. Progressively increased right atrial pacing shows 2:1 intra-Hisian block in the upper panel succeeded by complete intra-Hisian block in the lower three panels, with no ventricular response. With interruption of pacing (bottom panel) and resumption at a slower rate, normal albeit delayed intra-Hisian conduction is restored

may be produced by bundle branch or fascicular lesions (Krikler, 1971) is beyond the scope of this survey, and correlation of anatomical lesions with so-called 'hemiblocks' is imprecise but the presence of bilateral bundle branch lesions indicates a risk of development of complete heart block (Fig. 5.22). Such lesions may take the form of right bundle branch block complicated by marked axis deviation, left more often than right; there is some evidence that left bundle branch block complicated by marked left axis deviation is often found in the presence of extensive bilateral conduction system disease (Spurrell, Krikler and Sowton, 1972). Intracardiac electrography is an essential diagnostic and prognostic tool under these circumstances (Puech, 1975).

Precisely what transforms partial to complete heart block is not always clear but some important observations have recently been made in relation to rate-related block. This is of particular importance when parts of the intraventricular conducting system are already blocked, so that the production of block in the remaining fascicle leads to complete interruption of conduction between the atria and ventricles. Bradycardia-dependent block may be induced by premature beats (Coumel et al, 1971); these may prolong the T–P intervals so that the beat subsequent to the extrasystole finds the re- maining fascicle refractory. It has been suggested by Rosenbaum et al (1973) that tachycardia-induced block is related to supraventricular beats falling in

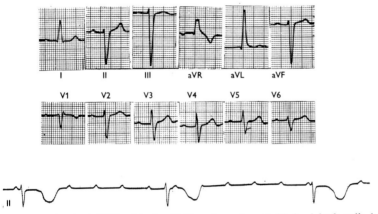

Figure 5.22 Twelve-lead ECGs showing P–R prolongation (0.28 s), right bundle branch block and marked left axis deviation, indicating bilateral bundle branch lesions; bottom panel shows complete heart block in same patient, with slow ventricular response and QRS pattern slightly different from that in sinus rhythm

phase 3 of the action potential and bradycardia-dependent block to beats reaching the tissue during spontaneous diastolic depolarisation; both these factors would inhibit further conduction. The clinical demonstration of bradycardia-dependent block induced, and then dispelled by premature beats, spontaneous or induced, has been well documented by Castellanos et al (1975). This very situation is seen in Figure 5.23, where this phenomenon is seen at the level of the AV node or bundle of His rather than within the intraventricular conducting system, as judged by the surface ECG.

TACHYARRHYTHMIAS

The diagnostic approach to tachyarrhythmias is depicted in Figure 5.24, which is a diagnostic tree that can be applied to most electrocardiograms in which the heart rate is increased. There are exceptions that cannot be fitted in, but the vast majority of clinically important rhythm disturbances can be identified in this way.

Atrioventricular Dissociation

This is a term that gives rise to considerable confusion, and if often mis-applied to heart block. It is proposed here to utilise a simple and widely applicable meaning for the term, in that the atria and the ventricles are

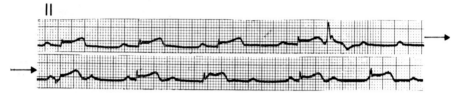

Figure 5.23   First four beats in upper panel show first-degree AV block; extrasystole (ventri-cular, or junctional with aberration) induces high-grade block, almost complete, with capture in third and last beats of bottom panel. ST segment elevation reflects acute inferior infarction

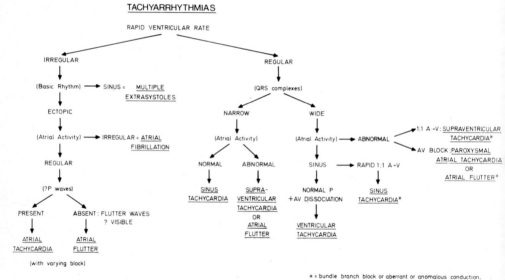

Figure 5.24   Flow diagram showing analysis of tachyarrhythmias (reprinted with permission from Krikler, 1974)

independently activated without there being any interference in anterograde conduction from the upper to the lower chambers. Atrioventricular dis-sociation may arise if the rate of discharge of a superior pacemaker is slowed, necessitating the functioning of a junctional escape mechanism; alternatively, the basic sinoatrial rate of discharge may be unaffected but the normal junctional pacemaker is enhanced and discharges more rapidly than the SA node and at times usurps the control of ventricular depolarisation. It is the latter which is of the greatest importance; previously it tended to occur in a number of infections especially rheumatic fever, but it is now usually seen in non-paroxysmal junctional tachycardia which may complicate inferior wall myocardial infarction, or when the junctional pacemaker activity is enhanced by drugs, notably digitalis. At times atrioventricular dissociation occurs without evident reason in the absence of clinical evidence of depression of SA nodal function (Fig. 5.25).

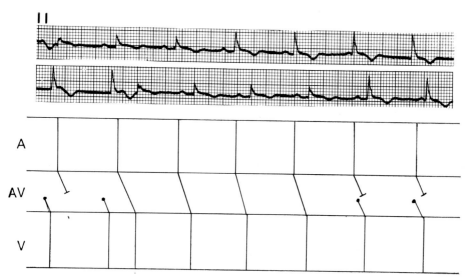

Figure 5.25 ECG, continuous strips of lead II, showing AV dissociation. The ladder diagram refers to the bottom panel, and shows two junctional escape beats preceding sinus P waves, the second P wave capturing the AV node and leading to four normally conducted beats before junctional acceleration produces AV dissociation again. Differentiation is aided by the slightly aberrant morphology of junctional beats and the fact that the P–R intervals of conducted beats are at the upper limit of normal

Apart from its occurrence as a primary situation, AV dissociation is clearly important when the ventricles are activated independently due to paroxysmal tachycardia. It is the hallmark of paroxysmal ventricular tachycardia; the usual situation is for the SA node to continue to function independently at its slower inherent rate, the faster ventricular ectopic focus or re-entry mechanism producing more rapid depolarisation of the heart. Whatever the mechanism, be it isolated AV dissociation (Fig. 5.25) or ventricular tachycardia causing dissociated atrial and ventricular activity (Fig. 5.26), suitably timed supraventricular impulses may find the AV node and His–Purkinje tissue conductive, and may capture the ventricles for one or more beats, until the distal pacemaker recaptures activity. The capture may be complete or may result in a fusion beat (Krikler, 1974). As will be seen later, ventricular tachycardia may not always show this type of dissociation, and a certain number of cases, especially when the tachycardia is relatively slow, display 1:1 ventriculo-atrial conduction (Wellens and Lie, 1975).

Extrasystoles

The occasional supplementary beat, arising in the atria or ventricles, will not increase the rate of the heart though several such beats occurring at frequent intervals may produce some irregularity of which the patient is aware. Indeed, the patient may well be aware of only isolated extra beats, and their significance may require more detailed investigation.

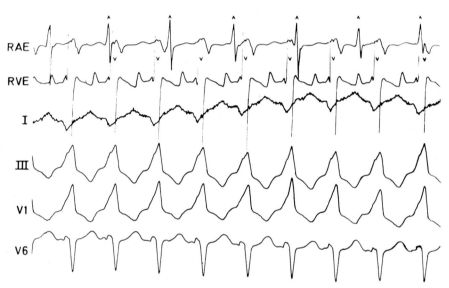

Figure 5.26 Intracardiac and surface ECGs in ventricular tachycardia, showing AV dissociation

The term ectopic beat is sometimes applied to extrasystoles to indicate their origin other than in the sinoatrial node, though the occurrence of SA nodal extrasystoles has been postulated (Langendorf and Mintz, 1946). If they occur early in the cycle, as a result of an active mechanism, they are premature beats; and if they occur late in the cycle, due to failure of formation of a proximal impulse, as escape beats. They may further be classified on the basis of their origin, in the atria, AV junctional area, or ventricles. Considerable controversy and little precise information exists as to the mechanism of extrasystoles; it has been suggested that they may occur because of localised enhanced automatic activity or because of local re-entry phenomena (see p.114).

Atrial extrasystoles characteristically show the same QRS configuration at sinus beats, but are preceded by a different-looking P wave, and the P–R interval may be different (Fig. 5.27); sometimes it may be possible to note the formation of atrial extrasystoles in two different sites (Fig. 5.28). The QRS complexes are not always narrow but can be widened, which may reflect aberrant conduction of an especially early atrial extrasystole because a bundle branch, usually the right, is still refractory (Fig. 5.29); as can also

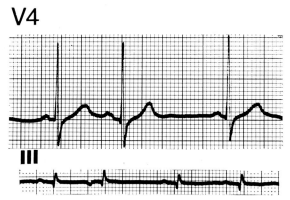

Figure 5.27 Upper panel: the first and third beats are normal sinus beats; the second beat shows a P wave of different configuration with a longer P–R interval, and is an atrial extrasystole. In lower panel the first, third and fourth are sinus beats; second beat is an atrial extrasystole with an inverted P wave

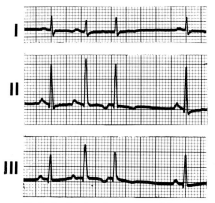

Figure 5.28 Simultaneous limb leads showing two atrial extrasystoles (second and third beats) with different P wave configurations

be seen in this illustration, if the atrial impulse formation is extremely early, only the ectopic P waves may be seen, onward transmission being blocked in both bundle branches, i.e. blocked atrial extrasystoles. As previously mentioned, sudden changes in rhythm may be due to concealed extrasystoles, and a possible explanation for the longer P–P interval between the third and fourth beats in Figure 5.11, as compared with the first two P–P spaces, may

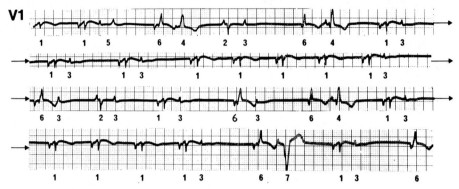

Figure 5.29 Continuous ECG from a patient with carcinoma of the bronchus. (1) sinus beats with normal conduction; (2) atrial extrasystoles with normal conduction; (3) blocked atrial extrasystoles; (4) atrial extrasystoles with right bundle branch aberration; (5) atrial extrasystoles with less marked right bundle branch block; (6) junctional escape beats with right bundle branch block; (7) atrial extrasystole with left bundle branch block

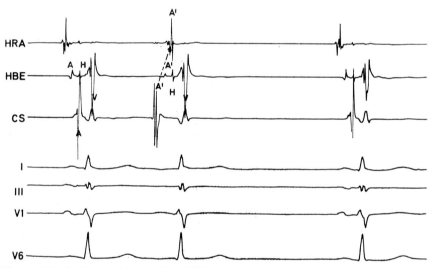

Figure 5.30 Surface and intracardiac ECGs showing that the second beat is a left atrial extrasystole, because the coronary sinus A' is earlier than those in HRA or HBE

be a concealed supraventricular extrasystole which was blocked both antegradely and retrogradely but which penetrated the sinoatrial node sufficiently to discharge it and reset it (Brat, 1975). While early beats may be aberrant or blocked, other factors may be responsible (Scherf and Schott, 1973).

P wave configurations are not necessarily a good index of the location of the extrasystole, as intra-atrial conduction disturbances may play a role, but intracardiac electrography can reveal the early origin of an extrasystole in one or other atrium (Fig. 5.30).

The diagnosis of junctional extrasystoles is often difficult, but can be made positively with the use of intracardiac recordings. On the surface ECG, the hallmark is the absence of a P wave (because it is buried within the QRS complex) or its presence immediately before or after the QRS complex, and showing a different morphology from that seen in sinus rhythm. Junctional

V1

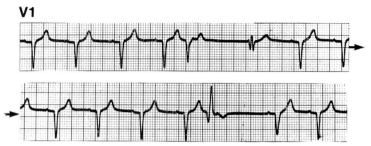

Figure 5.31   ECG showing junctional extrasystole (top panel, fifth beat: note retrograde P′), junctional escape beat with aberrant intraventricular conduction (sixth beat) and, in bottom panel, ventricular extrasystole with retrograde P′ (sixth beat)

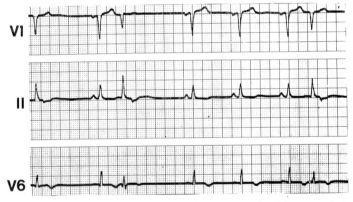

Figure 5.32   ECG showing 'main-stem' ventricular extrasystoles. The second, fourth, fifth and sixth are sinus beats; the first, third and seventh are ventricular extrasystoles showing basically the same QRS configuration (including initial vectors) as the sinus beats, with minimal widening; note retrograde atrial activation (P′ waves) in S–T segments

extrasystoles are most often seen as escape beats, complicating sinus suppression for any reason (Fig. 5.7), but a premature junctional beat is shown in Figure 5.31, followed by a junctional escape beat with aberration. The configuration of a junctional escape beat is also seen to resemble that of a sinus beat in Figure 5.9; the QRS complexes are identical, but there is no preceding P wave and only a very narrow interval between His bundle activation (which may be retrograde) and ventricular activation in the junctional beat.

Ventricular extrasystoles range in importance from the occasional annoying 'bump' to hazardous forerunners of more dangerous arrhythmias. They may arise in either ventricle. In narrow ('main-stem') extrasystoles, arising close to the origin of the normal conducting tissue, the configuration may resemble that of the normal QRS complexes (Fig. 5.32). Intracardiac electrography will confirm ventricular activation prior to that of the bundle of His, which is activated retrogradely, the two atria then being depolarised (Fig. 5.33). The clinical context will often be of the greatest importance in deciding on the significance of the extrasystoles, which again may be early or may reflect escape mechanisms. Retrograde conduction of ventricular extrasystoles to the atria is more frequent than generally recognised, but sometimes the degree of

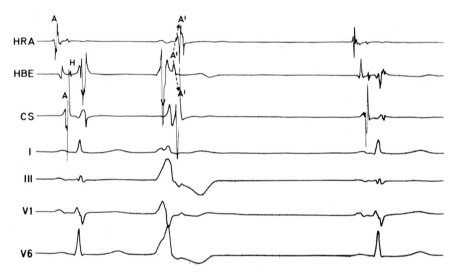

Figure 5.33   Intracardiac and surface ECGs showing ventricular extrasystole with simultaneous retrograde depolarisation of both atria following A′ in HBE

retrograde penetration is incomplete, only reaching the AV node and partially depolarising it; this reflects a form of *concealed conduction* (Langendorf and Pick, 1956), manifest at the end of a run of ventricular tachycardia by delayed antegrade conduction of the next sinus beat, shown by a prolonged P–R interval (Fig. 5.34). Not all P waves following ventricular extrasystoles are retrograde: some may be due to sinus activity with block to onward transmission because retrograde penetration of the ventricular extrasystole has rendered the AV node refractory (Fig. 5.35). As is well known, ventricular extrasystoles may occur regularly following each sinus beat in a fixed ratio (bigeminy) (Fig. 5.36), possibly a sign of digitalis intoxication though often occurring in ischaemic heart disease or without obvious reason.

Especially if there is some myocardial disease, e.g. ischaemia, particularly early ventricular extrasystoles, i.e. those occurring in relation to the peak of the T wave of the preceding sinus beats, may initiate ventricular tachy-arrhythmias (see below). An interesting form of apparently bidirectional ventricular extrasystolic activity (Fig. 5.37) may be seen in hypokalaemia and may be the herald of more serious arrhythmias (Curry et al, 1976).

It may be extremely difficult to distinguish between ventricular extra-systoles on the one hand and those of supraventricular origin in which there is an impairment of conduction down one of the bundle branches (usually the right) because of the earliness of that impulse. Typical criteria for dis-tinction have been laid down by Sandler and Marriott (1965) who suggest that the vast bulk of supraventricular extrasystoles with aberrant conduction

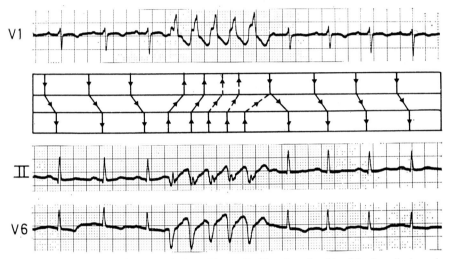

Figure 5.34 ECG showing ventricular tachycardia (five beats) with right bundle branch block pattern in V1, and P–R prolongation in the first sinus beat after the tachycardia, due to concealed retrograde conduction. Retrograde P waves can be seen after the first two beats of the tachycardia but not after the others

show typical right bundle branch block configuration, whereas ventricular extrasystoles show more bizarre features or a left bundle branch block pattern. This is a useful but by no means invariable rule, as is indicated in Figure 5.38 in which the second beat can be seen to reflect a ventricular extrasystole with an rsR' pattern in lead V1.

Parasystole

Parasystolic beats are sometimes confused with extrasystoles, but the distinction can usually be made on the surface electrocardiogram. With extrasystoles, the coupling interval between the first sinus beat and the ectopic beat is fixed; in parasystole it varies, and an interectopic interval can usually be calculated as a multiple of a common denominator. Furthermore,

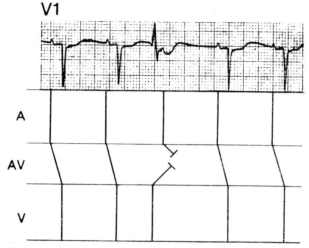

Figure 5.35   The first and last two beats are of sinus origin but the third beat is a ventricular extrasystole that is followed by an upright P wave which occurs at exactly the time the sinus impulse was due. Antegrade conduction from this third sinus beat is blocked by refractoriness in the AV node resulting from retrograde penetration by the ventricular extrasystole

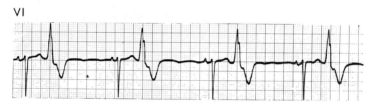

Figure 5.36   ECG showing bigeminy due to ventricular extrasystoles which show fixed coupling to the preceding sinus beat at an R–R′ interval of 480 ms

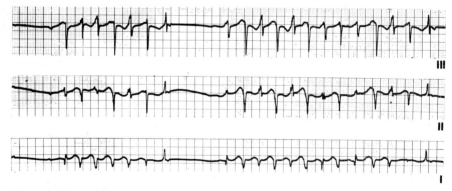

Figure 5.37   An ECG showing bidirectional ventricular tachycardia (140 beats/min) with AV dissociation, with a patient with hypokalaemia

VI

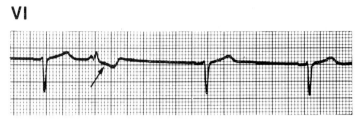

Figure 5.38   The first, third and fourth beats are normally conducted sinus impulses but the second is a ventricular extrasystole showing an rsR′ pattern with the retrograde P′ indicated by the arrow

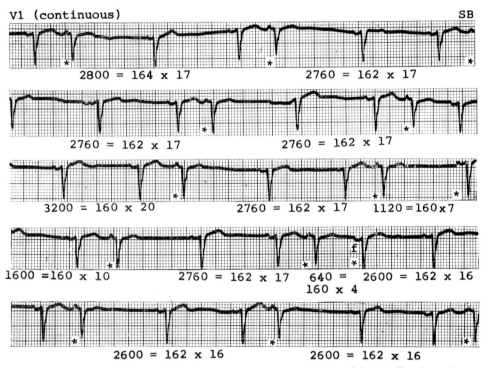

Figure 5.39   Atrial parasystole (parasystolic beats shown by asterisks): coupling intervals are multiples of 162 ms

sometimes the parasystolic impulse falls in close relation to the sinus beat, producing a degree of fusion; in atrial parasystole (Fig. 5.39) the fusion is between the ectopic and the sinus P waves. In ventricular parasystole, on the other hand, fusion will be seen as a QRS complex intermediate in form between that of the extrasystole and that of the sinus beat (Fig. 5.40). It has been suggested that many parasystolic foci, which manifest themselves as only occasional ectopic beats, may nevertheless represent an underlying tachycardia in the focus, with a high degree of exit block preventing appear-

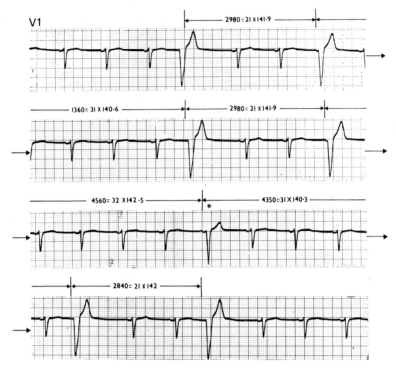

Figure 5.40   ECG showing ventricular parasystole with coupling intervals in multiples of approximately 141 ms; the asterisk in the third row indicates a fusion beat

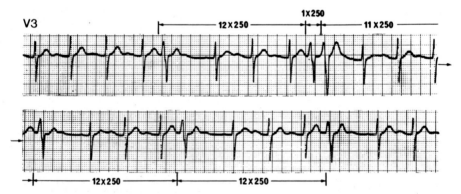

Figure 5.41   Tracing from a healthy young woman with recurrent palpitations showing ventricular parasystole. Note that the interectopic interval is a multiple of 250 ms, i.e. there is ventricular parasystolic tachycardia at a rate of 240/min; this is masked by high degree exit block around the focus

ance of a tachycardia except at intervals (Fig. 5.41). Atrial and junctional parasystole are much less often seen (Figs. 5.39, 5.42) than the ventricular arrhythmia.

The mechanism of parasystole is uncertain, but there does appear to be a degree of protection which enables the impulse to discharge and enter the rest of the myocardium (except when it is refractory) but with physiological characteristics which bar the sinus impulse from entering and discharging the parasystolic focus. It is often but not invariably found in diseased hearts; the same focus can behave both extrasystolically and parasystolically at different times (Schamroth, 1971).

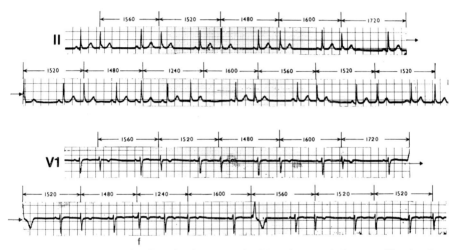

Figure 5.42 ECG showing junctional parasystole. Here the ectopic beats, unlike the sinus beats, are not preceded by P waves except fortuitously at abnormally short P–R intervals e.g. the last two parasystolic beats in lead II and the last parasystolic beat in V1. In V1, the sixth and tenth ectopic beats are conducted with right bundle branch aberration, and the eighth (f) shows fusion with the sinus impulse. The interectopic intervals are all multiples of approximately 64 ms

Paroxysmal Tachycardia

A series of regular repeated beats, exceeding three or four in number, constitutes paroxysmal tachycardia and these may arise in the atrium or ventricle or may reflect a mechanism involving the AV node alone or in association with an anomalous pathway. Paroxysmal tachycardia may either arise from re-entry or as a series of ectopic beats, so-called ectopic atrial or ventricular tachycardia, though it is not always possible even with the use of intracardiac electrography to distinguish this phenomenon from a minute localised re-entry circuit (see below).

Enhanced rate of discharge of an ectopic pacemaker within the myocardium under pathological circumstances may reflect changes in depolarisation so that a series of beats is produced more rapidly (Krikler, 1974); on the other hand, where two alternative pathways exist for an impulse to be conducted, relative block in one may enable an impulse to pass down the other and then prevent the first pathway responding to further proximal impulses, though it can be re-entered distally during recovery from the refractoriness. This is best exemplified in the AV node, in which fibres may have different electrophysiological properties rendering the situation more likely; and if the impulse travels down the blocked pathway again, a circus movement may be set up. This is the characteristic feature of so-called paroxysmal supraventricular junctional tachycardia, which is often miscalled paroxysmal atrial tachycardia, the inciting mechanism is usually the occurrence of a premature

V2

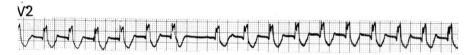

Figure 5.43   Ectopic atrial tachycardia (130/min) with spontaneous cessation, and resumption after a single sinus beat

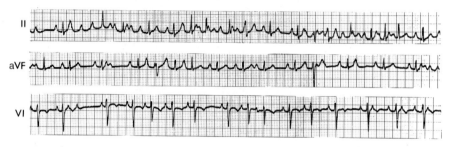

Figure 5.44   ECG showing chaotic atrial rhythm. The P waves vary considerably in configuration and conducted beats show varying P–R intervals; many P waves are blocked

beat, atrial or ventricular, which causes unidirectional block in one pathway. A similar situation occurs when the AV node is bypassed by an anomalous tract, e.g. the bundle of Kent in the Wolff–Parkinson–White syndrome: tachycardias are particularly likely to occur because the two tissues have different conducting and refractory properties, and this imbalance makes them particularly likely to respond in this way to suitably timed extrasystoles, whether occurring spontaneously or artificially induced during an electrophysiological study (Curry, 1975).

In *paroxysmal ectopic atrial tachycardia* (Fig. 5.43) the atria fire rapidly, and 1:1 conduction may take place, but varying degrees of block are more common because the AV node is less able to conduct efficiently at rates exceeding 150/min; the block may be spontaneous (Fig. 5.1) or induced by carotid sinus pressure (Krikler, 1974). Such tachycardias often reflect the presence of digitalis intoxication, but this is by no means invariable and a number of other disorders including cardiac ischaemia and cardiomyopathy may be responsible. When the P waves vary in morphology, and the P–R intervals are irregular, multifocal or chaotic tachycardia may be seen (Fig. 5.44).

Atrial Flutter

Atrial flutter is best considered here, as a more rapid regular atrial tachy-cardia more consistently showing AV block, usually 2:1; both the degree of block and thus the display of the flutter waves can be enhanced by vagal measures (Fig. 5.45). In the usual form, atrial activation (whether originating in a focus or a re-entry circuit) is caudocranial, but uncommonly the activation is reversed and the P wave morphology more in keeping with that in atrial tachycardia (Puech, Latour and Grolleau, 1970).

VI

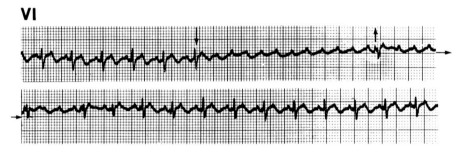

Figure 5.45 Atrial flutter with 2:1 AV response; carotid sinus pressure was applied at the first arrow and lifted at the second; there was transient depression of AV nodal conduction with a subsequent gradual return to the previous conduction sequence. During the inhibition of conduction to the ventricles, the flutter waves can be clearly seen

Atrial Fibrillation

The total irregularity of the ventricular response, with no constancy whatsoever between R–R intervals, and the absence of organised atrial activity in the form of detectable P or flutter (F) waves, is the hallmark of this condition. Atrial activity may be barely visible with fine fibrillation (f) waves (Fig. 5.46) but, especially but not invariably in cases of recent origin, coarse f waves may be evident (Fig. 5.47). It is now being recognised more and more that, in addition to the usual causes of atrial fibrillation, e.g. mitral valve disease, ischaemic heart disease, thyrotoxicosis, or less often atrial septal defect and constrictive pericarditis, a substantial proportion in ap-parently normal subjects arise on the basis of sinoatrial disease, and it may not be possible, on the surface ECG, to exclude the presence of an un-suspected pre-excitation syndrome, either the Lown–Ganong–Levine syn-drome (Schamroth and Krikler, 1967) or the Wolff–Parkinson–White syn-drome (Fig. 5.48). In the latter situation the syndrome is usually (but by no

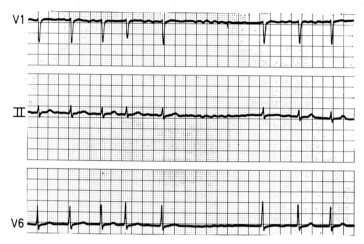

Figure 5.46   ECG with simultaneous leads showing atrial fibrillation: very minor fluctuations in the baseline can be seen in V1 and II and the ventricular response is totally irregular

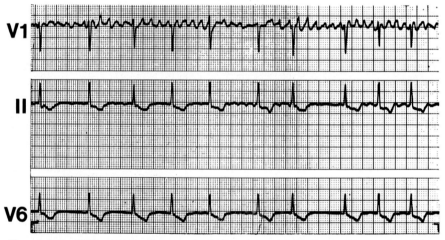

Figures 5.47   ECG with simultaneous leads showing atrial fibrillation with coarse baseline activity best seen in V1

means invariably) recognisable on the surface ECG (Krikler, 1975); usually during atrial fibrillation, conduction takes place down the anomalous pathway with occasional beats negotiating the AV node and producing narrow QRS complexes (Fig. 5.48b); but at other times the fibrillation may occur exclusively down the AV node and give no hint of the presence of pre-excitation (Fig. 5.48c). Conduction of incessant fibrillating atrial stimuli down the bypass into unprotected ventricular muscle, without the interposition of the AV node to act as a delaying mechanism, can lead to ventricular fibrillation (Dreifus et al, 1971).

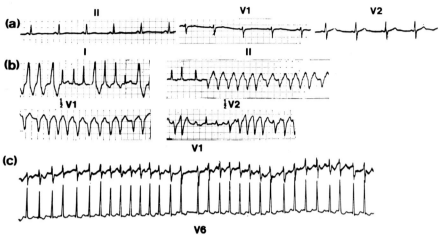

Figure 5.48 ECGs taken (a) in sinus rhythm, with minimal evidence of Wolff–Parkinson–White syndrome; (b) atrial fibrillation, with conduction down anomalous pathway (broad bizarre complexes) or AV node (narrow complexes); (c) atrial fibrillation with exclusive nodal conduction

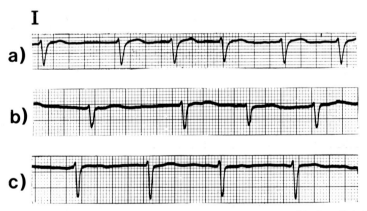

Figure 5.49 ECGs showing atrial fibrillation (a) prior to treatment; (b) after digitalisation; (c) digitalis intoxication with regularisation of ventricular response

Under normal circumstances, in chronic atrial fibrillation the diagnosis is easy, and digitalis may be used in the management to control the ventricular rate by increasing the refractoriness of the AV node. Paradoxically, an undue degree of regularity (Fig. 5.49) may result from excessive digitalis treatment.

Reciprocating Supraventricular Tachycardias

In AV junctional tachycardia, the subject is classically a healthy individual with no underlying cardiac disease, who has attacks of tachycardia of sudden onset and offset, and precise regularity (in the majority of cases). During such attacks the QRS complexes are usually identical to those found in sinus rhythm (Fig. 5.50); sometimes attacks occur almost incessantly, induced by frequent atrial extrasystoles (Fig. 5.51). This situation may complicate the Wolff–Parkinson–White syndrome, or other forms of pre-excitation, the anomalous pathway possibly being utilised in this disorder (Fig. 5.52) in different ways. In sinus rhythm, conduction is down both the AV node/His

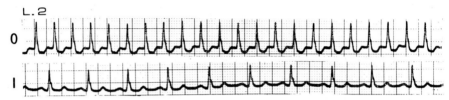

Figure 5.50   ECG (lead II) from a 62-year-old woman prone to repeated attacks of paroxysmal tachycardia. The QRS configurations are identical in the upper and lower panels, the upper showing paroxysmal supraventricular (AV junctional) tachycardia (190 beats/min); lower panel, sinus rhythm at 90 beats/min.

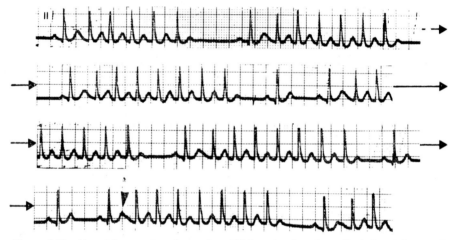

Figure 5.51   Almost-incessant reciprocating AV junctional tachycardia induced by atrial extrasystoles (note arrow in bottom panel)

axis and the bypass, producing a fusion complex (Fig. 5.52a, b); if the bypass were absent or blocked, the impulse would pass exclusively down the normal pathways, producing the situation seen in Figure 5.52c; on the other hand, blockage of the normal pathway will produce exclusive conduction down the anomalous pathway, yielding a broad bizarre QRS complex as in Figure 5.52b.

The usual form of circus movement tachycardia in the Wolff–Parkinson–White syndrome comprises anterograde conduction down the normal pathways and retrograde conduction up the anomalous bypass. Thus the QRS complex, previously widened by the fusion appearances, now becomes narrow and of different configuration (Figs. 5.52c, 5.53). Tachycardia in the reverse direction with conduction down the anomalous pathway and back up the normal tracts is much less frequently recognised and potentially more serious because of the more rapid rate at which the ventricles may be stimulated without the inter- position of the AV nodal delaying mechanism in the anterograde direction; as compared with the appearances during sinus rhythm, the evidence of pre- excitation becomes very much greater and quite altered, as in Figure 5.52b.

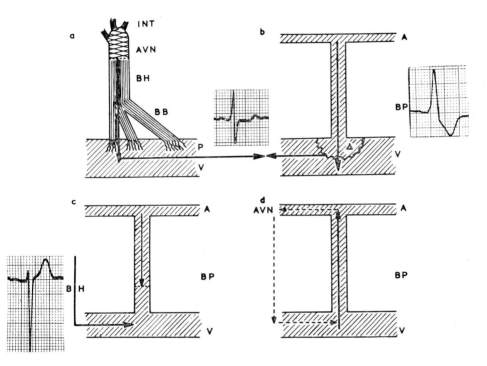

Figure 5.52   Diagram to show pathways in WPW syndrome; for discussion, see text. Re- printed with permission from Krikler (1974)

A newly understood mechanism relates the onset of AV reciprocating tachycardia to the production of unilateral block by an increase in the heart rate (shortening P–P cycles) of critical degree rather than extrasystoles (Coumel et al, 1970), and this can occur with AV nodal tachycardias (Fig. 5.54) as well as in pre-excitation (Krikler et al, 1976). Not all apparently pure AV nodal tachycardias do in fact exclusively involve the AV node; pre-excitation may never be detected in sinus rhythm as in the patient shown in Figure 5.55 with recurrent supraventricular tachycardia but may be de- tected after termination of the tachycardia by verapamil (Fig. 5.56) or be demonstrated by electrophysiological study (Spurrell, Krikler and Sowton, 1974; Krikler, 1975).

5

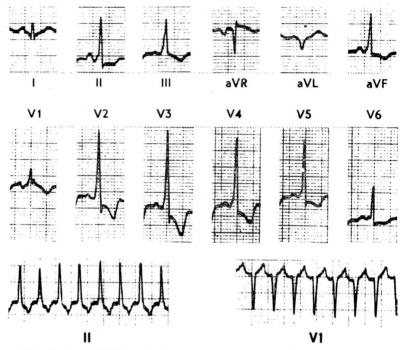

Figure 5.53   Twelve-lead ECGs showing WPW syndrome with short PR (see V5), wide QRS and delta wave (slurred onset of R waves well seen in II, aVF and V4–6). Bottom panels: paroxysmal tachycardia with narrow QRS complexes followed by retrograde P′ waves

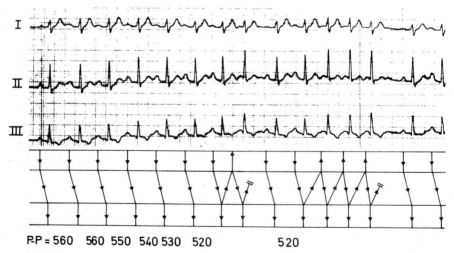

Figure 5.54   Simultaneous ECG leads showing initiation of reciprocating AV nodal echo or re-entry tachycardia with shortening of the spontaneous P–P cycles to 520 ms

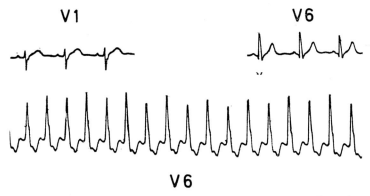

Figure 5.55   The upper two panels show V1 and V6 in sinus rhythm, with no abnormality. The bottom panel, V6, shows paroxysmal supraventricular tachycardia with left bundle branch block

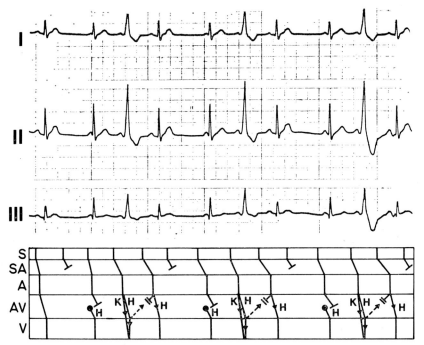

Figure 5.56   Same case as Figure 5.55. The paroxysmal tachycardia was stopped by intravenous verapamil. As indicated in the ladder diagram, the first, fourth, seventh and tenth QRS complexes reflect sinus beats conducted exclusively down the normal pathways; the second, fifth and eighth, junctional escape beats with normal conduction, with the focus firing prior to possible excitation from the preceding P waves: and the third, sixth and ninth are sinus beats showing the pre-excitation pattern. In addition, there is second-degree sinoatrial (Wenckebach, type I) block

Finally, there is now good evidence that re-entry can involve the SA node (Narula, 1974) and we have studied several patients with paroxysmal reciprocating sinus tachycardia. In this disorder, the P wave morphology is similar to that of sinus beats, sudden onset and cessation are observed (Fig. 5.57) and intracardiac studies confirm the initiation and termination of the

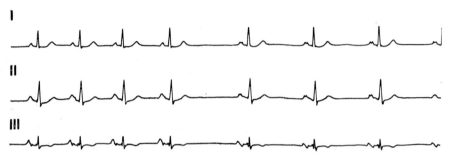

Figure 5.57 ECG showing spontaneous termination of reciprocating sinus tachycardia (P wave morphology resembles that in sinus rhythm)

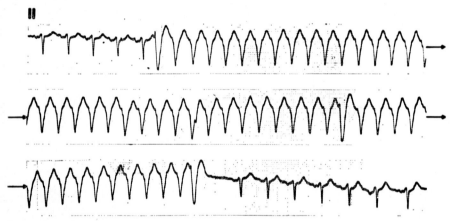

Figure 5.58 Reciprocating ventricular tachycardia initiated by extrasystole falling on T wave of fifth sinus beat (vulnerable phase): QRS morphology in tachycardia is slightly different from extrasystoles that initiate, fall during and terminate the arrhythmia

arrhythmia by suitably timed premature stimuli applied to the area of the SA node (Curry et al, 1976b).

Paroxysmal Ventricular Tachycardia

Ventricular tachycardia must be distinguished from supraventricular tachycardia with aberration: right bundle branch block usually points to the latter, but this is not invariable (Fig. 5.34, p. 109).

This serious disturbance may also occur on the basis of enhanced ectopic activity or re-entry. It has been suggested by Wellens, Lie and Durrer (1974) that in the acute stages of myocardial infarction tachycardias tend to reflect the former but in those appearing after some days, re-entry circuits may have become established. A re-entry origin is suggested on the surface ECG when tachycardia is initiated by a ventricular extrasystole the form of which varies somewhat from the configuration seen during tachycardia, and also when a similar extrasystole also terminates it (Figs. 5.58, 5.59); in both cases the tachycardia complicated the development of cardiac aneurysm and was controlled by its resection. If AV dissociation can be demonstrated (Figs. 5.26, 5.59), the ventricular origin is supported, but 1:1 VA conduction can confuse the issue in ventricular tachycardia (Wellens and Lie, 1975).

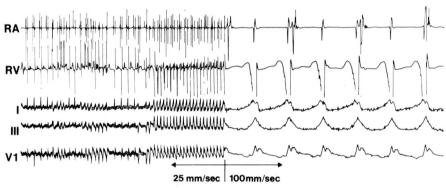

RA

RV

I

III

V1

25 mm/sec | 100mm/sec

Figure 5.59 Surface and intracardiac ECGs of a patient with repeated attacks of ventricular tachycardia associated with a ventricular aneurysm. In the tracing taken at a paper speed of 25 mm/s, sinus rhythm is interrupted by ventricular extrasystoles with two runs of ventricular tachycardia of different morphology from each other, initiated by R waves falling on the T waves of preceding sinus beats. The QRS configuration is better seen at a fast paper speed (100 mm/s), when the atrial activity (see RA lead) can be seen to be quite dissociated from the ventricular activity displayed in the RV and surface leads

Torsade de pointes

Under this heading we refer to a variety of ventricular tachycardias of uncertain mechanism but in which a particular form of re-entry is postulated (Slama et al, 1973). Recognised under a variety of names including transient ventricular fibrillation, cardiac ballet, etc., the hallmark of this disorder is a ventricular tachycardia in which there is phasic alteration in the axis of the QRS complexes, which seem to twist and turn (Fig. 5.60). Attacks are often self-limited, but may be associated with faintness or loss of consciousness and may lead to ventricular fibrillation. Among aetiological factors are significant bradycardias, most particularly high-degree AV or SA block (Fig. 5.61), though other important potential causes include electrolyte disturbance (hypokalaemia, hypomagnesaemia), drugs (quinidine, prenylamine, phenothiazines), and cardiac ischaemia, especially in the context of Prinzmetal's

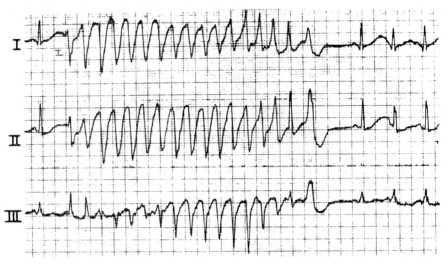

Figure 5.60   ECG showing torsade de pointes. Note the Q–T prolongation in the sinus beats and the onset of the arrhythmia with a late extrasystole falling after the apex of the first sinus T wave. In the three leads, the QRS complexes in tachycardia appear to undulate and the episode is terminated by an extrasystole of different configuration

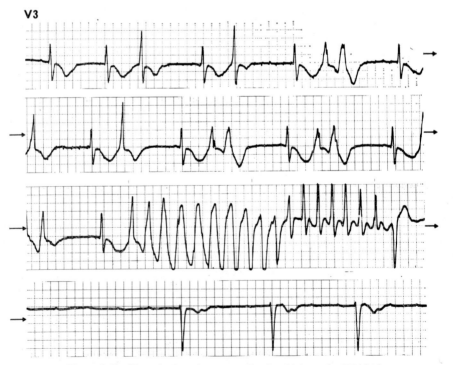

Figure 5.61   Torsade de pointes complicating high-grade AV block

variant angina (Chiche, Haiat and Steff, 1974). A number of otherwise un-explained cases may well be due to variants of hereditary syndromes in which the QT interval is prolonged, with or without deafness (Jervell and Lange-Nielsen, 1957; Ward, 1964).

Recognition of the arrhythmia as being different from conventional types of ventricular tachycardia is important (Krikler and Curry, 1976). Attacks tend to be induced by ventricular extrasystoles occurring relatively late in the cardiac cycle, as might be expected to occur when the QT interval of the preceding sinus beat is prolonged. Drugs that help conventional forms of ventricular tachycardia may aggravate matters by prolonging repolarisation; besides correcting the underlying factor, urgent action such as electroversion may be required. In a long episode where the patient is extremely ill either the

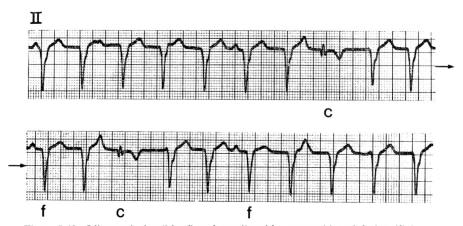

Figure 5.62   Idioventricular ('slow') tachycardia with capture (c) and fusion (f) beats

infusion of isoprenaline or the institution of rapid right atrial pacing may be effective.

Idioventricular tachycardia

Enhanced activation of a ventricular focus, beating more rapidly than is usually the case with ventricular escape beats, e.g. 70 to 110 beats/min, often tend to complicate acute myocardial infarction but may occur quite indepen-dently of this cause, and for long periods, with no obvious reason. This is sometimes an escape mechanism with an enhanced ventricular focus but it may be an active process that usurps control of the ventricles, and may commence, terminate, or be interrupted by fusion beats rising normally in the SA node (Fig. 5.62). It may be difficult, without intracardiac recordings, to distinguish between a focus of ventricular origin from one high in the His–Purkinje system that is conducted with aberration because it starts in one bundle branch system, being conducted rapidly down that fascicle but more slowly retrogradely and then into the others.

Benign ventricular tachycardia

Repetitive attacks of ventricular tachycardia causing few symptoms are by no means uncommonly seen in young people. The patient may have no symptoms at all and the pulse irregularity lead to the recording of an ECG and great concern, with an unpleasant diagnostic and prognostic situation

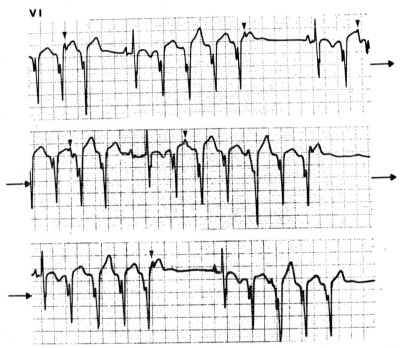

Figure 5.63   Repetitive idiopathic ventricular tachycardia in an apparently well young man: paroxysms are separated by single sinus beats only, and independent atrial activity can be seen (arrows)

unless the disorder is recognised. Such repetitive attacks have been described by Gallavardin (1922) and Parkinson and Papp (1947).

In this syndrome, episodes of tachycardia may be rare but often occur frequently, perhaps separated by only one or more sinus beats (Fig. 5.63); episodes may, as in other forms of ventricular tachycardia, be interrupted by fusion or capture beats (Fig. 5.64). The tachycardia tends to be relatively slow, rarely disabling the patient or preventing him or her from engaging in vigorous exertion; termination may be spontaneous, or occasionally, due to retrograde conduction into the AV node, by capture with an echo beat (Fig. 5.65). The underlying mechanism for such an episode may be para-

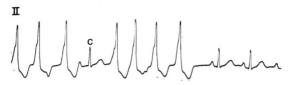

Figure 5.64 Idiopathic ventricular tachycardia interrupted by a capture beat (c); AV dissociation is clearly evident

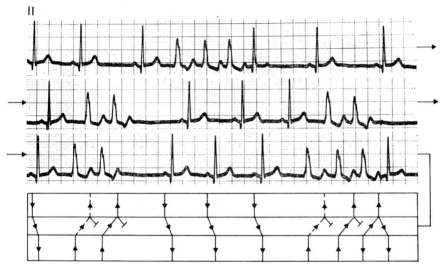

Figure 5.65 Idiopathic ventricular tachycardia (continuous recording) with ladder diagram below bottom panel to indicate termination of attack by ventricular capture by sinus impulse

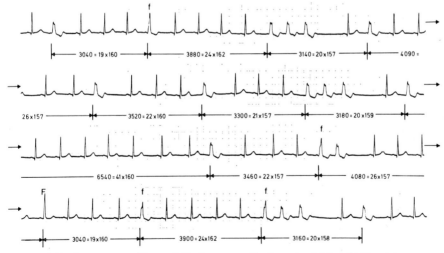

Figure 5.66 Same case as Figure 5.65. A parasystolic focus (multiple of 160 ms) is seen to initiate attacks of tachycardia

systolic (Fig. 5.66), and failure to respond to conventional measures is almost a hallmark of the disorder: indeed, the patients more often suffer toxic effects than benefit from the vigorous antiarrhythmic therapy given to treat the electrocardiographic abnormality. However, although apparently benign, the position is rarely recognised in those of middle age or beyond, suggesting either that it disappears by that stage of life, or that the course is potentially dangerous.

ACKNOWLEDGEMENT

We gratefully acknowledge support for these studies from the British Heart Foundation.

REFERENCES

American Heart Association (1967) Committee on electrocardiography. Recomendations for standardisation of leads and of specifications for instruments in electrocardiography and rectorcardiography. *Circulation*, **35**, 383.

Barold, S. S. & Friedberg, H. D. (1974) Second degree atrioventricular block. A matter of definition. *American Journal of Cardiology*, **33**, 311.

Brat, A. (1975) Concealed AV junctional extrasystoles simulating second-degree sinoatrial block. *British Heart Journal*, **37**, 449.

Castellanos, A., Khuddus, S. A., Sommer, L. S., Sung, R. J. & Myerburg, R. J. (1975) His bundle recordings in bradycardia-dependent AV block induced by premature beats. *British Heart Journal*, **37**, 570.

Chiche, P., Haiat, R. & Steff, P. (1974) Angina pectoris with syncope due to paroxysmal atrioventricular block: role of ischaemia. Report of two cases. *British Heart Journal*, **36**, 577.

Childers, R. W., Arnsdorf, M. F., De la Fuente, D. J., Gambetta, M. & Svenson, R. (1973) Sinus nodal echoes: clinical case report and canine studies. *American Journal of Cardiology*, **31**, 220.

Cohen, S. I., Smith, L. K., Aoresty, J. M., Voukydis, P. & Morkin, E. (1975) Atrioventricular conduction in patients with clinical indications for transvenous cardiac pacing. *British Heart Journal*, **37**, 583.

Cohn, A. E. & Lewis, T. (1912) Auricular fibrillation and complete heart block. *Heart*, **4**, 15.

Coumel, Ph., Motté, G., Gourgon, R., Fabiato, A., Slama, R. & Bouvrain, Y. (1970) Les tachycardies supraventriculaires par rythme réciproque en dehors du syndrôme de W.P.W. *Archives des Maladies du Coeur et des Vaisseaux*, **67**, 23.

Coumel, Ph., Fabiato, A., Waynberger, W., Motte, G., Slama, R. & Bouvrain, Y. (1971) Bradycardia-dependent atrioventricular block. Report of two cases of AV block elicited by premature beats. *Journal of Electrocardiology*, **4**, 168.

Curry, P. L. V. (1975) Fundamentals of cardiac arrhythmias. In *Cardiac Arrhythmias, the Modern Electrophysiological Approach*, ed. Krikler, D. M. & Goodwin, J. F., p. 39. London: W. B. Saunders.

Curry, P. V. L., Fitchett, D., Stubbs, W. & Krikler, D. M. (1976a) Ventricular arrhythmias and hypokalaemia. *Lancet*, **2**, 231.

Curry, P. V. L., Callowhill, E. & Krikler, D. M. (1976b) Paroxysmal re-entry sinus tachycardia. *British Heart Journal*, **38**, 311.

Damato, A. N., Schnitzler, R. N. & Lau, J. H. (1973) Recent advances in the bundle of His electrogram. In *Progress in Cardiology*, ed. Yu, P. N. & Goodwin, J. F., Vol. IV, p. 181. Philadelphia: Lea & Febiger.

Dreifus, L. S., Haiat, R., Watanabe, Y., Arriaga, J. & Reitman, N. C. (1971) Ventricular fibrillation, a possible mechanism of sudden death in patients with the Wolff–Parkinson–White syndrome. *Circulation*, **43**, 520.

Gallavardin, L. (1922) Extrasystolie ventriculaire à paroxysmes tachycardiques prolongés. *Archives des Maladies du Coeur et des Vaisseaux*, **15**, 298.

Jervell, A. & Lange-Nielsen, F. (1957) Congenital deaf-mutism, functional heart disease with prolongation of the Q–T interval, and sudden death. *American Heart Journal*, **54**, 59.

Krikler, D. M. (1971) Disturbances in intracardiac conduction. *British Journal of Hospital Medicine*, **5**, 164.

Krikler, D. M. (1974) A fresh look at cardiac arrhythmias. *Lancet*, **1**, 851, 913, 974, 1034.

Krikler, D. M. (1975) The Wolff–Parkinson–White and related syndromes. I. Presentations and implications. In *Cardiac Arrhythmias, the Modern Electrophysiological Approach*, ed. Krikler, D. M. & Goodwin, J. F., p. 144. London: W. B. Saunders.

Krikler, D. M. & Curry, P. V. L. (1976) Torsade de pointes, an atypical ventricular tachycardia. *British Heart Journal*, **38**, 117.

Krikler, D. M. & Macfarlane, P. W. (1974) Editorial: Standards for electrocardiographs. *British Heart Journal*, **36**, 945.

Krikler, D. M., Curry, P. V. L., Attuel, P. & Coumel, Ph. (1976) 'Incessant' tachycardias in Wolff–Parkinson–White syndrome. I. Initiation without antecedent extrasystoles or PR lengthening, with reference to reciprocation after shortening of cycle length. *British Heart Journal*, **38**, 885.

Krikler, D. M., Curry, P. V. L., Coumel, Ph. & Oakley, C. M. (1977) Wolff–Parkinson–White syndrome obscured by left bundle branch block. *European Journal of Cardiology*, **5**, 49.

Kulbertus, H. E. & Demoulin, J.-C. (1975) The conduction system; anatomical and pathological aspects. In *Cardiac Arrhythmias, the Modern Electrophysiological Approach*, ed. Krikler, D. M. & Goodwin, J. F., p. 16. London: W. B. Saunders.

Langendorf, R. & Mintz, S. S. (1946) Premature systoles originating in the sino-auricular node. *British Heart Journal*, **8**, 178.

Langendorf, R. & Pick, A. (1956) Concealed conduction. Further evaluation of a fundamental aspect of propagation of the cardiac impulse. *Circulation*, **13**, 381.

Latour, H. & Puech, P. (1957) *L'Electrocardiographie Endocavitaire*. Paris: Masson.

Lev, M., Silverman, J., Fitzmaurice, F. M., Paul, M. H., Cassels, D. E. & Miller, R. A. (1971). Lack of connection between the atria and the more peripheral conduction system in congenital atrioventricular block. *American Journal of Cardiology*, **27**, 481.

Lewis, T. (1910) On the electrocardiographic curves yielded by ectopic beats arising in the walls of the auricles and ventricles. *British Medical Journal*, **1**, 750.

MacKenzie, J. (1892) Pulsations in the veins with a description of a new method for graphically recording them. *Journal of Pathology and Bacteriology*, **1**, 53.

Mandel, W. J., Hayakawa, H., Allen, H. N., Danzig, R. & Kermaier, A. I. (1972) Assessment of sinus node function in patients with the sick sinus syndrome. *Circulation*, **46**, 761.

Medvedowsky, J. L., Barnay, C., Delaage, M., Nicolai, P. & Chostakoff, F. (1975) Etude de la fonction sinusale: résultats préliminaires. *Archives des Maladies du Coeur et des Vaisseaux*, **68**, 225.

Narula, O. S. (1974) Sinus node re-entry, a mechanism for supraventricular tachycardia. *Circulation*, **50**, 1114.

Narula, O. S., Samet, P. & Javier, R. P. (1972) Significance of the sinus node recovery time. *Circulation*, **45**, 140.

Parkinson, J. & Papp, C. (1947) Repetitive paroxysmal tachycardia. *British Heart Journal*, **8**, 241.

Puech, P. (1975) Atrioventricular block: the value of intracardiac recordings. In *Cardiac Arrhythmias: the Modern Electrophysiological Approach*, ed. Krikler, D. M. & Goodwin, J. F., p. 81. London and Philadelphia: W. B. Saunders.

Puech, P. & Grolleau, R. (1972) *L'activite du faisceau de His normale et pathologique*. Paris: Sandoz.

Puech, P., Latour, H. & Grolleau, R. (1970) Le flutter et ses limites. *Archives des Maladies du Coeur et des Vaisseaux*, **63**, 116.

Rosenbaum, M. B., Elizari, M. V., Levi, R. J. & Nau, G. J. (1973) Paroxysmal atrioventricular block related to hypopolarisation and spontaneous diastolic depolarisation. *Chest*, **63**, 678.

Sandler, I. A. & Marriott, H. J. L. (1965) The differential morphology of anomalous ventricular complexes of RBBB type in lead V1. Ventricular ectopy versus aberration. *Circulation*, **31**, 551.

Schamroth, L. (1971) *The Disorders of Cardiac Rhythm*. Oxford: Blackwell.

Schamroth, L. & Friedberg, H. D. (1969) Wedensky facilitation and the Wedensky effect during high-grade A–V block in the human heart. *American Journal of Cardiology*, **23**, 893.

Schamroth, L. & Krikler, D. M. (1967) The problem of lone atrial fibrillation. *South African Medical Journal*, **41**, 502.

Scherf, D. & Schott, A. (1973) *Extrasystoles and Allied Arrhythmias*, 2nd edn. London: Heinemann.

Scherlag, B. J., Lau, S. H., Helfant, R. H., Berkowitz, W. D., Stein, E. & Damato, A. N. (1969) Catheter technique for recording His bundle activity in man. *Circulation*, **39**, 13.

Schuilenburg, R. M. & Durrer, D. (1975) Problems in the recognition of conduction disturbances in the His bundle. *Circulation*, **51**, 68.

Short, D. S. (1954) The syndrome of alternating bradycardia and tachycardia. *British Heart Journal*, **16**, 208.

Slama, R., Waynberger, M., Motté, G. & Bouvrain, Y. (1969) La maladie rythmique auriculaire. Etude clinique, électrique et évolutive de 43 observations. *Archives des Maladies du Coeur et des Vaisseaux*, **62**, 297.

Slama, R., Motté, G. & Coumel, Ph. (1971) *Les Blocs Auriculoventriculaires*. Paris: Bailliere.

Slama, R., Coumel, Ph., Motté, G., Jourgon, R., Waynberger, M. & Touche, S. (1973) Tachycardies ventriculaires et torsades de pointes. Frontieres morphologique entre les dysrythmies ventriculaires. *Archives des Maladies du Coeur et des Vaisseaux*, **66**, 1401.

Spurrell, R. A. J., Krikler, D. M. & Sowton, E. (1972) Study of intraventricular conduction times in patients with left bundle branch block and left axis deviation in patients with left bundle branch block and normal QRS axis using His bundle electrograms. *British Heart Journal*, **34**, 1244.

Spurrell, R. A. J., Krikler, D. M. & Sowton, E. (1974) Retrograde invasion of the bundle branches producing aberration of the QRS complexes during supraventricular tachycardia studied by programmed electrical stimulation. *Circulation*, **50**, 487.

Steeg, C. N., Krongrad, E., Davachi, F., Bowman, F. O., Jr, Malm, J. R. & Jersony, W. M. (1975) Postoperative left anterior hemiblock and right bundle branch block following repair of tetralogy of Fallot: clinical and etiologic considerations. *Circulation*, **51**, 1026.

Strauss, H. C., Saroff, A. L., Bigger, J. T., Jr & Jiardina, E. G. V. (1973) Premature atrial stimulation as a key to the understanding of sinoatrial conduction in man. *Circulation*, **47**, 86.

Ward, O. C. (1964) A new familial cardiac syndrome in children. *Journal of the Irish Medical Association*, **54**, 103.

Wellens, H. J. J., Lie, K. I. & Durrer, D. (1974) Further observations on ventricular tachycardia as studied by electrical stimulation of the heart: chronic recurrent ventricular tachycardia and ventricular tachycardia during acute myocardial infarction. *Circulation*, **49**, 647.

Wellens, H. J. J. & Lie, K. I. (1975) Ventricular tachycardias: the value of programmed electrical stimulation. In *Cardiac Arrhythmias, the Modern Electrophysiological Approach*, ed. Krikler, D. M. & Goodwin, J. F., p. 182. London: W. B. Saunders.

6

DRUG THERAPY IN THE MANAGEMENT OF CARDIAC TACHYARRHYTHMIAS

C. R. Kumana

A number of considerations enter into the management of tachyar-rhythmias:

(a) Making an accurate diagnosis.

(b) Removal of precipitating or aggravating factors if possible.

(c) Deciding on whether or not the arrhythmia warrants treatment in the context of the particular clinical situation prevailing. This requires a sound understanding in the use of potentially beneficial drugs, since to embark on a course of treatment with these agents, their likely benefit should outweigh the risks associated with their use.

(d) Awareness of approaches to management other than the use of drugs. These include d.c. shock, programmed stimulation with pacemakers, surgical division of specialised conduction pathways or myocardium, as well as surgical excision of cardiac tissue.

Accurate Diagnosis

It is probably a valid 'clinical' truism to assert that 'the only object of diagnosis is treatment', using the word treatment in its widest sense, including offering a prognosis. It is also a fact that different groups of arrhythmias respond differently to drug therapy, so the importance of accurate diagnosis cannot be over-emphasised. Thus, the recognition of an ectopic ventricular escape rhythm, such as the so-called accelerated idioventricular rhythm, or even premature beats when the basic ventricular rate is slow requires that the main treatment be directed at the slow heart rate and not at the ventricular ectopics. Similarly, to mistake supraventricular tachycardias with aberrant ventricular conduction for ventricular tachycardia can lead to unnecessary and troublesome failure of treatment since unsuitable drugs might be used. Under some circumstances, it may also be useful to distinguish between reciprocal tachycardias and tachycardias due to rapidly discharging ectopic foci, as well as to distinguish between premature beats with fixed coupling intervals and those due to parasystole.

Deciding Whether or Not an Arrhythmia Warrants Treatment, and if so, What Approach to Treatment is Necessary

Treatment and/or suppression of any particular cardiac arrhythmia is only warranted if the consequent improvement in symptoms, morbidity and mortality outweigh the risks and inconvenience of treatment. There is little doubt that arrhythmias producing symptoms warrant treatment. Regrettably, for many relatively asymptomatic and seemingly benign arrhythmias, reliable information as to the need for treatment is not available and physicians often have to decide intuitively whether or not to treat any particular patient.

VENTRICULAR TACHYARRHYTHMIAS

There is general agreement that arrhythmias associated with acute cardio-vascular insults have a poor prognosis if untreated. For example, after cardiac infarction, many preventable deaths are probably due to ventricular tachy-arrhythmias and treatment of these is thought to reduce mortality (Lown et al, 1967, 1969). Distinction between parasystolic ventricular premature beats and those with a fixed coupling interval is generally regarded as academic, prognosis depending on their nearness in time to an acute cardiac event. Nevertheless, there is evidence that under some circumstances, such as in the late postinfarction period, parasystolic ectopics may be the more benign (Kotler et al, 1973). If treatment for ventricular premature beats is to be undertaken, there is very little information on whether any particular drug is as effective against parasystolic beats as against non-parasystolic (i.e. coupled ectopics).

The role of prophylactic antiarrhythmic therapy after myocardial infarction is a matter of some controversy (Koch-Weser, 1971a; Darby et al, 1972; Church and Biern, 1972; Lie et al, 1974b). The alternative approach is to administer antiarrhythmic drugs after cardiac infarction only in the event of the development of certain so-called warning arrhythmias (R-on-T, multifocal and runs of three or more ventricular ectopic beats or five or more premature ventricular beats per minute). Clarification of this issue is proceeding and depends on a number of points. Firstly, conventional electrocardiographic monitoring, even in specialised units, may not be efficient at detecting (and consequently treating) warning arrhythmias as compared to detection by computer (Vetter and Julian, 1975). Secondly, as primary ventricular fibrilla-tion is the important arrhythmia causing mortality, it becomes logical to determine whether 'warning' arrhythmias really do occur more frequently in patients going on to develop primary ventricular fibrillation than in those not developing this complication. That early in the course of myocardial infarction the predictive value of these so-called warning arrhythmias has come under suspicion (Lawrie et al, 1968; Lie, Wellens and Darrer, 1974a) is of con-siderable importance. Finally, regardless of the incidence of dangerous arrhythmias amongst those treated prophylactically and those treated electively, overall mortality and morbidity must also be considered.

As to premature ventricular beats unassociated with any acute cardiac event, even if they are exceedingly frequent, treatment does not seem to be warranted if they do not become more frequent with exercise. If their frequency increases during exercise, it is thought advisable to avoid strenuous exercise, but the need for any other form of therapy is debatable (*British Medical Journal*, 1973).

SINUS TACHYCARDIA

This requires that treatment be directed at the cause. The heart rate seldom exceeds 150 beats/min except in rare instances such as thyrotoxic crisis, when it may be useful to facilitate treatment by administering beta-adrenoceptor blocking drugs together with antithyroid medication (see p. 190). In general, it is a sound policy to assume that sinus tachycardia is a physiological response and that therefore attempts to suppress it could be harmful.

SUPRAVENTRICULAR TACHYCARDIAS

In these tachycardias (atrial tachycardia, atrial fibrillation, atrial flutter, AV junctional tachycardia), the conduction pathways often fail to propagate every proximal impulse so that the ventricular rate is frequently much slower than the basic rate of the tachycardia. Such dissociation of the ventricles is a physiological protective phenomenon, and when it fails the rapid ventricular rate consequent on 1 to 1 conduction may lead to serious haemodynamic disturbance and distress. It should also be realised that some of the drugs conventionally used in their treatment may actually be responsible for precipitating or aggravating these tachycardias. In particular, junctional tachycardias and paroxysmal atrial tachycardia with AV dissociation may result from digoxin overdose or sensitivity. Apart from being manifestations of cardiac disease, supraventricular tachycardias may also be features of extracardiac diseases such as thyrotoxicosis or chest infections. Whenever these tachycardias are paroxysmal and infrequent, treatment need not be initiated till their onset. When frequent paroxysms occur, it may prove worthwhile attempting to suppress their recurrences by continuous therapy.

Before recourse to drugs, measures to increase vagal tone such as carotid sinus pressure, Valsalva's manoeuvre, eyeball pressure or straining as at stool should be tried and may occasionally abolish the tachycardia. In any case, even transient dramatic slowing of the ventricular rate (whether by abolishing the tachycardia or by increasing AV block) can be taken as proof that the tachycardia is supraventricular in origin. Similarly, treatment with i.v. edrophonium used as in myasthenia (2 mg test dose, then 8 mg) may also be effective, and though it may cause transient gastrointestinal symptoms lasting a few minutes, hospital admission may nevertheless be obviated. Patients can sometimes be taught some of these manoeuvres so that they can abolish their own tachycardias. Atrial fibrillation and ventricular tachycardias do not show dramatic rate changes after these manoeuvres.

The definitive treatment of these arrhythmias involves two alternative approaches. The first of these is to restore and maintain sinus rhythm. This is most easily achieved if the factors responsible for the tachycardias (e.g. thyrotoxicosis, mitral stenosis, chest infection) have been corrected. If not, it may still be possible to maintain sinus rhythm using continuous treatment with drugs, though relapse rates are likely to be high. The second approach, which is mainly applicable when the factors producing these arrhythmias have not or cannot be removed, is to ensure that the ventricular rate does not become excessive and uncontrolled even though sinus rhythm is not restored. The haemodynamic disturbance and symptoms associated with a rapid ventricular rate would then be reduced, though the benefits of a normal sequence of cardiac activation would be lacking.

As *atrial flutter* is difficult to convert to either sinus rhythm or atrial fibrillation using drugs, recourse to d.c. shock should be relatively early. If the fundamental cardiac abnormality continues, a supraventricular tachycardia would be expected to recur, but it might do so in the form of atrial fibrillation which is more likely to be amenable to control by drugs. Treatment with drugs is generally more successful against *atrial tachycardia, atrial fibrillation and AV junctional tachycardias*. Digoxin usually slows the ventricular rate by increasing AV block or by converting atrial tachycardia (and rarely flutter) to atrial fibrillation, but may occasionally restore sinus rhythm; whilst beta blocking drugs may also restore sinus rhythm or slow the ventricular rate.

In the presence of atrial fibrillation or any other supraventricular tachycardia refractory to drugs, synchronised d.c. defibrillation may be used electively to restore sinus rhythm whenever a complete cure of the arrhythmia is indicated. It may also be used in an emergency when drugs have failed to control the ventricular rate, realising that any restoration of sinus rhythm may be temporary and with the hope that any further supraventricular tachycardia might be more amenable to drug treatment.

WOLFF–PARKINSON–WHITE SYNDROME

This condition is associated with two groups of tachycardias. Commonly, a reciprocating tachycardia occurs involving the AV node and normal specialised conduction system as the antegrade pathway and involving retrograde conduction in the accessory pathways. More rarely when atrial fibrillation or flutter develop, rapid conduction through the accessory pathway may give rise to very rapid ventricular rates or even ventricular fibrillation. The use of continuous therapy as opposed to therapy for each bout of tachycardia must depend on the frequency and severity of the above-mentioned arrhythmias and on the effectiveness of the drugs (e.g. β-blockers, verapamil, disopyramide) used in any particular patient. There has been a single case report of digoxin possibly precipitating ventricular fibrillation when given to treat a tachycardia associated with Wolff–Parkinson–White syndrome (Dreifus et al, 1971); nevertheless, that patient was eventually managed on continuous digoxin therapy in association with other drugs to prevent relapses of tachycardia.

Remediable Precipitating or Aggravating Factors

A fairly comprehensive list of remediable factors is given below:

1. Anatomically remediable—mitral stenosis, constrictive pericarditis, myxoma, etc.
2. Sympathetic stimulation involved—CATS (caffeine, alcohol, tobacco, stress); anoxia; excessive supportive treatment with catecholamines.
3. Hypertension.
4. Metabolic—e.g. hypokalaemia (rarely hyperkalaemia), thyrotoxicosis (especially crisis), hypercalcaemia, phaeochromocytoma, etc.
5. Drugs—especially digoxin, tricyclic antidepressants, phenothiazines, fluorocarbons, halothane, chloroform, and the so-called 'antiarrhythmic drugs' themselves.

SYMPATHETIC STIMULATION

Many of these factors exert their influence either by increasing the exposure of the heart to catecholamines or by sensitising it to their actions. On the basis of animal work, it has been suggested that excessive myocardial sympathetic activity accentuates Ca^{2+} influx into cells, leading to cell necrosis as well as to recognisable arrhythmias. Anoxia per se and anoxic myocardium round a cardiac infarct are both likely to provoke catecholamine release which might in turn contribute to the production of cardiac arrhythmias. There is also evidence that thyrotoxic patients have increased sensitivity to catecholamines, it being known that blockade of adrenergic neurones or the β-adrenoceptors in particular relieve many of the clinical features of thyrotoxicosis (Turner, 1974). Many anaesthetic agents are also thought to affect the heart in a similar way.

TRICYCLIC ANTIDEPRESSANTS

Some of the peripheral actions of tricyclic antidepressants resemble those of anticholinergic drugs. In the central nervous system, they interfere with reuptake of amines into intraneuronal stores and thus increase the free concentrations of these substances at receptors. It is interesting to speculate whether they also have similar properties outside the central nervous system. Since the 1960s, reports have suggested that these drugs used in normal or only slightly excessive doses might give rise to various heart blocks, ventricular premature beats, supraventricular and ventricular tachycardias and even ventricular fibrillation. Such abnormalities usually disappeared on withdrawing treatment and returned after a variable period when patients were rechallenged with their drug. Young persons appeared to be particularly sensitive. Since there is a relatively high incidence of cardiac disease in the general population, appraisal of these reports was difficult and there is some confusion as to the place of these drugs in patients having ischaemic heart disease.

Scottish workers (Moir et al, 1972; Moir, Dingwall-Fordyce and Weir, 1973) undertook an investigation using hospital-based computerised drug information and monitoring systems. They found no significant difference in the incidence of sudden deaths amongst hospital patients receiving amitriptylene and a group of matched control patients. However, a significant excess of sudden deaths was noted in patients with cardiac disease also receiving amitriptylene compared to control patients with cardiac disease not receiving the drug and otherwise well matched. When the study was extended to cover outpatient follow-up, an excess of sudden deaths was only revealed in those cardiac patients receiving amitriptylene who were also more than 70 years old. These findings need to be interpreted with care. Firstly, the control group of cardiac patients differed from the test group not only by virtue of not receiving amitriptylene, but also presumably by not being depressed. Secondly, in both the inpatient and outpatient studies, overall mortality in the two groups was similar, so that if patients on amitriptylene had a higher incidence of sudden death, then the control group must have had a higher incidence of insidious death. A report from the Boston Collaborative Drug Surveillance Program (1972) did not confirm the Scottish findings. However, their investigation had not distinguished between different antidepressant drugs, included patients with hypertension, and in general their control patients had not been strictly matched.

It is recommended that regular electrocardiograms should be undertaken on all patients receiving these agents. That their peripheral (cardiac) actions might well be akin to their central actions is supported by the observation that some tachyarrhythmias arising after overdosage with tricyclic antidepressants respond promptly to β-blocking drugs (Freeman and Loughhead, 1973). However, there would be little point in administering any given β-blocking agent concurrently with an antidepressant unless it could be established that the latter's therapeutic central action would not also be negated. It needs to be seen whether some tricyclic antidepressants will indeed turn out to be free of cardiovascular side effects (Pitts, 1969). Alternative treatment such as electroconvulsive therapy should also be considered more readily in vulnerable patients.

PHENOTHIAZINES

Anecdotal reports implicate phenothiazines as a possible cause of cardiac damage giving rise to tachyarrhythmias and heart blocks (Alexander and

Nino, 1969). That they produce reversible electrocardiographic changes (T-waves becoming flat, bifid and occasionally inverted, slight prolongation of QTc) in some individuals is undoubted (Huston and Bell, 1966). Such changes, which are mainly changes in T-vector amplitude rather than axis, can be completely or incompletely reversed by taking potassium supplements or by overnight fasting (Alvarez-Mena and Frank, 1973). The phenothiazines have also been incriminated as a cause of death resulting from cardiac arrhythmias (Kelly, Fay and Laverty, 1963; Giles and Modlin, 1968); however the precise role of these drugs with respect to sudden, 'autopsy negative' deaths which are a recognised occurrence in schizophrenics is uncertain (*Lancet*, 1966; Peele and von Loetzen, 1973).

FLUOROCARBON AEROSOL PROPELLANTS

Animal work as well as the occurrence of sudden deaths in glue sniffers suggest that inhalation of very high concentrations of fluorocarbons may give rise to ventricular tachyarrhythmias. However, the greatest hazard from these substances may occur in asthmatics when together with sympathomimetic agents they are inhaled in excess (*Lancet*, 1975).

HYPOKALAEMIA

According to the theory of Hodgkin and Huxley, the resting membrane potential across excitable membranes is proportional to log of the ratio of intracellular potassium ion (K^+) concentration to extracellular K^+ concentration. As the extracellular K^+ concentration is very low in relation to the intracellular K^+ concentration, it follows that a given absolute change in K^+ concentration outside cell membranes produces a relatively large change in the ratio when compared to that accompanying a similar change in intracellular K^+ concentration. Thus for most practical purposes, it is the extracellular K^+ concentration which is likely to be critical whatever happens to intracellular or total body potassium, both of which are difficult to measure. Low plasma K^+ concentrations affect the myocardial cell membranes so as to facilitate the onset of ventricular premature beats and ventricular fibrillation, and also sensitise the heart to some of the toxic effects of digoxin. It is of interest that a number of recent reports (Dargie et al, 1974; Wilkinson et al, 1975) have doubted the need to administer potassium supplements routinely when K^+ losing diuretics such as frusemide and thiazides are being used in hypertensive patients. Nevertheless, it is likely that patients with oedema due to heart failure or cirrhosis may be excessively sensitive to the plasma potassium lowering properties of these diuretics and require appropriate supplements, and it would seem safest to monitor plasma potassium levels in all patients receiving these agents. It is also prudent to check plasma potassium values whenever ventricular tachyarrhythmias occur, not only as hypokalaemia may contribute to their presence, but also as drugs such as lignocaine may not be fully effective unless the plasma K^+ concentration is kept well up within the normal range (Pamintuan, Dreifus and Watanabe, 1970).

Electrical and Surgical Approaches

Electrical defibrillation of the heart is the only reliable treatment of ventricular fibrillation. When used with some form of general anaesthetic with appropriate timing of the shock, it is also the treatment of choice whenever it is considered desirable to convert atrial fibrillation or any other refractory tachycardia to sinus rhythm. Other sophisticated electrophysiological techniques, though less well known, are proving useful in the study of antiarrhythmic drugs, and are giving rise to exciting advances in the diagnosis and treatment of tachyarrhythmias.

In evaluating the influence of antiarrhythmic drugs, it is useful to be able to control heart rate so that actions on other aspects of cardiac performance can be assessed independently. By using atrial and ventricular pacing and also by initiating reciprocal tachycardias, effects on antegrade and retrograde conduction can be determined. By delivering accurately timed premature stimuli, the effects of drugs on refractory period can also be assessed.

RECIPROCAL TACHYCARDIAS

During any tachycardia appropriately placed intra and extracardiac recording electrodes can reveal whether or not activation of the ventricles is always preceded by activation of the His bundle, or whether atrial activation is independent of ventricular activation. The use of some further measures can be helpful in deciding whether any given paroxysmal tachycardia is likely to be due to a rapidly discharging ectopic focus or to a reciprocal rhythm. Reciprocal tachycardias are thought to arise whenever there are two or more possible pathways, conventionally denoted alpha (α) and beta (β), by which activation of distal tissues can occur and when one pathway (β) has a longer refractory period than the other. If a premature beat occurs while only one pathway (β) is refractory, activation proceeds along the other pathway (α) of short refractory period but long conduction time. Provided the first pathway (β) is no longer refractory when the impulse conducted relatively slowly through the other pathway (α) excites the distal tissues, the β pathway may be activated retrogradely, to restimulate the whole circuit and initiate a tachycardia. A premature beat arising during a tachycardia could make a section of the pathway refractory, preventing the passage of the next circulating impulse with the result that the tachycardia would be terminated when the anterograde and retrograde activation fronts meet. It is likely that such circuits may involve two pathways within the AV junction itself or any combination of either of the following: AV junction and His–Purkinje system (usually the anterograde pathway) with myocardium or accessory conduction pathways as in pre-excitation. Characteristically, such reciprocal tachycardias may be initiated and terminated by suitably timed artificial premature beats, and furthermore, premature beats which fail to terminate the tachycardia are followed by less than full compensatory pauses (Wellens, Schuilenburg and Durrer, 1972). Mapping studies, accurately timing the onset of activation over the epicardium, allow more precise location of accessory AV pathways and re-entry mechanisms in WPW syndrome and in certain ventricular tachycardias (Durrer and Roos, 1967; Spurrell et al, 1975). It is possible that similar reciprocal mechanisms may be involved in the pathogenesis of both atrial and ventricular fibrillation.

Most tachycardias associated with pre-excitation situations such as the WPW syndrome are reciprocal in nature, usually involving antegrade conduction via the normal AV junction and retrograde conduction via an accessory pathway. A minority of tachycardias, however, are due to a dangerously rapid ventricular rate or ventricular fibrillation, which may occur when the patient develops atrial fibrillation or atrial flutter. It is presumed that the potential for a rapid ventricular response to these atrial tachycardias occurs whenever the refractory period of the abnormal bypass becomes very short in response to repetitive stimulation.

DRUGS

Drugs which selectively increase refractoriness in the less refractory of two hypothetical pathways (α) relative to the other pathway (β), could prevent the initiation of a reciprocal tachycardia by premature beats. Thus it is thought that verapamil may be used in the management of reciprocal tachycardias associated with WPW syndrome, since it selectively increases refractoriness of the AV junction (anterograde pathway), but not of the abnormal bypass (see p. 141). It should also be appreciated that regardless of their actions on the normal AV junction, drugs may also have independent and important actions on the accessory pathway; for example, quinidine-like drugs usually increase refractoriness and suppress such conduction, which may at least partly explain their role in countering reciprocal tachycardias involving the accessory pathways and preventing very rapid ventricular rates associated with atrial fibrillation and flutter (Wellens and Durrer, 1974; *British Medical Journal*, 1974). It should not be forgotten that in some patients, these drugs can actually promote arrhythmias (Wellens and Durrer, 1974), probably by creating an imbalance in the conduction properties of alternative pathways. In some patients, digitalis decreases the refractoriness in accessory pathways, and can hence predispose to dangerously rapid ventricular rates in the presence of atrial fibrillation, flutter or tachycardia (Dreifus et al, 1971). Paradoxically, drugs which selectively accelerate conduction in one hypothetical pathway might also prove useful in abolishing reciprocal tachycardias, since the impulse may then reach distal tissues when they are still refractory to stimulation.

PACING AND SURGERY

From what has been discussed, it follows that when reciprocal tachycardias prove difficult to manage conservatively, pacemakers could be used to deliver suitably timed premature beats in order to terminate the tachycardias. So-called 'chronic overdrive pacing' can also be undertaken (Johnson et al, 1974), since it seems likely that at faster heart rates inequalities in the refractoriness of alternative pathways through which the cardiac impulse is conducted may sometimes be eliminated, hence preventing re-entry. Provided the re-entry pathways are accurately known, it may also be feasible to interrupt them surgically so as to effect a radical cure (Durrer and Roos, 1967; Spurrell et al, 1975). Alternatively, the normal His–Purkinje pathway may be interrupted, but then a pacemaker would be required, and patients with WPW syndrome who develop atrial tachycardias would still be prone to a dangerously rapid ventricular rate if the refractoriness of their bypass was unduly short (Dreifus et al, 1971).

Surgical excision of rapidly discharging ectopic foci, such as are thought to occur in ventricular aneurysms, may also be useful (Thind, Blakemore and Zinsser, 1971). However, without detailed study, re-entry mechanisms in the margin of such aneurysms cannot be excluded, and the cures resulting from aneurysmectomy may have been due to interruption of re-entry circuits (Spurrell et al, 1975).

CLASSIFICATION OF ANTIARRHYTHMIC DRUGS

There is no entirely satisfactory way of grouping drugs used in the treatment of cardiac arrythmias just as there is no entirely simple and practical way of categorising the arrhythmias themselves. Based on the work of Vaughan Williams (1975) and other research workers (Krikler, 1974a; Naylor, 1976) on electrophysiological and allied properties of cardiac tissue, it has been proposed that the drugs be divided into different classes as shown below. Reference to Figure 6.1 may clarify some of the mechanisms postulated.

Class I. Drugs which reduce the rate of rise of the action potential (Fig. 6.1) slow conduction and increase the refractory period of myocardial cells as well as having other actions, e.g. quinidine, procainamide, disopyramide, ajmaline, lignocaine, mexiletine, phenytoin and propranolol (in high concentrations only).

Bigger (1974) drew attention to some electrophysiological properties of phenytoin and lignocaine which distinguished them from other drugs in class I. Both these drugs enter and act on the central nervous system, may give rise to sympathetic stimulation, seem not to interfere with AV conduction and may be useful in treating arrhythmias associated with digoxin toxicity.

Class II. β-Blockers and other sympatholytic drugs such as bretylium.

Class III. Drugs producing changes analogous to the effects of hypothyroidism, prolonging the duration of the action potential (Fig. 6.1) and hence also the refractory period. These drugs are useful in treating AV junctional dysrhythmias as in WPW syndrome. Examples include amiodorone and a β-blocker, sotalol—producing this effect in high concentrations.

Class IV. Drugs acting on calcium ions at the cell membrane. The coupling of electrical activation to mechanical activation appears to be Ca^{2+} dependent. These drugs deplete available Ca^{2+} stores at the cell membranes, block Ca^{2+}

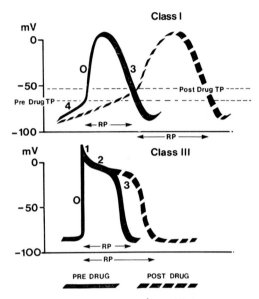

Figure 6.1   Diagrammatic representation of transmembrane cardiac action potential recorded by intra-cellular electrodes. *Class I drug* (shown to be acting on a cell with automatic behaviour, e.g. from SA node) reduces rate of rise of action potential (phase 0) and interferes with propagation of impulse so as to slow conduction, reduces rate of diastolic depolarisation (phase 4) and may (as shown here) reduce the threshold potential (TP). These actions tend to increase the duration of the refractory period (RP). Reduction in the rate of rise of the action potential may block conduction to adjacent cells completely or merely slow conduction. It should be appreciated that some of these drugs may alter the timing of the refractory period quite apart from prolonging it. *Class III drug* (shown to be acting on a non-automatic myocardial cell. Note absence of phase 4 diastolic depolarisation, phase 0 depolarisation is initiated by arrival of an impulse from adjacent regions). The drug lengthens action potential duration resulting in an increased refractory period (RP)

entry across membranes, which is particularly important for activation and conduction in the AV node, and depress contractility, e.g. verapamil, disopyramide, prenylamine; they are effective against AV junctional re-entry tachycardias (e.g. in WPW syndrome).

To understand the mode of action of the class IV drugs, it is important to appreciate that Ca^{2+} ions play different roles in the function of cardiac and skeletal muscle. Although the action potential is largely attributable to entry of Na^+ ions into myocardial cells, the final rise to peak and the plateau is associated with an influx of Ca^{2+} ions (held in the cell membrane). The latter probably trigger the release of still greater amounts of Ca^{2+} ions from stores (e.g. in the sarcoplasmic reticulum) within the cell, and these Ca^{2+} ions are thought to produce the coupling of electrical and mechanical systole (Nayler, 1973). It appears that verapamil and to a less extent disopyramide reduce the availability of Ca^{2+} ions in the cell membrane (Nayler and Szeto, 1972; Nayler, 1976). There is speculation that these drugs may suppress extra-systoles dependent on Ca^{2+} influx if these exist; by interfering with the conversion of electrical to mechanical activity, theoretically at least these drugs would be expected to have a negative inotropic effect. It is of interest that ouabain has converse actions on membrane Ca^{2+} in doses which exert a positive inotropic effect (Nayler, 1973).

A major shortcoming of this classification is its lack of practical relevance to the clinician. Also the properties of some drugs overlap into different classes whilst others defy classification. Besides, it may be incorrect to assume that in vitro studies on the cardiac tissues of animals necessarily reflect the way in which these drugs act on the diseased hearts of living humans, and it is also unlikely that the actions of each drug on different types of cardiac tissue (e.g. sino-atrial node, atrial muscle, AV node, working ventricular muscle, Purkinje system, accessory AV pathway such as the bundle of Kent) would necessarily be the same.

It has often been assumed that the actions of antiarrhythmic agents are reversibly linked to the concentrations of the unbound drug in contact with myocardial tissues. It follows that in investigating the clinically important mode of action of these drugs using isolated preparations, their concentrations in the surrounding media should be of the same order as plasma concentrations encountered during therapy. Thus the class I actions of propranolol are unlikely to be clinically relevant since the concentrations required to demonstrate class I effect (Coltart and Meldrum, 1971) are about a hundred-fold greater than those encountered in the plasma of patients receiving routine doses for β-adrenergic blockade. Furthermore, investigators often fail to consider the extent of protein binding of these drugs in plasma. For example, propranolol is highly protein bound and therefore class I activity encountered in vitro occurs at about 1000 times the concentrations of free non-protein bound propranolol encountered clinically.

In vitro experiments can take no account of active drug metabolites formed in distant tissues such as the liver, but these may have important roles in the control of arrhythmias. For example, both the acetylated metabolite of procainamide and the hydroxylated metabolite encountered after oral doses of propranolol (see Table 6.1, p. 144) are active and are formed in the liver.

It is now realised that tachyarrhythmias may result from rapidly discharging ectopic foci or from abnormal circus movement of electrical activity. It follows that drugs could be classified according to whether by their action on rhythmicity, they were effective against tachycardias due to rapidly discharging ectopic foci or whether they interfered with reciprocal tachycardias by their actions on conduction and refractoriness or both. It would be important to discover on what particular cardiac tissue these agents had their main actions, and whether anterograde and/or retrograde impulse propagation were equally affected, since if all pathways were affected in the same manner, circus tachycardias would not be abolished. Furthermore, this kind of information would allow selection of the most suitable drug to suppress ectopically discharging foci or reciprocal mechanisms at any particular location. Till such time as detailed information about different drugs becomes available and, more importantly, till it becomes practical to classify routinely encountered arrhythmias according to their basic mode of production, an empirical classification will continue to remain the most satisfactory.

The beneficial effects of drugs in tachyarrhythmias may be explained as follows:

1. Propagation from rapidly discharging ectopic foci might be prevented by blocking conduction from them or rendering distal cardiac tissue refractory.
2. The initiation and propagation of re-entry tachycardias could be prevented in an exactly analogous way by blocking conduction in the reciprocal circuit or making some part of it refractory.
3. During normal sinus rhythm, unequal refractoriness in alternative pathways may be the result of conduction along one of them being faster than the other. One of the pathways would be expected to have a shorter and earlier refractory period, and a drug which could slow conduction in one of the pathways without slowing conduction in the other might equalise refractoriness in the two pathways and thus prevent re-entry tachycardias.

On the other hand, in some circumstances, agents having these same actions might slow conduction along alternative pathways unequally so as to render only one of them refractory, and in so doing, they might actually facilitate the development of re-entry (see p. 138).

PHARMACOKINETICS

Pharmacokinetics refers to the way in which the body handles drugs over a period of time. It should be realised that for any particular drug there are usually species differences, and that even within any single species very considerable differences in drug handling can occur due to genetic and other factors. In patients it is usually only practical to obtain blood and urine for measurement of drug levels and then to extrapolate as to the handling of the drug by the body as a whole. Whether in research or in a service capacity, there are two broad applications of pharmacokinetics: bio-availability determination and pharmacodynamics.

Bio-availability

Absorption and systemic availability

To check on the amount of drug capable of reaching the tissues, the concentration of drug and/or metabolites in plasma and in urine may be measured both after single doses administered by different routes as well as after regular maintenance doses. Inadequate absorption and/or excessive metabolism of orally administered drugs can then be discerned. It should be realised that inadequate absorption can be due to improper formulation of the preparation, gastrointestinal disorder in the patient or failure to take tablets. It is now apparent that the bio-availability of the same doses of any drug taken orally by the same subjects may differ substantially depending on the formulation of the drug. For the sake of consistency a case can be made out for prescribing these drugs by their trade names rather than their approved names, and this is likely to be particularly important when specialised sustained release formulations (discussed later) are to be used. The way in which a drug is

Table 6.1 Metabolism of antiarrhythmic drugs

	Quinidine	Procainamide	Propranolol	Phenytoin	Lignocaine
Metabolism	Hydroxylation	Acetylation	Hydroxylation	Parahydroxy-lation, glucuronide conjugation	Oxydative de-ethylation, hydrolysis
Protein binding	>60%	15%	90%	>50%	80%
Renal excretion	20–50%	50–60%	<1%	<5%	5%

After Bigger (1972) and Kessler (1974).

eliminated in healthy individuals frequently allows the physician to anticipate the way in which it is handled in disease states. Such predictions must of necessity be confirmed, and as a general rule it is important to appreciate and investigate possible alterations in drug distribution and/or protein binding which may also occur in disease states or when other drugs are being administered.

Metabolism

It should be remembered that drugs which are substantially eliminated by metabolism frequently also show substantial protein binding in plasma, and hence they may be subject to displacement from binding proteins by other drugs. They may also be affected by drugs which give rise to liver enzyme induction or inhibition. Occasionally the extent of elimination by metabolism is much greater after oral than after intravenous administration. This may be due to metabolism in the gut or gut wall or hepatic metabolism when a high concentration of the drug is carried to the liver in the portal vein (first pass effect). Common antiarrhythmic drugs predominantly eliminated by metabolism are listed in Table 6.1.

Renal function

Table 6.2 summarises the influence of renal function on the elimination of some commonly used antiarrhythmic drugs. It will be noted that drugs which are normally predominantly metabolised may sometimes show enhanced elimination in renal failure, as if, in uraemia, the burden of eliminating toxic substances gives rise to non-specific hepatic enzyme induction. It should also be realised that in heart failure or when there is a low blood pressure, renal and/or hepatic perfusion may be reduced so that abnormal retention of these drugs may occur. Drug metabolites tend to be more water-soluble than their parent compounds, and are more likely to be cleared by the kidneys. If these metabolites possess activity or toxicity their accumulation in renal failure might have clinical significance even though there may be no accumulation of the parent drug.

Table 6.2   Elimination of antiarrhythmic drugs

Elimination impaired in renal failure	Elimination unaffected or even enhanced in renal failure
Procainamide[a]	Lignocaine[a]
Practolol[b]	Phenytoin[a]
Digoxin[c]	Quinidine[a]
	Digitoxin[c]
	Propranolol[a]
	Acebutolol[d]

From [a]Kessler (1974).
[b]Eastwood, Curtis and Smith (1975).
[c]See p. 437.
[d]Kaye (1975).

Drug elimination and urine pH

Apart from diurnal variations, wide person to person variation in urine pH has been noted to occur in normal subjects as well as in coronary care unit patients (Elliot, Sharp and Lewis, 1959; Kiddie et al, 1974; Kiddie, 1975). It is therefore important to appreciate whether and to what extent alterations in urinary pH might affect the elimination of any particular antiarrhythmic drug.

The excretion of a drug in urine may be pH dependent if its pK_a value (the pH at which equal quantities of drug are in the ionised and the unionised form) lies between about 4 and 9, so that either predominantly ionised or non-ionised forms of the drug can exist depending on the prevailing hydrogen ion concentration. It has often been assumed that non-ionised substances in the glomerular filtrate are invariably able to diffuse out of the renal tubular lumen and so account for pH dependent renal excretion. This cannot be the whole explanation since propranolol and practolol have very similar pK_a values (i.e. similar tendency to ionise at different pH values), yet only propranolol shows pH dependent urinary excretion (Kaye, Robinson and Turner, 1973). It is likely that the high lipid solubility of propranolol as opposed to practolol might account for these differences, so that adequate lipid solubility

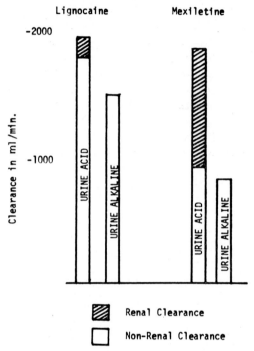

Figure 6.2   Influence of urine pH on the clearance of lignocaine and mexiletine

Table 6.3   Relevance of urinary pH to elimination of antiarrhythmic drugs

Urinary pH	Antiarrhythmic drug	Reference
Urinary excretion dependent on pH (enhanced in acid)	Mexiletine Quinidine	Kiddie et al, 1974 Gerhardt et al, 1969[a]
Urinary excretion independent of pH	Procainamide Practolol Atenolol Disopyramide Acebutolol	Bellet, 1971 Kaye et al, 1973 Kaye, 1974 Kaye, 1975 Kaye, 1975
Unimportant pH-dependent urinary excretion—as drug largely eliminated by metabolism	Lignocaine Propranolol Phenytoin Quinidine	Kiddie, 1975 Kaye et al, 1973 Woodbury and Swinyard, 1972 Kessler, 1974

[a] Applies to metabolites as based on the use of a non-specific assay.

and appropriate pK_a values both appear to be prerequisites for pH dependent urinary elimination.

Kiddie (1975) has shown that it is important to consider pH dependent excretion in relation to the total extent of renal and non-renal drug elimination. During conditions of optimal urinary excretion for lignocaine (i.e. urine acid), urinary clearance accounts for less than 10 per cent of its total clearance from plasma. Therefore, even though renal elimination of the drug virtually ceases when urine becomes alkaline (since lignocaine is highly lipid soluble and has a pK_a value of 7.9), only a slight reduction in total clearance occurs. In contrast with mexiletine (a recently introduced antiarrhythmic drug), renal clearance accounts for about 50 per cent of its total clearance when acid urine is being produced, but when urine becomes alkaline and its renal clearance is virtually abolished, a marked influence on total elimination becomes evident (Fig. 6.2).

The relevance of urinary pH to the elimination of some of the commonly used antiarrhythmic drugs has been summarised in Table 6.3.

Pharmacodynamics

Pharmacodynamics is the interpretation of response to a drug in terms of its pharmacokinetics. Relevant pharmacokinetic data typically consist of plasma (or serum or blood) concentrations, and the implication is that measurement of these drug levels may be more predictive of effect than drug dosage. Clearly, if simple plasma-level/effect relationships can be shown to exist, then titrating the dose to obtain a given plasma level would help reduce the variation in predicted response. The marketed preparations of several antiarrhythmic drugs consist of racemic mixtures, and in many instances only one stereo-isomeric form has appreciable therapeutic activity, which means that half the administered drug may have no clinical value though it could still contribute to side effects and toxicity and hence reduce the margin between safe and toxic drug doses.

Although pharmacokinetics are accessible to direct and relatively simple chemical analysis, for several reasons the relationships of plasma drug concentrations to antiarrhythmic and toxic effects are very difficult to verify.

1. The proper parameters of therapeutic effect and toxicity are hard to decide and are often selected arbitrarily, e.g. complete or partial abolition of arrhythmia, effects on the ECG such as QT prolongation.

2. Measurement of biological effect at any given time is imprecise; arrhythmias being subject to spontaneous changes independent of therapy.

3. Established tachyarrhythmias which are dangerous or distressing preclude the use of placebo where active drug or other forms of therapy are available. Therefore, the precise efficacy of these drugs can only be measured in prophylactic studies. Plasma levels needed for prophylaxis may differ from those needed for active treatment.

4. Prophylactic studies are formidable to organise since to attain satisfactory arrhythmia detection rates, continuous electrocardiographic monitoring is desirable together with appropriate ancillary back-up facilities.

5. The importance of drug distribution and drug metabolites have to be

considered, and hence after single doses there is frequently insufficient evidence to establish valid plasma-level/effect relationships.

6. Antiarrhythmic effect may be irreversible, as, for example, the termination of a reciprocal tachycardia. In that event, the tachycardia would not necessarily reappear when the plasma level of the drug falls away. Therefore, to obtain valuable information, the nature of the arrhythmia and the way in which it is conventionally described should be accurately known, and it may be necessary to study a large number of arrhythmias.

7. Concentration/effect relationships as measured may not be linear, and with increasing plasma levels of some drugs, effect might increase to an optimal level and then decrease.

For these reasons it should be realised that evidence on which concentration/effect or concentration/toxicity relationships is based may be weak. What can be approximately defined are the plasma drug concentrations on regular maintenance therapy which are usually associated with successful treatment or toxicity in a particular group of patients and using a given method of drug assay. In many instances active or inactive drug metabolites are also present in the plasma and may or may not be measured by the assay. These sometimes depend on the route and duration of drug administration (Coltart and Shard, 1970; Cleveland and Shard, 1972). When assays are highly specific, any particular patients who metabolise drugs differently from the general population may have different 'drug concentration/effect relationships'. Individual variations in these relationships may also be considerable. Plasma protein binding can change both as a result of disease states and after administration of other drugs, so that once again drug concentration/effect relationships might differ. With some drugs, the relationship between their plasma concentrations as measured and the extent of any given type of cardiac action does not invariably remain the same. For example, after single oral doses of practolol, cardiac β-adrenergic blocking activity associated with a given plasma level of drug seems to increase over a few hours after administration of a single oral dose (Kumana and Kaye, 1974). Similarly, it has been shown that using some assays to measure quinidine, the cardiac effects of single doses of the drug may not correlate directly with serum levels obtained (Edwards, Hancock and Saynor, 1974). Whether due to the drug taking time to reach receptors, to formation of active metabolites not measured with the parent drug, formation of inactive metabolites not distinguished by the drug assay or to any other reason, the presence of changing relationships adds to imprecision.

It follows that too much reliance must not be placed on plasma level estimations in the face of contrary clinical evidence. Despite all these problems pharmacodynamics have been very useful in devising satisfactory dosage schedules quite apart from any usefulness they may have in helping to prescribe appropriate doses of therapeutic agents for individual patients.

INDIVIDUAL DRUGS

Quinidine, Procainamide and Lignocaine (General Remarks)

These agents are the standard drugs used in the treatment of ventricular premature beats and ventricular tachycardias, and they also have some beneficial influence on supraventricular tachycardias. Their pharmacological properties, clinical characteristics and their pharmacokinetics have been reviewed by Bigger (1972), Jewitt (1975) and Kessler (1974). These drugs have a number of properties in common which may help to explain their antiarrhythmic activity as well as some of their side effects and toxicity. They may be listed as follows:

1. *Negative chronotropism* (reduction of cardiac automaticity). This probably occurs by virtue of reducing the rate of phase 4 depolarisation, thus depressing ectopic pacemaker tissue. This action may predispose to bradycardia and asystole.

2. *Negative inotropism* (decreased force of contraction of cardiac muscle). This may predispose to heart failure.

3. *Decreased conduction in excitable tissues.* This results in prolongation of effective refractory periods and hence may interfere with the propagation of re-entry tachycardias and rapidly discharging ectopic pacemaker activity. Compatible with this action, these drugs are local anaesthetics and sometimes give rise to disorders of cardiac conduction. (Lignocaine has very little effect on this kind on the heart.)

4. *Positive chronotropism.* Paradoxically, these drugs may predispose towards the development of tachycardias (sinus tachycardia, supraventricular and ventricular tachycardias and ventricular fibrillation). This may be due to their having atropine-like properties resulting in the blockade of efferent vagal nerve endings and/or their ability to sensitise tissues to catecholamines by interfering with the reuptake of these amines into stores. In addition, re-entry tachycardia may be facilitated (see p. 139).

In the doses used conventionally, quinidine manifests these properties more than procainamide and lignocaine manifests them least of all. It is therefore not surprising that amongst these three drugs quinidine is regarded as the most effective and the most dangerous; whilst lignocaine is regarded as the safest and produces the least degree of prolongation in the various electrocardiographic intervals (e.g. QRS and QT). However, the comparative superiority of any one of these drugs must be open to some doubt since they cannot be strictly compared under all circumstances. In at least one double blind study conducted on patients with healed myocardial infarction, quinidine was no more effective than procainamide in treating premature ventricular beats (van Durme, Bogaert and Rosseel, 1974). It is of interest that quinidine and procainamide also have vasodilator properties, though lignocaine vasoconstricts; a fact which is evident from the blanching of skin round intra-dermal injections of lignocaine compared to erythema surrounding similar injections of procaine. Thus, lignocaine in itself rarely gives rise to hypo-tension, whilst hypotension is common after procainamide given intra-venously, and quinidine even when it is given by mouth. Apart from these pharmacological characteristics, a number of other features unique to each, govern the choice of drug in any particular clinical situation.

Lignocaine (Xylocaine, Lidocaine)

This highly lipid soluble local anaesthetic is generally used intravenously to treat acute ventricular tachyarrhythmias, especially those occurring after myocardial infarction or cardiac surgery. It may also be given to prevent the recurrence of ventricular fibrillation after electroversion (d.c. shock).

It is administered intravenously as a slow bolus injection (100 mg) repeated if necessary, and concurrently an intravenous infusion (1–2 mg/min) is usually commenced. The plasma level declines after the bolus injection and rises again to plateau in about 6 h as the drug accumulates from the infusion (Fig. 6.3). Recurrence of ventricular arrhythmias in the intervening period, corresponding to the saddle-shaped fall in plasma lignocaine, can be appro-priately treated with a further bolus (Bassan, Weinstein and Mandel, 1974). If the arrhythmia continues to be troublesome, the dose of lignocaine in the infusion can be increased after additional bolus doses to 3, 4 or more milligrams per minute till control is achieved, or till signs of toxicity appear, in which case another agent should be tried.

Plasma level determinations have little practical application in routine management since results do not become available for several hours after sampling, allowing time for levels to change drastically, and urgent clinical features have immediate and overriding importance. The drug is largely eliminated by hepatic metabolism and it has a half life of about $1\frac{1}{2}$ h (Boyes et al, 1971). In heart failure and cardiogenic shock, when hepatic blood flow is likely to be reduced, the drug may accumulate and a reduction in dosage may become necessary. Furthermore, as the time to reach steady state plasma levels is a function of half life, it may take several hours longer than normal for plateau concentrations to occur if the loading dose is omitted.

Lignocaine has the advantage over quinidine and procainamide in that it is a safe drug with little or no proven cardiovascular toxicity, even though it is administered intravenously (Harrison, Sprouse and Morrow, 1963; Schumacher et al, 1968). In addition, it is eliminated rapidly, and as it is administered intravenously, it enables rapid adjustment of therapy as and when required. On the other hand, a very substantial first pass effect (Boyes et al, 1971) and its very rapid elimination make it unsuitable for oral therapy. Overdosage with lignocaine (Åstrom, 1971) manifests as CNS toxicity (lightheadedness, confusion, twitching, paraesthesiae in the mouth and extremities, fits, respiratory arrest). The occurrence of fits can be treated with intravenous diazepam, but this leads to hypotension and therefore it is advisable to reduce the dose of lignocaine or continue treatment with an alternative agent whenever CNS signs appear.

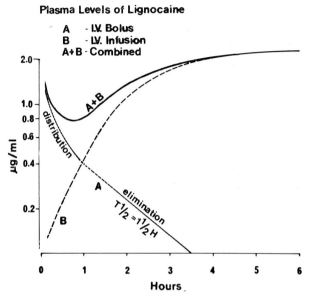

Plasma Levels of Lignocaine

A   - I.V. Bolus
B   - I.V. Infusion
A+B - Combined

Figure 6.3 Diagrammatic illustration of plasma lignocaine levels occurring after an i.v. bolus injection (A) during an i.v. infusion (B) and when both are administered concurrently (A+B). Patients frequently experience lightheadedness, deafness and oral parathesiae during or soon after a single i.v. bolus, and at the same time their ventricular tachyarrhythmias often subside. However, over the next 10 to 30 min, as the plasma lignocaine level begins to fall off sharply (coincident with drug distribution throughout the body), arrhythmias often recur and the central nervous symptoms abate. Such observations are in keeping with the notion that lignocaine rapidly enters the brain and heart (being well-perfused tissues with a relatively high affinity for the drug), and that some of it subsequently leaves these tissues to become redistributed (Benowitz, 1974). It follows that i.v. bolus injections should not be given very rapidly lest they give rise to fits

Procainamide (Pronestyl)

Like lignocaine, procaine is metabolised rapidly and enters the central nervous system to cause toxicity, but differs from it in being a vasodilator drug. On the other hand, procainamide (PCA) which is the amide analogue of procaine has similar properties to procaine, but is not eliminated so rapidly and does not give rise to CNS toxicity to any extent (Mark et al, 1951).

PCA is usually administered orally (loading dose 1 g followed by 375 mg 3-hourly or 500 mg 4-hourly), suitable adjustments being made for extremes of body weight and variations in plasma levels (Koch-Weser and Klein, 1971; Shaw et al, 1974). Treatment is rarely continued for more than two to four weeks. Intravenous PCA (repeated 100 mg boluses every 5 min) is only rarely resorted to for the treatment of ventricular tachyarrhythmias, as by this route sensitive individuals are liable to develop hypotension particularly after repeated doses (Harrison et al, 1963; Kayden et al, 1951; Giardina, Heisenbuttel and Bigger, 1973). For this reason, PCA is usually given orally even when it is used in acute situations. In coronary care unit patients with acute myocardial infarction Koch-Weser et al (1969) found oral PCA was superior to placebo in the prevention of ventricular arrhythmias. Oral PCA may also be used when it is considered desirable to continue antiarrhythmic treatment in the weeks after patients leave the coronary care unit when they are being mobilised and no longer have intravenous drips.

PCA is well absorbed from the gut, peak plasma levels occurring about 1 h after an oral dose, and it has an elimination half life of about $3\frac{1}{2}$ h (Koch-Weser, 1971b; Shaw et al, 1974). About 60 per cent is excreted unchanged in urine, and it is likely that the remainder is largely metabolised at least partly to an active metabolite, N-acetylprocainamide (Kessler, 1976). Contrary to earlier assertions based on animal work (Weily and Genton, 1972), studies in human volunteers show that its excretion in urine is independent of urinary pH (Meyer, Kaye and Turner, 1974). The elimination of PCA is impaired in renal failure (Koch-Weser, 1971a; Weily and Genton, 1972). In heart failure, PCA absorption may be delayed or incomplete (Shaw et al, 1974) but toxic levels may still occur since heart failure leads to renal insufficiency and increased procainamide retention as well as to a decreased apparent volume of distribution of the drug (Koch-Weser, 1971a). Under such circumstances, measurement of plasma levels may be very useful.

PCA has the advantage over lignocaine in that it has fairly good systemic availability when given by mouth and that it does not produce central nervous system toxicity to any extent. Nevertheless, there are a number of disadvantages and special problems associated with its use. These include gastrointestinal intolerance, skin rashes, and the risk of hypotension, particularly when the drug is given by intravenous injection. The above-mentioned shortcomings are not encountered commonly and are relatively unimportant compared to two other unique disadvantages which are major obstacles to maintenance therapy with the drug.

To ensure that plasma levels always remained within the proposed therapeutic range of 4 to 8 μg/ml (Fig. 6.4), it has been found necessary to administer the conventional PCA tablets every 3 to 4 h (Koch-Weser and Klein, 1971; Shaw et al, 1974). Administration of the same daily dose by means of larger less frequent aliquots allows plasma levels to become ineffective near the end of each dosing interval. On the other hand, using the same reduced dosing frequency, low levels could be avoided by using larger individual doses (i.e. increasing the total daily dose), but then levels would become toxic soon after each dose. This frequent dosing is a major inconvenience since it disturbs sleep in patients who are supposed to be resting, doses can be accidentally omitted in busy medical wards, and the regime is not suitable for use outside hospital. It may be feasible, however, to avoid frequent dosing by using sustained release PCA preparations provided their kinetics are well understood (Fremstad et al, 1973), since by prolonging the time over which each dose would be absorbed, larger individual doses could be given without plasma drug concentrations becoming ineffective (Fig. 6.5). The validity of a well-defined range of therapeutic plasma levels for all situations may however be open to some doubt since individual differences may be critical, and also in some circumstances the beginning of the 'therapeutic' range may well be lower than that defined above (van Durme et al, 1974).

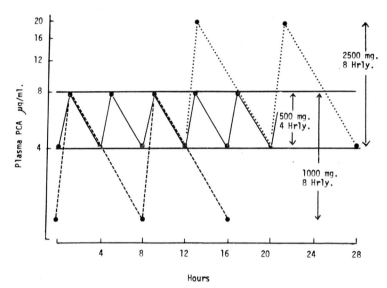

Figure 6.4 Procainamide dosage schedules. The horizontal lines define the 'therapeutic range' of plasma concentrations. Hypothetical plasma levels for a patient taking 500 mg of PCA every 4 h are represented by the continuous line. The same daily dose administered at less frequent intervals (1000 mg 8-hourly) results in levels becoming excessively low near the end of each dosing interval (– – –). Using 8-hourly administration, these low levels could be avoided by increasing each dose, but then levels become toxic soon after dosing (......)

A further major problem associated with the long-term use of PCA is the development of a syndrome clinically and serologically akin to systemic lupus erythematosus. After treatment with PCA for one year, virtually all patients develop a rise in antinuclear antibody titre, and more than 10 per cent are liable to develop symptoms (Kosowsky et al, 1973). The clinical features associated with this syndrome include joint pains, pyrexia, myalgia, weight loss, fatigue, headaches, rashes, pleuropulmonic involvement, pericarditis and various other abnormalities (Blomgren, Condemi and Vaughan, 1972). Patients developing the frank illness manifest earlier and higher rises of anti-nuclear factor. This syndrome differs from classical systemic lupus erythematosus in that the characteristic renal involvement (wire loop lesion of the glomerulus) does not occur and therefore prognosis tends to be much better and all its manifestations are substantially reversible once administration of the drug is stopped. Furthermore, the syndrome has no special predisposition for females, and the predominant antinuclear factor is usually not an anti-DNA antibody as in classical systemic lupus erythematosus (Hughes, Cohen and Christian, 1971). Haptene formation is likely to play a part in this syn-

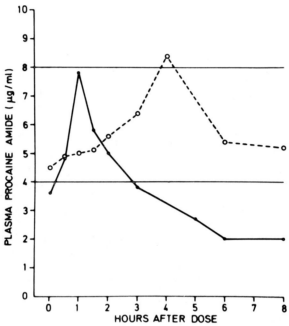

Figure 6.5 Unpublished data from the study of Shaw et al (1975), on a hospital inpatient who was treated with conventional procainamide (Pronestyl 500 mg 4-hourly) for one week and subsequently treated with a sustained release formulation (Cardiorytmin Retard 1200 mg 8-hourly for one week). The figure shows the plasma levels obtained in the 8 h after the final dose of each formulation and shows that they only remain in the therapeutic range during the first 4 h or so after Pronestyl (——), but remain more or less in the therapeutic range throughout the 7 h after the sustained release formulation (– – –), thus indicating the feasibility of using sustained release procainamide

drome. As it occurs with such a high frequency the use of PCA on a long-term basis has largely been abandoned.

Quinidine

The dextroisomer of quinine has been the prototype of anti-arrhythmic drugs. Though originally given to treat atrial arrhythmias, the doses required were usually so high that its use in this respect has been superseded by other safer drugs and by electroversion. However, it still has a place in the management of ventricular tachyarrhythmias, particularly when other drugs have not been successful and when prolonged treatment is deemed necessary. It may also have some use in preventing the recurrence of atrial arrhythmias after d.c. shock. As a rule, the drug is given only by mouth since the risks of side effects and toxicity become unacceptable with parenteral administration. When conventional quinidine is being used, it is safest to give a test dose (125 mg) lest patients are excessively sensitive to the drug, and provided no gastrointestinal intolerance, hypotension or arrhythmia occur, regular main-tenance treatment (400 mg 8-hourly or 6-hourly) may be commenced. Sus-tained release preparations (e.g. Kinidin durules) smooth out the normal absorption peaks and are less liable to produce gastrointestinal or cardio-vascular complications (Cramer, Varanuskas and Werkö, 1964), and they have therefore gained acceptance for routine use. They also have the advantage that use of a test dose before starting treatment is less important, and that they need only be administered twice or thrice daily.

Quinidine pharmacokinetics have been well reviewed by Kessler (1974) and by Regardh (1973). The drug appears to be well absorbed and has a half life of about 6 to 8 h. In plasma, it is about 85 per cent bound to protein, and it is usually presumed that the remaining unbound fraction correlates better with therapeutic effect and toxicity than the total plasma level. It is of interest that protein binding of quinidine in plasma is reduced in cirrhosis and other hypoalbuminaemic states, but is normal in cardiac and renal failure. Up to about one-seventh of any oral dose may appear as unchanged drug in urine; the remainder being metabolised to more water-soluble but less active metabolites. The plasma levels encountered depend on the specificity of the assay method used. Using fairly specific assays, therapeutic concentrations range from 2.5 to 5 $\mu g/ml$, the range being higher with less specific assays which also measure metabolites. When specific assays are being used, quinidine elimination is found to be unaffected in the presence of cardiac or renal failure. The small fraction of unchanged quinidine in urine virtually dis-appears when the urine becomes alkaline.

Though regarded as more effective than PCA and lignocaine, controlled studies to substantiate this claim are lacking. At least one double-blind trial in patients convalescing from myocardial infarction found quinidine not to be superior to PCA (van Durme et al, 1974). In contrast to both lignocaine and PCA, quinidine is not eliminated very rapidly, and unlike lignocaine, its systemic availability is reasonable when it is given by mouth, and therefore of the three drugs, it is the most suitable for oral administration. Unlike PCA, prolonged treatment is not associated with a high incidence of any special complication such as systemic lupus erythematosus.

Despite these advantages, it has a high incidence of mild and serious undesirable effects (Cramer, 1968; Bigger, 1972; Lindsay, 1973), which limit its use very considerably. Adverse effects include thrombocytopenia, fever, skin rashes and cinchonism (tinnitus, deafness, vertigo, vomiting and various types of visual impairment), all of which are rare. On the other hand, gastro-intestinal disturbance is common and affects up to 30 per cent of all patients. The cardiovascular toxicity of quinidine gives much more cause for concern. Apart from a tendency occasionally to produce hypotension or cardiac failure, it may itself be responsible for cardiac arrhythmias (various AV blocks, bundle branch blocks and intraventricular blocks, sinus tachycardia, ventricular and supraventricular tachycardias, ventricular fibrillation and asystole). Syncopal spells and sudden deaths are reported to occur in patients taking relatively small doses to prevent the recurrence of atrial arrhythmias after electrical cardioversion. These manifestations have been presumed to be due to tachycardias, asystole or ventricular fibrillation, and may have arisen

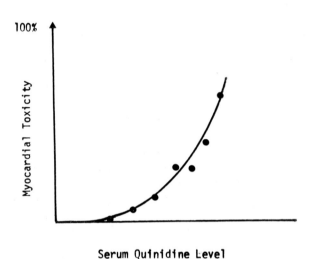

Figure 6.6   Relationship of myocardial toxicity to serum levels of quinidine. By myocardial toxicity is meant the development of cardiac signs requiring cessation of therapy. (Modified from Sokolow and Ball (1956) and presented by permission of the American Heart Association)

directly from taking the drug. It now seems that quinidine treatment after d.c. countershock may only have a marginal influence in preventing the recurrence of atrial fibrillation, and there is real doubt whether anything is to be gained from using it for such a purpose (Lindsay, 1973).

It remains a matter of speculation why patients on quinidine who are apparently well should develop these complications so abruptly. A clue may be provided by the relationship of myocardial toxicity to serum levels (Fig. 6.6). At high normal serum levels, small incremental increases may produce a great increase in toxicity. Spontaneous variation of urine pH to alkaline might result in slight accumulation of quinidine and perhaps considerable accumulation of potentially toxic metabolites. If the metabolic elimination of quinidine is subject to a degree of saturation kinetics at high serum levels, the rise in serum level occurring when urine was alkaline might become compounded. A combination of these factors could produce acute quinidine toxicity. It may therefore be worthwhile checking that the plasma or serum levels of quinidine in patients on regular therapy remain below the toxic range.

Physicians and anaesthetists should also be aware that quinidine has neuromuscular blocking properties which may at least partly explain the weakness complained of by some patients who are taking the drug. More important, however, is the recognition that potentiation of depolarising and non-depolarising muscle relaxants may occur (Schmidt, Vick and Sedore, 1965), so that in the presence of quinidine, the need for additional post-operative respiratory support should be anticipated (Way, Katzung and Larson, 1967).

Phenytoin (Epanutin, Dilantin)

In 1950, this anticonvulsant was shown to have antiarrhythmic activity in the presence of experimental myocardial infarction (Harris and Kokernot, 1950). It is now generally used intravenously when lignocaine has been unsuccessful in the treatment of a ventricular tachyarrhythmia, and it is especially indicated in digitalis-induced tachycardias.

When being administered intravenously, the conventional preparation must be made up freshly in its appropriate diluent (40 per cent propylene glycol and 10 per cent ethanol in water, pH 12). Doses of 50 to 250 mg may be administered slowly over 5 to 10 min, ensuring that the needle tip is free in the lumen of the vein. A ready mixed parenteral preparation made by Parke-Davis is now available. Lest precipitation occurs, phenytoin prepared for intravenous use should not be added to other intravenous solutions.

Due to its complicated pharmacokinetics (discussed later), the prescribing of phenytoin requires special care. When the drug is not previously present in a patient's body, regular continuous administration (whether by i.v. infusion or by mouth) takes time to achieve therapeutic steady state concentrations and become effective. Once effective, however, small increases in dosage can give rise to very high concentrations and toxicity. It is therefore especially important to use relatively large loading doses on commencing therapy and continue treatment on small maintenance doses. Thus, 250 mg of the drug may be given intravenously over the first 10 min and subsequently a slow infusion of phenytoin may be continued. Phenytoin infusions containing 750 mg of the drug in 450 ml of saline are marketed in West Germany under the name of 'Phenhydan'. On oral maintenance treatment of 400 mg of phenytoin daily, Bigger, Schmidt and Kutt (1968) found that adequate plasma levels were only reached after about one week. However, by giving doses of about 1 g on the first day, then 500 to 600 mg on day two and subsequently 400 mg daily, adequate plasma levels and effectiveness could reasonably be expected to ensue from 24 h.

When prescribing phenytoin, physicians should be guided by clinical evidence of effectiveness and toxicity rather than by its serum levels. Nevertheless, an understanding of its pharmacokinetics can be of great help when doses need to be adjusted. The fact that the drug obeys saturation (not first order) kinetics has important consequences with respect to prescribing of the drug. If the elimination of phenytoin were expressed in absolute terms, with increasing doses (and increasing serum concentrations), the rate of elimination would increase to a maximum and no further. This means that elimination rate expressed as a function of the serum concentration would be high at low concentrations and vice versa. For this reason, determination of phenytoin half life in the accepted sense is not possible. However, in epileptics receiving long-term maintenance therapy with phenytoin, Houghton and Richens (1974a) have shown that the half life of radioactively labelled phenytoin increases with increasing serum concentrations of the drug. Furthermore, with saturation kinetics, one would predict that when serum concentrations are low (low maintenance doses), a given incremental increase in daily dose should produce only small increases in serum level, as the eliminating enzymes can cope with additional drug. Whereas when serum concentrations are high (high maintenance doses) and the metabolising enzymes virtually saturated, the same incremental dosage increase should produce sharp rises in serum level which may reach well into the toxic range. This expected pattern of serum phenytoin levels in association with different maintenance doses has actually been confirmed in individual patients (Fig. 6.7), and is the basis for current prescribing habits.

Phenytoin is highly protein bound and lipid soluble, and is largely metabolised in the liver by parahydroxylation and then glucuronidation and excreted in the urine conjugated to glucuronic acid. It is also likely that therapeutic effect correlates best with the unbound phenytoin concentration. Because of these properties, it displays important interactions with other drugs, and its handling may also be altered in diseased states. These interactions may be listed as follows:

1. Decrease in drug bound to plasma protein
   e.g.—aspirin, phenylbutazone, sulphafurazole
   —low plasma albumen, uraemia
2. Elimination enhanced (presumably due to liver enzyme induction)
   e.g.—phenobarbitone, carbamazepine
   —renal failure
3. Elimination inhibited (presumably liver enzyme activity reduced)
   e.g.—INAH, dicoumarol, chloramphenicol, sulthiame
   —liver disease such as hepatitis, cirrhosis, halothane anaesthesia.

The influence of benzodiazepines on liver enzymes is very small, and self-induction by phenytoin is also unlikely to be important in view of its saturation kinetics. Pheneturide (a second-line antiepileptic drug) which is sometimes administered to patients already on phenytoin appears to be one of the most powerful known inducing agents of liver enzymes (Latham et al, 1973), and yet for some reason, it actually inhibits phenytoin elimination (Houghton and Richens, 1976b). Such paradoxes underline the complexity of phenytoin metabolism and emphasise the difficulties of anticipating serum levels. Genetic factors also appear to affect the rate of phenytoin metabolism, and some racial groups have a high incidence of relatively slow metabolisers. The subject of phenytoin handling has been reviewed by Kessler (1974).

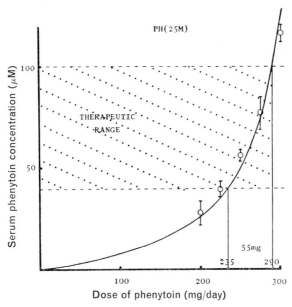

Figure 6.7 Serum phenytoin concentration in a 25-year-old male epileptic patient receiving phenytoin at several different daily doses. Each point represents the mean±s.d. of three to eight separate estimations on a given dose. The curve drawn through the points was fitted to the Michaelis–Menten equation by computer. The horizontal dotted lines represent the upper and lower limits of the therapeutic range of the laboratory. From the computer plot, it can be seen that a dose of 235 mg daily would produce a serum concentration at the lower limit of the therapeutic range in this patient, while a dose of 290 mg would be required to produce a level at the upper limit. The enzyme metabolising phenytoin would be totally saturated at 344 mg daily. (Modified from Richens (1974) and reproduced with his permission)

As a result of animal work (Sasyniuk and Ogilvie, 1975), it is thought that phenytoin decreases cardiac automaticity, and this property might explain its mode of action in digitalis induced tachyarrhythmias. The drug has been effective in the treatment of ventricular premature beats and ventricular tachycardias due to a wide variety of causes, whether or not patients were receiving digitalis, and it has also been effective against digitalis induced supraventricular tachycardias (Bigger et al, 1968; Eddy and Singh, 1969; Rosen, Lisak and Rubin, 1967). As a result of intravenous studies (Bigger et al, 1968) it has been found that control of ventricular tachyarrhythmias is usually achieved when plasma levels range from 10 to 18 μg/ml, there being a critical effective level for most patients. However, even in the presence of 'adequate' dosing and 'adequate' plasma levels, one group found it to be of no value in suppressing ventricular tachyarrhythmias occurring from 3 days to 15 months after cardiac infarction (Stone, Klein and Lown, 1971). Toxicity (nystagmus, ataxia and vertigo, drowsiness, dysarthria, nausea and rarely vomiting) becomes common when plasma levels exceed 20 μg/ml, though some patients show signs of intoxication at lower levels. Individual patients, however, may need higher levels, and may be able to tolerate them. Relatively slight and short-lived myocardial depression (left ventricular dp/dt falling and end diastolic pressure rising) without hypotension, has been noted to occur in patients with heart disease, given intravenous boluses of the drug at cardiac catheterisation (Lieberson et al, 1967). Electrophysiological studies (Sasyniuk and Ogilvie, 1975) suggest that low phenytoin concentrations may actually increase the rate of phase 0 depolarisation and hence conduction velocity and membrane responsiveness, especially in the presence of low extracellular potassium concentrations, cardiac glycosides, hypoxia and other forms of stress. This may account for the reported improvement of AV conduction occurring in digitalised and non-digitalised patients, even though in atrial fibrillation and flutter, ventricular rates usually fall (Helfant et al, 1967). For these reasons, it should be realised that theoretical hazards involved in using phenytoin for digitalis toxicity include:

(a) Reduction in rhythmicity before improvement in AV conduction leading to very slow heart rates.

(b) Improvement in AV conduction in the presence of PAT 'with block' before reduction in automaticity, thus resulting in 1:1 conduction.

Verapamil (Cordilox, Isoptin)

Originally introduced for the treatment of angina, verapamil has been shown to have useful antiarrhythmic properties. It may be administered intravenously (5–10 mg) or orally (40–160 mg 6-hourly), though experience in the management of arrhythmias using the latter route has not been well documented. Its pharmacokinetics in man need elucidation, but there is evidence that active metabolites similar to those occurring in dogs may be formed (McIlhenny, 1971).

It has proved effective in slowing the ventricular rate in atrial fibrillation and atrial flutter even in digitalised patients (Bender et al, 1966; Shamroth, Krikler and Garrett, 1972). Conversion of atrial flutter to sinus rhythm occurs occasionally (Shamroth et al, 1972), furthermore AV junctional tachycardias and paroxysmal supraventricular tachycardias associated with WPW syndrome also respond favourably (Bender et al, 1966; Shamroth et al, 1972). The drug appears to have been successful where the tachycardias had been resistant to other drugs and even d.c. shock (Oram et al, 1971). By virtue of slowing conduction and increasing refractoriness in the normal AV junctional pathway (Roy, Spurrell and Sowton, 1974), it is likely that the drug can suppress reciprocal tachycardias involving this pathway, including those associated with WPW syndrome. On the other hand, there seems to be no consistent effect on refractoriness and only minimal effects on conduction in the anomalous pathway in WPW syndrome (Spurrell, Krikler and Sowton, 1974), and hence, in most of these patients, there is no untoward risk of increasing the ventricular rate and precipitating ventricular fibrillation should AF or atrial flutter develop. After verapamil, sinus tachycardia may be slowed, from which it may be inferred that it affects the SA node (Shamroth et al, 1972). The drug is no longer regarded as having β-blocking or quinidine-like actions.

Hypotension and aggravation of cardiac failure have not been a problem following the usual recommended doses (Bender et al, 1966; Shamroth et al, 1972). However, there is a very real risk of precipitating asystole, bradycardia or hypotension when the drug is used in combination with β-blocking drugs, particularly when the latter have been administered prior to verapamil (Krikler, 1974b), and lest it leads to severe bradycardia, it should be administered cautiously in patients with the bradycardia–tachycardia syndrome (Krikler, 1974b).

Disopyramide (Rythmodan, Norpace)

Though recently introduced into the UK and North America, this drug with wide ranging antiarrhythmic activity has been in use in France for several years (Desruelles et al, 1967; Granier, 1968). It is currently made in capsule form (dose 100 mg every 8 h up to 200 mg every 6 h) and an i.v. preparation is also likely to become available. The drug has an elimination half life of about 5 to 7 h, and it is largely excreted in urine, about 25 per cent being metabolised when given by mouth or intravenously (Ranney et al, 1971).

Using recommended doses, its main advantages over drugs such as quinidine are its relative lack of side effects and its usefulness both in supraventricular and ventricular tachyarrhythmias. By increasing the effective refractory period of atria and ventricles, it is especially indicated in the suppression of atrial and ventricular extrasystoles and the termination of supraventricular and ventricular tachycardias due to reciprocal rhythms, and because it increases refractoriness in anomalous AV pathways, it may safely and usefully be administered to suppress tachycardias associated with Wolff–Parkinson–White syndrome (Spurrell et al, 1975). Several reports suggest that the drug may prove useful in treating tachyarrhythmias which have proved resistant to conventional drugs (Conway et al, 1973; Poletti et al, 1971), and there have been double-blind controlled trials indicating that it may have prophylactic value after cardiac infarction (Vismara, Mason and Amsterdam, 1974; Besterman et al, 1975).

Side effects appear to be few and relatively unimportant and include gastrointestinal disturbance (nausea, vomiting, diarrhoea and abdominal pain), mild anticholinergic effects (hesitancy and retention of urine, dry mouth, dry eyes, blurred vision and presumably a risk of precipitating glaucoma), hypotension and skin rashes (Roussel Laboratories Ltd, 1974). The drug has been described to give rise to prolongation of all the electro-cardiographic intervals particularly the P–R interval (Ranney et al, 1971), but bradycardia has only been reported to occur very occasionally (Besterman et al, 1975). In the doses usually administered, heart failure does not figure as an important complication despite adverse haemodynamic effects having been demonstrated at cardiac catheterisation (Befeler et al, 1973; Jensen, Sigurl and Uhrenholt, 1975).

Amiodarone

Though originally introduced as an antianginal agent by Belgian and French workers, this drug was soon recognised to have beneficial effects on a wide range of supraventricular and ventricular tachyarrhythmias (Schepdael and Solvay, 1970). It is reported to be highly effective in preventing and treating refractory tachyarrhythmias associated with Wolff–Parkinson–White syndrome (Rosenbaum et al, 1974). Since it is effective against reciprocal tachycardias associated with this syndrome it has been surmised that it may increase the refractoriness of the normal AV junction and specialised con-duction pathways. Presumably, a different mechanism is responsible for its action in preventing atrial fibrillation and the associated very rapid ventricular rates. The drug may take several days to become effective (usual oral dose 300–600 mg/day). Characteristically, the ECG shows QT prolongation and the appearance of U waves.

It may give rise to gastrointestinal disturbance, atropine resistant brady-cardias, as well as AV and intraventricular heart blocks, and therefore brady-cardia and bundle branch block constitute relative contraindications to its use. Two other unique complications probably related to dosage and duration of therapy are of great interest. Micro-deposits of pigment appear in the cornea and skin of some patients. The corneal deposits disappear on cessation of therapy, and when small, produce no important visual symptoms. It is claimed that the corneal deposits can be avoided without recurrence of ar-rhythmias by discontinuing the drug for about one week every one to two months. Nevertheless, regular slit lamp examination is advisable. Deposits in the skin are responsible for pseudocyanotic discoloration of exposed parts, which may be preceded by photosensitivity. These undesirable effects have been well discussed by Rosenbaum and collaborators (1974) and by Delage, Laggage and Huard (1975).

It is also of interest to speculate whether the actions of this iodinated drug (namely antianginal effect, bradycardia, prolongation of action potential duration and corrected QT interval) occur through inducing hypothyroidism. Clinically, however, hypothyroidism is not evident, T$_3$ resin uptake is normal as are T$_3$ and T$_4$ levels, though not surprisingly the PBI tends to be high (Prichard, Singh and Hurley, 1975).

Bretylium Tosylate

This compound, which was originally introduced as an adrenergic neurone blocking hypotensive, has been found to be effective against many ventricular tachyarrhythmias refractory to more conventional antiarrhythmic drugs (Bernstein and Koch-Weser, 1972), and is reported to be of use in treating patients with ventricular fibrillation resistant to multiple d.c. shocks before and after lignocaine administration (Holder et al, 1973).

Although tolerance to its antihypertensive effects is the rule, this does not seem to be the case with respect to its antiarrhythmic properties. However, its long-term use is accompanied by a very high incidence of persistent parotid pain and prolonged therapy is therefore unacceptable in the majority of cases. Hence, it is mainly used parenterally in treating acute arrhythmias (about 5 mg/kg, i.m. or i.v. every 6–8 h). So long as patients remain recumbent, its main side effect (namely hypotension) can be limited to some extent. Nausea and vomiting often occur after intravenous administration.

After intramuscular administration, suppression of premature ventricular beats occurs several hours after peak plasma concentrations of the drug, whilst its hypotensive effect also occurs somewhat earlier (Romhilt and Fowler, 1975). On the other hand, it seems that refractory ventricular fibrillation may respond within a few minutes, so that the drug may well act in several different ways. When adrenergic neurone blocking drugs are first introduced into the body they are thought to release catecholamines from tissue stores and then prevent their subsequent reaccumulation. This may explain why tachyarrhythmias may actually be aggravated when therapy is first initiated, and pretreatment with β-adrenergic blocking agents to circumvent this possibility has been recommended. Because of its side effects the use of bretylium is usually restricted to refractory situations.

Other Antiarrhythmic Drugs

Antiarrhythmic properties have been claimed for a large number of agents, many of which may have antianginal actions as well (e.g. β-adrenergic blockers, verapamil, amiodorone, prenylamine, perhexiline). Some of these claims remain to be substantiated in man. It has also been claimed that treatment with lipid lowering agents early after myocardial infarction reduces ventricular tachyarrhythmias (Rowe, Neilson and Oliver, 1975). Similarly, the tranquillising drugs (e.g. diazepam, chlordiazepoxide) may also have a beneficial influence against ventricular arrhythmias, and there are anecdotal reports of ventricular tachycardias promptly responding to intravenous doses of these drugs. As to how they may act and their exact clinical significance in arrhythmia management, little is known. Other less well-known and relatively recently introduced antiarrhythmic agents are discussed in the following section.

As already mentioned, *mexiletine* (a lignocaine analogue) has the advantage over lignocaine in that it is effective against ventricular tachyarrhythmias when given by mouth as well as intravenously (Talbot et al, 1973; Campbell et al, 1975), but it has inconstant pharmacokinetics depending on urinary pH (Kiddie et al, 1974). Dose-related toxic side effects include paraesthesiae and central nervous system symptoms as well as hypotension and various bradycardias and heart blocks. Just how much its clinical use will be tempered because of its pH-dependent urinary excretion and the practicality of controlling urine pH remains to be seen. In one double-blind trial involving patients recovering from cardiac infarction, mexiletine was as effective as procainamide (500 mg every 4 h) in suppressing ventricular rhythm disorders, and had the advantage of less frequent (8-hourly) dosing (Campbell et al, 1975).

Aprindine, a newly introduced local anaesthetic agent, appears to be promising, and compares favourably with procainamide and quinidine (van Durme, 1974). The drug may be given intravenously and orally. Overdosage may result in central nervous system side effects.

Ajmaline, a rauwolfia alkaloid given parenterally or by mouth is reported to be effective against a wide range of tachyarrhythmias (Blacow, 1973). It does not give rise to untoward haemodynamic disturbances, at least after single i.v. doses, but abnormalities of conduction have been noted to occur especially in digitalised patients (Saetre, Ahlmark and Ahlberg, 1974).

The antihistaminic drug, *antazoline*, whether administered i.v. or orally is effective against ventricular and supraventricular tachyarrhythmias, especially when induced by digitalis (Sotomayer, 1963; Dreifus, Rebbino and Watanabe, 1964; Bellet, 1971). Unlike quinidine or procainamide, hypotension is not a frequent complication even after intravenous use. Reported side effects include lightheadedness, drowsiness, gastrointestinal upset, involuntary movements, fits, peppermint taste in the mouth, and hot flushes. Heart blocks and cardiac failure constitute relative contraindications to its use.

Animal work (Schuster et al, 1973) indicates that the *dimethyl quaternary derivative of propranolol* has powerful, long-lasting antiarrhythmic properties despite being devoid of local anaesthetic and β-blocking activity. It has been shown to counteract or prevent ventricular tachyarrhythmias induced by digitalis, coronary occlusion and electrical stimulation, whilst appearing to have a higher margin of safety (with respect to myocardial depression) than propranolol. It is currently being investigated in man.

Of the drugs widely in use, it will be noted that none of them is ideally suited for long-term treatment of ventricular tachyarrhythmias. The less well-known and relatively recently introduced products must still be regarded as on trial, while a search for other promising agents still continues. In the event of a safer drug emerging, it is unrealistic to imagine it will be a panacea for all patients with ventricular arrhythmias. Whatever the outcome of further research, an element of controversy is bound to ensue. On the one hand, there will always be protagonists of prophylactic therapy, and opposing them will be those drawing attention to what has been termed a 'medical nemesis' (Illich, 1975).

REFERENCES

Alexander, C. S. & Nino, A. (1969) Cardiovascular complications in young persons taking psychotropic drugs. *American Heart Journal*, **78**, 757–769.

Alvarez-Mena, S. C. & Frank, M. J. (1973) Phenothiazine-induced T-wave abnormalities: effects of overnight fasting. *Journal of the American Medical Association*, **224**, 1730–1733.

Åstrom, A. (1971) General pharmacology and toxicology of lidocaine, in the treatment of ventricular arrhythmias. In *Proceedings of a Symposium held in Edinburgh in September, 1970*, ed. Scott, D. B. & Julian, D. G., pp. 128–140. Edinburgh and London: Livingstone.

Bassan, M. M., Weinstein, S. R. & Mandel, W. J. (1974) Use of Lidocaine by continuous infusion. *American Heart Journal*, **87**, 302–303.

Befeler, B., Castellanos, A., Wells, D. E., Vagueiro, C., Yeh, B. K. & Myerburg, R. J. (1973) Electrophysiological effects of disopyramide phosphate, a new anti-arrhythmic agent. *American Journal of Cardiology*, **31**, 119.

Bellet, S. (1971) Antihistaminic drugs. In *Clinical Disorders of the Heart Beat*, 3rd edn, pp. 1135–1137. Philadelphia: Lea and Febiger.

Bender, F., Kojima, N., Reploh, H. F. & Oelman, G. (1966) Ventricular tachycardia due to auricular fibrillation and auricular flutter, supraventricular tachycardia. *Medizinische Welt.* **20**, 1120–1123.

Benowitz, N. L. (1974) Clinical applications of the pharmacokinetics of lidocaine. In *Cardiovascular Drug Therapy*, ed. Melmon, K. L., pp. 81–82. Philadelphia: Davis.

Bernstein, J. G. & Koch-Weser, J. (1972) Effectiveness of bretylium tosylate against refractory ventricular arrhythmias. *Circulation*, **45**, 1024–1034.

Besterman, E. M. M., Jennings, G. L., Jones, M. B., Kidner, P. H., Model, D. G. & Turner, P. P. (1975) A double-blind study on the effect of oral disopyramide (Rythmodan) in the prophylaxis of arrhythmias following acute myocardial infarction. *British Journal of Clinical Pharmacology*, **2**, 186P.

Bigger, J. T. (1972) Arrhythmias and anti-arrhythmic drugs. In *Advances in Internal Medicine*, Vol. 18, pp. 251–281, ed. Stollerman, G. H. Chicago: Year Book Medical Publishers.

Bigger, J. T., Schmidt, D. H. & Kutt, H. (1968) Relationship between the plasma level of diphenylhydantoin sodium and its cardiac anti-arrhythmic effects. *Circulation*, **38**, 363–374.

Blacow, N. W. (1973) Ajmaline. *Martindale, The Extra Pharmacopeoia*, 26th edn, p. 1570. London: The Pharmaceutical Press.

Blomgren, S. E., Condemi, J. J. & Vaughan, J. H. (1972) Procainamide-induced lupus erythematosus. *American Journal of Medicine*, **52**, 338–348.

Boston Collaborative Drug Surveillance Program (1972) Adverse reactions to the tricyclic anti-depressant drugs. *Lancet*, **1**, 529–531.

Boyes, R. N., Scott, D. B., Jebson, P. J., Godman, M. J. & Julian, D. G. (1971) Pharmacokinetics of Lidocaine in man. *Clinical Pharmacology and Therapeutics*, **12**, 105–116.

British Medical Journal (1973) Significance of ectopic beats. **2**, 191–192.

British Medical Journal (1974) Surgery in Wolff–Parkinson–White syndrome. **4**, 547–548.

Campbell, N. P. S., Chaturvedi, N. C., Kelly, J. G., Strong, J. E., Shanks, R. G. & Partridge, J. F. (1973) Mexiletine (Kö-1173) in the management of ventricular dysrhythmias. *Lancet*, **2**, 404–407.

Campbell, R. W. F., Dolder, M. A., Prescott, L. F., Talbot, R. G., Murrary, A. & Julian, D. G. (1975) Comparison of procainamide and mexiletine in prevention of ventricular arrhythmias after acute myocardial infarction. *Lancet*, **1**, 1257–1259.

Church, G. & Biern, R. (1972) Prophylactic lidocaine in acute myocardial infarction. *Circulation*, **46**, Suppl. 2, 139.

Cleaveland, C. R. & Shand, D. G. (1972) Effect of route of administration on the relationship between beta-adrenergic blockade and plasma propranolol level. *Clinical Pharmacology and Therapeutics*, **13**, 181–185.

Coltart, D. J. & Meldrum, S. J. (1971) The effect of racemic propranolol, dextro-propranolol and racemic practolol on human and canine cardiac transmembrane action potential. (Beta blockade and cardiac action potential.) *Archives of Internal Pharmacodynamics and Therapeutics*, **192**, 188–197.

Coltart, D. J. & Shand, D. G. (1970) Plasma propranolol levels in the quantitative assessment of beta-adrenergic blockade in man. *British Medical Journal*, **3**, 731–734.

Conway, J. F., Bottomley, K., Wakeley, E. J. & Duff, R. S. (1973) Disopyramide in cardiac arrhythmias—an initial appraisal. *Journal of International Medical Research*, **1**, 105–114.

Cramer, G. (1968) Early and late results of conversion of atrial fibrillation with quinidine. *Acta medica scandinavica*, Suppl., 490–495+.

Cramer, G., Varanuskas, E. & Werko, L. (1964) A new form of administration for quinidine, durules. *Nordisk Medicin*, **71**, 130.

Darby, S., Bennett, M. A., Cruickshank, J. C. & Pentecost, B. C. (1972) Trial of combined intramuscular and intravenous lignocaine in prophylaxis of ventricular tachyarrhythmias. *Lancet*, **1**, 817–819.

Dargie, H. J., Boddy, K., Kennedy, A. C., King, P. C., Read, P. R. & Ward, D. M. (1974) Total body potassium in long-term frusemide therapy; is potassium supplementation necessary? *British Medical Journal*, **4**, 316–319.

Delage, C., Lagace, R. & Huard, J. (1975) Pseudocyanotic pigmentation of the skin induced by amiodarone: a light and electron microscopic study. *Canadian Medical Association Journal*, **112**, 1205–1208.

Desruelles, J., Gerard, A., Ducatillon, P. & Herbaux, A. (1967) Our first clinical trials on disopyramide (H. 3292) in cardiac rhythm troubles. *Therapie*, **22**, 937–944.

Dreifus, L. S., Rebbino, M. D. & Watanabe, Y. (1964) Newer agents in the treatment of cardiac arrhythmias. *Medical Clinics of North America*, **48**, 371–387.

Dreifus, L. S., Haiat, R., Watanabe, Y., Arriago, J. & Reitman, N. (1971) Ventricular fibrillation. A possible mechanism of sudden death in patients with Wolff–Parkinson–White syndrome. *Circulation*, **43**, 520–527.

van Durme, J. P., Bogaert, M. G. & Rosseel, M. T. (1974) Comparison of the therapeutic effectiveness of aprindine, procainamide and quinidine in chronic ventricular dysrhythmias. *British Journal of Clinical Pharmacology*, **1**, 461–466.

Durrer, D. & Roos, J. P. (1967) Epicardial excitation of the ventricle in a patient with Wolff–Parkinson–White syndrome (type B). *Circulation*, **35**, 15–21.

Eastwood, J. B., Curtis, J. R. & Smith, R. B. (1975) Pharmacodynamics of practolol in chronic renal failure. *British Medical Journal*, **4**, 320–323.

Eddy, J, D. & Singh, S. P. (1969) Treatment of cardiac arrhythmias with phenytoin. *British Medical Journal*, **4**, 270–273.

Edwards, I. R., Hancock, B. W. & Saynor, R. (1974) Correlation between plasma quinidine and cardiac effect. *British Journal of Clinical Pharmacology*, **1**, 455–459.

Elliot, J. S., Sharp, R. F. & Lewis, L. (1959) Urinary pH. *Journal of Urology*, **81**, 339–343.

Freeman, J. W. & Loughhead, M. G. (1973) Beta-blockade in the treatment of tricyclic antidepressant overdosage. *Medical Journal of Australia*, **1**, 1233–1235.

Fremstad, D., Dahl, S., Jacobsen, S., Lunde, P. K. M., Nadland, K., Marthense, A. A., Waaler, T. & Landmark, K. H. (1973) A new sustained-release tablet formulation of procainamide. *European Journal of Clinical Pharmacology*, **6**, 251–255.

Gerhardt, R. E., Knouss, R. F., Thyrum, P. T., Luchi, R. J. & Morris, J. (1969) Quinidine excretion in aciduria and alkaluria. *Annals of Internal Medicine*, **71**, 927–933.

Giardina, E. V., Heissenbuttel, R. H. & Bigger, J. T. (1973) Intermittent intravenous procaine amide to treat ventricular arrhythmias—correlation of plasma concentration with effect on arrhythmia, electrocardiogram and blood pressure. *Annals of Internal Medicine*, **78**, 183–193.

Giles, T. D. & Modlin, R. K. (1968) Death associated with ventricular arrhythmia and thioridazine hydrochloride. *Journal of the American Medical Association*, **205**, 108–110.

Granier, J. (1968) A new anti-arrhythmic, disopyramide. *Presse Medicale*, **76**, 1605–1606.

Harris, A. S. & Kokernot, R. H. (1950) Effects of diphenylhydantoin sodium upon ectopic ventricular tachycardia in acute myocardial infarction. *American Journal of Physiology*, **163**, 505–516.

Harrison, D. C., Sprouse, J. H. & Morrow, A. G. (1963) The anti-arrhythmic properties of lidocaine and procaine-amide. Clinical and physiological studies of their cardiovascular effects in man. *Circulation*, **28**, 486–491.

Helfant, R. H., Lau, S. H., Cohen, S. I. & Damato, A. N. (1967) Effects of diphenylhydantoin on atrioventricular conduction in man. *Circulation*, **36**, 686–691.

Holder, D. A., Sniderman, A. D., Fraser, D. G. & Fallen, E. L. (1975) Experience with bretylium tosylate by a mobile resuscitation team. *Circulation*, **51**, **52**, Suppl. 2.

Houghton, G. W. & Richens, A. (1974a) Rate of elimination of tracer doses of phenytoin at different steady state serum phenytoin concentrations in epileptic patients. *British Journal of Clinical Pharmacology*, **1**, 155–161.

Houghton, G. W. & Richens, A. (1974b) The effect of benzodiazepines and pheneturide on phenytoin metabolism in man. *British Journal of Clinical Pharmacology*, **1**, 344.

Hughes, G. R. V., Cohen, S. A. & Christian, C. L. (1971) Anti-DNA activity in systemic lupus erythematosus. *Annals of Rheumatic Diseases*, **30**, 259–264.

Huston, J. R. & Bell, G. E. (1966) The effect of thioridazine hydrochloride and chlorpromazine on the electrocardiogram. *Journal of the American Medical Association*, **198**, 16–20.

Illich, I. (1975) *Medical Nemesis*. London: Calder and Boyars.

Jensen, G., Sigurd, B. & Uhrenholt, A. (1975) Haemodynamic effects of intravenous disopyramide in heart failure. *European Journal of Clinical Pharmacology*, **8**, 167–173.

Jewitt, D. E. (1975) Anti-arrhythmic drugs and their mechanisms of action. In *Modern Trends in Cardiology*, ed. Oliver, M. F., Vol. 3, pp. 341–355. London and Boston: Butterworths.

Johnson, R. A., Hutter, A. M., Jr, Desanctis, R. W., Yurchak, P. M., Leinbach, R. C. & Harthorne, J. W. (1974) Chronic overdrive pacing in the control of refractory ventricular arrhythmias. *Annals of Internal Medicine*, **80**, 380–383.

Kayden, H. J., Steele, J. M., Mark, L. C. & Brodie, B. B. (1951) The use of procaine amide in cardiac arrhythmias. *Circulation*, **4**, 13–22.

Kaye, C. M. (1974) The influence of urine pH on the renal excretion of I.C.I. 66082 in man. *British Journal of Clinical Pharmacology*, **1**, 513–514.

Kaye, C. M. (1975) Personal communication.

Kaye, C. M., Robinson, D. G. & Turner, P. (1973) The influence of urine pH on the renal excretion of practolol and propranolol. *British Journal of Pharmacology*, **49**, 155.

Kelly, H. G., Fay, J. E. & Laverty, S. G. (1963) Thioridazine hydrochloride (Mellaril): its effect on the electrocardiogram and a report of two fatalities with electrocardiographic abnormalities. *Canadian Medical Association Journal*. **89**, 546–554.

Kessler, K. M. (1974) Individualisation of dosage of anti-arrhythmic drugs. *Medical Clinics of North America*, **58**, 1019–1026.

Kiddie, M. A. (1975) Studies on the absorption, distribution and elimination of some cardiac anti-dysrhythmic drugs in man (unpublished work).

Kiddie, M. A., Kaye, C. M., Turner, P. & Shaw, T. R. D. (1974) Influence of urinary pH on elimination of mexiletine. *British Journal of Clinical Pharmacology*, **1**, 229–232.

Koch-Weser, J. (1971a) Anti-arrhythmic prophylaxis in acute myocardial infarction. *New England Journal of Medicine*, **285**, 1024–1025.

Koch-Weser, J. (1971b) Pharmacokinetics of procainamide in man. *Annals of the New York Academy of Sciences*, **179**, 370–382.

Koch-Weser, J. & Klein, S. W. (1971) Procainamide dosage schedules, plasma concentrations and clinical effects. *Journal of the American Medical Association*, **215**, 1454–1460.

Koch-Weser, J., Klein, S. W., Foo-Canto, L. L., Kastor, J. A. & DeSanctis, R. W. (1969) Anti-arrhythmic prophylaxis with procainamide in acute myocardial infarction. *New England Journal of Medicine*, **281**, 1253–1260.

Kosowsky, B. D., Taylor, J., Lown, B. & Ritchie, R. F. (1973) Long-term use of procaine amide following acute myocardial infarction. *Circulation*, **47**, 1204–1210.

Kotler, M. N., Tabatznik, B., Mower, M. M. & Tominaga, S. (1973) Prognostic significance of ventricular ectopic beats with respect to sudden death in the late post-infarction period. *Circulation*, **47**, 959–966.

Krikler, D. M. (1974a) A fresh look at cardiac arrhythmias; therapy. *Lancet*, **1**, 1034–1037.

Krikler, D. (1974b) Verapamil in cardiology. *European Journal of Cardiology*, **2**(1), 3–10.

Kumana, C. R. & Kaye, C. M. (1974) An investigation of the relationship between beta-adrenoceptor blockade and plasma practolol concentration in man. *European Journal of Clinical Pharmacology*, **7**, 243–248.

Lancet (1975) Fluocarbon aerosol propellants. **1**, 1073–1074.

Lancet (1966) Sudden death and phenothiazines. **2**, 740.

Latham, A. N., Millbank, C., Richens, A. & Rowe, D. J. F. (1973) Liver enzyme induction by anti-convulsant drugs and its relationship to disturbed calcium and folic acid metabolism. *Journal of Clinical Pharmacology*, **13**, 337–342.

Lawrie, D. M., Higgins, M. R., Godman, M. J., Oliver, M. F., Julian, D. G. & Donald K. W. (1968) Ventricular fibrillation complicating acute myocardial infarction. *Lancet*, **2**, 523–528.

Lie, K. I., Wellens, H. J. & Durrer, D. (1974a) Characteristics and predictability of primary ventricular fibrillation. *European Journal of Cardiology*, **1**, 379–384.

Lie, K. I., Wellens, H. J., Van Capelle, F. J. & Durrer, D. (1974b) Lidocaine in the prevention of primary ventricular fibrillation. *New England Journal of Medicine*, **291**, 1324–1326.

Lieberson, A. D., Schumacher, R. R., Childress, R. H., Boyd, D. L. & Williams, J. F. (1967) Effect of diphenylhydantoin on left ventricular function in patients with heart disease. *Circulation*, **36**, 692–699.

Lindsay, J. (1973) Quinidine and countershock: a reappraisal. *American Heart Journal*, **85**, 141–143.

Lown, B., Fakhro, A. M., Hood, W. B. & Thorn, G. W. (1967) The coronary care unit: new perspectives and directions. *Journal of the American Medical Association*, **199**, 188–198.

Lown, B., Kosowsky, B. D. & Klein, M. D. (1969) Pathogenesis, prevention and treatment of arrhythmias in myocardial infarction. *Circulation*, **39, 40**, Suppl. IV, 261–270.

Mark, L. C., Kayden, J. J., Steele, J. M., Cooper, J. R., Berli, I., Rovenstine, E. A. & Brodie, B. B. (1951) The physiological disposition and cardiac effects of procaine amide. *Journal of Pharmacology and Experimental Therapeutics*, **102**, 5–15.

McIlhenny, H. M. (1971) Metabolism of ^{14}C verapamil. *Journal of Chemistry*, **14**, 1178–1184.

Meyer, W., Kaye, C. M. & Turner, P. (1974) A study of the influence of pH on the buccal absorption and renal excretion of procainamide. *European Journal of Clinical Pharmacology*, 287–289.

Moir, D. C., Cornwell, W. D., Dingwall-Fordyce, I., Crooks, J., O'Malley, K., Turnbull, M. J. & Weir, R. D. (1972) Cardiotoxicity of amitriptylene. *Lancet*, **2**, 561–564.

Moir, D. C., Dingwall-Fordyce, I. & Weir, R. D. (1973) Medicines evaluation and monitoring group. A follow-up study of cardiac patients receiving amitriptylene. *European Journal of Clinical Pharmacology*, **6**, 98–101.

Nayler, W. G. (1973a) An effect of ouabain on the superficially located stores of calcium in cardiac muscle cells. *Journal of Molecular and Cellular Cardiology*, **5**, 101–110.

Nayler, W. G. (1973b) Regulation of myocardial function—a subcellular phenomenon. *Journal of Molecular and Cellular Cardiology*, **5**, 213–219.

Nayler, W. G. (1976) Personal communication.

Nayler, W. G. & Szeto, J. (1972) Effect of verapamil on contractility, oxygen utilisation and calcium exchangeability in mammalian heart muscle. *Cardiovascular Research*, **6**, 120–128.

Oram, S., Catley, P. F., Livesley, B. & Kidner, P. H. (1971) An anti-dysrhythmic agent. *British Medical Journal*, **4**, 113.

Pamintuan, J. C., Dreifus, L. S. & Watanabe, Y. (1970) Comparative mechanism of anti-arrhythmic agents. *American Journal of Cardiology*, **26**, 512–519.

Peele, R. & von Loetzen, I. S. (1973) Phenothiazine deaths: a critical review. *American Journal of Psychiatry*, **130**, 306–309.

Pitts, N. E. (1969) The clinical evaluation of Doxepin—a new psychotherapeutic agent. *Psychosomatics*, **10**, 164–171.

Poletti, T., Aquaro, G., D'Arrigo, A. & Pavia, M. (1971) Anti-arrhythmic activity of disopyramide in comparison with that of quinidine. *Bolletino dela Sociata Italiana di Cardiologica*, **16**, 591–600.

Prichard, D. A., Singh, B. N. & Hurley, P. J. (1975) Effects of amiodarone on thyroid function in patients with ischaemic heart disease. *British Heart Journal*, **37**, 856–860.

Ranney, R. E., Dean, R. R., Karim, A. & Radzialowski, F. M. (1971) Disopyramide phosphate: pharmacokinetic and pharmacologic relationships of a new anti-arrhythmic agent. *Archives Internationales de Pharmacodynamie et de thérapie*, **191**, 162–188.

Regardh, C. G. (1973) Relationship between pharmacokinetics and pharmacodynamics of quinidine. In *Proceedings of the Cardiology Conference, Gotenberg, Sweden, 1973*, pp. 115–123. Astra Chemicals Ltd.

Richens, A. (1974) Drug estimation in the treatment of epilepsy. *Proceedings of the Royal Society of Medicine*, **67**, 1228.

Romhilt, D. W. & Fowler, N. O. (1975) Bretylium tosylate. In *Drugs in Cardiology*, ed. Donoso, E., Vol. 1, pp. 80–90. New York and London: Grune and Stratton.

Rosenbaum, M. B., Chiale, P. A., Ryba, D. & Elizari, M. V. (1974) Control of tachyarrhythmias associated with Wolff–Parkinson–White syndrome by amiodarone hydrochloride. *American Journal of Cardiology*, **34**, 215–223.

Rosen, M., Lisak, R. & Rubin, I. L. (1967) Diphenylhydantoin in cardiac arrhythmias. *American Journal of Cardiology*, **20**, 674–678.

Roussel Laboratories Ltd (1974) Personal communication.

Rowe, M. J., Neilson, J. M. M. & Oliver, M. F. (1975) Control of ventricular arrhythmias during myocardial infarction by antilipolytic treatment using a nicotinic acid analogue. *Lancet*, **1**, 295–300.

Roy, P. R., Spurrell, R. A. J. & Sowton, E. (1974) The effect of verapamil on the cardiac conduction system in man. *Postgraduate Medical Journal*, **50**, 270–275.

Saetre, H., Ahlmark, G. & Ahlberg, G. (1974) Haemodynamic effects of ajmaline in man. *European Journal of Clinical Pharmacology*, **7**, 253–257.

Sasyniuk, B. I. & Ogilvie, R. I. (1975) Anti-arrhythmic drugs: electrophysiological and pharmacokinetic considerations. *Annual Review of Pharmacology*, **15**, 131–155.

Schamroth, L., Krikler, D. M. & Garrett, C. (1972) Immediate effects of intravenous verapamil in cardiac arrhythmias. *British Medical Journal*, **1**, 660–662.

Schepdael, J. V. & Solvay, H. (1970) Etude Clinique de l'amiodarone dans les toubles du rhythme cardiaque. *Presse Médicale*, **78**, 1849–1850.

Schmidt, J. L., Vick, N. A. & Sadove, M. S. (1963) The effect of quinidine on the action of muscle relaxants. *Journal of the American Medical Association*, **183**, 669–671.

Schumacher, R. R., Lieberson, A. D., Childress, R. H. & Williams, J. F. (1968) Haemodynamic effects of lidocaine in patients with heart disease. *Circulation*, **37**, 965–972.

Schuster, D. P., Benedict, R. L., Nancy, L. N., Michael, N. M., Raymond, E. C. & Frank, J. K. (1973) The anti-arrhythmic properties of UM-272, the dimethyl quarternary derivative of propranolol. *Journal of Pharmacology and Experimental Therapeutics*, **184**, 213–227.

Shaw, T. R. D., Kumana, C. R., Royds, R. B., Padgham, C. M. & Hamer, J. (1974) Use of plasma levels in evaluation of procainamide dosage. *British Heart Journal*, **36**, 265–270.

Shaw, T. R. D., Kumana, C. R., Kaye, C. M., Padgham, C., Kaspi, T. & Hamer, J. (1975) Procainamide absorption studies to test the feasibility of using a sustained-release preparation. *British Journal of Clinical Pharmacology*, **2**, 515-519.

Sokolow, M. & Ball, R. L. (1956) Factors influencing conversion of atrial fibrillation with special reference to serum quinidine. *Circulation*, **14**, 568–583.

Sotomayer, L. L. (1963) A clinical evaluation of the anti-arrhythmic properties of antazoline. *American Journal of Cardiology*, **2**, 646–653.

Spurrell, R. A. J., Krikler, D. M. & Sowton, E. (1974) Effects of verapamil on electrophysiological properties of anomalous atrioventricular connection in Wolff–Parkinson–White syndrome. *British Heart Journal*, **36**, 256–264.

Spurrell, R. A. J., Thorburn, C. W., Camm, J., Sowton, E. & Deuchar, D. C. (1975) Effects of disopyramide on the electrophysiological properties of specialised conduction system in man and on the accessory atrioventricular pathway in the Wolff–Parkinson–White syndrome. *British Heart Journal* **37**, 861–867.

Spurrell, R. A. J., Yates, A. K., Thorburn, C. W., Sowton, G. E. & Deuchar, D. C. (1975) Surgical treatment of ventricular tachycardia after epicardial mapping studies. *British Heart Journal*, **37**, 115–126.

Stone, N., Klein, M. D. & Lown, B. (1971) Diphenylhydantoin in the prevention of recurring ventricular tachycardia. *Circulation*, **43**, 420–427.

Talbot, R. G., Clark, R. A., Nimmo, J., Neilson, J. M. M., Julian, D. G. & Prescott, L. F. (1973) Treatment of ventricular arrhythmias with mexiletine (Kö 1173). *Lancet*, **2**, 399–403.

Thind, G. S., Blakemore, W. S. & Zinsser, H. F. (1971) Ventricular aneurysmectomy for the treatment of recurrent ventricular tachyarrhythmia. *American Journal of Cardiology*, **27**, 690–694.

Turner, P. (1974) Beta-adrenergic receptor blocking drugs in hyperthyroidism. *Drugs*, **7**, 48–54.

Vaughan Williams, E. M. (1975) Anti-dysrhythmic drugs—their mode of action. In *Contraction and Relaxation of the Myocardium*, ed. Nayler, W. G. London: Academic Press.

Vetter, N. J. & Julian, D. G. (1975) Comparison of arrhythmia computer and conventional monitoring in coronary care unit. *Lancet*, **1**, 1975.

Vismara, L. A., Mason, D. T. & Amsterdam, E. A. (1974) Disopyramide phosphate, clinical efficacy of a new oral anti-arrhythmic drug. *Clinical Pharmacology and Therapeutics*, **16**, 330–335.

Way, W. L., Katzung, B. G. & Larson, C. P. (1967) Recurarisation with quinidine. *Journal of the American Medical Association*, **200**, 153–154.

Weily, H. S. & Genton, E. (1972) Pharmacokinetics of procainamide. *Archives of Internal Medicine*, **130**, 366–369.

Wellens, H. J. J. & Durrer, D. (1974) Effect of procainamide, quinidine and ajmaline in the Wolff–Parkinson–White syndrome. *Circulation*, **50**, 114–120.

Wellens, H. J. J., Schuilenburg, R. M. & Durrer, D. (1972) Electrical stimulation of the heart in patients with ventricular tachycardia. *Circulation*, **46**, 216–226.

Wilkinson, P. R., Issler, H., Hesp, R. & Raffery, E. B. (1975) Total body and serum potassium during prolonged thiazide therapy for essential hypertension. *Lancet*, **1**, 759–762.

Woodbury, D. M. & Swinyard, E. A. (1972) Diphenylhydantoin absorption, distribution and excretion in anti-epileptic drugs, ed. Woodbury, D. M., Penry, M. D. & Schmidt, R. P., pp. 113–126. New York: Raven Press.

7
THERAPEUTIC USES OF
β-ADRENERGIC BLOCKING DRUGS

John Hamer

ANGINA PECTORIS

The hypothesis which led to the development of β-adrenergic blocking drugs for treatment of angina pectoris on the basis of the evidence (Raab, 1945) that increased sympathetic activity played a part in the production of this symptom has been amply confirmed in controlled studies of exercise tolerance (Hamer and Sowton, 1966) and in clinical trials (Sharma and Taylor, 1973; Prichard and Gillam, 1971), although the precise mechanism of action is still under discussion.

The early observation of slowing of the heart rate after β-adrenergic blockade in patients with angina suggested an obvious cause for the less easy production of angina of effort. However, early objective studies (Hamer and Sowton, 1966) showed that angina after the drug did not occur at precisely the same heart rate as in the untreated state, suggesting that other factors were playing a part and leading to the widely held *hypothesis* that angina occurred at a critical level of *myocardial oxygen consumption*. The reduction in heart rate, systolic blood pressure and myocardial contractility produced by β-adrenergic blockade might be expected to reduce the myocardial oxygen consumption for a given degree of physical exercise, so improving the exercise tolerance limit for angina. The alternative suggestion that the longer diastolic periods associated with bradycardia would allow greater diastolic coronary blood flow was negated by the finding that an increased duration of systole prevented the usual increase in diastolic time with bradycardia induced by β-adrenergic blockade (Hamer, 1975).

Nevertheless, the myocardial oxygen consumption hypothesis never carried great conviction because of the increase in duration of systole and the increase in heart size (Crawford et al, 1975), probably indicating left ventricular dilatation (Hamer and Fleming, 1969); both factors which will tend to increase myocardial oxygen consumption after β-adrenergic blockade. A careful analysis by Taylor (1975) has shown that heart rate is by far the most important determinant of the onset of angina under different conditions, giving support to the widespread use of atrial pacing to determine the angina threshold in evaluation of patients (Balcon, Maloy and Sowton, 1968). However, direct calculation of myocardial oxygen consumption based on coronary sinus flow measurements show no change after β-adrenergic blockade (Stephens et al, 1976) if the heart rate is held constant by pacing.

The diastolic hypothesis

An alternative explanation refers to the changes in the diastolic performance of the left ventricle (Amende et al, 1975).

The uptake of Ca ions by the Ca pump enzyme of the sarcoplasmic reticulum is apparently critically sensitive to hypoxia, and in angina local ischaemia leads to impairment of relaxation, a partial contracture, which is a factor in the rise of left ventricular end-diastolic pressure found at the onset of angina. The relaxation process is shown by in vitro studies of sarcoplasmic reticulum from animal hearts to be under autonomic control and a reduced sympathetic drive to relaxation after β-adrenergic blockade may reduce the tendencies for ischaemic contracture to occur in diastole (Harris, 1975).

This *diastolic hypothesis* seems a more suitable explanation of the response to β-adrenergic blockade in angina and bradycardia may be only a marker of drug action, although it is difficult to exclude a part played by the fall in exercise heart rate on myocardial oxygen consumption.

The major side-effect of removal of normal cardiac sympathetic drive is the production of congestive heart failure in patients with left ventricular disease of such a degree that increased sympathetic activity is needed to maintain adequate performance. For this reason, β-adrenergic blocking drugs are usually avoided in treating the unusual patient with angina in the presence of mild congestive heart failure or left ventricular disease evident as cardiac enlargement in the chest radiograph (but see p. 173).

Subsidiary properties of β-adrenergic blocking drugs

These include

(a) quinidine-like activity (membrane stabilising effect) possessed by propranolol, oxprenolol and several other well-known agents in large dose, or

(b) intrinsic sympathomimetic activity (ISA) (partial agonist effect) possessed by oxprenolol, pindolol, practolol amongst others,

(c) cardioselectivity, acting particularly on cardiac and to a lesser extent on bronchial and peripheral vascular β-adrenergic receptors, possessed by practolol, metopolol and atenolol, and

(d) class III anti-arrhythmic effect of Vaughan Williams (prolongation of action potential and so of refractory period) possessed by sotalol in high concentration.

The subsidiary properties of the β-adrenergic blocking drugs play little part in the response in angina. It seems clear that quinidine-like activity (membrane stabilising effect) is irrelevant to the response of angina or the production of congestive heart failure, even with the largest doses used in clinical practice, as when failure occurs it is seen with relatively small doses and is unlikely to appear at later increases in the dose if smaller doses are tolerated without disturbance (Prichard, 1976). Although some studies show practolol to be as effective as propranolol (Coltart, 1971), there is a progressive response to increasing doses of propranolol (Prichard and Gillam, 1971) and comparative study trials using graded doses show propranolol to be more effective (Prichard, 1975). Differing subsidiary properties do not fundamentally alter the effectiveness of β-adrenergic blocking drugs in appropriate doses in angina (Taylor, Thadani and Sharma, 1973).

Cardioselectivity

Cardioselectivity carries the advantage that effective cardiac β-adrenergic blockade is unlikely to cause troublesome bronchoconstriction in asthmatic subjects and there may be less reduction in cardiac output, perhaps as a peripheral venoconstrictor effect is avoided (Gibson, 1974).

The necessary withdrawal of the oral preparation of practolol because of serious side-effects on prolonged treatment (Wright, 1975) has left a serious gap in the therapeutic armamentarium, although several other cardioselective agents are being currently assessed, e.g. metoprolol (Betaloc, Astra or Lepressor, Geigy), and atenolol (Tenermin, ICI); unfortunately, the otherwise promising Pfizer drug (tolamolol) has been withheld because of carcinogenic effects in animals. The side-effects of dry eye leading to blindness, rash and various other disturbances of serous membranes, seem to be confined to practolol therapy, and suggestions of association of those reactions with other β-adrenergic blocking drugs are at present unconvincing.

Intrinsic sympathomimetic activity (ISA) (partial agonist effect)

ISA does not seem to interfere with the response, and oxprenolol for instance is also effective (Taylor et al, 1973), suggesting that it is removal via the CNS of exogenous stimulation of the heart, such as effort or emotional stress, that is the major important factor rather than the level of intrinsic sympathetic tone. ISA may minimise the tendency to increase airways obstruction in susceptible subjects. There is also a less well-substantiated suggestion that the presence of ISA reduces the risk of heart failure, although it seems to minimise the fall in cardiac output (Grandjean and Rivier, 1968). In considering treatment with β-adrenergic blocking drugs in patients with a tendency to congestive heart failure, it is unwise to rely on the suggestion that drugs with cardioselectivity or ISA are less likely to cause this problem. Although, in the marginal situation, Crawford et al (1975) report that patients limited by dyspnoea rather than angina after propranolol may show an improvement in exercise tolerance when digitalis glycosides are added to the treatment with some reduction in heart size, these findings cannot be extrapolated to the treatment of patients with frank congestive heart failure, either with pulmonary or systemic venous congestion. Fortunately, angina is rare in this situation, but the suggestion that treatment may be given in such

patients if failure is prevented with digitalis, with or without diuretic treatment, is open to doubt as the degree of β-adrenergic blockade needed to
improve angina will certainly lead to some impairment of myocardial contractility, which will accentuate any tendency to failure and which is unlikely
to be counteracted by the relative slight effect of digitalis glycosides in
improving contractility (Ogden, Selzer and Cohn, 1969; Davidson and
Gibson, 1973; Cohn et al, 1975). In this situation, β-adrenergic blocking
drugs have little to offer the patient and angina of effort may be relieved by
reduced physical activity, which will in itself be beneficial for congestive
heart failure. Attempts to maintain normal activity under these circumstances
are inappropriate.

Concern is often expressed that the reduction in cardiac output produced
by β-adrenergic blocking drugs will have a deleterious effect by reducing
perfusion of vital organs. However, in the absence of heart failure the reduction in blood flow is not critical and tissue oxygenation is maintained by
increased extraction of oxygen in the tissues so that venous oxygen saturation
falls (Hamer and Sowton, 1966); there is much reserve in this mechanism
which is the usual response in normal subjects approaching the limits of
exercise tolerance. Although maximal exercise may be limited in this way by
treatment with β-adrenergic blocking drugs and may be a consideration in
the use of these agents in fit, normal subjects—for instance, to treat anxiety—
it is unlikely to be important in the management of patients with ischaemic
heart disease. The coronary circulation which normally operates near to
maximal oxygen extraction is little disturbed by the treatment and seems to
adjust to the metabolic requirements of the myocardium, even in the presence
of coronary artery disease (Stephens et al, 1975). The sensation of easy
fatigue frequently noted by relatively fit and active subjects on propranolol
may be related to the limitation of cardiac output as it seems less troublesome
with drugs having cardioselectivity (e.g. practolol) or ISA (e.g. oxprenolol).

It is best to begin treatment gradually with small doses, as other effects of
β-adrenergic blockade may limit the dose that can be used. Severe bradycardia may lead to faintness, and is usually evident in the ECG as severe
sinus slowing as the usual escape pacemakers may also be suppressed by the
drug. There is a possibility that a slow heart rate may accentuate angina as
has been described with bradycardia in other circumstances (Fowler et al,
1969) and this could lead to mistaken persistence with treatment. On the
other hand, the heart rate at rest may not be a good guide to the response as
it is modified by other factors, such as vagal tone (often low with patients who
have been athletic in youth), and the exercise heart rate is a better guide to the
limit of treatment (Jackson, Atkinson and Oram, 1975).

A fall in blood pressure may also cause problems, but is unlikely to be
troublesome unless there is cerebral vascular disease. In so far as part of the
beneficial effect is due to reduction in the load on the left ventricle, this
change may be regarded as part of the therapeutic response. If symptomless,

neither bradycardia nor hypotension need prevent the use of adequate doses of β-adrenergic blocking drugs.

It is usual to begin with small doses, such as propranolol 10 mg four times a day, in case of undue sensitivity, and the dose can be increased to 40 mg four times a day in a few days. Doses of this order are often effective, but there is evidence of progressive benefit with larger doses, so it is reasonable to increase the dose to the limits of tolerance.

Stopping treatment with β-adrenergic blocking drugs may lead to a dangerous exacerbation of symptoms (Diaz et al, 1974; Mizgala and Counsell, 1974) after the drug has been excreted. In many patients this effect is due to an increase in the customary level of activity as a result of the beneficial effect of treatment, but the occurrence of such problems in hospital in patients awaiting cardiac surgery suggests that the heart may be more susceptible to external influences under these circumstances. The biological and effective half-life of propranolol is such that the β-adrenergic blocking effect is lost after about 48 h (Faulkner et al, 1973; Coltart et al, 1975). However, the problems of operating during β-adrenergic blockade may have been exaggerated as the need for a larger dose of isoprenaline to overcome the competitive blockade and produce β-adrenergic stimulation if necessary would not seem to be a major one for the sophisticated anaesthetist. However, it is difficult to exclude the possibility of long-term changes in myocardial function analogous to those described by Vaughan Williams et al (1975) in growing rabbits in which heart weight is reduced without change in contractility or response to isoprenalone; such a process might prevent the usual compensatory hypertrophy in ischaemic heart disease with myocardial damage and make the heart less able to withstand the effects of cardiac surgery. Trinitrin may usually be continued in patients on β-adrenergic blocking drugs and there is some evidence of a synergistic effect (MacAlpin, Kattus and Winfield, 1965).

Angina in Patients with Normal Coronary Arteries

A high proportion of patients with classical angina of effort are found at coronary arteriography to have normal coronary arteries (Herman, Cohn and Gorlin, 1973). This situation seems particularly common in middle-aged women and is said to carry a good prognosis. The mechanism is in doubt. Some have postulated disease of the small coronary arteries, but none has been demonstrated. A myocardial abnormality has been shown in some patients in biopsy specimens (Richardson et al, 1974). Coronary artery spasm, as suggested for Prinzmetal's angina (see later) (*British Medical Journal*, 1975), remains a possibility. Another suggestion (Eliot and Bratt, 1969) is an abnormality of the dissociation of oxyhaemoglobin reducing the availability of oxygen to the myocardium; changes of this type could arise as a functional disturbance from alterations in the plasma, and as propranolol in large doses has been shown to have the opposite effect on oxyhaemoglobin a therapeutic action in this way is a theoretical possibility (Lichtman et al, 1974).

A further possibility is that there is an overactive left ventricle having an excessive myocardial oxygen consumption that cannot be satisfied even by normal coronary arteries. Evidence to support this view is provided by the finding of an unusually large ejection fraction (Mamohansingh and Parker, 1975). Provided a minor variant of hypertrophic obstructive cardiomyopathy is excluded this raises the possibility that excessive sympathetic stimulation, perhaps on the basis of an anxiety state, might be the fundamental disturbance. It seems likely that many different entities are included in this group and careful individual evaluation of each patient is needed to plan optimal treatment.

Sometimes these patients show a therapeutic response to β-adrenergic blocking drugs (Donsky et al, 1975), as might be expected in the hyper-dynamic group (Mamohansingh and Parker, 1975), and this treatment should be given a trial. As ECG changes may be seen in these patients there seems no way to distinguish this group short of coronary arteriography.

Patients with a billowing mitral valve (non-ejection systolic click and mitral systolic murmur) may have angina and ECG changes with normal coronary arteries, and coronary artery spasm secondary to the tension on the papillary muscle is suggested as the mechanism (Barlow and Pocock, 1975). β-Adrenergic blocking drugs do not relieve coronary artery spasm as the β-sympathetic innervation of the coronary arteries is vasodilator, α-adrenergic blockade would be more appropriate (Yasua et al, 1974).

ACUTE CORONARY INSUFFICIENCY

Several conditions associated with prolonged attacks of anginal pain without infarction are included under this heading, sometimes referred to as 'intermediate coronary syndrome'.

1. Severe attacks of angina from sudden anaemia or hypotension as in gastrointestinal haemorrhage; corrected by transfusion.
2. Severe angina of effort or at rest or on recumbency (angina decubitus) in severe aortic stenosis; indicating a need for early valve replacement.
3. Preinfarction angina. Increased frequency and more prolonged episodes of angina, often with rest pain, leading up to cardiac infarction. Frequent in retrospect in patients with established infarction.
4. Similar exacerbation of symptoms suggestive of impending infarction and probably related to deterioration of coronary artery disease.
5. Prinzmetal's variant form of angina with local ST segment elevation during attacks of rest pain, often at night. Some of these patients have no coronary artery disease.
6. Rudimentary cardiac infarction (East and Oram, 1948); transient T-wave inversion, usually V_3 and V_4.

7. Subendocardial shell infarction. Often seen after prolonged hypotension or myocardial stress as a result of critical impairment of blood supply to the inner layers of the myocardium by penetrating arteries from the superficial plexus of major coronary vessels.

Both these situations (6 and 7) are in fact myocardial infarction, but are not transmural and are therefore without the characteristic ECG changes.

The usual problem is that cardiac infarction seems likely, though many of these patients settle down with medical treatment and the prognosis is not in fact as bad as might be thought (Fulton et al, 1972). Coronary arteriography with a view to possible corrective grafts might be thought a reasonable approach once the severe symptoms have subsided. β-Adrenergic blocking drugs may be effective probably on the basis of reducing the load on the myocardium, and may help to reduce the disturbance while definitive treatment is being considered.

In *Prinzmetal's angina*, which is characterised by angina at rest with preservation of exercise capacity and local ST segment elevation in the ECG (MacAlpin et al, 1973), coronary artery spasm is postulated (Yasua et al, 1974) particularly in those patients showing normal coronary arteries, or minimal disease, unrelated to the area of ischaemia. On this basis, β-adrenergic blocking drugs might be thought to be contraindicated unless cardioselective, as the β-sympathetic supply to the coronary arteries is vasodilator and blockade might accentuate constriction. In fact, although some patients deteriorate (King et al, 1973) and others find equivocal results (MacAlpin et al, 1973), these drugs have been found to produce a favourable response in some patients (Donsky et al, 1975). So, either spasm is not a constant mechanism in this group, or the metabolic effects of ischaemia swamp the autonomic responses in the coronary arteries as in conventional angina, where no difference can be found between propranolol and the cardioselective drug, atenolol (Stephens et al, 1976).

MYOCARDIAL INFARCTION

Several possible uses of β-adrenergic blocking drugs in cardiac infarction are suggested.

1. To abolish the early increase in sympathetic tone.
2. Prevention of potentially fatal ventricular arrhythmias from:

    (a) direct effect on ventricular ectopic foci
    (b) prevention of release of free fatty acids which have an adverse effect on ventricular ectopic foci.

3. Minimising the extent of infarction by reducing left ventricular oxygen consumption, partly as a result of action 1.

4. Rapid control of supraventricular tachyarrhythmias, will also influence 3 (see later, p. 189).
5. As long-term treatment to prevent late mortality at reinfarction through mechanisms 1 and 2.

Prevention of Ventricular Arrhythmias

Pantridge et al (1974) have demonstrated that patients seen early after cardiac infarction, using a coronary ambulance service, often show severe autonomic disturbances. The changes after anterior infarction are mainly an increase in sympathetic activity, shown by an undue tachycardia or a rise in blood pressure; but after posterior infarction, increased vagal activity predominates. The brisk tachycardia seen after atropine in some of these patients suggests that sympathetic tone may also be increased in this group, and Mulholland and Pantridge (1974) recommend the combination of atropine and the un-complicated β-adrenergic blocker sotalol to remove all these autonomic influences and avoid extremes of either bradycardia or tachycardia, which may have adverse effects on the relation of myocardial oxygen consumption to supply.

Conventional anti-arrhythmic drugs, such as lignocaine, are relatively ineffective in the early stages of myocardial infarction, as seen with a coronary ambulance service, and sympathetic influences may be more important at this stage in producing dangerous ventricular ectopic rhythms and ventricular fibrillation. One suggested mechanism is by producing increased dispersion of the recovery period through the focal effect of stimulation via the neurogenic sympathetic nervous system (Han and Moe, 1964), thereby facilitating re-entry phenomena leading to ventricular fibrillation. An alternative possibility is that late after-potentials due to Ca ion currents, which occur when the normal Na ion action potential is prevented by loss of the resting membrane potential as K ions leak from the damaged cell (Gettes, 1975), are potentiated by sympathetic activity as catecholamines produce similar after-potentials. β-Adrenergic blockade may reduce the risk of these arrhythmias by removing the sympathetic component of the synergistic process.

A similar mechanism is probably responsible for the beneficial effect of β-adrenergic blocking drugs in patients with recurrent syncope due to ventricular arrhythmias associated with a long Q–T interval ('repolarisation cardiomyopathy'), sometimes associated with congenital deafness (Jervell and Lange Nielson syndrome) in which a disturbance of myocardial sympathetic innervation is suspected (Schwartz, Periti and Malliani, 1975).

The quinidine-like activity (membrane stabilising effect) of some β-adrenergic blocking drugs seems irrelevant to their anti-arrhythmic action at usual doses, as the concentrations needed for this action are several orders greater than those producing β-adrenergic blockade (Barrett, 1973). The scattered reports of anti-arrhythmic effects with the dextro-isomers, which have in the main a quinidine-like action only (Howitt et al, 1965; Sowton et al, 1970), may be attributed to incomplete separation from the laevo-isomer, the minor β-adrenergic blocking effect of the dextro-isomer, or the effects of transient high blood levels after intravenous injection.

Release of free fatty acids mediated by sympathetic stimulation of fat stores has been suggested as a possible effect producing arrhythmias after myocardial infarction. The suggestion is that a direct effect of free fatty acids, e.g. the increased myocardial oxygen consumption needed to metabolise fatty acids rather than glucose, accentuates the effects of myocardial ischaemia (Oliver, 1975).

Although the initial subdivision of β-adrenergic blocking drugs as cardio-selective included the metabolic receptors with the cardiac ones as β_1 receptors (Lands et al, 1967), the best known cardioselective agent, practolol, has little effect on release of free fatty acids. As practolol is relatively effective in the control of postinfarction arrhythmias, it seems likely that an action preventing liberation of free fatty acids from fat stores is not of major importance. Block of release of fatty acids may accentuate exercise hypoglycaemia in diabetics on β-adrenergic blocking drugs, and non-cardioselective β-adrenergic blocking treatment is contraindicated in this group of patients (Lloyd-Mostyn and Oram, 1975).

The good response with reduction in late sudden deaths in survivors of cardiac infarction on practolol (A Multicentre International Study, 1975) confirms the suggestion that increased sympathetic activity contributes to the early mortality of cardiac infarction. Presumably, practolol is acting to prevent early arrhythmic deaths at reinfarction. Similar responses have been demonstrated in less extensive trials with other β-adrenergic blocking drugs (Wilhelmsson et al, 1974; Fox et al, 1975).

It is tempting to link the particular benefit from practolol in survivors of anterior infarction with the evidence that increased sympathetic activity is particularly frequent with infarcts in this location (Pantridge et al, 1974). The location of coronary artery disease in a particular patient might predispose to further infarction in the same general area as a previous lesion (Lindén, 1974).

Reduction in Size of Infarction

The experimental work of Braunwald and Maroko (1974) strongly suggested that in situations of critically impaired myocardial blood supply a reduction in myocardial oxygen consumption might limit the extent of myocardial necrosis. Many interventions aimed to reduce the load on the left ventricle have been tested in this respect, and among the more successful has been β-adrenergic blockade (Backer, Ferreira and Thomas, 1975; Lancet, 1974). A major benefit in this way arises from the reduction in heart rates after β-adrenergic blockade, especially if there is a sinus tachycardia from sympathetic stimulation, or a supraventricular tachyarrhythmia (see later, p. 187).

A fall in blood pressure and in the velocity of myocardial contraction may augment the response, but any increase in left ventricular volume by increasing total wall tension in systole from the Laplace relationship would tend to have the opposite effect, as would an increase in the duration of systole. The benefit must result from a net favourable balance from the effects on rate, blood pressure and contractility against the adverse effect of an increase in left ventricular volume or in the duration of systole.

There is evidence that β-adrenergic blocking drugs reduce the extent and severity of ST segment elevation in an area of infarction, and this response has been regarded as evidence that the extent of myocardial damage is reduced, a suggestion supported by other evidence of reduction in release of myocardial enzymes.

This response lends support to the routine use of β-adrenergic blocking drugs in the early stages of myocardial infarction as the anti-arrhythmic effect will be combined with further expected benefit in terms of reduction in size of infarction. Such early treatment may play a part in reducing the incidence of potentially fatal complications, such as cardiogenic shock and left ventricular failure, that result from extensive myocardial damage.

The main danger of β-adrenergic blockade early in myocardial infarction is the production of acute left ventricular failure from the withdrawal of necessary sympathetic drive from a damaged ventricle operating under stress. Unfortunately, relatively small doses of β-adrenergic blockers may have this effect. Propranolol has a particularly bad reputation in this respect and must be used with great caution; doses of 1 to 2 mg intravenously, repeated as indicated from the response, up to 5 or 10 mg seems reasonable. Mulholland and Pantridge (1974) recommend sotalol which has been thought to have relatively little effect on contractility in an animal study (Brooks et al, 1971) and has an additional property, the class III anti-arrhythmic effect of Singh and Vaughan Williams (1970), with prolongation of the action potential, which may improve contractility, although this is not supported by studies in man (Gibson, Hoy and Sowton, 1974) and there is little evidence of less tendency to produce left ventricular failure in clinical use. Cardioselective agents are thought to have less effect on contractility, as are drugs with ISA (partial agonist effect). Practolol, with both these properties, is still available as an intravenous preparation in spite of the serious toxicity in long-term oral use. A dose of 5 to 10 mg intravenously is generally satisfactory. Other cardioselective drugs without ISA just coming into clinical use are atenolol and metoprolol. Of the non-cardioselective agents with ISA, the best known in Britain is oxprenolol, but pindolol and alprenolol, widely used in other countries, are similar. Presumably the therapeutic effect relies more on the elimination of exogenous sympathetic stimulation which outweighs the effect of ISA in countering some of the abolition of resting sympathetic tone.

HYPERTENSION

A number of different mechanisms are proposed to account for the effectiveness of β-adrenergic blocking drugs in hypertension. The discovery of the response caused some surprise as the peripheral effect of the non-cardioselective agents (generally propranolol) used at first might be expected to increase peripheral resistance (Frohlich et al, 1968).

The existence of a subgroup of hypertensives particularly dependent on sympathetic overactivity has long been suspected, and there is evidence that some patients have mild borderline hypertension on a neurogenic basis, perhaps as a psychosomatic disturbance. α-Sympathetic activity will increase the peripheral resistance and the β-sympathetic will boost plasma renin levels and the cardiac output (Julius, Ester and Randall, 1975). A group of labile hypertensives with raised cardiac output have evidence of increased sympathetic activity acting mainly on venous tone (Safar et al, 1975). That more than a raised cardiac output is involved is shown by the relative failure of propranolol in 'hyperkinetic' hypertension; the high cardiac output and tachycardia are reduced with relief of symptoms, but the blood pressure remains raised (Ibrahim et al, 1975). There is evidence, from raised plasma catecholamines (de Quattro and Chan, 1972) of a general increase in sympathetic activity in hypertension, suggesting that sympathetic nervous activity is involved in the maintenance of the raised blood pressure.

Haemodynamic Effects

Although the acute response of the blood pressure to an intravenous dose is modest, the effect of larger doses to produce plasma levels corresponding to those used in treating hypertension has not been tested as it is usual to increase the dose gradually, eliminating patients responding easily or showing side-effects, before using larger doses (Conway, 1975). The haemodynamic response may involve a peripheral readjustment to the surges of cardiac output produced by sympathetic stimulation, with eventually a fall in peripheral resistance (Prichard and Gillam, 1966). The end result is a smooth control of blood pressure with retention of reflex peripheral vascular control, a situation described by Prichard and Gillam (1966) as 'resetting the baroceptors'. The absence of any postural fall in blood pressure (Prichard et al, 1970) is a great advantage over other agents, such as ganglion-blocking drugs, which are difficult to manage because of the profound postural fall in BP with effective treatment. The reduced heart weight observed in growing rabbits on β-adrenergic blocking drugs (Vaughan Williams et al, 1975) may be an indication of a general effect, which by preventing hypertrophy might limit the cardiac response in hypertension.

The modest fall in cardiac output produced by β-adrenergic blocking drugs is usually well tolerated and compensated by an increase in extraction of oxygen in the tissues, but there is evidence that renal function may deteriorate in patients with hypertension and chronic renal failure (Warren, Swainson and Wright, 1974) and treatment with β-adrenergic blocking drugs may be contraindicated in this group.

Action on Renin Secretion

The secretion of renin by the juxtaglomerular apparatus of the kidney is under autonomic control and is prevented by β-adrenergic blocking drugs. Plasma renin levels are raised in many patients with hypertension and it has been suggested (Bühler et al, 1973) and denied (Doyle et al, 1973) that renin produces the vascular damage characteristic of severe hypertensive states.

Although Bühler et al (1973) claim that patients with high or normal plasma renin levels respond better to β-adrenergic blocking drugs than those with low renin levels, others have found it difficult to correlate response with renin level before treatment (Leonetti et al, 1975; Morgan et al, 1975), and the improvement in blood pressure does not always coincide with a fall in the plasma renin (Morgan et al, 1975). Renin secretion responds to small plasma concentrations of β-adrenergic blocking drugs, but much higher levels may be needed for a hypotensive response (Leonetti et al, 1975). Although Koch-Weser (1975) suggested that cardioselective β-adrenergic blocking drugs did not block plasma renin release, more recent evidence (Bühler et al, 1975) shows that this is not the case and the renin release mechanism must be regarded as a β_1-receptor although located peripherally (Hamer, 1976). Bühler et al (1975) also suggest that agents with strong partial agonist effect (ISA), such as pindolol, which reduce blood pressure without change in basal plasma renin (Morgan et al, 1975), may be effective by blocking renin release in response to stimuli such as the upright exercise used in their study. Taylor et al (1976) and Lohmöller and Frohlich (1975) confirmed that the subsidiary properties of various β-adrenergic blocking drugs did not affect the effectiveness of these agents in hypertension.

Central Action

The undoubted central effects of many β-adrenergic blocking drugs, such as propranolol, which may produce minor sedation and bizarre dreams led to the suggestion that the fall in blood pressure was also produced by a central action (Dollery et al, 1973). The cerebral β-adrenergic receptors may mediate vasoconstriction so a fall in blood pressure would be expected from an action at this site (Conway, 1975). A problem with the central hypothesis is that drugs, such as practolol and atenolol (Hansson et al, 1975), thought from their chemical properties to be unlikely to cross the blood–brain barrier, seem as effective as other β-adrenergic blocking agents in the treatment of hypertension.

A Unifying Hypothesis

The low renin hypertensives are thought to have suppression of renin secretion by high levels of circulating aldosterone, as in Conn's syndrome, or of another as yet unidentified mineralocorticoid, or by abnormal sensitivity to normal levels of aldosterone activity, perhaps as a late stage in hypertensive disease. These patients may respond to β-adrenergic blocking drugs by a separate mechanism, even if suppression of renin secretion accounts for some of the response in the patients with higher plasma renin activities.

Hollifield et al (1976) have presented evidence that an early response to propranolol correlated with renin suppression may be followed by a later further fall in blood pressure probably through the mediation of another mechanism requiring larger doses, such as a central effect or an augmentation of the acute haemodynamic response. Such a hypothesis would explain the failure of correlation between suppression of plasma renin and fall in blood pressure. It might be expected that patients with normal or raised plasma renin activity would show some response to modest doses of β-adrenergic blocking drugs, although large doses might produce a further response and may be needed to control the patients with low or suppressed plasma renin activity, who might in any case be expected to respond better to diuretic therapy or aldosterone antagonists (Karlberg et al, 1976; MacGregor and Dawes, 1975).

The combination of diuretic therapy with β-adrenergic blocking drugs has a synergistic effect in the treatment of hypertension. The objection that renin secretion is accentuated by diuretic therapy is countered by the evidence that this effect is lost in a few months with continued treatment (Bourgoignie, Catanzaro and Perry, 1968).

Initial very small doses, such as propranolol 10 mg 6-hourly, are used by some to test for hypersensitivity—for instance, severe bradycardia (see earlier, p. 174)—but 40 mg 6-hourly will generally be effective and should suppress plasma renin. Very large doses of the order of 1 or 2 g a day may be reached by gradual increases over several months before a response is attained.

Bradycardia is the usual limiting factor, but central side-effects such as drowsiness or nightmares may prevent intensive treatment. Congestive heart failure is accentuated by β-adrenergic blocking drugs and evidence of early failure or radiographic cardiac enlargement should be regarded as a contra-indication to this treatment, which is at its best in the otherwise fit and active hypertensive. When failure is accentuated this seems to be a phenomenon of the early stages of the dose regimen rather than a response to very large doses, so that if moderate doses are accepted without failure it is unlikely to appear during progression to a high dose level (Prichard, 1976).

7

EFFECTS IN MYOCARDIAL DISEASE

The usually unwanted effects of β-adrenergic blocking drugs on myocardial performance can be turned to advantage in some situations. In *hypertrophic obstructive cardiomyopathy*, the dynamic outflow tract obstruction is increased by isoprenaline and reduced by β-adrenergic blockade. There is some evidence that the abnormal myocardial tissue in this condition is related to the sympathetic nervous system (Goodwin, 1974). The symptomatic improvement of these patients on β-adrenergic blocking drugs may be in part related to relief of obstruction on this basis, but there is also evidence that the diastolic compliance of the hypertrophied and necessarily stiff left ventricle is improved by β-adrenergic blockade (Webb-Peploe et al, 1971). Relief of arrhythmias, which may be in part responsible for episodes of syncope or for sudden death, is a further benefit of treatment (Hardarson et al, 1973). Treatment seems to put the patient back a year or two in the progress of the natural history of the condition, but eventually obstructive symptoms or pulmonary congestion from the resistance to filling of the stiff left ventricle will return. Although practolol has been reported as particularly favouring diastolic relaxation, there seems little firm evidence to favour any particular β-adrenergic blocking drug in this condition.

A similar situation is evident in *Fallot's tetralogy* where a response was detected much earlier in the history of β-adrenergic blockade. The dynamic outflow tract in tetralogy of Fallot may constrict to produce the syncopal episodes or cyanotic spells frequent in severe cases of this condition. These attacks may be fatal and are a prime indication for surgical treatment. As a temporary measure they may be treated by β-adrenergic blocking drugs which cause the outflow tract to relax and relieve the obstruction to pulmonary blood flow.

In the inherited cardiomyopathies with long Q–T interval (*repolarisation cardiomyopathy*), which may be associated with congenital deafness and is accompanied by repeated attacks of ventricular tachycardia or fibrillation (p. 178) which may produce syncope, an imbalance of sympathetic innervation of the heart is suspected, and a favourable response to β-adrenergic blocking drugs is reported (Schwartz et al, 1975).

The recent report that patients with *congestive heart failure* due to myocardial disease may respond to small doses of β-adrenergic blocking drugs (Waagstein et al, 1975) may be related to an improvement in myocardial diastolic compliance. The situation of the sympathetic nervous system in the failing myocardium is unusual in that there is evidence of high circulating and urinary concentrations of catecholamines but the myocardial concentrations are reduced, suggesting intense general sympathetic stimulation but exhaustion of the myocardial stores. Synthesis in the myocardium is also impaired. Under these circumstances there may be myocardial hypersensitivity to circulating catecholamines (Rutenberg and Spann, 1973) and an effect of β-adrenergic blockade may be evident at doses below those that precipitate severe failure. It is said that the difficulty is to establish treatment and if the patient can be maintained on small doses without deterioration there is improvement in the long term (Waagstein et al, 1975). Alternative or additional effects may be the reduction in a more than compensatory tachycardia which is wasteful of myocardial oxygen consumption or suppression of excessive renin secretion and consequent hyperaldosteronism which is frequent in patients with congestive heart failure maintained on diuretic treatment after elimination of oedema (Nicholls et al, 1974).

Acute Central Nervous System Effects

The ECG changes found in *subarachnoid haemorrhage*, including flat T-waves and prolonged Q–T interval, are abolished by β-adrenergic blocking drugs (Cruickshank, Neil-Dwyer and Lane, 1975). As these changes probably indicate sympathetically mediated myocardial stress they may have an adverse effect on prognosis, and a clinical trial has been suggested. Similar responses are seen if the ECG changes are produced by other causes of raised intracranial pressure (Jochuk et al, 1975).

ECTOPIC RHYTHMS RELATED TO SYMPATHETIC NERVOUS ACTIVITY

In some situations ectopic rhythms, generally ventricular ectopic beats or more serious disturbances, occur in relation to sympathetic stimulation, either as an isolated phenomenon as in anxiety states, or by potentiating the effect of other noxious agents, such as anaesthetic gases or digitalis overdosage. The situation in this group is similar to that found in myocardial infarction (see above, p. 178) where hypoxia and sympathetic stimulation may have potentiating effects, and similarly more serious ectopic rhythms may be seen leading eventually to cardiac arrest from ventricular fibrillation. In other circumstances, increased sympathetic activity may be generated by drug treatment as in overdosing with tricyclic antidepressants or by disease as in phaeochromocytoma (see later, p. 192).

Anxiety Ectopic Beats

The frequent palpitation associated with anxiety may be due to sinus tachycardia but is frequently related to ventricular ectopic beats which seem to occur in a normal heart under these circumstances. The potentiating effects of caffeine and its analogues in tea or coffee, or of alcohol may be blamed, but these added factors are not a necessary accompaniment of ventricular ectopic beats. These rhythm disturbances are generally benign in that more serious problems do not follow. If cardiac infarction should occur these patients may be at greater risk of ventricular fibrillation than patients without associated ventricular ectopic beats, so specific therapy may be indicated on these grounds in apparently susceptible patients. In many patients relief of the anxiety or psychotropic drugs may be in themselves sufficient to eliminate the disturbance, but in others persistent symptoms may justify the use of β-adrenergic blocking drugs to eliminate ectopic beats and relieve the associated discomfort; this treatment may lead to improvement in the underlying anxiety state (see later, p. 191).

Anaesthetic Gases

The tendency to ventricular ectopic activity, most obvious with chloroform, seems to be shared to some extent by the less toxic halogenated hydrocarcon gases, such as trichlorethylene (Trilene) and halothane (Fluothane) and also by cyclopropane. The effects arise partly by synergism with increased sympathetic activity under anaesthesia and are relieved by β-adrenergic blockade, although this approach must be used with caution as the first step in preventing arrhythmias is to provide full oxygenation and avoid CO_2 retention while taking care to keep the concentration of the potentially toxic anaesthetic gas to a minimum. It is thought that halothane and cyclopropane sensitise the myocardium to the effects of sympathetic stimulation (Davis, Temple and Murphy, 1969; Wit, Hoffman and Rosen, 1975).

This action may be mediated by an effect on the slow inward Ca ion current as the anaesthetic gases may interfere with the Ca ion stores in the external basement layer of the cardiac cell membrane (Naylor and Sebra-Gomez, 1975) and potentiate the effect of catecholamines on the Ca ion current.

Digitalis Toxicity

Much debate has been generated by the demonstration in animals that ventricular ectopic rhythms due to digitalis toxicity are abolished by β-adrenergic blocking drugs. In some studies large doses of drugs with quinidine-like action were used. However, other studies suggest that a response may occur with smaller doses or with drugs not having a quinidine-like effect; so it seems clear that there is some potentiation between digitalis effect and sympathetic activity to produce the ectopic rhythm. The evidence (Gillis, Pearle and Levitt, 1975) that large doses of digitalis exert a sympathomimetic effect by an action in the central nervous system is in line with this suggestion. This situation is evident in man where relatively small, i.e. conventional, doses of β-adrenergic blocking drugs may abolish ventricular ectopic beats due to digitalis effect. The more usual autonomic effects of digitalis involve a direct enhancement of vagal tone and sensitisation of carotid baroreceptors to produce vagal activation and sympathetic withdrawal, producing a major reflex depression of AV node function (Gillis et al, 1975). For this reason, treatment of digitalis-induced arrhythmias with β-adrenergic blocking drugs is *not recommended* as the summated effect of the two drugs on conduction at the AV node may lead to AV block associated with suppression of escape pacemakers, so that dangerous or inconvenient *asystole* may follow suppression of the ectopic beats: lignocaine or epanutin with minimal or contrary effects on AV conduction are to be preferred in the treatment of digitalis ectopic arrhythmias.

A possible mechanism for the summation of effects between digitalis and sympathetic stimulation is that both digitalis and catecholamines produce late spontaneous diastolic depolarisation mediated by the inward Ca ion current which may initiate ventricular ectopic rhythms. Such a summation of effect has been observed in Purkinje fibres (Tse and Han, 1974).

Overdosage with Tricyclic Antidepressant Drugs

The cocaine-like action of the tricyclic antidepressants preventing uptake of catecholamines, which leads to increased tissue catecholamine concentrations, are generally thought to contraindicate the simultaneous use of β-adrenergic blocking drugs as α-adrenergic responses would be enhanced. However, some patients with tricyclic overdose present with serious and recurrent ventricular ectopic disturbances and β-adrenergic blockade may then be of therapeutic value (Freeman and Loughead, 1973).

The association between treatment with tricyclic antidepressant drugs and sudden death, particularly in patients with coronary artery disease, may have a similar basis, and coincident treatment with β-adrenergic blocking drugs may be an advantage, although care will be needed to detect and eliminate any evidence of excessive α-adrenergic activity, such as a rise in blood pressure, and control of coincident associated hypertension may be a problem.

SUPRAVENTRICULAR TACHYCARDIAS

Junctional Re-entry Tachycardias

Recent evidence suggests that most repetitive supraventricular tachycardias in apparently normal subjects are due to re-entry mechanisms involving the AV node. The situation is clearest in *Wolff–Parkinson–White* (*WPW*) *syndrome* in which an anomalous communication between the atria and the ventricles (the bundle of Kent), usually placed laterally in the AV groove, allows re-entry of the impulse to the atria, so producing a tachycardia. A similar re-entry process may occur with other anomalous fibres in the region of the AV node (Fig. 7.1). In patients not showing the anomalous connections junctional tachycardias may be produced by a re-entry mechanism utilising two parallel pathways of differing properties (conduction velocity and refractory period) within the meshwork of the AV node itself. In any case, the pathway of the re-entry tachycardia will involve the AV node. The specialised electrical properties of the cells of the AV node, slow conduction due to depolarisation by the slow inward Ca ion current which is under autonomic influence, makes them particularly responsive to β-adrenergic blocking drugs which are often effective in terminating an attack. In the long term these drugs may prevent recurrent episodes by changing the

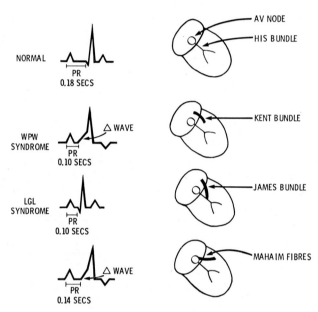

Figure 7.1 Possible abnormal atrioventricular communications which may give rise to pre-excitation or re-entry phenomena producing paroxysmal tachycardia. Diagrams show the normal conducting system (top) and three situations in which abnormal pathways can allow rapid re-entry of the activation process to the atria, producing a junctional tachycardia. The bundle of Kent (Wolff–Parkinson–White (WPW) syndrome) and the James bundle (Lown–Ganong–Levine (LGL) syndrome) bypass the AV node, giving a short P–R interval in the ECG during normal rhythm. The bundle of Kent (WPW) and Mahaim fibres allow abnormal entry of the activation process to the ventricles, giving a slurred onset to the QRS complex (delta (Δ) wave) during normal rhythm. Junctional tachycardia in patients without anomalous connections, may arise by a re-entry process in parallel pathways within the AV node. (Reproduced, with permission, from Hamer, 1975, *An Introduction to Electrocardiography*, Pitman Medical Publishing Co. Ltd, Tunbridge Wells, Kent.)

properties of the re-entry pathway or preventing the atrial or ventricular ectopic beats which, falling outside the refractory period of the pathway, may initiate the tachycardia. In patients with attacks associated with episodes of anxiety, this treatment may be particularly appropriate (Dighton, 1976). In patients with anomalous AV connections (e.g. WPW syndrome) the major risk of conduction of fast atrial arrhythmias, such as atrial fibrillation (AF) or an early atrial ectopic beat to the ventricles through an anomalous connection of short refractory period and high conducting velocity, with the possible risk of induction of ventricular fibrillation if the impulse falls in the vulnerable period of a previous beat (R-on-T phenomenon), is not prevented by this treatment except in so far as initiating atrial ectopic beats are sup-

♂ 62 after AVR

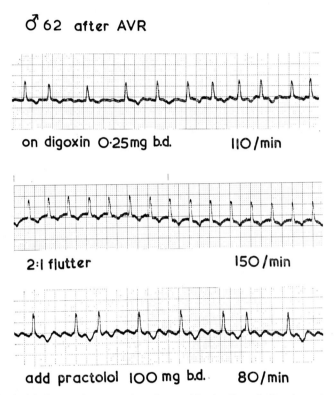

on digoxin 0·25mg b.d.   110/min

2:1 flutter   150/min

add practolol 100 mg b.d.   80/min

Figure 7.2   Atrial flutter, demonstrating the combined effect of digoxin and propranolol. The patient, a man aged 62, developed atrial flutter a few days after aortic valve replacement. All ECGs are lead II. The *top tracing* shows the situation before the onset of flutter. There is atrial fibrillation with a ventricular rate of 110/min on digoxin 0.25 mg b.d. This dose had given good control preoperatively, the relatively rapid rate is probably due to the effect of postoperative stress. The *middle tracing* shows atrial flutter without change in digoxin dose, giving an inconvenient ventricular rate of 150/min (a 2:1 response). The *lower tracing* shows the effect of adding practolol 100 mg b.d. Ventricular rate is reduced to 80/min with an irregular ventricular response. Further convalescence was uneventful

pressed. Additional or alternative drugs or surgical division of the anomalous pathway must therefore be considered.

Atrial Flutter and Fibrillation (AF)

The relatively slow onset of action of digitalis glycosides in atrial fibrillation make these drugs unsuitable for the urgent control of AF in acute situations, as in cardiac infarction or at cardiac catheterisation. Intravenous practolol, slowly up to 10 mg, will usually produce quick control of the ventricular rate before the action of concurrent digitalis glycosides can become effective, although if there is distress from the rapid ventricular rate, as may occur in cardiac infarction shock or in mitral stenosis, the immediate effect of electro-version may be preferred.

Atrial flutter is a notoriously difficult rhythm to control with digitalis glycosides as near toxic doses may be needed to produce the optimal 4:1 block of the flutter needed to produce a ventricular rate of 80 to 100/min, and even so exercise is likely to provoke an improvement in AV conduction to double the ventricular rate by the return of a 2:1 response. Advantage may be taken of the summation of effect of digitalis glycoside and β-adrenergic blocking drugs on AV conduction to produce an optimal response while avoiding the toxic effect of either agent.

A conventional dose of digitalis plus β-adrenergic blockade will usually give adequate control (Fig. 7.2) and prevent the improvement in conduction on exercise which is mediated by sympathetic stimulation. Similar considerations apply to some patients with atrial fibrillation where control at rest is difficult and tachycardia on exercise may be troublesome. The situation can be improved by combining β-adrenergic blockade with digitalis treatment; care must be taken that the reduction in myocardial contractility produced by β-adrenergic blockade does not accentuate congestive heart failure, but in some patients a satisfactory regime can be established on this basis.

THYROTOXICOSIS

Many of the changes produced by thyrotoxicosis are mediated by sympathetic stimulation, and the circulatory effects may be abolished by β-sympathetic blockade; these drugs replacing reserpine which has been used for this purpose in the past. The reduction in tachycardia and in cardiac output produced by these drugs may eliminate many of the symptoms of thyrotoxicosis (Turner, 1974; McDevitt, 1976). Tremor may improve as do other forms of tremor in anxiety or idiopathic tremor (see later, p. 191). Prompt satisfactory control of thyrotoxicosis may be achieved and this therapeutic approach can be used while awaiting the effects of definitive treatment; such as antithyroid drugs (e.g. carbimazole) or radioactive iodine. This regime has also been used with iodine as a preliminary to thyroidectomy with satisfactory results.

Control of sinus tachycardia in thyrotoxicosis is generally achieved and is a useful guide to dosage. In atrial fibrillation the effect of digitalis treatment will usually be needed to control the ventricular rate, but the summation of effect on the AV node may reduce the dose of digitalis needed.

PSYCHIATRIC DISTURBANCES

Anxiety States

The relief of palpitation from sinus tachycardia or ectopic beats may have a general beneficial effect in anxiety by removing a feed-back mechanism produced by these symptoms which may in themselves lead to anxiety. Tremor is also relieved with similar benefit.

Some consider that a central effect of those drugs (Conway, 1975) may act to improve anxiety states, although such a response is likely to be confined to those which penetrate the central nervous system, such as propranolol (Suzman, 1976), rather than the less lipid-soluble drugs, such as practolol, which do not but are nevertheless effective in anxiety (Benn, Turner and Hicks, 1972).

Tremor

The improvement of tremor in anxiety states and in thyrotoxicosis has led to trial of these drugs in other forms of tremor. Essential tremor both in younger and older subjects responds, and anecdotal evidence of improved marksmanship on the rifle range may have a similar basis. The rhythmic movements of Parkinson's disease are however less affected. The effect is a local one, mediated by β receptors in skeletal muscle and the same mechanism is responsible for the tremor produced by β-sympathetic agonists (Watson and Richens, 1974).

Schizophrenia

Reports are beginning to appear of a beneficial effect of centrally acting β-adrenergic blocking drugs, such as propranolol, in schizophrenia (Yorkston et al, 1976). A recently demonstrated inhibition of central effect of serotonin may be responsible (Green and Grahame-Smith, 1976). Although full study is needed to reach definite conclusions, early work gives ground for optimism. Large does are generally required and cardiovascular side-effects, such as symptomatic bradycardia and hypotension, may eliminate some patients before therapeutic doses can be reached. Large doses introduced suddenly may produce a paradoxical hypertensive reaction.

Drug Addiction

Narcotic withdrawal in addicts is said to be facilitated by β-adrenergic blocking drugs. The benefit is partly by removing the sympathetically mediated effects of narcotic withdrawal, but a central contribution may also be present in the response as heroin euphoria is said to be prevented by propranolol and the craving after withdrawal attenuated (Grosz, 1974).

Propranolol has also been found useful in the withdrawal phase of chronic alcoholism, either by suppressing a hyperkinetic circulatory response or by a central action decreasing tension (Carlsson, 1976).

PHAEOCHROMOCYTOMA

The excessive catecholamine secretion of these tumours is evident as both α- and β-adrenergic stimulation. Alpha effects predominate in the nor-adrenaline secreting ectopic tumours and play a major role in tumours of the adrenal medulla which tend to secrete adrenaline also. Beta sympathetic effects are mainly found in this group and include sinus tachycardia, ectopic rhythms and excessive myocardial contraction contributing to focal necrosis, which is probably in part related to the α effect on the coronary arteries (i.e. vasoconstriction). A major problem in the control of the β-adrenergic mani-festations with specific blocking drugs is that such treatment necessarily potentiates the effect of α-adrenergic stimulation and may allow a dangerous hypertensive paroxysm, leading to acute coronary insufficiency, probably from the combination of effects on the coronary arteries and the greatly increased load on the left ventricle. Even small doses of β-adrenergic blocking drugs may provoke a serious reaction.

β-Adrenergic blocking drugs are not therefore suitable as primary treatment for angina or hypertension in patients with phaeochromocytoma. An adverse reaction to such treatment is not a good way to diagnose this condition.

The primary treatment of phaeochromocytoma should therefore be with α-adrenergic blocking drugs, such as the relatively long-acting phenoxy-benzamine, phentolamine or parenteral thymoxamine. Preoperative pre-paration with these drugs will allow restoration of the reduced circulating blood volume, which is secondary to the prolonged vasoconstriction, to increase the safety of surgical removal of the tumour and will control the hypertension. When this treatment is established, β-adrenergic blocking drugs can be used to control specific features such as tachycardia.

During operation, blood pressure will be controlled by α-adrenergic blocking drugs, and β-adrenergic blocking drugs can be kept in reserve to control any episode of tachycardia or ventricular ectopic rhythm provoked for instance by handling the tumour. After the operation, careful withdrawal of the α-sympathetic blocking drugs is needed to avoid hypotension. For this reason short-acting agents (phentolomine or thymoxamine) are usually preferred to cover the operative period.

PERIPHERAL VASOCONSTRICTION

The peripheral vasoconstrictor effect of the non-cardioselective β-adrenergic blocking drugs may produce cold extremities as a side-effect of treatment in angina or hypertension, particularly in susceptible subjects, such as patients with Raynaud's phenomenon. Advantage has been taken of this action in the treatment of migraine where a useful effect is obtained (Bøgesen, 1976).

REFERENCES

A Multicentre International Study (1975) Improvement in progress of myocardial infarction by long-term beta-adrenoceptor blockade using practolol. *British Medical Journal*, **3**, 735.

Amende, J., Coltart, D. J., Krayenbuhl, H. P. & Rutishauser, W. (1975) Assessment of left ventricular contraction and relaxation in patients with coronary heart disease. *European Journal of Cardiology*, **3**, 37.

Backer, L. C., Ferreira, R. & Thomas, H. (1975) Effect of propranolol and isoprenaline in experimental myocardial ischaemia. *Cardiovascular Research*, **9**, 178.

Balcon, R., Maloy, W. C. & Sowton, E. (1968) Clinical use of atrial pacing test in angina pectoris. *British Medical Journal*, **3**, 91.

Barlow, J. B. & Pocock, W. A. (1975) The problem of non-ejection systolic clicks and associated mitral systolic murmurs. Emphasis on the billowing mitral valve syndrome. *American Heart Journal*, **90**, 636.

Barrett, A. M. (1973) The pharmacology of beta-adrenoceptor antagonists. In *Recent Advances in Cardiology*, 6th edn, ed. Hamer, J. Edinburgh and London: Churchill Livingstone.

Benn, J. A., Turner, P. & Hicks, D. C. (1972) Beta-adrenergic receptor blockade with practolol in treatment of anxiety. *Lancet*, **1**, 814.

Bøgesen, S. E. (1976) Treatment of migraine with propranolol. *Postgraduate Medical Journal*, **52**, Suppl. 4, 163.

Bourgoignie, J. J., Catanzaro, F. T. & Perry, H. H. (1968) Renin–angiotension–aldosterone system during chronic thiazide therapy of benign hypertension. *Circulation*, **37**, 27.

Braunwald, E. & Maroko, P. R. (1974) Reduction of infarct size—an idea whose time (for testing) has come. *Circulation*, **50**, 206.

British Medical Journal (1971) Prinzmetal's variant angina. **2**, 298.

Brooks, H., Banes, J. S., Dalen, J. F. & Dexter, L. (1971) Cardiovascular and contractile responses to non-depressant beta-adrenergic blockade. *American Journal of Physiology*, **221**, 138.

Bühler, F. R., Laragh, J. H., Vaughan, E. D., Brunner, H. R., Gavros, H. & Baer, L. (1973) The antihypertensive action of propranolol: specific antirenin responses in high and normal renin essential, real, renovascular and malignant hypertension. *American Journal of Cardiology*, **39**, 511.

Bühler, F. R., Marbet, G., Patel, U. & Burkart, F. (1975) Renin-suppressing potency of various beta-adrenergic blocking agents at supine rest and during upright exercise. *Clinical Science and Molecular Medicine*, **48**, 615.

Carlsson, C. (1976) Propranolol in the treatment of alcoholism: a review. *Postgraduate Medical Journal*, **52**, Suppl. 4, 166.

Cohn, K., Selzer, A., Kersh, E. S., Karpren, L. S. & Goldschlager, N. (1975) Variability of haemodynamic responses to acute digitalisation in chronic cardiac failure due to cardiomyopathy and coronary artery disease. *American Journal of Cardiology*, **35**, 461.

Coltart, D. J. (1971) Comparison of effects of propranolol and practolol on exercise tolerance in angina pectoris. *British Heart Journal*, **33**, 62.

Coltart, D. J., Cayen, M. N., Stinson, E. B., Goldman, R. H., Davies, R. O. & Harrison, P. C. (1975) Investigation of the safe withdrawal period for propranolol in patients scheduled for open heart surgery. *British Heart Journal*, **37**, 1228.

Conway, J. (1975) Beta-adrenergic blockade and hypertension. In *Modern Trends in Cardiology*, ed. Oliver, M. F., Vol. 3, p. 376. London and Boston: Butterworth.

Crawford, M. H., Le Wintor, M. M., O'Rourke, R. A., Karliner, J. S. & Ross, J. (1975) Combined propranolol and digoxin therapy in angina pectoris. *Annals of Internal Medicine*, **83**, 449.

Cruickshank, J. M., Neil-Dwyer, G. & Lane, J. (1975) The effect of oral propranolol upon the ECG changes occurring in subarachnoid haemorrhage. *Cardiovascular Research*, **9**, 236.

Davidson, C. & Gibson, D. (1973) Clinical significance of positive inotropic action of digoxin in patients with left ventricular disease.. *British Heart Journal*, **35**, 970.

Davis, L. D., Temple, J. V. & Murphy, G. R. (1969) Epinephrine-cyclopropane effects on Purkinje's fibers. *Anesthesiology*, **36**, 369.
de Quattro, V. & Chan, S. (1972) Raised plasma catecholamines in some patients with primary hypertension. *Lancet*, **1**, 806.
Diaz, R., Somberg, J., Freeman, E. & Levitt, B. (1974) Myocardial infarction after propranolol withdrawal. *American Heart Journal*, **88**, 257.
Dighton, D. H. (1976) The autonomic features of supraventricular tachycardia. *British Heart Journal*, **38**, 319.
Dollery, C. T., Lewis, P. J., Muers, M. G. & Reid, J. L. (1973) Central hypotensive effect of propranolol in the rabbit. *British Journal of Pharmacology*, **45**, 343P.
Donsky, M. S., Harris, M. D., Curry, G. C., Blonquist, C. G., Willerson, J. T. & Mullins, C. B. (1975) Variant angina pectoris: a clinical and arteriographic spectrum. *American Heart Journal*, **89**, 571.
Doyle, A. E., Jerums, G., Johnston, C. J. & Louis, W. J. (1973) Plasma renin levels and vascular complications in hypertension. *British Medical Journal*, **2**, 206.
East, T. & Oran, S. (1948) Cardiac pain with recovery of the T wave. *British Heart Journal*, **10**, 263.
Eliot, R. S. & Bratt, G. (1969) The paradox of myocardial ischaemia and neurosis in young women with normal coronary arteriograms. Relation to abnormal hemoglobin–oxygen dissociation. *American Journal of Cardiology*, **23**, 633.
Faulkner, S. L., Hopkins, J. T., Boerth, R. C., Young, J. L., Jellett, L. B., Nies, A. S., Bender, H. W. & Shand, D. G. (1973) Time required for complete recovery from chronic propranolol therapy. *New England Journal of Medicine*, **289**, 607.
Fowler, P. B. S., Ikram, H., Maini, R. N., Makey, A. R. & Kirkham, J. S. (1969) Bradycardiac angina: haemodynamic aspects and treatment. *British Medical Journal*, **1**, 92.
Fox, K. M., Chopra, M. P., Portal, R. W. & Aber, C. P. (1975) Long-term beta blocker: possible protection from myocardial infarction. *British Medical Journal*, **1**, 117.
Freeman, J. W. & Loughead, M. G. (1973) Beta blockade in the treatment of tricyclic antidepressant overdosage. *Medical Journal of Australia*, **60**, 1233.
Frohlich, E. D., Tarazi, R. C., Duston, H. P. & Page, I. H. (1968) The paradox of beta-adrenergic blockade in hypertension. *Circulation*, **37**, 417.
Fulton, M., Duncan, B., Lutz, W., Morrison, S. L., Donald, K. W., Kerr, F., Kirby, B. T., Julian, D. G. & Oliver, M. F. (1972) Natural history of unstable angina. *Lancet*, **1**, 860.
Gettes, L. S. (1975) Electrophysiologic basis of arrhythmias in acute myocardial ischaemia. In *Modern Trends in Cardiology*, ed. Oliver, M. F., Vol. 3, p. 219. London and Boston: Butterworths.
Gibson, D. G. (1974) Pharmacodynamic properties of β-adrenergic receptor blocking drugs in man. *Drugs*, **7**, 8.
Gibson, D., Hoy, J. & Sowton, E. (1974) Comparison of haemodynamic effects of oxprenolol (Trasicor), alprenolol (Aptin) and sotalol (MJ 1999) in man. *British Heart Journal*, **32**, 553P.
Gillis, R. A., Pearle, D. L. & Levitt, B. (1975) Digitalis: a neuro-excitatory drug. *Circulation*, **52**, 739.
Goodwin, J. F. (1974) Prospects and predictions for the cardiomyopathies. *Circulation*, **50**, 216.
Grandjean, F. & Rivier, J. L. (1968) Cardio-circulatory effects of beta-adrenergic blockade in organic heart disease. Comparison between propranolol and CIBA 39089 Ba. *British Heart Journal*, **30**, 50.
Green, A. R. & Grahame-Smith, D. G. (1976) (−)-propranolol inhibits the behavioural responses of rats to increased 5-hydroxy-tryptamine in the central nervous system. *Nature*, **262**, 594.
Grosz, H. J. (1974) Effect of propranolol on active users of heroin. *Lancet*, **1**, 612.
Hamer, J. (1975) W. G. Smith Memorial Lecture given in Perth, Western Australia, June 1975.
Hamer, J. (1976) Renin and beta-adrenergic blockade: the mechanism of the hypotensive effect. *British Journal of Clinical Pharmacology*, **3**, 425.
Hamer, J. & Fleming, J. (1969) Action of propranolol on left ventricular contraction in aortic stenosis when a fall in heart rate is prevented by atropine. *British Heart Journal*, **6**, 670.
Hamer, J. & Sowton, E. (1966) Effect of propranolol on exercise tolerance in angina pectoris. *American Journal of Cardiology*, **18**, 354.

Han, J. & Moe, G. K. (1964) Non-uniform recovery of excitation in ventricular muscle. *Circulation Research*, **14**, 44.

Hansson, L., Åberg, H., Karlberg, B. E. & Westerland, A. (1975) Controlled study of atenolol in treatment of hypertension. *British Medical Journal*, **3**, 367.

Hardarson, T., de la Calzada, C. S., Curiel, R. & Goodwin, J. F. (1973) Prognosis and mortality of hypertrophic obstructive cardiomyopathy. *Lancet*, **2**, 1462.

Harris, P. (1975) A theory concerning the course of events in angina and myocardial infarction. *European Journal of Cardiology*, **3**, 157.

Herman, M. V., Cohn, P. F. & Gorlin, R. (1973) Angina-like chest pain without identifiable cause. *Annals of Internal Medicine*, **29**, 445.

Hollifield, J. W., Sherman, K., Zuagg, R. V. & Shand, D. G. (1976) Proposed mechanism of propranolol's hypotensive effect in essential hypertension. *New England Journal of Medicine*, **295**, 68.

Howitt, G., Husainy, M., Rowland, D. T., Logan, W. F., Shanks, R. G. & Evans, M. G. (1965) The effect of the dextro-isomer of propranolol on sinus and cardiac arrhythmias. *American Heart Journal*, **76**, 736.

Ibrahim, M. M., Tarazi, R. C., Dustan, H. P., Bravo, E. L. & Gifford, R. W. (1975) Hyperkinetic heart in severe hypertension: a separate clinical hemodynamic entity. *American Journal of Cardiology*, **35**, 667.

Jackson, G., Atkinson, L. & Oram, S. (1975) Reassessment of failed beta-blocker treatment in angina pectoris by peak-exercise heart-rate measurements. *British Medical Journal*, **3**, 616.

Jochuk, S. T., Ramon, P. S., Clerk, P. & Kalbaq, R. M. (1975) Electrocardiographic abnormalities associated with raised intracranial pressure. *British Medical Journal*, **1**, 242.

Julius, S., Ester, M. D. & Randall, O. S. (1975) Role of the autonomic nervous system in mild human hypertension. *Clinical Science and Molecular Medicine*, **48**, 2435.

Karlberg, B. E., Kågedal, B., Tegler, L. & Tolagen, K. (1976) Renin concentrations and effects of propranolol and spironolactone in patients with hypertension. *British Medical Journal*, **1**, 251.

King, M. J., Zir, L. M., Kaltman, A. J. & Fox, A. C. (1973) Variant angina associated with angiographically demonstrated coronary artery spasm and REM sleep. *American Journal of Medical Science*, **265**, 419.

Koch-Weser, J. (1975) Non-beta-blocking actions of propranolol. *New England Journal of Medicine*, **293**, 988.

Lancet (1974) Beta-blockade and size of acute myocardial infarction. **2**, 813.

Lands, A. M., Arnold, A., McAuliff, J. P., Ludena, F. P. & Brown, J. G. (1967) Differentiation of receptor systems activated by sympathomimetic amines. *Nature*, **211**, 597.

Leonetti, G., Meyer, G., Terzoli, L., Zanchetti, A., Bianchetti, G., di Salle, E., Morselli, P. L. & Chidsey, C. A. (1975) Hypotensive and renin-suppressing activities of propranolol in hypertensive patients. *Clinical Science and Molecular Medicine*, **48**, 491.

Lichtman, M. A., Cohen, J., Murphy, M. S., Kearnes, E. A. & Whitback, A. A. (1974) Effect of propranolol on oxygen binding to hemoglobin in vitro and in vivo. *Circulation*, **49**, 881.

Lindén, V. (1974) Anterior and inferior myocardial infarction. Comparison with regard to some diseases and background factors. *British Heart Journal*, **36**, 1092.

Lloyd-Mostyn, R. H. & Oram, S. (1975) Modification by propranolol of cardiovascular effects of induced hypoglycaemia. *Lancet*, **1**, 1213.

Lohmöller, G. & Frohlich, E. D. (1975) A comparison of timolol and propranolol in essential hypertension. *American Heart Journal*, **891**, 437.

MacAlpin, R. N., Kattus, A. A. & Winfield, M. E. (1965) The effect of a β-adrenergic-blocking agent (Nethalide) and nitroglycerine on exercise tolerance in angina pectoris. *Circulation*, **31**, 869.

MacAlpin, R. N., Kattus, A. A. & Alvaro, A. B. (1973) Angina pectoris at rest with preservation of exercise capacity. Prinzmetal's variant angina. *Circulation*, **47**, 946.

McDevitt, D. G. (1976) Propranolol in the treatment of thyrotoxicosis. *Postgraduate Medical Journal*, suppl. 4, 157.

MacGregor, G. A. & Dawes, P. (1975) Antihypertensive effect of propranolol and spironolactone in relation to plasma angiotensin II. *Clinical Science and Molecular Medicine*, **19**, 18P.

Mamohansingh, P. & Parker, J. O. (1975) Angina pectoris with normal coronary arteriograms: hemodynamic and metabolic responses to atrial pacers. *American Heart Journal*, **90**, 635.

Mizgala, H. F. & Counsell, J. (1974) Acute coronary syndromes following abrupt cessation of oral propranolol therapy. *Circulation*, **49, 50**, Suppl., 111–33.

Morgan, T. O., Roberts, R., Carney, S. L., Louis, W. J. & Doyle, A. E. (1975) β-Adrenergic receptor blocking drugs, hypertension and plasma renin. *British Journal of Clinical Pharmacology*, **2**, 159.

Mulholland, H. C. & Pantridge, J. F. (1974) Heart rate changes during movement of patients with acute myocardial infarction. *Lancet*, **1**, 1244.

Naylor, W. G. & Sebra-Gomez, R. (1975) Excitation–contraction coupling in cardiac muscle. *Progress in Cardiovascular Disease*, **18**, 75.

Nicholls, M. G., Espiner, E. A., Donald, R. A. & Hughes, H. (1974) Aldosterone and its regulation during diuresis in patients with gross congestive heart failure. *Clinical Science and Molecular Medicine*, **47**, 301.

Ogden, P. C., Selzer, A. & Cohn, K. E. (1969) The relationship between the inotropic and dromotropic effects of digitalis: the modulation of these effects by autonomic influences. *American Heart Journal*, **77**, 628.

Oliver, M. F. (1975) The vulnerable ischaemic myocardium and its metabolism. In *Modern Trends in Cardiology*, ed. Oliver, M. F., Vol. 3, p. 250. London and Boston: Butterworth.

Pantridge, J. F. (1974) Mobile coronary care units. In *Prospects in the Management of Ischaemic Heart Disease*, ed. Muir, J. R. p. 36. Horsham, England: CIBA Laboratories.

Pantridge, J. F., Webb, S. W., Adgey, A. A. J. & Geddes, J. S. (1974) The first hour after the onset of acute myocardial infarction. *Progress in Cardiology*, **3**, 172.

Prichard, B. N. C. (1976) Propranolol in the treatment of angina. *Postgraduate Medical Journal*, **52**, supplement 4, 35.

Prichard B. N. C., Shinebourne, L., Fleming, J. & Hamer, J. (1970) Haemodynamic studies in hypertensive patients treated by oral propranolol. *British Heart Journal*, **32**, 236.

Prichard, B. N. C. & Gillam, P. M. S. (1966) Propranolol in hypertension. *American Journal of Cardiology*, **18**, 387.

Prichard, B. N. C. & Gillam, P. M. S. (1971) Assessment of propranolol in angina pectoris. Clinical dose–response curve and effect on electrocardiogram at rest and on exercise. *British Heart Journal*, **33**, 473.

Raab, W. (1945) Adreno-sympathogenic heart disease (neurohormonal factors in pathogenesis and treatment). *Annals of Internal Medicine*, **28**, 1010.

Richardson, P. J., Livesley, P., Oram, S., Olsen, E. G. T. & Armstrong, P. (1974) Angina pectoris with normal coronary arteries. *Lancet*, **2**, 677.

Rutenberg, H. L. & Spann, J. F. (1973) Alterations of cardiac sympathetic neurotransmitter activity in congestive heart failure. *American Journal of Cardiology*, **32**, 472.

Safar, M. J., Landor, G. M., Weiss, Y. A. & Milliez, P. L. (1975) Vascular reactivity to norepinephrine and haemodynamic parameters in borderline hypotension. *American Heart Journal*, **89**, 480.

Schwartz, P. J., Periti, M. & Malliani, A. (1975) The long Q–T syndrome. *American Heart Journal*, **89**, 378.

Sharma, B. & Taylor, S. H. (1973) A critical review of the symptomatic, electrocardiographic and circulatory effects of beta-receptor antagonists in angina pectoris. In *New Perspectives in Beta-Blockade*, ed. Barley, D. M., Frier, J. H., Rondel, R. K. & Taylor, S. H., p. 129. Horsham, England: CIBA Laboratories.

Singh, P. N. & Vaughan Williams, E. M. (1970) A third class of anti-arrhythmic action. Effects on atrial and ventricular intracellular potentials and other pharmacological action on cardiac muscle. *British Journal of Pharmacology*, **39**, 675.

Sowton, E., Bennett, D., Smith, E., Balcon, R. & Gibson, D. (1970) Antidysrhythmic effects of beta-blocking drugs. In *Symposium on Cardiac Arrhythmias*, ed. Sandoe, E., Flensted-Jensen, E., & Olesen, K. H. Sodertälje: AB Astra.

Stephens, J., Hamer, J., Hayward, R. & Ead, H. (1975) The effect of selective and non-selective beta-blockade on the coronary circulation in man. *British Heart Journal*, **38**, 311.

Suzman, M. M. (1976) Propranolol in the treatment of anxiety. *Postgraduate Medical Journal*, **52**, Suppl. 4, 168.

Taylor, S. H. (1975) Pathophysiology of angina pectoris. Presented at *National Conference on Cardiology*, London, December 1975.

Taylor, S. H., Davidson, C., Singleton, W. & Thadani, V. (1976) A comparison of the antihypertensive effectiveness of beta-adrenoreceptor antagonists with differing pharmacological properties. *British Heart Journal*, **38**, 313.

Taylor, S. H., Thadani, V. & Sharma, B. (1973) Comparison of the symptomatic, electrocardiographic and circulatory effects of propranolol, oxprenolol and practolol in angina pectoris. In *New Perspectives in Beta-Blockade*, ed. Barley, D. M., Frier, J. H., Rondel, R. K. & Taylor, S. H., p. 177. Horsham, England: CIBA Laboratories.

Tse, W. W. & Han, J. (1974) Interaction of epinephrine and ovabovine on automaticity of Purkinje fibres. *Circulation Research*, **34**, 777.

Turner, P. (1974) β-Adrenergic receptor blocking drugs in hyperthyroidism. *Drugs*, **7**, 48.

Vaughan Williams, E. M., Raine, A. E. G., Cabrero, A. A. & Whyte, J. M. (1975) The effects of prolonged β-adrenoreceptor blockade on heart weight and cardiac intracellular potential in rabbits. *Cardiovascular Research*, **9**, 579.

Waagstein, F., Hjalmarson, A., Varnauskas, E. & Wallentin, J. (1975) Effect of chronic beta-adrenergic receptor blocked in congestive cardiomyopathy. *British Heart Journal*, **37**, 1022.

Warren, D. J., Swainson, C. D. & Wright, N. (1974) Deterioration in renal function after beta-blockade in patients with chronic renal failure and hypertension. *British Medical Journal*, **2**, 193.

Watson, J. M. & Richens, A. (1974) The effects of salbutamol and terbutaline on physiological tremor, bronchial tone and heart rate. *British Journal of Clinical Pharmacology*, **1**, 223.

Webb-Peploe, M. M., Croxson, R. S., Oakley, C. M. & Goodwin, J. F. (1971) Cardioselective beta-adrenergic blockade in hypertrophic obstructive cardiomyopathy. *Postgraduate Medical Journal*, **47**, Suppl., 93.

Wilhelmsson, C., Vedin, J. A., Wilhelmsson, L., Tibblin, G. & Warkö, L. (1974) Reduction of sudden deaths after myocardial infarction by treatment with alprenolol. *Lancet*, **2**, 1157.

Wit, A. L., Hoffman, B. F. & Rosen, M. R. (1975) Electrophysiology and pharmacology of cardiac arrhythmias. IX. Cardiac electrophysiologic effects of beta-adrenergic stimulation and blockade. *American Heart Journal*, **70**, 521, 665.

Wright, P. (1975) Untoward effects associated with practolol administration. *British Medical Journal*, **1**, 595.

Yasua, H., Tanyama, M., Shimanoto, M., Kato, H., Tanako, S. & Akiyama, F. (1974) Role of autonomic nervous system in the pathogenesis of Prinzmetal's variant form of angina. *Circulation*, **50**, 834.

Yorkston, N. J., Zaki, S. A., Themen, J. F. A. & Havard, C. V. H. (1976) Safeguards in the treatment of schizophrenia with propranolol. *Postgraduate Medical Journal*, **52**, suppl. 4, 175.

8
AETIOLOGY OF HYPERTENSION
C. R. W. Edwards

It is now clear that arterial hypertension does not have a single cause. Conventionally, hypertension is classified on the basis of its aetiology into a primary, idiopathic category, usually referred to as essential hypertension, and a secondary group including patients with phaeochromocytoma, renovascular disease or adrenocortical hyperactivity. However, it is now becoming obvious that even patients with essential hypertension do not belong to a homogeneous group. Various authors have, for example, further classified these patients into low renin, normal renin and high renin groups, and have suggested that this classification has important implications for treatment.

It is a truism, all too commonly forgotten, that to understand hypertension requires an understanding of the mechanisms controlling normal blood pressure. Thus a full review of recent advances in the aetiology of hypertension would cover humoral factors affecting blood pressure such as angiotensin, catecholamines, serotonin, prostaglandins, mineralocorticoid steroids and salt; factors affecting blood vessel reactivity and elasticity, peripheral resistance, blood viscosity, plasma and extracellular fluid volume, cardiac output, and neural control mechanisms. However, to aid digestion I have chosen to structure this review on the basis of classifying hypertensive diseases into those associated with high, normal or low plasma renin activity. This approach emphasises the major advances that have been made in the diagnosis and treatment of angiotensinogenic hypertension and also highlights the progress of steroid chemistry that has led to the isolation of mineralocorticoid steroids, other than aldosterone, that may play a role in the genesis of certain types of essential hypertension. This chapter, therefore, encompasses a review of these advances and an indication as to whether or not they constitute anything more than a ripple on the Gaussian distribution curve of the hypertensive population.

HYPERTENSION ASSOCIATED WITH ELEVATED PLASMA RENIN ACTIVITY

The idea that the kidneys may play a part in the genesis of certain types of hypertension originated from the observations of Richard Bright (1827) in patients with nephritis. Further support for the association came from the demonstration by Tigerstedt and Bergman (1898) of the pressor action of a crude kidney extract and the discovery by Goldblatt et al (1934) that clamping the renal artery of a dog with subsequent removal of the opposite kidney produced a chronic elevation in blood pressure. This led to the demonstration of the renin–angiotensin system (Braun-Menendez et al, 1939; Page and Helmer, 1940). These workers showed that a renal enzyme, renin, acts on a substrate, angiotensinogen (an α_2-globulin produced by the liver), to form a decapeptide, angiotensin I, which is then broken down by a converting enzyme to an octapeptide, angiotensin II. Despite the fact that this is a potent pressor agent there has been considerable controversy as to whether it has a direct role in renal hypertension or acts indirectly by stimulating the production of aldosterone.

Inhibitors of the Renin–Angiotensin System

Several methods have been used to inhibit the renin–angiotensin system and thus determine its importance in the maintenance of hypertension. Eide and Aars (1969) found that immunisation of rabbits with an angiotensin II protein conjugate did not prevent the development of renal hypertension. This was despite the fact that high titre antisera were produced which blocked the effect of injected angiotensin II. This suggested that the pressor action of angiotensin was not responsible for the hypertension in these animals. However, subsequent work has shown that this method produces a less effective blockade than other chemical inhibitors, possibly because angiotensin II may be generated at a site that is inaccessible to the angiotensin antiserum (Thurston and Swales, 1974).

Recently the introduction of two new peptides that inhibit the renin–angiotensin system has helped to clarify the role of angiotensin. One of these is a nonapeptide, isolated from the venom of the South American pit viper, which inhibits the enzyme that converts angiotensin I to angiotensin II. Gavras and his colleagues (1974) showed that a single intravenous injection of this inhibitor lowered blood pressure in patients with renovascular hypertension. At the same time there was a rise in plasma renin activity and a fall in plasma aldosterone. In contrast, the second peptide called saralasin is a competitive antagonist of angiotensin II. This compound differs by only two amino acids from angiotensin II (Pals et al, 1971). Infusion of this drug has been shown to lower blood pressure in patients with hypertension associated with elevated plasma renin activity, such as malignant or advanced renovascular hypertension (Brunner, Gavras and Laragh, 1973). This drug may not only be of considerable therapeutic value in the emergency treatment of such patients but may also be of diagnostic use. Streeten and his colleagues (1975) found that infusion of saralasin blocked the hypertensive effect of angiotensin II in normal subjects. To investigate whether the drug could be used to identify patients with 'angiotensinogenic' hypertension they infused saralasin into 60 hypertensive subjects. In 16 of these patients the drug lowered the blood pressure. Radiographic investigation of 10 patients in this group showed that 9 had a renal artery stenosis. Other studies showed that this group was also characterised by elevated peripheral and renal vein plasma renin activity. In the four patients subjected to surgery nephrectomy produced a moderate or excellent response. These initial results suggest that infusion of this drug could be used as a screening procedure but obviously further experience is necessary before the role of saralasin in predicting patients that may respond to renovascular surgery is established.

Primary Reninism

This important syndrome of hypertension associated with a tumour of the juxtaglomerular apparatus was first described by Robertson and his colleagues in 1967. Since then several other cases have been described (Kihara et al, 1968; Eddy and Sanchez, 1971; Bonnin, Hodge and Lumbers, 1972; Conn et al, 1972; Schambelan and Biglieri, 1972). The majority of the patients have been less than 25 years old and have had severe hypertension with moderate hypokalaemia, elevated plasma renin activity and increased aldosterone secretion. Renal arteriography has shown that the vasculature is normal and in some cases has identified the tumour in the cortex. Selective renal vein catheterisation has shown elevated plasma renin activity in the venous blood coming from the kidney containing the tumour. Following nephrectomy the blood pressure has been lowered to normal levels. Histology of the tumour is that of a haemangiopericytoma, and electron microscopy has shown typical renin granules containing diamond and rhomboid-shaped crystalline inclusions, identical with those seen in normal juxtaglomerular cells (Conn et al, 1972). Extraction of the tumours has demonstrated that they contain up to 100 times the normal kidney content of renin, and further proof of renin synthesis has been provided by immunofluorescent and tissue culture studies.

Secondary Reninism

Diuretic therapy

The commonest cause of an elevated level of plasma renin activity in patients with hypertension is treatment with diuretics, in particular those of the benzothiadiazine group. In some patients the plasma renin activity and angiotensin II levels return to normal within a few weeks of starting treatment (Bourgoignie, Catanzaro and Perry, 1968; Catt et al, 1971) but in others the levels remain elevated for more than 12 months (Brown et al, 1972).

Renal artery stenosis and intrinsic renal disease

The hypertension of a significant number of patients with unilateral renal artery stenosis or renal disease responds to surgical treatment either by nephrectomy or corrective renovascular surgery. The main problem has been to determine those patients that may benefit from surgery. The possible use of inhibitors of the renin–angiotensin system has been discussed but this is at present in an experimental stage. The usefulness of renal vein renin activity measurements to determine the functional significance of a renal artery stenosis was first reported by Judson and Helmer (1965). Other studies have confirmed the importance of this technique. Amsterdam and his colleagues (1969) showed that if the ratio of the plasma renin activity values on the affected to unaffected sides was greater than 2.5:1 the outcome of surgery was likely to be good. Using this value the prognostic accuracy was 90 per cent as compared to 46 per cent using the results of the intravenous pyelogram, 50 per cent for divided renal function studies and 62 per cent for peripheral venous renin activity.

Stockigt and his collaborators (1972) measured renal vein renin activity in 110 patients with suspected renal hypertension, 78 of whom had renal artery stenosis while 32 had other abnormalities including unilateral hydronephrosis, segmental renal infarction and intrarenal vascular malformations. Of this group 41 were treated surgically. The results in this group showed that a renal vein renin activity ratio greater than 1.5:1 was useful in predicting a satisfactory response. Laragh's group have suggested that a better prediction can be obtained using a scoring system based on three criteria—abnormally high peripheral plasma renin activity in relation to sodium excretion, complete suppression of renin secretion from the contralateral uninvolved kidney and an abnormally increased renal vein renin content relative to arterial renin from the ischaemic kidney (Vaughan et al, 1973).

Experimental studies in animals have shown that when one renal artery is constricted and hypertension results the kidney on the side of the stenosis is spared vascular damage. Wilson and Byrom (1939) suggested that damage to the untouched kidney might be responsible for maintaining hypertension when the renal artery clip was removed. An analogous situation may occur in man. Three cases have now been described in whom renovascular surgery for a unilateral renal artery stenosis did not relieve hypertension but the blood pressure was lowered by removal of the contralateral kidney (Thal, Grage and Vernier, 1963; Miller and Phillips, 1968; McAllister et al, 1972).

Malignant hypertension

Elevated levels of plasma renin activity, angiotensin II and aldosterone are found in most patients with malignant hypertension. This has been well reviewed by Glaz and Vecsei (1971). The extremely high levels of renin are associated with low plasma sodium levels in contrast to the normal or elevated plasma sodium found in Conn's syndrome (Brown et al, 1965, 1966). The high aldosterone secretion is not altered by changes in sodium intake (Laragh et al, 1960), and results in excessive potassium loss with hypokalaemia. Successful therapy for the hypertension results in lowering of plasma renin activity and aldosterone, and return of the plasma electrolytes to normal (Gill et al, 1964). This is thought to be due to resolution of the vascular changes in the small vessels of the kidney that have inappropriately stimulated the release of renin. The key to the distinction between malignant hypertension and Conn's syndrome is measurement of plasma renin activity. In the future, however, it would seem likely that infusion of an inhibitor of the renin–angiotensin system such as saralasin would be the most immediate method of confirming the diagnosis of 'angiotensinogenic' hypertension and would provide an effective and safe method of lowering the blood pressure.

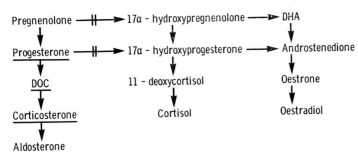

Figure 8.1 Pathways of adrenocortical steroid biosynthesis indicating the block produced by 17α-hydroxylase enzyme deficiency

HYPERTENSION ASSOCIATED WITH LOW PLASMA RENIN ACTIVITY

Congenital or Familial Causes of Low-renin Hypertension

17α-Hydroxylase deficiency syndrome

In 1966 Biglieri, Herron and Brust described a new syndrome resulting from defective 17-hydroxylation in both the adrenals and the gonads (Fig. 8.1). This defect results in inadequate cortisol secretion and hence, via the negative feedback mechanism, increased ACTH secretion. The resulting excess secretion of corticosterone and deoxycorticosterone produces a mineralocorticoid excess syndrome characterised by hypertension and a hypokalaemic alkalosis.

As the enzyme defect is also present in the gonads these patients cannot synthesise androgens or oestrogens. Thus the women have had primary amenorrhoea and the men have been pseudohermaphrodites. The aldosterone secretion rate in this syndrome is low and it was suggested that there might be a second biosynthetic defect. Bricaire and his colleagues (1972) found a five-fold elevation of the secretion rate of 18-hydroxycorticosterone (18-OH-B) with undetectable aldosterone suggesting that the defect was due to

18-OH-dehydrogenase deficiency with failure of conversion of 18-hydroxy-corticosterone to aldosterone.

Since the initial case report several further examples of this enzyme deficiency have been recognised in both females (Goldsmith, Solomon and Horton, 1967; Mills et al, 1967; Mallin, 1969; Linquette, Dupont and Racadot, 1971; Tronchetti, Materazzi and Franchi, 1973) and males (New, 1970; Mantero et al, 1971; Bricaire et al, 1972; Alvarez, Cloutier and Hayles, 1973; Kershnar, Borut and Kogut, 1973). Glucocorticoid replacement therapy lowers plasma deoxycorticosterone and corticosterone levels and usually results in restoration of a normal blood pressure. The suppressed plasma renin activity usually rises with glucocorticoid therapy. In some cases this has been associated with a rise in aldosterone secretion (Goldsmith et al,

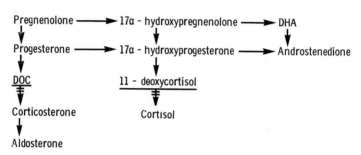

Figure 8.2 Pathways of adrenocortical steroid biosynthesis indicating the block produced by 11β-hydroxylase enzyme deficiency

1967; Mills et al, 1967; New, 1970) but in others the low aldosterone secretion has continued. The changes that have been reported in aldosterone secretion suggest that there may not be a second enzyme defect and that the low aldosterone secretion may relate to the prolonged suppression of the renin–angiotensin system.

11β-Hydroxylase deficiency syndrome

Eberlein and Bongiovanni (1956) described an eight-year-old female pseudohermaphrodite with congenital adrenal hyperplasia and hypertension. Detailed steroid studies showed that there was a deficiency of the 11β-hydroxylase enzyme. This led to deficient cortisol secretion, elevation of ACTH by the negative feedback control and thus excessive secretion of deoxycorticosterone, 11-deoxycortisol and adrenal androgens (Fig. 8.2). These patients are thus clinically distinct from those with the 17α-hydroxylase deficiency syndrome in that they are both virilised and hypertensive.

Liddle's syndrome

In 1963 Grant Liddle and his colleagues described a familial renal disorder simulating primary hyperaldosteronism but with negligible aldosterone secretion. The affected individuals had hypertension and a hypokalaemic alkalosis. The electrolyte abnormality could not be corrected by treatment with the mineralocorticoid antagonist spironolactone but the patients did respond to triamterene which inhibits renal tubular ionic transport. Thus the abnormality seems to be an unusual tendency of the kidneys to conserve sodium and lose potassium even when mineralocorticoid secretion is low.

Primary Hyperaldosteronism

This syndrome was first described by Conn in 1955 and has been classified into four different types (Biglieri, Stockigt and Schambelan, 1972): (1) primary aldosteronism due to an adrenal adenoma, (2) idiopathic hyperaldosteronism in which there is bilateral hyperplasia of the zona glomerulosa (Davis et al, 1967; Katz, 1967), (3) indeterminate hyperaldosteronism in which aldosterone secretion is suppressed by the administration of deoxycorticosterone (unlike the other types of primary hyperaldosteronism) (Biglieri et al, 1967) and (4) glucocorticoid-remediable hyperaldosteronism (Sutherland, Ruse and Laidlaw, 1966; Salti et al, 1969).

Separation of the four types

It is obviously important to make a definitive diagnosis and distinguish between these different types before any operative procedure. Failure to find an adenoma has occurred in up to 50 per cent of cases with suspected primary hyperaldosteronism subjected to surgery (George et al, 1970). In addition, whereas patients with idiopathic hyperaldosteronism respond well to treatment with spironolactone (Brown et al, 1972a), they may not respond to bilateral adrenalectomy (Biglieri et al, 1972).

All types of primary hyperaldosteronism are characterised by hypertension, hypokalaemia, excess aldosterone secretion and low plasma renin activity. In general, the electrolyte abnormalities tend to be more marked in patients with aldosterone producing adenomas as compared with the other types (Biglieri et al, 1972). The development of satisfactory radioimmunoassays for measuring plasma aldosterone has been a major factor in facilitating both the making of the diagnosis and the differential diagnosis. The majority of these assays have used antisera with slight cross-reactivity with cortisol and have required tedious and time-consuming paper chromatographic or other techniques to separate aldosterone (Edwards and Landon, 1976). Recently more specific assays have been developed which do not require long purification procedures and thus have an increased sample capacity (Vetter, Vetter and Siegenthaler, 1973; McKenzie and Clements, 1974).

Peripheral venous plasma levels of aldosterone are elevated in patients with primary hyperaldosteronism (Mayes et al, 1970; Horton and Finck, 1972; Vetter et al, 1973; Ganguly et al, 1973), and do not suppress after giving deoxycorticosterone (Biglieri et al, 1967) or fludrocortisone (Horton, 1969) with the exception of patients with indeterminate hyperaldosteronism. The effect of posture on plasma aldosterone levels is very helpful in distinguishing between patients with an adrenal adenoma and those with idiopathic adrenocortical hyperplasia. Ganguly and his colleagues (1973) measured plasma aldosterone levels in recumbent patients with suspected primary hyperaldosteronism at 08.00 hours and again at 12.00 hours after 4 h standing. In patients with an aldosterone-producing adenoma the plasma aldosterone levels fell during the course of the morning in contrast with the rise

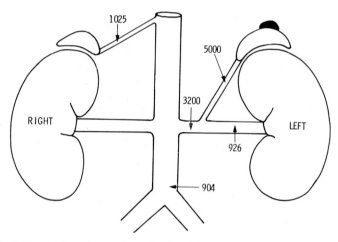

Figure 8.3 Differential venous catheter study with measurement of plasma aldosterone levels (pg/ml) in adrenal vein samples in a patient with primary hyperaldosteronism due to a left adrenal adenoma

found in patients with idiopathic hyperplasia. The fall found in the patients with adenomas reflects the fact that the adenoma appears to be ACTH-responsive and thus its output of aldosterone falls during the morning in keeping with reduced ACTH secretion.

The differential diagnosis can also be made by measuring plasma aldosterone levels in adrenal venous blood. If there is an adrenal tumour the side with the lesion has a much higher level whereas, in idiopathic hyperplasia high levels are found on both sides (Melby et al, 1967; Horton and Finck, 1972; Nicolis et al, 1972). An example of a typical differential venous catheterisation study is given in Figure 8.3. A high level of plasma aldosterone was found in the left adrenal vein with a slightly lower level in the part of the left renal vein between the junction of the left adrenal vein and the inferior vena cava. The level in the right adrenal vein was not significantly different from that found in the inferior vena cava. At operation a left adrenal adenoma was found.

The introduction of adrenal scanning after administration of radioactive iodocholesterol has been a considerable advance in making a diagnosis of either an aldosterone or a cortisol producing adenoma (Lieberman et al, 1971). The [131]I-19-iodocholesterol is selectively localised in the tumour. A typical adrenal scan done in a patient with a left-sided aldosterone producing adenoma is shown in Figure 8.4.

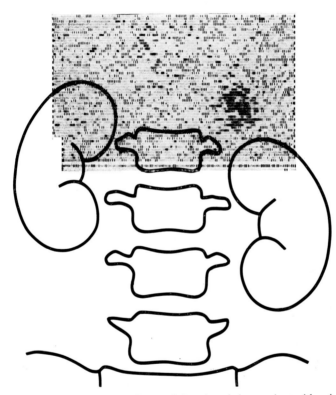

Figure 8.4 Radioactive iodocholesterol scan of the adrenals in a patient with primary hyper-aldosteronism due to a left adrenal adenoma

Low-renin Essential Hypertension

Two major and opposing schools of thought exist concerning the aetiology of this condition. One group feels that low-renin essential hypertension is a separate diagnostic entity and is probably due either to excessive production of an unidentified mineralocorticoid steroid or to enhanced sensitivity to the normal circulating aldosterone levels. The other group concludes that this is not a separate diagnostic category, that there is no evidence of excess mineralocorticoid activity as judged by measurement of extracellular fluid and plasma volume, and that plasma renin activity falls with age.

Evidence in favour of cryptic mineralocorticoid excess

Several groups have postulated that the syndrome of low-renin essential hypertension might be due to the excess production of an unknown mineralocorticoid. To further investigate this Woods and his co-workers (1969) carried out a double-blind study of the antihypertensive effect of aminoglutethimide, a drug that inhibits the conversion of cholesterol to pregnenolone. They found that this drug lowered the blood pressure of patients with low-renin essential hypertension but not of patients with normal-renin essential hypertension. Since this study many groups have looked for the unknown mineralocorticoid. So far small groups of patients with excess production of deoxycorticosterone, 18-hydroxydeoxycorticosterone, corticosterone and 16β-hydroxydehydroepiandrosterone have been described. The relevance of the steroid production to the hypertension is, however, still unclear as most of the steroids found are only weak mineralocorticoids.

Evidence suggesting that low-renin essential hypertension is not a separate diagnostic group

Padfield and his colleagues (1975) studied plasma renin concentration in 81 patients with essential hypertension. They were unable to distinguish a subpopulation of patients with low-renin levels and therefore used an arbitrary dividing line to define a low-renin group. No attempt was made to distinguish two populations by dynamic tests such as diuretic administration. Patients with low-renin hypertension were significantly older than patients with normal plasma renin. They concluded that the low-renin group was not a separate diagnostic category and that plasma renin falls with age in essential hypertension. A prospective study of this problem by Aurell, Pettersson and Berglund (1975) also failed to distinguish a subpopulation of patients with low-renin hypertension. This important study was based on an epidemiological survey of 50-year-old men in Göteborg, Sweden. Every third man of this age was asked to participate. The subjects were then classified into a normotensive and hypertensive group. Plasma renin activity in the normotensive and untreated hypertensives was normally distributed with slight skewness to the right. There was no evidence of a separate population with 'low-renin' hypertension. The mean plasma renin activity in the hypertensive group was slightly but not significantly lower than that of the normotensive reference group. They suggested that the renin changes in essential hypertension may be secondary to the pressure changes.

This problem has also been investigated by measuring plasma and extracellular fluid volumes in patients with low-renin hypertension and postulated mineralocorticoid excess (Schalekamp et al, 1974) and total exchangeable sodium and potassium (Padfield et al, 1975). Unlike patients with primary hyperaldosteronism these patients had normal plasma and extracellular fluid volumes and also no increase in total exchangeable sodium. However, the low renin group had significantly lower exchangeable potassium values and contained five patients with persistent hypokalaemia. Plasma aldosterone and deoxycorticosterone levels were normal and the authors suggest that there may be cryptic or intermittent mineralocorticoid excess. On the basis of the serum and exchangeable potassium levels, therefore, there does seem to be a separate diagnostic group and all these patients had low plasma renin concentrations.

The incidence and diagnosis of low-renin essential hypertension

Part of the confusion over the identification of a low-renin group has arisen because of the widely differing tests that have been used. In 14 studies reviewed by Drayer, Kloppenborg and Benraad (1975), each involving at least 50 hypertensive patients, the percentage of subjects with low-renin hypertension has varied from 12 to 46 per cent (Helmer, 1965; Creditor and Loschky, 1967; Ledingham, Bull and Laragh, 1967; Granger, Boucher and Genest, 1968; Jerums and Doyle, 1969; Channick, Adlin and Marks, 1969; Doyle and Jerums, 1970; Gunnels et al, 1970; Adlin, Marks and Channisk, 1972; Crane, Harris and Nokus, 1972; Brunner, Sealy and Laragh, 1973; Mrozeck, Finnerty and Catt, 1973; Tuck et al, 1973; Kloppenborg et al, 1973). Some authors have just measured basal plasma renin activity, whilst others have used sodium restriction and the upright posture. The latter involves hospital admission and many groups have, therefore, relied on screening patients after oral or intravenous diuretics. Drayer and his colleagues (1975) compared three methods of stimulating renin release—five days of sodium restriction followed by 3 h ambulation, frusemide stimulation (140 mg in 18 h) followed by ambulation and five days of chlorthalidone with 3 h ambulation. They showed that in 11 normotensive control subjects and 20 hypertensive patients the outpatient chlorthalidone test identified the same subgroups of patients as having low- or normal-renin hypertension as did the inpatient sodium restriction test. However, the frusemide test did not identify the same renin-suppressed hypertensive group as did sodium restriction.

Deoxycorticosterone

In 1972 Brown and his colleagues from Glasgow described a syndrome of isolated deoxycorticosterone excess (Brown et al, 1972c). They measured plasma deoxycorticosterone (DOC) levels in 31 hypertensive patients and found persistently high levels in six patients. These six were all in a group of 21 patients that had low plasma renin concentrations, and no patient with a normal renin concentration had a persistently elevated DOC level. Intermittent hypokalaemia was found in these six patients. Five of the patients with high DOC levels were treated successfully with spironolactone but no fall in blood pressure was found in three patients treated with dexamethasone.

The biochemical findings in these patients were similar to those found in the 17α-hydroxylase or 11β-dehydrogenase deficiency syndromes with the exception of aldosterone secretion which was normal in the isolated DOC excess syndrome but low in the congenital enzyme deficiency syndromes. The cause of the excess DOC secretion was unknown but at least one of the patients was thought to have an adrenocortical tumour. Even though the plasma DOC levels were only modestly raised it was suggested that the hypertensive effects of DOC may be disproportionate to its actions on sodium and potassium excretion. This may also explain why further studies have failed to show an increased plasma or extracellular fluid volume in these patients.

Cope and Loizou (1975) developed a radioimmunoassay for deoxycorticosterone and used it to measure DOC excretion in normal, hypertensive and hypokalaemic subjects. In 14 subjects with essential hypertension and normal plasma electrolytes the DOC excretion was not significantly different from that in normal subjects. Similar results were found in 10 out of 12 patients with Cushing's syndrome due to pituitary-dependent bilateral adrenocortical hyperplasia. However, eight out of nine patients with hypokalaemia had elevated urinary DOC levels and of these six were hypertensive. One of these patients had a confirmed aldosterone secreting tumour and DOC excretion returned to normal after excision of the tumour. Another patient with hypertension and hypokalaemia had the ectopic ACTH syndrome due to a pancreatic carcinoma. The remaining four hypertensive patients were thought to have hyperplasia of the zona glomerulosa. Other groups have reported similar results using different methodology. DOC secretion appears to be frequently elevated in patients with aldosterone producing tumours and may play a role in the development of the hypertension (Biglieri et al, 1968; Nolten et al, 1968). Similarly, high secretion rates have been reported in the ectopic ACTH syndrome (Biglieri et al, 1968; Schambelan, Slaton and Biglieri, 1971).

18-Hydroxy-11-deoxycorticosterone (18-OH-DOC)

Production of this steroid by the human adrenal was first shown in 1964 by Carballeira and Venning, and this was confirmed by de Nicola and Birmingham in 1968. It has been suggested that this is the steroid responsible for the genesis of two types of experimental hypertension in rats. Birmingham MacDonald and Rochefort (1968) found that 18-OH-DOC was the main steroid secreted by the enucleated adrenal in adrenal regeneration hypertension and Rapp and Dahl (1971) reported elevated 18-OH-DOC secretion in rats genetically susceptible to salt-induced hypertension.

Melby, Dale and Wilson (1971) isolated 18-OH-DOC from human adrenal vein blood and also measured its secretion rate in man. Administration of ACTH increased 18-OH-DOC secretion up to 20-fold but the secretion rate was not altered by angiotensin infusion. In patients with essential hypertension and normal plasma renin activity the excretion of the 18-OH-DOC metabolite 18-OH-tetrahydro-DOC (18-OH-TH-DOC) was found to be normal (Melby et al, 1972). However, patients with suppressed plasma renin activity had a highly significant elevation of urinary 18-OH-TH-DOC. The administration of spironolactone to 22 of the 30 patients studied produced a significant reduction in blood pressure and in 60 per cent spironolactone reduced the blood pressure into the normal range. This contrasted with the poor results of spironolactone therapy in the group of patients with normal plasma renin activity. Another interesting finding was that administration of dexamethasone to five of the patients with elevated 18-OH-DOC secretion produced a lowering of blood pressure in four patients and three of these became normotensive. Further investigation of other types of low-renin hypertension showed that 18-OH-DOC secretion was also elevated in ACTH-dependent Cushing's syndrome, the 17α-hydroxylase deficiency syndrome and also primary hyperaldosteronism.

16α,18-Dihydroxy-deoxycorticosterone

Dale and Melby (1973) studied steroidogenesis in vitro using the adrenals from normal subjects and a patient with low-renin essential hypertension. They found that all the adrenals converted 1,2-^{3}H-18-hydroxy-deoxycorticosterone to a more highly hydroxylated material which they identified as being 16α,18-dihydroxy-deoxycorticosterone. However, the yield of this steroid was much higher in the incubations with the adrenal tissue from the patient with low-renin hypertension than with the adrenals from the normal subjects. The mineralocorticoid activity of the compound as measured using sodium transport across the toad bladder or with the rat bioassay was insignificant. However, further experiments have shown that this compound can potentiate the effect of aldosterone (Melby and Dale, 1975). If this can be confirmed in man it may indicate that this steroid could be important in the genesis of low-renin hypertension.

Corticosterone

In 1968 Fraser and his colleagues reported studies on a patient with a corticosterone-secreting adrenocortical tumour. The patient presented with headaches, muscle weakness and ankle oedema and was found to be hypertensive and hypokalaemic. Plasma steroid studies showed that the plasma levels of aldosterone and cortisol were normal but corticosterone levels were 25 to 50 times normal. At laparotomy an adrenal carcinoma was found and removal of this restored the electrolytes to normal and produced a temporary remission of her clinical condition. Apart from this patient there have been very few cases of isolated corticosterone excess producing hypertension described and there does not seem to be a syndrome related to isolated corticosterone overproduction in patients with essential hypertension.

16β-Hydroxy-dehydroepiandrosterone (16β-OH-DHEA)

Liddle and Sennett (1975) found that urine from patients with low-renin essential hypertension contained more mineralocorticoid activity, as measured by bioassay using adrenalectomised rats, than could be accounted for by the known mineralocorticoid steroids present. Using chromatographic methods they were able to isolate the unknown mineralocorticoid activity. This was then analysed by mass spectroscopy and found to contain 16β-OH-DHEA and its 16-oxo-17β-ol isomer. The mineralocorticoid activity of these steroids was investigated using synthetic compounds and found to be only one-fortieth of that of aldosterone. The mineralocorticoid activity of both the natural and the synthetic steroids could be blocked by spironolactone. They thought that these steroids probably had clinical significance as 15 out of 15 patients with low-renin essential hypertension had an elevated 24 h urinary excretion of the steroids as compared to only 1 out of 14 patients with normal or high plasma renin activity. The importance of this research is, however, unclear. There appears to be a discrepancy between the amount of unknown mineralocorticoid activity in the urine of these patients and the modest increase in excretion of the weakly mineralocorticoid 16β-OH-DHEA and its isomer. Funder and his colleagues (1975) have examined the affinity of binding of this steroid for the rat kidney mineralocorticoid receptors and found that it was less than 0.1 per cent that of aldosterone. They also looked at a series of related compounds including 16α-OH-DHEA, 16β-OH-DHEA monosulphate and 16β-OH-DHEA diacetate and found that they also had negligible affinity for the aldosterone receptor.

Exogenous mineralocorticoid

Liquorice contains the ammonium salt of glycyrrhizic acid and this substance has an action like aldosterone. Occasionally ingestion of large amounts of liquorice can produce hypokalaemia and hypertension. The clinical picture simulates primary hyperaldosteronism but can be distinguished by finding low aldosterone secretion. The hypertension and hypokalaemia are corrected by stopping liquorice or treatment with spironolactone (Borst et al, 1950; Salassa, Mattox and Rosevear, 1962; Conn, Rovner and Cohen, 1968; Holmes et al, 1970). A similar condition can also occur in patients with peptic ulcers on treatment with carbenoxalone sodium, a derivative of glycyrrhetinic acid (Holmes et al, 1970; Davies, Rhodes and Calcraft, 1974).

Adrenocorticotrophic Hormone-induced Hypertension

Coghlan and his colleagues (1972) found that intramuscular administration of ACTH to sheep for five days resulted in a significant increase in the systemic arterial pressure. Urinary sodium retention occurred during the first two to three days but this was followed by a natriuresis. Plasma potassium levels fell in contrast to an increase in plasma sodium. ACTH stimulated increased secretion of cortisol, corticosterone, deoxycortisol and deoxy-corticosterone. However, infusion of these steroids alone or in combination did not reproduce the ACTH-induced hypertension (Scoggins et al, 1973). The changes in plasma electrolytes, however, closely resembled those found with ACTH. It would therefore seem possible that there may be an unknown steroid that can produce hypertension in the sheep. Recent work with in-fusions of 18-hydroxydeoxycorticosterone into sheep has shown that this can produce hypertension but does not seem to reproduce the results seen with ACTH administration. Obviously these studies may be of considerable relevance to man, in particular to the genesis of hypertension in Cushing's disease and the ectopic ACTH syndrome.

Hypertension Associated with Pregnancy or Oral Contraceptive Therapy

Pregnancy

High blood pressure in association with pregnancy may be the result of pre-existing hypertension or renal disease, or relate to pre-eclamptic toxaemia. However, the classic triad of hypertension, proteinuria and oedema which constitutes pre-eclamptic toxaemia may include patients with essential hyper-tension, as oedema is more common in pregnant hypertensive subjects and proteinuria more frequently found in pregnancy in patients with essential hypertension (Thomson, Hytten and Billewicz, 1967; Beilin, Redman and Bonnar, 1974). The two major organs that are thought to be related to the development of hypertension in pregnancy are the uterus and the kidney. However, even the uterus does not appear to be essential as toxaemia may occur with extra-uterine pregnancy (Baehler et al, 1975).

Several theories have been advanced in an attempt to explain how the uterus and placenta may affect the kidney and produce hypertension. These theories have been well reviewed recently (*Lancet*, 1975), and include the release of thromboplastic material into the maternal circulation, excessive production of mineralocorticoid steroids, increased production of renin by the chorion and decreased placental prostaglandin synthesis.

Evidence favouring intravascular coagulation secondary to the release of thromboplastic material has been adduced from renal biopsy studies on pregnant women. Eighteen out of 50 specimens had fibrinogen-like material in the glomeruli and these patients had pre-eclamptic toxaemia (Morris et al, 1964). In addition, infusion of thromboplastin into rabbits produced glo-merular lesions which on both light and electron microscopy are identical to those found in patients with toxaemia (Vassalli, Simon and Rouiller, 1963). These results suggested that toxaemia might be due to degeneration of trophoblastic tissue with release of thromboplastin into the maternal circula-tion. However, they beg the question as to what is the primary event that initiates the placental dysfunction.

Gordon and his colleagues (1976) have recently carried out a large prospective study to establish the true incidence of intravascular coagulation in pre-eclampsia and to determine whether it is a primary or secondary event. They used a sensitive and precise radioimmunoassay to measure one of the terminal degradation or core fragments of fibrinogen, fragment E. Elevated levels were found in only 2.5 per cent of mild and moderate cases, and in 30 per cent of severe cases. However, these changes occurred after and not before the onset of clinical signs suggesting that the coagulation changes and fibrin deposition are not the primary event.

Excess mineralocorticoid secretion leading to salt retention was one of the most attractive early hypotheses. Aldosterone secretion is markedly increased during normal pregnancy (Watanabe et al, 1963). However, this appears to be a compensatory increase to offset the natriuretic effect of increased progesterone secretion (Ehrlich et al, 1962). Weir and his colleagues (1973) measured plasma renin, angiotensin II and aldosterone in patients with pre-eclamptic toxaemia and showed that the levels were all decreased in comparison to normal pregnancy. These results contrasted with those of Gordon and his co-workers (1969) who carried out a prospective study. They showed that the mean level of plasma renin activity of 10 women who subsequently developed toxaemia was about 60 per cent higher than in 48 women with normal pregnancies. More recently Symonds and his colleagues (1975) have shown a highly significant correlation between diastolic blood pressure and plasma angiotensin II levels. These patients were studied at term and this may explain the different results obtained by Weir et al (1973) at an earlier stage of pregnancy.

Several studies have suggested that renin may be produced by the utero-placental unit. Gross and his colleagues (1964) showed that there was a pressor substance similar to renin in normal rabbit placentae as well as in the uteri of intact and nephrectomised rabbits. Subsequently, Ferris, Gorden and Mulrow (1967) found that the renin content of the pregnant rabbit uterus was about three times the amount found in both kidneys. Further work has shown that the release of uterine renin is unaffected by physiological changes which normally suppress the release of renin from the kidney. However, uterine ischaemia can release angiotensin II into the uterine vein (Smith, Selinger and Stevenson, 1969). Support for the concept that the human uteroplacental unit could release renin came from studies in four patients with toxaemia who had higher levels of renin activity in the samples of uterine vein blood taken at caesarean section than in the uterine artery (Bell, 1973). It would seem likely that the chorion is the main source of renin in the uteroplacental unit (Skinner, Lumbers and Symonds, 1968). At the present moment it is unclear whether these changes in uterine renin secretion are part of the primary disease process or simply secondary to ischaemia. Another interesting possibility is that the hypertension of pregnancy might be due to a failure of production of a vasodepressor substance. Speroff (1973) suggested that toxaemia could result from either inadequate placental prostaglandin production or to a loss of response to prostaglandins or to a combination of both. This was based on the findings of Ryan and his colleagues (1969) who demonstrated that extracts of human placental tissue contained a substance similar to prostaglandin E which lowered blood pressure. Placentae from toxaemic patients contained less of this material than normal placentae.

Despite the large amount of research devoted to it the riddle of hypertension in pregnancy remains. However, with the advent of new diagnostic and therapeutic weapons such as the angiotensin II blocking drugs it would seem likely that major advances will be made.

Oral contraceptives

Many studies have shown that blood pressure rises in women on oral contraceptives. In a four year controlled prospective study carried out by Weir and his colleagues (1971, 1974) of women taking oestrogen–progestogen oral contraceptives the mean systolic blood pressure rose by 14.2 mmHg and the diastolic by 8.5 mmHg. After stopping the pill blood pressure returned to pretreatment levels within three months. It would seem likely that this rise is related to the oestrogenic component of the pill as no rise in blood pressure has been found in women taking progestogens alone (MacKay, Khoo and Adam, 1971; Spellacy and Birk, 1972) but has been observed with oestrogen therapy alone (Lim et al, 1970).

The mechanism whereby oestrogens produce a rise in blood pressure has been extensively investigated. In 1967 Laragh and his colleagues showed that oral contraceptives produced a striking and sustained increase in plasma renin substrate concentration and suggested that in the presence of an increased substrate concentration less renin would be required to produce a given amount of angiotensin. However, the relevance of these observations to the development of hypertension was unclear as the same changes occurred in treated normotensive women. A possible mechanism was suggested by Saruta and his colleagues (1970). They carried out a prospective study and found that 10 of 56 previously normotensive women became hypertensive during administration of an oestrogen containing oral contraceptive. The plasma renin concentration fell slightly in those patients whose blood pressure did not increase but was significantly greater in those whose blood pressure rose with treatment. On the basis of this they suggested that there might be a failure of the normal feedback suppression of angiotensin on the juxta-glomerular cell and hence renin release.

Detailed study of the components of the renin–angiotensin system in women during oral contraceptive therapy by Catt and his colleagues (Catt, Cain and Menard, 1972) showed that plasma renin substrate and renin activity increased to about three times the basal value in contrast to plasma renin concentration which was reduced by about 50 per cent. Angiotensin II levels were markedly elevated. Serial measurements showed that the levels rose within the first week of therapy and remained high during treatment for up to three months. None of the patients became hypertensive during treatment but the group as a whole showed a significant increase in blood pressure. The fall of plasma renin concentration suggested that in these patients high blood angiotensin II levels did lead to suppression of renin secretion.

A detailed study of changes in the renal circulation of women who developed hypertension on the pill has been carried out by Boyd, Burden and Aber (1975). All patients showed abnormalities of the peripheral renal arteries on angiography and these were most commonly attenuated, tortuous and reduced in number with wide-angled bifurcations. Renal biopsies showed glomerular sclerosis with periglomerular thickening. Three out of the five patients showed arteriolar changes with intimal proliferation and medial hyperplasia. These angiographic changes are not similar to those seen in essential hypertension and presumably relate directly to the oral contraceptive therapy. Two further patients remained hypertensive after a pregnancy complicated by hypertension. They were put on to an oral oestrogen–progestogen immediately after the pregnancy and developed diffuse intravascular coagulation with elevated concentration of fibrin degradation products and intrarenal microthrombi on renal biopsy. Stopping the oral contraceptive resulted in a fall in blood pressure to normal, disappearance of the fibrin degradation products and improvement in renal function.

OTHER AETIOLOGICAL FACTORS

Role of Catecholamines

Even though phaeochromocytoma is a rare cause of hypertension it should be looked for in all patients with hypertension. In particular the diagnosis should be excluded in patients with paroxysmal hypertension or diseases known to be associated with an increased incidence of phaeochromocytoma such as medullary carcinoma of the thyroid and neurofibromatosis. This subject has recently been well reviewed by Wolf (1974).

The role of catecholamines in the genesis of essential hypertension is a much more controversial subject, some authors suggesting that there is increased catecholamine secretion whilst others have found it to be normal. Part of this controversy probably relates to methodological problems in the assay of catecholamines and also to the type of patients that have been studied. However, using specific assay methods there does seem to be some evidence indicating sympathetic overactivity in essential hypertension. Doyle, Louis and Geffen (1973) measured plasma noradrenaline, adrenaline and dopamine β-hydroxylase (an enzyme released from sympathetic nerve terminals and the adrenal medulla) in 31 patients with essential hypertension. The plasma levels of noradrenaline and dopamine β-hydroxylase correlated closely with the level of diastolic blood pressure. They concluded that in essential hypertension the elevated blood pressure was sustained by increased activity of the sympathetic nervous system.

Labile hypertension

Extensive studies have been carried out to determine the role of catechol-amines in patients with labile hypertension. Kuchel and his colleagues (1973) investigated 28 patients with labile hypertension and were able to classify them into two groups: one with a normal pulse rate response to standing and the other with an excessive response. These two groups could be distinguished not only from each other but also from normal subjects and patients with stable hypertension. The group with a normal pulse rate response had an increased supine urinary noradrenaline excretion but a normal plasma nor-adrenaline level. This contrasted with the second group which had an elevation of both plasma and urinary noradrenaline. Those patients with stable hypertension had normal urinary noradrenaline and usually normal plasma noradrenaline. These results stress the difficulty of drawing conclusions from studies based on urinary catecholamines alone.

Dopamine is an important neurotransmitter not only in the central but also in the peripheral nervous system. Cuche and his colleagues (1975) measured the urinary excretion of homovanillic acid, the main metabolite of dopamine, in normotensive subjects and patients with either labile or stable hypertension. The mean homovanillic acid excretion was $314 \, \mu g/4$ h in the normotensive subjects and was significantly greater in patients with labile hypertension (mean $2506 \, \mu g/4$ h, $P < 0.001$) or stable hypertension (mean $795 \, \mu g/4$ h, $P < 0.01$). They concluded that this was further evidence of sympathetic hyperactivity in patients with labile hypertension. However, little is known of the role that dopamine might play in these patients.

Neurogenic Hypertension

Several pieces of evidence suggest that neurogenic mechanisms may be important in the aetiology of certain types of hypertension. In the rat, for example, with renovascular hypertension the ablation of sympathetic nerve fibres by 6-hydroxydopamine or immunosympathectomy can lower the blood pressure to normal (Grewal and Kaul, 1971). Similar results have been obtained in the rat made hypertensive by unilateral nephrectomy and treat-ment with deoxycorticosterone acetate and salt (Finch, 1971; De Champlain and Van Amerigan, 1972). These experiments indicate that the sympathetic nervous system plays a key role in the development of different types of hypertension. Dickinson (1965) has suggested that the neurogenic component of renal hypertension might be due to functional constriction of cerebral arteries and arterioles possibly by angiotensin. He argues that the rise in blood pressure that occurs is the normal adaptation of the body to an increase in cerebrovascular resistance. Essential hypertension could be due to an analogous situation in which the increased cerebrovascular resistance was due to atheroma affecting the arteries supplying the hind-brain.

Role of Prostaglandins

Prostaglandins A, E and F have been extracted from renal medullary tissue in many different animal species. Prostaglandins A and E increase renal blood flow and urinary sodium excretion (Johnston, Hertzog and Lauler, 1967; Lee, 1972). Zusman and his colleagues (1973) measured prostaglandin A in plasma samples from normal subjects and patients with essential hypertension. In the normal subjects the plasma levels varied with sodium intake being lowered by a high sodium diet and increased by salt depletion. In the hypertensive patients the circulating prostaglandin A levels were significantly lower than those in normal subjects. Whether these lower levels are simply secondary to the hypertension or indicate a deficiency which contributes to the development of the hypertension is unknown.

Role of Heredity and Environment

It would seem likely that essential hypertension is caused by the interaction of multiple genetic and environmental factors. Blood pressure measurements in the population show a unimodal distribution suggesting that there is not a distinct group of patients with an inherited form of hypertension (Hamilton et al, 1954). However, as suggested by Dickinson (1965) this lack of a separate peak of blood pressure which might correspond to a 'disease' called essential hypertension could be explained by supposing that the disease is due to a graded rather than an all-or-none defect, and that this defect is extremely common in the population.

In addition to the genetic factors blood pressure also seems to be affected by age, sex, body weight, salt intake and stress. In most Western societies blood pressure tends to increase with age in about 70 per cent of the population. In primitive communities, however, this rise with age may not occur (Maddocks, 1961) and pressure may fall with age (Sinnett and Whyte, 1973). The hormonal environment may also be important, blood pressure usually being higher in males than females. Morrison and Pickford (1971), for example, demonstrated that testosterone enhanced the development of experimental hypertension in animals infused with angiotensin and noradrenaline. The association of obesity with hypertension has been noted in studies on both adults and children (Froment et al, 1970). It is, however, possible that this may relate not just to a high calorie but also to a high salt intake. The role of salt alone in the genesis of hypertension is unknown. Epidemiological studies have shown that some communities with a very high salt intake such as the Japanese island of Northern Honshu have a very high incidence of hypertension and its cerebrovascular complications (Dahl, 1960).

In contrast Sinnett and Whyte (1973) found a very low incidence of hypertension in a community with a mean sodium excretion of less than 15 mEq/day. However, these effects could be unrelated to salt and result from other dietary factors (Denton, 1973). In addition studies in Western communities have shown little relationship between salt intake and hypertension, and severe restriction of sodium intake is necessary to lower blood pressure in hypertensive subjects.

The Role of Sensitising Factors

Mizukoshi and Michelakis (1972) suggested that the plasma of hypertensive patients contained a sensitising factor which increased the vascular sensitivity to angiotensin II and noradrenalone. In an attempt to further characterise this factor plasma samples from normotensive subjects, patients with malignant hypertension and dogs with renovascular hypertension were fractionated by gel-filtration and ion exchange chromatography (Michelakis et al, 1975). The sensitising activity was only found in the plasma of hypertensive patients and hypertensive dogs, and was located in three main fractions. The chromatography studies suggested that the molecular weight of the factor was between 1000 and 20 000 and that it was probably an acidic protein distinct from angiotensin I and II.

SUMMARY

Despite the fact that a large number of different causes of hypertension have been discovered, there is as yet very little information about their epidemiological importance. This is partly due to the limited application of specialised techniques of investigation. However, even when these techniques are applied to an unselected hypertensive population the yield may be low. For example, out of 252 patients found to be hypertensive in a Scottish screening survey none had primary hyperaldosteronism. This contrasts with a 13 per cent incidence of this syndrome found by the same clinicians using identical methods amongst patients referred to the Medical Research Council blood pressure unit. Obviously what is now required is a similar screening programme in which the mineralocorticoids other than aldosterone are measured in an unselected hypertensive population. Such a programme appears to be warranted as it has implications in terms of management of the hypertension. The same consideration applies to the measurement of plasma renin activity. In future it would seem likely that this will be part of the routine investigation of hypertension and this may be considerably facilitated by the development of a direct radioimmunoassay for renin. It would also seem probable that inhibitors of the renin–angiotensin system such as saralasin will be used as a diagnostic test to detect patients with angiotensinogenic hypertension. However, even in patients with this type of hypertension, the precise mechanism for the development of the high blood pressure is obscure as the peripheral plasma renin activity is often normal. As in many other types of hypertension there appears to be a complex interaction between what appears to be the primary cause and other mechanisms such as the neurogenic control, the renal handling of sodium and possible sensitising factors.

REFERENCES

Adlin, E. K., Marks, A. D. & Channick, B. J. (1972) Spironolactone and hydrochlorothiazide in essential hypertension. *Archives of Internal Medicine*, **130**, 855–858.

Alvarez, M. N., Cloutier, M. D. & Hayles, A. B. (1973) Male pseudohermaphroditism due to 17-hydroxylase deficiency in two siblings. *Paediatric Research*, **7**, 325.

Amsterdam, E. A., Couch, N. P., Christlieb, A. R., Harrison, J. H., Crane, C., Dobrzinsky, S. J. & Hickler, R. B. (1969) Renal vein renin activity in the prognosis of renovascular hypertension. *American Journal of Medicine*, **47**, 860–868.

Aurell, M., Pettersson, M. & Berglund, G. (1975) Renin–angiotensin system in essential hypertension. *Lancet*, **2**, 342–345.

Baehler, R. W., Copeland, W. E., Stein, J. H. & Ferris, T. F. (1975) Plasma renin and aldosterone in an abdominal pregnancy with toxemia. *American Journal of Obstetrics and Gynecology*, **122**, 545–548.

Beilin, L. J., Redman, C. W. G. & Bonnar, J. (1974) In *Hypertension: its Nature and Treatment*, p. 99. CIBA.

Bell, C. (1973) Vasoactive substances in the circulation of the pregnant dog during acute fetal ischaemia. *American Journal of Obstetrics and Gynecology*, **117**, 1088–1092.

Biglieri, E. G., Herron, M. A. & Brust, N. (1966) 17-hydroxylation deficiency in man. *Journal of Clinical Investigation*, **45**, 1946–1954.

Biglieri, E. G., Slaton, P. E., Kronfield, S. J. & Schambelan, M. (1967) Diagnosis of an aldosterone producing adenoma in primary hyperaldosteronism: an evaluative manoeuvre. *Journal of American Medical Association*, **201**, 510–514.

Biglieri, E. G., Slaton, P. E., Schambelan, M. & Kronfield, S. J. (1968) Hypermineralo-corticoidism. *American Journal of Medicine*, **45**, 170–175.

Biglieri, E. G., Stockigt, J. R. & Schambelan, M. (1972) Adrenal mineralocorticoids causing hypertension. *American Journal of Medicine*, **52**, 623–632.

Birmingham, M. K., MacDonald, M. L. & Rochefort, J. G. (1968) In *Functions of the Adrenal Cortex*, ed. McKerns, K. W., Vol. 2, pp. 647–689. New York: Appleton.

Bonnin, J. M., Hodge, R. L. & Lumbers, E. R. (1972) A renin-secreting renal tumour associated with hypertension. *Australian and New Zealand Journal of Medicine*, **2**, 178–181.

Borst, J. G. G., Blomhert, G., Molhuysen, J. A., Gerbrandy, J., Turner, K. P. & de Vries, L. A. (1950) De uitscheiding van water en electrolyten gedurende het etmaal en onder invlocd van succus liquiritiae. *Acta clinica belgica*, **5**, 405–409.

Bourgoignie, J. J., Catanzaro, P. J. & Perry, H. M. (1968) Renin–angiotensin–aldosterone system during chronic thiazide therapy of benign hypertension. *Circulation*, **37**, 27–35.

Boyd, W. N., Burden, R. P. & Aber, G. M. (1975) Intrarenal vascular changes in patients receiving oestrogen-containing compounds—a clinical, histological and angiographic study. *Quarterly Journal of Medicine*. **175**, 415–431.

Braun-Menendez, E., Fasciolo, J. C., Leloir, L. F., Munoz, J. M. & Jaquini, A. (1939) *Hypertension Arterial Nefrogena*, pp. 173–183. Buenos Aires: Libreria y Editorial Al Ateneo.

Bricaire, H., Luton, J. P., Laudat, P., Legrand, J. C., Turpin, G., Corvol, P. & Lemmer, M. (1972) A new male pseudohermaphroditism associated with hypertension due to a block of 17α-hydroxylation. *Journal of Clinical Endocrinology and Metabolism*, **35**, 67–72.

Bright, R. (1827) *Reports of Medical Cases*, pp. 1–10. London: Longman, Reese, Orme, Brown, and Green.

Brown, J. J., Davies, D. L., Lever, A. F. & Robertson, J. I. S. (1965) Plasma renin concentration in human hypertension. II. Renin in relation to aetiology. *British Medical Journal*, **2**, 1215–1219.

Brown, J. J., Davies, D. L., Lever, A. F. & Robertson, J. I. S. (1966) Renin and angiotensin. A survey of some aspects. *Postgraduate Medical Journal*, **42**, 153–176.

Brown, J. J., Fraser, R., Lever, A. F. & Robertson, J. I. S. (1972a) Hypertension with aldosterone excess. *British Medical Journal*, **2**, 391–396.

Brown, J. J., Davies, D. L., Ferriss, J. B., Fraser, R., Haywood, E., Lever, A. F. & Robertson, J. I. S. (1972b) Comparison of surgery and prolonged spironolactone therapy in patients with hypertension, aldosterone excess, and low plasma renin. *British Medical Journal*, **2**, 729–734.

Brown, J. J., Fraser, R., Love, D. R., Ferriss, J. B., Lever, A. F., Robertson, J. I. S. & Wilson, A. (1972c) Apparently isolated excess deoxycorticosterone in hypertension. *Lancet*, **2**, 243–247.

Brunner, H. R., Gavras, H. & Laragh, J. H. (1973) Angiotensin-II blockade in man by Sar^1-Ala^8-angiotensin II for understanding and treatment of high blood pressure. *Lancet*, **2**, 1045–1048.

Brunner, H. R., Sealey, J. E. & Laragh, J. H. (1973) Renin sub-groups in essential hypertension. *Circulation Research*, **32–33**, Suppl. 1, 99–109.

Carballeira, A. & Venning, E. H. (1964) Conversion of steroids by chromaffin tissue. 1. Studies with a phaeochromocytoma. *Steroids*, **4**, 329–350.

Catt, K. J., Zimmet, P. Z., Cain, M. D., Cran, E., Best, J. B. & Coghlan, J. P. (1971) Angiotensin II blood levels in human hypertension. *Lancet*, **1**, 459–463.

Catt, K. J., Cain, M. D. & Menard, J. (1972) Radioimmunoassay studies of the renin–angiotensin system in human hypertension and during oestrogen treatment. In *Hypertension*, pp. 591–604. Berlin, Heidelberg, New York: Springer-Verlag.

Channick, B. J., Adlin, E. V. & Marks, A. D. (1969) Suppressed plasma renin activity in hypertension. *Archives of Internal Medicine*, **123**, 131–140.

Coghlan, J. P., Cran, E. J., Denton, D. A., Fan, S. K., McDougall, J. G., Oddie, C. J., Scoggins, B. A. & Simpson, P. (1972) The metabolic effects of ACTH in sheep. *Proceedings 15th Annual Meeting Endocrine Society of Australia*, No. 45.

Conn, J. W. (1955) Primary aldosteronism, a new clinical syndrome. *Journal of Laboratory and Clinical Medicine*, **45**, 3–17.

Conn, J. W., Rovner, D. R. & Cohen, E. L. (1968) Licorice-induced pseudoaldosteronism. Hypertension, hypokalaemia, aldosteronopenia and suppressed plasma renin activity. *Journal of the American Medical Association*, **205**, 492–496.

Conn, J. W., Cohen, E. L., Lucas, C. P., McDonald, W. J., Mayor, G. H., Blough, W. M., Eveland, W. C., Bookstein, J. J. & Lapides, J. (1972) Primary reninism. *Archives of Internal Medicine*, **130**, 682–696.

Cope, C. L. & Loizou, S. (1975) Deoxycorticosterone excretion in normal, hypertensive and hypokalaemic subjects. *Clinical Science and Molecular Medicine*, **48**, 97–105.

Crane, M. G., Harris, J. J. & Nokus, V. J. (1972) Hyporeninaemic hypertension. *American Journal of Medicine*, **52**, 457–466.

Creditor, M. C. & Loschky, U. K. (1967) Plasma renin activity in hypertension. *American Journal of Medicine*, **43**, 371–382.

Cuche, J. L., Kuchel, O., Barbeau, A. & Genest, J. (1975) Urinary homovanillic acid, dopamine and norepinephrine excretion in patients with essential hypertension. *Canadian Medical Association Journal*, **112**, 443–446.

Dahl, L. K. (1960) Possible role of salt intake in the development of essential hypertension. In *Essential Hypertension, an International Symposium*, ed. Bock, K. D. & Cottier, P. T., pp. 53–65. Berlin: Springer-Verlag.

Dale, S. L. & Melby, J. C. (1973) Isolation and identification of 16α,18-dihydroxydeoxycorticosterone from human adrenal gland incubations. *Steroids*, **21**, 617–632.

Davies, G. J., Rhodes, J. & Calcraft, B. J. (1974) Complications of carbenoxalone therapy. *British Medical Journal*, **3**, 400–402.

Davis, W. W., Newsome, H. H., Wright, L. D., Hammond, W. R., Easton, J. & Bartter, F. C. (1967) Bilateral adrenal hyperplasia as a cause of primary aldosteronism with hypertension, hypokalaemia and suppressed renin activity. *American Journal of Medicine*, **42**, 642–647.

De Champlain, J. & Van Amerigan, M. R. (1972) Regulation of blood pressure by sympathetic nerve fibres and adrenal medulla in normotensive and hypertensive rats. *Circulation Research*, **31**, 617.

De Nicola, A. F. & Birmingham, M. K. (1968) Biosynthesis of 18-hydroxydeoxycorticosterone from deoxycorticosterone-4-^{14}C by the human adrenal gland. *Journal of Clinical Endocrinology and Metabolism*, **28**, 1380–1383.

Denton, D. A. (1973) Sodium and hypertension. In *Mechanisms of Hypertension*, ed. Sambhi, M. P., pp. 46–54. Excerpta Medica, American Elsevier.

Dickinson, C. J. (1965) *Neurogenic Hypertension*. Oxford: Blackwell Scientific Publications.

Doyle, A. E. & Jerums, G. (1970) Sodium balance, plasma renin and aldosterone in hypertension. *Circulation Research*, **22–27**, Suppl. 2, 267–275.

Doyle, A. E., Louis, W. J. & Geffen, L. B. (1973) Plasma noradrenaline and dopamine beta hydroxylase in hypertension. In *Mechanisms of Hypertension*, ed. Sambhi, M. P., pp. 155–159. Excerpta Medica, American Elsevier.

Drayer, J. I. M., Kloppenborg, P. W. C. & Benraad, T. J. (1975) Detection of low-renin hypertension; evaluation of out-patient renin-stimulating methods. *Clinical Science and Molecular Medicine*, **48**, 91–96.

Eberlein, W. R. & Bongiovanni, A. M. (1956) Plasma and urinary corticosteroids in the hypertensive form of congenital adrenal hyperplasia. *Journal of Biological Chemistry*, **223**, 85–94.

Eddy, R. L. & Sanchez, S. A. (1971) Renin-secreting renal neoplasm and hypertension with hypokalaemia. *Annals of Internal Medicine*, **75**, 725–729.

Edwards, C. R. W. & Landon, J. (1976) In *Hormone Assays and their Clinical Application*, 4th edn, ed. Loraine, J. A. & Bell, T. Edinburgh: Churchill Livingstone.

Ehrlich, E. N., Laves, M., Lugibihl, K. & Landau, R. L. (1962) Progesterone–aldosterone interrelationships in pregnancy. *Journal of Laboratory and Clinical Medicine*, **59**, 588–595.

Eide, I. & Aars, H. (1969) Renal hypertension in rabbits immunised with angiotensin. *Nature*, **222**, 571.

Ferris, T. F., Gorden, P. & Mulrow, P. J (1967) Rabbit uterus as a source of renin. *American Journal of Physiology*, **212**, 698–702.

Finch, L. (1971) The neurogenic component in the experimental hypertensive rat. *Pharmacology*, **5**, 245.

Fraser, R., James, V. H. T., Landon, J., Peart, W. S., Rawson, A., Giles, C. A. & McKay, A. M. (1968) Clinical and biochemical studies of a patient with a corticosterone secreting adrenocortical tumour. *Lancet*, **2**, 1116–1120.

Froment, A., Milon, H., Vincent, M., Dupont, J. C. C. & Dupont, J. (1970) La pression artérielle chez l'enfant d'âge scolaire. Relation avec quelques variables. *Bulletin de l'Institut national de la Sante et de la recherche médicale*, **25**, 1237–1248.

Funder, J. W., Robinson, J. A., Feldman, D. & Wynne, K. N. (1975) The affinity of 16β-hydroxy-dehydroepiandrosterone for mineralocorticoid receptors. *Endocrinology*, **96**, Suppl., 54.

Ganguly, A., Melada, G. A., Luetscher, J. A. & Dowdy, A. J. (1973) Control of plasma aldosterone in primary aldosteronism; distinction between adenoma and hyperplasia. *Journal of Clinical Endocrinology and Metabolism*, **37**, 765–775.

Gavras, H., Brunner, H. R., Laragh, J. H., Sealey, J. E., Gavras, I. & Vukovich, R. A. (1974) An angiotensin converting-enzyme inhibitor to identify and treat vasoconstrictor and volume factors in hypertensive patients. *New England Journal of Medicine*, **291**, 817–821.

George, J. M., Wright, L., Bell, N. H. & Bartter, F. C. (1970) The syndrome of primary aldosteronism. *American Journal of Medicine*, **48**, 343–356.

Gill, J. R., George, J. M., Solomon, A. & Bartter, F. C. (1964) Hyperaldosteronism and renal sodium loss reversed by drug treatment for malignant hypertension. *New England Journal of Medicine*, **270**, 1088–1092.

Glaz, E. & Vecsei, P. (1971) In *Aldosterone*. International Series of Monographs in Pure and Applied Biology, Biochemistry Division, Vol. 6. Oxford: Pergamon Press.

Goldblatt, H., Lynch, J., Hanzal, R. F. & Summerville, W. W. (1934) Studies on experimental hypertension. I. The production of persistent elevation of systolic blood pressure by means of renal ischemia. *Journal of Experimental Medicine*, **59**(3), 347.

Goldsmith, O., Solomon, D. H. & Horton, R. (1967) Hypogonadism and mineralocorticoid excess. The 17-hydroxylase deficiency syndrome. *New England Journal of Medicine*, **277**, 673–677.

Gordon, R. D., Parsons, S. & Symonds, E. M. (1969) A prospective study of plasma renin activity in normal and toxemic pregnancy. *Lancet*, **1**, 347–349.

Gordon, Y. B., Ratky, S. M., Baker, L. R. I., Letchworth, A. T., Leighton, P. C., Sola, C. M. & Chard, T. (1976) Circulating levels of fibrin(ogen) degradation fragment E measured by radioimmunoassay in pre-eclampsia. *British Journal of Obstetrics and Gynaecology* **83**, 287–291.

Granger, P., Boucher, R. & Genest, J. (1968) L'aldosteronisme primaire. *Pathologie-Biologie,* **16**, 511–516.

Grewal, R. S. & Kaul, C. L. (1971) Importance of the sympathetic nervous system in the development of renal hypertension in the rat. *British Journal of Pharmacology,* **42**, 497.

Gross, F., Schaechtelin, G., Ziegler, M. & Berger, M. (1964) A renin-like substance in the placenta and uterus of the rabbit. *Lancet,* **1**, 914–916.

Gunnels, J. C., McGuffin, W. L., Robinson, R. R., Grim, C. E., Wells, S., Silver, D. & Glenn, G. F. (1970) Hypertension, adrenal abnormalities and alterations in plasma renin activity. *Annals of Internal Medicine,* **73**, 901–911.

Hamilton, M., Pickering, G. W., Roberts, J. A. F. & Sowry, G. S. C. (1954) The aetiology of essential hypertension. *Clinical Science,* **13**, 11–35.

Helmer, O. M. (1965) The renin angiotensin system and its relation to hypertension. *Progress in Cardiovascular Diseases,* **8**, 117–118.

Holmes, A. M., Marrott, P. K., Young, J. & Prentice, E. (1970) Pseudohyperaldosteronism induced by habitual ingestion of liquorice. *Postgraduate Medical Journal,* **46**, 625–629.

Horton, R. (1969) Stimulation and suppression of aldosterone in plasma of normal men and in primary aldosteronism. *Journal of Clinical Investigation,* **48**, 1230–1236.

Horton, R. & Finck, E. (1972) Diagnosis and localisation in primary aldosteronism. *Annals of Internal Medicine,* **76**, 885–890.

Jerums, G. & Doyle, A. E. (1969) Renal sodium handling and responsiveness of plasma renin levels in hypertension. *Clinical Science,* **37**, 79–80.

Johnston, H. H., Herzog, J. P. & Lauler, D. P. (1967) Effect of prostaglandin E on renal hemodynamics, sodium and water excretion. *American Journal of Physiology,* **213**, 939–946.

Judson, W. E. & Helmer, O. M. (1965) Diagnostic and prognostic values of renin activity in renal venous plasma in renovascular hypertension. *Hypertension,* **13**, 79.

Katz, F. H. (1967) Primary aldosteronism with suppressed renin activity due to bilateral nodular hyperplasia. *Annals of Internal Medicine,* **67**, 1035–1042.

Kershnar, A. K., Borut, D. & Kogut, M. D. (1973) 17-Hydroxylase deficiency mimicking testicular feminisation. *Pediatric Research,* **7**, 329.

Kihara, I., Kitamura, S., Hoshino, T., Seida, H. & Watanabe, T. (1968) A hitherto unreported vascular tumour of the kidney: a proposal of 'juxtaglomerular cell tumour'. *Acta pathologica japonica,* **18**, 197–206.

Kloppenborg, P. W. C., Benraad, H. B., Drayer, J. I. M. & Benraad, Th. J. (1973). Defective 'turn off' of aldosterone secretion by sodium loading, especially in 'low renin' hypertension. *Netherlands Journal of Medicine,* **16**, 52.

Kuchel, O., Cuche, J. L., Hamet, P., Barbeau, A., Boucher, R. & Genest, J. (1973) Catecholamines, cyclic adenosine monophosphate and renin in labile hypertension. In *Mechanisms of Hypertension,* ed. Sambhi, M. P., pp. 160–175. Excerpta Medica, American Elsevier.

Lancet (1975) Hypertension in pregnancy, **2**, 487–489.

Laragh, J. H., Ulick, S., Januszewicz, V., Deming, Q. B., Kelley, W. G. & Lieberman, S. (1960) Aldosterone secretion and primary and malignant hypertension. *Journal of Clinical Investigation,* **39**, 1091–1106.

Laragh, J. H., Sealey, J. E., Ledingham, J. G. G. & Newton, M. A. (1967) Oral contraceptives. Renin, aldosterone and high blood pressure. *Journal of American Medical Association,* **201**, 918–922.

Ledingham, J. G. G., Bull, M. B. & Laragh, J. H. (1967) The meaning of aldosterone in hypertensive disease. *Circulation Research,* **20–21**, Suppl. 2, 177–186.

Lee, M. R. (1972) Renin-secreting kidney tumours. *Lancet,* **2**, 254–255.

Liddle, G. W., Bledsoe, T. & Coppage, W. S. (1963) A familial renal disorder simulating primary aldosteronism but with negligible aldosterone secretion. *Transactions of the Association of American Physicians,* **66**, 199–213.

Liddle, G. W. & Sennett, J. A. (1975) New mineralocorticoids in the syndrome of low-renin essential hypertension. *Journal of Steroid Biochemistry,* **6**, 751–753.

Lieberman, L. M., Beierwaltes, W. H., Conn, J. W., Ansari, A. N. & Nishiyama, H. (1971) Diagnosis of adrenal disease by visualisation of human adrenal glands with 19-iodo-cholesterol-^{131}I. *New England Journal of Medicine*, **285**, 1387–1393.

Lim, Y. L., Lumbers, E. R., Walters, W. A. W. & Whelan, R. F. (1970) Effects of oestrogens on the human circulation. *Journal of Obstetrics and Gynaecology of the British Common-wealth*, **77**, 349–355.

Linquette, M., Dupont, A. & Racadot, A. (1971) Deficit en 17-hydroxylase. A propos d'une observation. *Annales d'Endocrinologie*, **32**, 574.

MacKay, E. V., Khoo, S. H. & Adam, R. R. (1971) Contraception with a six-monthly injection of progestogen. *Australian and New Zealand Journal of Obstetrics and Gynaeco-logy*, **11**, 148–156.

Maddocks, I. (1961) Possible absence of essential hypertension in two complete Pacific Island populations. *Lancet*, **2**, 396–399.

Mallin, S. R. (1969) Congenital adrenal hyperplasia secondary to 17-hydroxylase deficiency. Two sisters with amenorrhoea, hypokalaemia, hypertension and cystic ovaries. *Annals of Internal Medicine*, **70**, 69–75.

Mantero, F., Busnardo, B., Riondel, A., Veyrat, R. & Austoni, M. (1971) Hypertension artérielle, alcalose hypokaliémique et pseudo-hermaphrodisme male par deficit en 17 alpha-hydroxylase. *Schweizerische medizinische Wochenschrift*, **101**, 38–43.

Mayes, D., Furuyama, S., Kem, D. C. & Nugent, C. A. (1970) A radioimmunoassay for plasma aldosterone. *Journal of Clinical Endocrinology and Metabolism*, **30**, 682–685.

McAllister, R. G., Michelakis, A. M., Oates, J. A. & Foster, J. M. (1972) Malignant hyper-tension due to renal artery stenosis. *Journal of the American Medical Association*, **221**, 865–868.

McKenzie, J. K. & Clements, J. A. (1974) Simplified radioimmunoassay for serum aldo-sterone utilising increased antibody specificity. *Journal of Clinical Endocrinology and Metabolism*, **38**, 622–627.

Melby, J. C., Spark, R. F., Dale, S. L., Egdahl, R. H. & Kahn, P. C. (1967) Diagnosis and localisation of aldosterone-producing adenomas by adrenal vein catheterisation. *New England Journal of Medicine*, **277**, 1050–1056.

Melby, J. C., Dale, S. L. & Wilson, T. E. (1971) 18-hydroxy-deoxycorticosterone in human hypertension. *Circulation Research*, **28/29**, Suppl. 2, 143–152.

Melby, J. C., Dale, S. L., Grekin, R. J., Gaunt, R. & Wilson, T. E. (1972) 18-hydroxy-11-deoxycorticosterone (18-OH-DOC) secretion in experimental and human hypertension. *Recent Progress in Hormone Research*, **28**, 287–351.

Melby, J. C. & Dale, S. L. (1975) Adrenal steroidogenesis in 'low renin' or hyporeninemic hypertension. *Journal of Steroid Biochemistry*, **6**, 761–766.

Michelakis, A. M., Mizukoshi, H., Huang, C., Murakami, K. & Inagami, J. (1975) Further studies on the existence of a sensitising factor to pressor agents in hypertension. *Journal of Clinical Endocrinology and Metabolism*, **41**, 90–96.

Miller, H. C. & Phillips, C. E. (1968) Subsequent nephrectomy of the contralateral kidney for recurrent renovascular hypertension. *Surgery, Gynecology and Obstetrics*, **127**, 1274–1280.

Mills, I. H., Wilson, R. J., Tait, A. D. & Cooper, H. R. (1967) Steroid metabolic studies in a patient with 17-hydroxylase deficiency. *Journal of Endocrinology*, **38**, xix–xx.

Mizukoshi, H. & Michelakis, A. M. (1972) Evidence for the existence of a sensitising factor to pressor agents in the plasma of hypertensive patients. *Journal of Clinical Endocrinology and Metabolism*, **34**, 1016–1024.

Morris, R. H., Vassalli, P., Beller, F. K. & McCluskey, R. T. (1964) Immunofluorescent studies of renal biopsies in the diagnosis of toxaemia of pregnancy. *Obstetrics and Gynecology*, **24**, 32–46.

Morrison, J. F. & Pickford, M. (1971) Sex differences in the changes in sympathetic nerve activity when arterial pressure is raised by infusion of angiotensin and noradrenaline. *Journal of Physiology (London)*, **216**, 69–85.

Mrozeck, W. J., Finnerty, F. A. & Catt, K. J. (1973) Lack of association between plasma renin and history of heart attack or stroke in patients with essential hypertension. *Lancet*, **2**, 464–468.

New, M. I. (1970) Male pseudo-hermaphroditism due to 17-alpha-hydroxylase deficiency. *Journal of Clinical Investigation*, **49**, 1930–1941.

Nicolis, G. L., Mitty, H. A., Modlinger, R. S. & Gabrilove, J. L. (1972) Percutaneous adrenal venography. *Annals of Internal Medicine*, **76**, 899–909.

Nolten, W., Vecsei, P., Kohler, M., Purjesz, I. & Wolff, H. P. (1968) Untersuchungen uber sekretion und stoffwechsel von DOC am gesunden und kranken. *Verhandlung der Deutschen Gesellschaft fur Inneren Medizin*, **74**, 1218–1220.

Padfield, P. L., Brown, J. J., Lever, A. F., Schalekamp, M. A. D., Beevers, D. G., Davies, D. L., Robertson, J. I. S. & Tree, M. (1975) Is low-renin hypertension a stage in the development of essential hypertension or a diagnostic entity? *Lancet*, **1**, 548–550.

Page, I. H. & Helmer, O. M. (1940) A crystalline pressor substance, angiotonin, resulting from the reaction between renin and renin activator. *Journal of Experimental Medicine*, **71**, 29–42.

Pals, D. T., Masucci, F. D., Denning, G. S., Sipos, F. & Fessler, D. C. (1971) Role of the pressor action of angiotensin II in experimental hypertension. *Circulation Research*, **29**, 673–681.

Rapp, J. P. & Dahl, L. K. (1971) 18-hydroxy-deoxycorticosterone secretion in experimental hypertension in rats. *Circulation Research*, **28/29**, Suppl. 2, 153–159.

Robertson, P. W., Klidjian, A., Harding, L. K., Walters, G., Lee, M. R. & Robb-Smith, A. H. T. (1967) Hypertension due to a renin-secreting renal tumour. *American Journal of Medicine*, **43**, 963–976.

Ryan, W. L., Coronel, D. M. & Johnson, R. J. (1969) A vasodepressor substance of the human placenta. *American Journal of Obstetrics and Gynecology*, **105**, 1201–1206.

Salassa, R. M., Mattox, V. R. & Rosevear, J. W. (1962) Inhibition of the mineralocorticoid activity of licorice by spironolactone. *Journal of Clinical Endocrinology and Metabolism*, **22**, 1156–1159.

Salti, I. S., Ruse, J. L., Stiefel, M., De Larne, N. C. & Laidlaw, J. C. (1969) Non-tumorous 'primary' aldosteronism. 1. Type relieved by glucocorticoid (glucocorticoid-remediable hypertension). *Canadian Medical Association Journal*, **101**, 1–10.

Saruta, T., Saade, G. A. & Kaplan, N. M. (1970) A possible mechanism for hypertension induced by oral contraceptives—diminished feedback suppression of renin release. *Archives of Internal Medicine*, **126**, 621–626.

Schambelan, M., Slaton, P. E. & Biglieri, E. G. (1971) Mineralocorticoid production in hyperadrenocorticism: role in pathogenesis of hypokalaemic alkalosis. *American Journal of Medicine*, **51**, 299–303.

Schambelan, M. & Biglieri, E. G. (1972) Regulation and significance of hyper-reninaemia from renin-secreting tumor. *Clinical Research*, **20**, 439.

Schalekamp, M. A., Lebel, M., Beevers, D. G., Fraser, R., Kolsters, G. & Birkenhager, W. H. (1974) Body-fluid volume in low-renin hypertension. *Lancet*, **2**, 310–311.

Scoggins, B. A., Coghlan, J. P., Cran, E. J., Denton, D. A., Fan, S. K., McDougall, J. G., Oddie, C. J., Robinson, P. M. & Shulkes, A. A. (1973) Experimental studies on the mechanism of adrenocorticotrophic hormone-induced hypertension in the sheep. *Clinical Science and Molecular Medicine*, **45**, 2695–2715.

Sinnett, P. F. & Whyte, H. M. (1973) Epidemiological studies in a total highland population, Tukisenta, New Guinea. Cardiovascular disease and relevant clinical electrocardiographic, radiological and biochemical findings. *Journal of Chronic Diseases*, **26**, 265–290.

Skinner, S. L., Lumbers, E. R. & Symonds, E. M. (1968) Renin concentrations in human fetal and maternal tissues. *American Journal of Obstetrics and Gynecology*, **101**, 529–533.

Smith, R. W., Selinger, H. E. & Stevenson, S. F. (1969) The uteroplacental complex. Its role in alterations of renin activity. *American Journal of Obstetrics and Gynecology*, **105**, 1129–1131.

Spellacy, W. N. & Birk, S. A. (1972) The effect of intrauterine devices, oral contraceptives, oestrogens and progestogens on blood pressure. *American Journal of Obstetrics and Gynecology*, **112**, 912–919.

Speroff, L. (1973) Toxemia of pregnancy—mechanism and therapeutic management. *American Journal of Cardiology*, **32**, 582–591.

Stockigt, J. R., Collins, R. D., Noakes, C. A., Schambelan, M. & Biglieri, E. G. (1972) Renal vein renin in various forms of renal hypertension. *Lancet*, **1**, 1194–1197.

Streeten, D. H. P., Anderson, G. H., Freiberg, J. M. & Delakos, T. G. (1975) Use of an angiotensin II antagonist (Saralasin) in the recognition of 'angiotensinogenic' hypertension. *New England Journal of Medicine*, **292**, 657–662.

Sutherland, D. J. A., Ruse, J. L. & Laidlaw, J. C. (1966) Hypertension, increased aldosterone secretion, and low plasma renin activity relieved by dexamethasone. *Canadian Medical Association Journal*, **95**, 1109–1119.

Symonds, E. M., Pipkin, F. B. & Craven, D. J. (1975) Changes in the renin–angiotensin system in primigravidae with hypertensive disease of pregnancy. *British Journal of Obstetrics and Gynaecology*, **82**, 643–650.

Thal, A. P., Grage, T. B. & Vernier, R. L. (1963) Function of the contralateral kidney in renal hypertension due to renal artery stenosis. *Circulation*, **27**, 36–43.

Thomson, A. M., Hytten, F. E. & Billewicz, W. Z. (1967) The epidemiology of oedema during pregnancy. *Journal of Obstetrics and Gynaecology of the British Commonwealth*, **74**, 1–10.

Thurston, H. & Swales, J. D. (1974) Action of angiotensin antagonists and antiserum upon the pressor response to renin: further evidence for the local generation of angiotensin II. *Clinical Science*, **46**, 273–276.

Tigerstedt, R. & Bergman, P. G. (1898). Niere und Kreislauf. *Skandinavisches Archiv fur Physiologie*, **8**, 223–271.

Tronchetti, F., Materazzi, F. & Franchi, F. (1973) Troubles surréno-ovariens par deficits enzymatiques. In *Actualités endocrinologiques* 13ème série. Paris: L'Expansion édit.

Tuck, M. L., Williams, G. H., Cain, J. P., Sullivan, J. M. & Dluhy, R. G. (1973) Relation of age, diastolic pressure and known duration of hypertension to presence of low renin essential hypertension. *American Journal of Cardiology*, **32**, 637–642.

Vassalli, P., Simon, G. & Rouiller, C. (1963) Production of ultra-structural glomerular lesions resembling those of toxaemia of pregnancy by thromboplastin infusion in rabbits. *Nature*, **199**, 1105–1106.

Vaughan, E. D., Buhler, F. R., Laragh, J. H., Sealey, J. E., Baer, L. & Bard, R. H. (1973) Renovascular hypertension: renin measurements to indicate hypersecretion and contra-lateral suppression, estimate renal plasma flow and score for surgical curability. *American Journal of Medicine*, **55**, 402–414.

Vetter, W., Vetter, H. & Siegenthaler, W. (1973) Radioimmunoassay for aldosterone without chromatography. 2. Determination of plasma aldosterone. *Acta endocrinologica*, **74**, 548–557.

Watanabe, M., Mecker, C. I., Gray, M. J., Sims, E. A. H. & Solomon, S. (1963) Secretion rate of aldosterone in normal pregnancy. *Journal of Clinical Investigation*, **42**, 1619–1631.

Weir, R. J., Briggs, E., Browning, J., Mack, A., Naismith, L., Taylor, L. & Wilson, E. (1971) Blood pressure in women after one year of oral contraception. *Lancet*, **1**, 467–470.

Weir, R. J., Brown, J. J., Fraser, R., Kraszewski, A., Lever, A. F., McIlwaine, G. M., Morton, J. J., Robertson, J. I. S. & Tree, M. (1973) Plasma renin, renin substrate, angiotensin II and aldosterone in hypertensive disease of pregnancy. *Lancet*, **1**, 291–294.

Weir, R. J., Briggs, E., Mack, A., Naismith, L., Taylor, L. & Wilson, E. (1974) Blood pressure in women taking oral contraceptives. *British Medical Journal*, **1**, 533–535.

Wilson, C. & Byrom, F. B. (1939) Renal changes in malignant hypertension. *Lancet*, **1**, 136–139.

Wolf, R. L. (1974) Phaeochromocytoma. *Clinics in Endocrinology and Metabolism*, **3**, 609–621.

Woods, J. W., Liddle, G. W., Stant, E. G., Michelakis, A. M. & Brill, A. B. (1969) Effect of an adrenal inhibitor in hypertensive patients with suppressed renin. *Archives of Internal Medicine*, **123**, 366–370.

Zusman, R. M., Spector, D., Caldwell, B. V., Speroff, L., Schneider, G. & Mulrow, P. J. (1973) The role of prostaglandin A in the regulation of sodium balance and blood pressure in man. In *Mechanisms of Hypertension*, ed. Sambhi, M. P., pp. 274–277. Excerpta Medica, American Elsevier.

9

TREATMENT OF HYPERTENSION

B. N. C. Prichard   J. Tuckman

The present discussion of antihypertensive drugs is divided into five sections: diuretics, adrenergic neurone inhibiting drugs (bethanidine, debrisoquine and guanethidine), α-methyldopa, clonidine and β-adrenoceptor blocking drugs. This is the approximate chronological order in which the agents were introduced. Diuretics are discussed first because they are not only used alone but often administered in combination with one of the other drugs. Beta-adrenergic blocking agents are considered last as they may have the most important role in the near future. In this regard there has been considerable recent interest in the use of peripheral vasodilators with β-blocking drugs and discussion of them is included in this section.

HYPERTENSIVE EMERGENCIES

Effective drugs for rapid control of severe hypertension have existed for more than a decade but the literature on this subject has been rather confused. Primarily, this is because some of the drugs have not been available to physicians in different countries. Another reason is that life-threatening hypertensive emergencies have not always commanded the degree of medical and nursing care which, for example, is readily given to even minor surgical operations. Thus, parenteral administration of drugs that require frequent measurements of blood pressure during one or two days has, in general, been considered an impracticable form of treatment and this has been responsible for the restricted appeal of sodium nitroprusside. A more recent reason for difficulty in obtaining comparative information on the efficacy of drugs in hypertensive emergencies is that the condition is now becoming much less common with the increasing awareness and earlier treatment of hypertension.

Intravenous infusions of sodium nitroprusside or rapid injections of diazoxide will adequately lower blood pressure within minutes in nearly all hypertensive crises (Finnerty, 1974; Gifford, 1975; Palmer and Lasseter, 1975a). Nitroprusside is effective in those rare patients who do not respond to diazoxide (AMA Committee on Hypertension, 1974). The use of both drugs, when administered correctly, does not cause deterioration of renal function, an important consideration when renal function is poor.

Nitroprusside

Intravenous sodium nitroprusside infusions predictively lower blood pressure in all types of hypertensive emergencies including that associated with phaeochromocytoma (AMA Committee on Hypertension, 1974). The antihypertensive effect appears within 30 s of administration of an adequate dose and the blood pressure rises to previous levels within 2 min after the infusion is stopped (Gifford, 1975). A convenient concentration is 100 mg/litre 5 per cent dextrose/water (100 μg/ml) but stronger solutions can be given in order to reduce the intake of fluid. The initial rate is usually 20 μg/min and it is gradually increased until the desired blood pressure is achieved. Most patients require 50 to 200 μg/min but a few have needed, rarely, more than 500 μg/min during short periods (Palmer and Lasseter, 1975a, b). After the proper rate has been determined the pressure remains reasonably stable and it is necessary to measure it only every 5 or 10 min. The drug has been commercially available in some countries since 1974 as a lyophilised powder in ampoules (Nipride; Hoffmann–LaRoche, USA), but otherwise it is easy and inexpensive to make up stock solutions from the sodium salt of nitro-ferricyanic acid, $Na_2[Fe(CN)_5NO].2H_2O$, i.e. sodium nitroprusside (AMA Committee on Hypertension, 1974). Since the agent is light sensitive and decomposes into toxic thiocyanate, the solution is put into dark-coloured glass bottles and stored in a refrigerator at non-freezing temperatures. For the same reason, the infusion bottle or syringe (in a pump) are covered with a dark cloth or aluminium foil. Only one adverse reaction has been observed during our 12 years of experience with the drug (Tuckman, unpublished observations): this was mild vertigo that disappeared within minutes after the infusion was discontinued. In two instances the infusion was continued for three to six weeks. If thiocyanate levels are too high in the blood they may cause nausea, anorexia, rashes, headaches, hypothyroidism and psychological disturbances (Page et al, 1955; Palmer and Lasseter, 1975a). If very large doses of nitroprusside are used or if it is given for more than three days, especially in those with poor renal function, blood thiocyanate levels should be measured and administration stopped if the concentration is higher than 12 mg/100 ml (Gifford, 1975). Sodium nitroprusside is a relatively difficult drug to use and, because of this, its application outside the US has been limited, simpler alternatives being preferred. However, it remains a useful reserve drug and, when properly used, produces a smooth and controlled reduction in blood pressure.

Diazoxide

Rapid intravenous injection of diazoxide between 10 and 15 s, to prevent neutralisation of the antihypertensive action by serum protein binding (Sellers and Koch-Weser, 1973), effectively reduces blood pressure in 95 per cent of patients with severe hypertension (Finnerty, 1974). The dose is 300 mg, except in children or exceptionally heavy individuals, to whom 5 mg/kg body weight are given. More than one injection is often required to produce continuous antihypertensive control and the second administration may be given about 20 min after the initial dose (Gifford, 1975). Eventually, a single injection will cause adequate falls in pressure for as long as 24 h (Finnerty, 1974). The drug should be used in combination with a loop diuretic, such as frusemide, to prevent sodium retention by diazoxide and to potentiate the antihypertensive effect of diazoxide. Although nitroprusside provides smoother reduction and control of the pressure, intermittent injections of diazoxide, in general, provide more 'practical' treatment because they do not require continuous monitoring of the patient (AMA Committee on Hypertension, 1974). However, that drug's abrupt action is not advised in patients who have symptoms of acute coronary or cerebrovascular insufficiency. Also, nitroprusside may be particularly suited for use in patients in whom the hypertensive crisis is associated with severe left ventricular failure (Cohn, 1973).

Alternative Agents

Other drugs are used in hypertensive emergencies. Those used in patients with advanced renal impairment are hydrallazine (i.m. 10–50 mg; i.v. 10–20 mg), α-methyldopa (i.v. 250–500 mg), clonidine (i.m., s.c. or i.v. 300–600 μg) or reserpine (i.m. 1–5 mg) (Onesti et al, 1971a; AMA Committee on Hypertension, 1974). All of them may fail to lower blood pressure adequately, the onset of effective action of α-methyldopa and reserpine may take two or more hours, while i.v. clonidine is associated with an initial pressor response. Hydrallazine causes a reflex tachycardia and increase in cardiac output that can produce angina pectoris or a myocardial infarction. Also, α-methyldopa, reserpine and clonidine produce marked sedation which complicates the assessment and further management of hypertensive encephalopathy.

Recently there have been reports of the efficacy of i.v. labetolol, the combined β- and α-adrenoreceptor blocking drug, in the treatment of severe hypertension (Rosei et al, 1975).

In patients with reasonably good renal function, other drugs which significantly reduce renal blood flow can be used as well. Intravenous guanethidine is useful but it causes an initial pressor response. Intramuscular or s.c. administration avoids that reaction but then the onset of the antihypertensive may be delayed several hours (Lee, 1966). The initial i.v. dose is 0.25 mg/kg body weight and, if this is inadequate, successive injections of 0.50 and 1.00 mg/kg are given at hourly intervals. Ganglion blocking drugs can also be used in these patients, such as an intravenous infusion of fast acting trimethaphan camsylate, Arfonad (in concentrations of 1–2 g/litre) or i.v. injections of the slower acting pentolinium tartrate, Ansolysen (0.50 mg/min; maximal dose about 10 mg).

Oral antihypertensive drugs should be started, whenever possible, on the same day that the parenteral agents are begun. In this manner the latter can usually be discontinued on the second or third day and treatment becomes much simpler.

If the emergency is one which permits a delay of 12 to 24 h for control of blood pressure then it is easier to use *oral* bethanidine in patients with reasonable renal function. The first administration is 25 mg and it can be doubled every 3 h until the dose reaches 200 mg. This treatment should include a diuretic. Oral debrisoquine is not recommended for this type of acute administration as large doses may cause prolonged hypertensive episodes lasting several hours (Luria and Freis, 1965).

DIURETICS

The introduction of chlorothiazide in 1957 was an extremely important advance in the treatment of hypertension. It not only controlled blood pressure in many patients when used alone but also potentiated the action of other antihypertensive drugs.

Thiazides

Chlorothiazide is a benzothiadiazine derivative as are most of the other oral diuretics that were synthesised after 1957. In some, another radical was substituted for the thiadiazine ring and in the case of chlorthalidone this was a phthalimidine nucleus. The benzothiadiazines and phthalimidines are classified as moderate diuretics (Davies and Wilson, 1975) and they have essentially equal antihypertensive activity (Cranston et al, 1963; Lund-Johansen, 1970; Degnbol, Dorph and Marner, 1973). They cause approximately the same maximal diuresis when given in large doses (Davies and Wilson, 1975), and this begins, reaches its peak and terminates about 2, 4 and 12 h after ingestion respectively for most of the drugs.

Long-acting derivatives
The diuresis caused by the longer acting benzothiadiazines, such as methyclothiazide, polythiazide and cyclothiazide may last 24 h and that after chlorthalidone for as long as 72 h (Bengtsson et al, 1975).

Biochemical effects
These agents bring about natriuresis by inhibiting sodium absorption in the cortical segment of the ascending loop of Henle. They also produce hypokalaemia and alkalosis as side effects because more sodium is absorbed in the distal convoluted tubule in exchange for potassium and hydrogen ions; the increased exchange results from the large amount of sodium delivered to the distal tubule and the secondary hyperaldosteronism induced by the

diuretics (Anderton and Kincaid-Smith, 1971; Dustan, Tarazi and Bravo, 1974).

Loop Diuretics

Frusemide and ethacrynic acid were introduced in 1963. Frusemide has a furfuryl radical in place of the thiadiazine ring but there is no obvious structural similarity between ethacrynic acid and the other drugs discussed previously. These agents are classified as 'potent' diuretics because they produce a much greater maximal diuresis than the benzothiadiazines and phthalimidines. The effect begins, reaches its peak and terminates within 30 min, 2 h and 4 to 6 h after ingestion (Anderton and Kincaid-Smith, 1971; Davies and Wilson, 1975). Frusemide and ethacrynic acid are also called loop diuretics because of their extensive action on the ascending loop of Henle, in which they inhibit the absorption of sodium from both the medullary and cortical segments. They are effective in patients with severe renal impairment and still cause a natriuresis in subjects with creatinine clearances which are 20 to 30 per cent of normal, in whom the moderate diuretics have little influence (Tarazi and Gifford, 1975).

Potassium-sparing Diuretics

Spironolactone, triamterene and amiloride were introduced between 1960 and 1966 and are classified as potassium-sparing diuretics. Spironolactone is an antagonist of aldosterone and is ineffective in adrenalectomised subjects. This is not true of triamterene or amiloride which act on the kidney independently of aldosterone. The three drugs inhibit Na–K exchange in the distal tubule and, since the amount of absorption of sodium at this site is relatively small, they are weak diuretics and also poor antihypertensive agents (Tarazi and Gifford, 1975). They are used in the treatment of hypertension primarily in combination with the other diuretics to prevent excessive hypokalaemia.

Mechanisms of the Antihypertensive Action

There is general agreement that the diuretics reduce plasma and extracellular volumes during the first week or two of administration, but until recently there was controversy whether this occurred in long-term treatment. However, from 1968, serial studies of hypertensive patients receiving only diuretics clearly showed that chronic treatment was associated with a decrease in plasma volume of 7 to 10 per cent (Hansen, 1968; Leth, 1970; Tarazi, Dustan and Frohlich, 1970), and a probable reduction of extracellular volume (Leth, 1970; Tarazi et al, 1970). These results are consistent with the widespread clinical observations that most patients have an increase in weight when the drugs are interrupted after long use (Tarazi et al, 1970).

Haemodynamic effects

Results from investigations in man on the short- and long-term effect of the diuretics on cardiac output are conflicting and indicate that it is unchanged or reduced and accompanied with respective decreases or elevations of peripheral vascular resistance (Davidov, Kakaviatos and Finnerty, 1967a; Lund-Johansen, 1970; Dustan et al, 1974; Tarazi and Gifford, 1975). None the less, these data from both the short- and long-term studies showed that the drugs reduced peripheral resistance; when the cardiac output did not fall there was an absolute decrease in resistance, and if reduced the rise in resistance was relatively less than that expected under other conditions in which there is no inhibition of sympathetic compensatory vascular tone. Indeed, there is considerable evidence that the diuretics diminish the effect of sympathetic activity on blood vessels (possibly due to decreased total exchangeable body sodium (Hansen, 1968)) and this may be why the rather small short- and long-term decrease of plasma volume of approximately 10 per cent and of total blood volume of only 5 per cent are associated with lowered arterial pressure. Therefore, several workers have proposed that the reduction in blood volume and the diminished peripheral resistance are both primary, simultaneous causal factors in the mechanism of the maintained antihypertensive action of the diuretics, when used alone or with other drugs which inhibit adrenergic activity (Dustan et al, 1974; Tarazi and Gifford, 1975). This view is supported by their clinical data which showed that the success of treatment was inversely correlated with blood volume.

Clinical Use

Some physicians use the diuretics as initial and sole therapy in most patients and if pressure is inadequately lowered they are combined with other drugs (Dustan et al, 1974). Others prefer to use the 'more potent' anti-hypertensive drugs alone and add a diuretic only when indicated (Prichard et al, 1968). This can reduce the number of patients exposed to more than one drug and lessens the risk of developing biochemical side effects from the diuretics.

The moderate diuretics, the benzothiadiazines and phthalimidines, are the diuretics of choice in antihypertensive treatment. They have relatively flat dose–response curves so that the same dose can be prescribed for nearly all patients without fear of causing exaggerated responses. There are a large number of these drugs but except for their different duration of action there is little reason to choose one from the other. Most should be given twice daily as their duration of action is about 12 h, and it is better to take the second dose early in the afternoon to avoid disturbing sleep by the diuresis. The longer acting drugs need be given only once a day and, of course, early in the morning. An optimal antihypertensive effect can usually be obtained with hydrochlorothiazide 50 mg bds, bendrofluazide 5 mg bds and cyclopenthiazide 0.5 mg bds. The daily dosages of the longer acting drugs are: chlorthalidone 100 mg and polythiazide 2 mg. Low salt diets are not necessary but patients should avoid a large intake as this will neutralise the antihypertensive effect of the medication (Winer, 1961).

The loop diuretics are not obviously superior to the benzothiadiazines and phthalimidines for routine treatment and their use can be more troublesome. The initial doses can cause inordinate responses in sensitive patients (Davidov et al, 1967a) and chronic large doses may cause unwanted levels of dehydration, particularly in the elderly and in hot climates. Also, as they are given three times a day, they often produce frequent periods of inconvenient copious diuresis. The loop diuretics are more effective in patients with moderate or severe renal impairment (Tarazi and Gifford, 1975) and frusemide is easier to use than ethacrynic acid as the latter often causes gastrointestinal disturbances. Convenient doses of frusemide are 40 or 80 mg tds, but doses of one or more grams have been used in patients with very poor renal function (Davies and Wilson, 1975). These large amounts may cause ototoxicity.

Spironolactone, triamterene and amiloride are mainly used with other diuretics to prevent unacceptable levels of hypokalaemia. Doses for this purpose are spironolactone 25 mg bds or qds, triamterene 100 mg bds and amiloride 5 mg bds. Patients receiving these drugs should be warned never to take potassium supplements unless specifically instructed and then only if frequent checks are made of the serum potassium concentrations. For the same reason, to avoid hyperkalaemia, these diuretics should not be used in patients with moderate or severe renal impairment unless they are under strict medical supervision.

Side Effects

Hypokalaemia

Some degree of hypokalaemia occurs in most patients who receive adequate antihypertensive doses of the diuretics. However, several workers doubt whether potassium supplements or potassium-sparing adjuvants need routinely be given to patients on chronic therapy (Dargie et al, 1974; Wilkinson et al, 1975) because it is now known that the diuretics do not usually cause excessive reductions of total body potassium (Edmonds and Jasani, 1972; Dargie et al, 1974). But patients on diuretics in hypertension clinics occasionally have very low concentrations of serum potassium and it cannot be ignored that potassium deficiency causes renal damage in man and animals (Relman and Schwartz, 1958). Thus, it would seem prudent to correct serum potassiums if they tend to be less than 3.0 to 3.5 mEq/litre (Dustan et al, 1974). In general, potassium supplements are preferable to the potassium-sparing diuretics. The latter are more expensive, more likely to cause side effects (other than perhaps gastrointestinal discomfort), and there is always a possibility they may produce hyperkalaemia. Potassium chloride, 8 or 16 mEq tds, provides adequate amounts of the ion for most patients, but supplements in forms other than the chloride will not efficiently correct the hypokalaemia. Measurements of serum or plasma potassium levels is best done one or two months after the diuretics are started and then at six-monthly intervals. If the patient also receives digitalis the measurements should be more frequent and the concentrations required somewhat higher. Potassium supplements rarely cause small-bowel ulceration and stenosis (Baker, Schrader and Hitchcock, 1964) and still more infrequently lesions of the oesophagus when passage is hindered by an obstruction such as an enlarged heart (Howie and Strachan, 1975). This complication is caused by the rapid discharge of concentrated potassium chloride into a small region of the gut, e.g. from enteric coated tablets, and the incidence is presumably less when slow release tablets are used.

Hyperuricaemia

The frequent hyperuricaemia associated with the diuretics is nearly always symptomless but it may produce clinical gout; primarily in those with a history of the condition (Dustan et al, 1974; Davies and Wilson, 1975). The plasma uric acid concentration is easily lowered in patients with good renal function with the uricosuric agent probenecid or with allopurinol in those with advanced renal impairment. It seems unnecessary to treat symptomless elevations of uric acid of 10 mg/100 ml or less in patients with good renal function and no history of gout (Dustan et al, 1974). It would appear wise, however, to keep the level below 8 mg/100 ml in those susceptible to gout and/or in patients with moderate or severe renal disease (Davies and Wilson, 1975; Tarazi and Gifford, 1975).

Hyperglycaemia

The diuretics sometimes cause hyperglycaemia and, rarely (primarily in prediabetic patients), frank diabetes. They are not contraindicated in diabetics (Tarazi and Gifford, 1975), and, in the uncommon event that they disturb the requirements for antihyperglycaemic agents, small appropriate elevations in the dosages of those drugs rectify the situation.

Other side effects

The moderate and loop diuretics produce other rare side effects. These include hypercalcaemia, thrombocytopenia, neutropenia and pancytopenia. They have also been associated with skin rashes, photosensitivity, acute haemorrhagic pancreatitis, acute pulmonary reactions, allergic interstitial nephritis and positive antinuclear factor tests (Davies and Wilson, 1975). The potassium sparing diuretics may cause gastrointestinal disturbances and spironolactone may produce gynaecomastia, impotence in males, and menstrual disorders (Davies and Wilson, 1975).

Nearly two decades of widespread use has shown that the diuretics cause very few clinically significant untoward reactions. They will no doubt continue to be used extensively in the future.

ADRENERGIC NEURONE INHIBITING DRUGS (ANID)

Mode of Action

Bethanidine, debrisoquine and guanethidine are selectively concentrated in the terminals of postganglionic sympathetic nerves and lower blood pressure by inhibiting the release of noradrenaline caused by action potentials. Guanethidine was the first of the three drugs used and it was quickly established in animals that single injections of large doses, by clinical standards, depleted the neurons of noradrenaline. Since this did not occur when bethanidine or debrisoquine were given, at least during short periods, some workers proposed that the antihypertensive effect of guanethidine, in man, was due to depletion of the transmitter from sympathetic nerves and that of the other drugs to inhibition of the 'physiological release' of noradrenaline (Abrams et al, 1964).

However, it is unlikely that the clinical action of adrenergic neurone inhibiting drugs (ANID) is dependent on exhaustion of noradrenaline. First, guanethidine inhibits release of noradrenaline during sympathetic stimulation long before it depletes nerves of the catecholamine (Boura and Green, 1965). Secondly, the doses of ANID used in man are much smaller than those needed to deplete animals of noradrenaline. Thirdly, effective antihypertensive treatment with ANID does not produce a complete sympathectomy. Patients are not incapacitated by postural hypotension and exercise causes large increases in cardiac work (Taylor et al, 1962; Chamberlain and Howard, 1964; Khatri and Cohn, 1970). And, lastly, i.v. tyramine induces obvious pressor responses in those on long-term guanethidine therapy, from the presumed release of endogenous noradrenaline (Cohn, Liptak and Freis, 1963).

Intravenous injections of ANID first release noradrenaline from the sympathetic nerves and produce a pressor response before they reduce blood pressure. In man, i.v. debrisoquine causes a large increase during 1 or 2 h (Abrams et al, 1964; Kakaviatos et al, 1964), guanethidine induces a moderate increase for several minutes, and bethanidine is associated with only a minimal elevation (Fewings et al, 1964; Johnston, Prichard and Rosenheim, 1964). As the pressor effects are not combined with an important decrease of the transmitter in sympathetic nerves it is not apparent how the three drugs differentially change the balance between neuronal noradrenaline synthesis, release, uptake, storage and monoamine deamination during this period. A relevant factor might be that bethanidine (Boura and Green, 1965) and debrisoquine (Pettinger et al, 1969) are monoamine oxidase (MAO) inhibitors, and, therefore, their concentration in the nerves could prevent inactivation of free (extravesicular) intraneural noradrenaline to vanillylmandellic acid.

Unfortunately, the hypothesis does not explain the greater elevation of pressure caused by guanethidine compared with bethanidine, since the former is not a MAO inhibitor (Furst, 1967).

It is not generally appreciated that large *oral* doses of debrisoquine cause severe elevations of blood pressure which can last several hours (Luria and Freis, 1965). There have not been reports that *oral* bethanidine increases blood pressure. It has also been found that subjects given debrisoquine showed increased pressor responses to oral and i.v. tyramine and that they experienced serious hypertensive reactions after eating Gruyère cheese and oral administration of phenylephrine (Abrams et al, 1964; Pettinger et al, 1969; Amery and Deloof, 1970; Aminu, D'Mello and Vere, 1970). Similar reports about possible clinical manifestations from MAO inhibitory activity of bethanidine in man, whether negative or positive, have not been published.

When noradrenaline is released by postganglionic action potentials its major pathways include direct stimulation of adrenergic receptors, metabolism by extraneuronal catechol-*o*-methyl transferase to normetanephrine, or uptake back into the nerves by an energy dependent pump (Iversen, 1973). The amount of uptake is an important factor which limits the level of cardiovascular stimulation; less uptake provides more transmitter at the receptors and vice versa. ANID also enter the nerves through the same membrane pump and are competitive antagonists of noradrenaline at this site. Therefore, they dangerously potentiate the pressor response to i.v. administered noradrenaline or to the endogenous release of the amine in patients with phaeochromocytoma. Similarly, tricyclic antidepressants affect the neuronal pump and by that means block entry of ANID into the sympathetic nerves and reduce their antihypertensive action (Mitchell et al, 1970).

Haemodynamic Effects

Studies of supine subjects at rest indicate that the lowering of blood pressure caused by ANID are associated with either average decreases in cardiac output or peripheral resistance or with simultaneous reductions of both measurements (Richardson et al, 1960; Novack, 1961; Cohn et al, 1963; Abrams et al, 1964; Villarreal et al, 1964; Onesti et al, 1969). Whether cardiac output or peripheral resistance fell below pretreatment values in the various investigations does not suggest that different haemodynamic mechanisms were responsible for the antihypertensive action, as some workers have argued. It merely indicated that under the conditions of study there was a relative difference between the decreases of the two variables, produced by sympathetic inhibition, from their expected levels. Normally, in untreated subjects a decrease in cardiac output is associated with a reflex increase in peripheral resistance and, conversely, a decrease in peripheral resistance would produce an elevation of cardiac output.

ANID characteristically cause postural hypotension. Again, there is controversy whether the drugs decrease cardiac output or peripheral resistance and analysis of the question has been particularly inadequate because the upright haemodynamic measurements have usually been compared with those obtained in the supine position. When untreated subjects change from a supine to an upright position there is a large shift of blood volume to the dependent veins, a decrease in cardiac output of 20 to 25 per cent and a compensatory reflex increase in peripheral resistance of approximately 30 per cent. If this is considered, the results from haemodynamic studies of ANID in upright subjects at rest show that they usually lower blood pressure largely by reducing peripheral resistance (Richardson et al, 1960; Abrams et al, 1964; Chamberlain and Howard, 1964; Villarreal et al, 1964; Onesti et al, 1966; Khatri and Cohn, 1970). They only slightly exaggerate the normal orthostatic decrease in cardiac output but they inhibit most of the usual 30 per cent compensatory increase of peripheral resistance. The data therefore suggest that ANID do not cause excessive peripheral venous pooling in upright patients at doses which produce tolerable degrees of postural hypotension.

An important aspect of treatment with ANID is that they cause exertional hypotension. Patients receiving the drugs perform exercise at much lower arterial pressures than do untreated hypertensive subjects, especially in upright positions. Also, the agents commonly reduce blood pressures during physical activity to levels below the resting, treated, measurements.

Haemodynamic studies of untreated subjects have shown that exercise produces a large fall of vascular resistance in the active limbs, an increase of arteriolar and venous vasoconstriction in other regions, a large elevation of cardiac output, and usually a small increase in mean arterial pressure. Only an approximate estimation can be made of the effects that ANID have on the haemodynamic changes of exercises because the few relevant studies were carried out under varied conditions. In these investigations the exercise, after administration of ANID, was associated with small increases or decreases of mean arterial pressure (compared with resting, treated, measurements) in both supine and upright positions (Taylor et al, 1962; Chamberlain and Howard, 1964; Khatri and Cohn, 1970) except in the study of a group of patients who were selected because they had moderate to large degrees of hypotension, even when supine (Dollery, Emslie-Smith and Shillingford, 1961). All results showed large average increases in cardiac output, including those from the subjects who had had the larger falls of arterial pressure. The data are not detailed enough to answer the question whether those patients with the greatest falls in pressure had smaller increases in cardiac output and/ or greater decreases of total peripheral resistance. In any event, these results indicate that patients treated with ANID still possess considerable cardiac reserve and can increase their external cardiac work (expressed as the product of cardiac output and mean arterial pressure) by at least 100 per cent.

Clinical Use

Guanethidine, bethanidine and debrisoquine have been used in the treatment of hypertension since 1959, 1961 and 1963 respectively. All are very effective antihypertensive drugs but unfortunately they also cause important side effects. Some workers have reported that one or another is better tolerated by patients, but the differences are clearly marginal except when guanethidine causes severe diarrhoea.

Details of management

Oral doses of guanethidine do not begin to lower arterial pressure until three days after treatment is started and it takes another two or three days before its maximal action occurs. This delay and the wide range of patients' sensitivities, between 10 and 1050 mg/day, means that it could require several months to determine an individual's correct antihypertensive dose. The maximal antihypertensive effect of oral bethanidine and debrisoquine is produced within 4 h of ingestion and subsides several hours later (Abrams et al, 1964; Johnston et al, 1964). Therefore, these two drugs can gain control of blood pressure within a day, when necessary, and they have to be given in divided daily doses, tds or qds. The range of patients' sensitivities to bethanidine varies between 10 and 1000 mg/day, and that reported for debrisoquine has been between 10 and 360 mg/day. Bethanidine and debrisoquine are both primarily excreted by the kidneys so that single oral doses can produce severe hypotensive episodes for as long as one or two days in subjects with poor renal function (Montuschi and Pickens, 1962).

If it is accepted that antihypertensive drugs provide good control when standing diastolic pressure is 100 mmHg or less, then ANID, often in combination with diuretics, achieved this result in approximately 40 to 80 per cent of patients in different investigations (Montuschi and Pickens, 1962; Johnston et al, 1964; Kitchen and Turner, 1966; Prichard et al, 1968; Adi, Eze and Anwunah, 1975).

Side effects and precautions

The most important and debilitating symptoms are from postural and exercise hypotension (Prichard et al, 1968) and these are aggravated by hot climates and working environments. Generally, ANID should not be used in patients who do heavy manual labour and they must not be given if dizziness and syncope might cause catastrophic accidents.

Another very serious side effect of ANID is that they disturb sexual functions in a majority of male patients (Prichard et al, 1968; Bauer et al, 1973; Adi et al, 1975). It therefore follows that they should only be used in young males when absolutely necessary and with understanding in older men.

Guanethidine causes loose watery stools in as many as two-thirds of patients (Prichard et al, 1968). In most this is only a nuisance but in others the bowel movements are so frequent, urgent and explosive that the drug is intolerable. Other side effects caused by ANID are usually of minor importance. Guanethidine produces an obvious bradycardia but this is rarely of clinical significance. The fluid retention that may be associated with the use of these three drugs is easily prevented or reversed in patients with adequate renal function by adding a diuretic to the antihypertensive regime. The drugs can also cause muscle weakness and stuffiness of the nose (Kitchen and Turner, 1966; Prichard et al, 1968).

There are other precautions which should be noted when using ANID. Since they reduce glomerular filtration rate (Richardson et al, 1960; Novack, 1961; Villarreal et al, 1964), they can precipitate frank uraemia in patients with advanced renal impairment; that effect is nearly always reversible when the drugs are discontinued. Also, the blood pressure will usually increase to near pretreatment levels within less than a day if bethanidine or debrisoquine are abruptly stopped and this might present a danger in those who take medications in an undisciplined manner. Under other circumstances the prolonged effect on blood pressure of guanethidine, for approximately three days, could be disadvantageous, for instance when it is necessary to stop or reduce dosages of antihypertensive drugs during the episodes of hypotension which are associated with haemorrhage, myocardial infarction, infection or trauma.

Finally, amphetamine, tricyclic antidepressants, and chlorpromazine inhibit the antihypertensive action of ANID and, conversely, serious hypotension may occur when these psychotropic agents are discontinued.

METHYLDOPA

Mode of Action

How α-methyldopa exerts its antihypertensive effect is not entirely clear but a central action seems probable (Laverty, 1973).

False transmitter hypothesis

It had been suggested by Day and Rand (1963) that α-methyldopa exerted its hypotensive action by being converted to α-methylnoradrenaline which then acts as a false transmitter when liberated at sympathetic nerve endings. However, α-methylnoradrenaline is about equipotent to noradrenaline in the cat and dog, and is only slightly less potent than noradrenaline on human smooth muscle. Although the acute administration of α-methyldopa depresses the function of sympathetic nerves, no effect was seen on the responses after chronic treatment (Haefely, Hürlimann and Thoenen, 1967).

Central action

A number of observations have suggested that the central nervous system is the site of action. A small dose of α-methyldopa injected into the vertebral artery produced a fall of blood pressure while intravenous administration produces no effect. Secondly, the administration of α-methyldopa into the vascularly isolated perfused cat brain caused a fall of blood pressure in the rest of the animal (Laverty, 1973). Thirdly, Baum, Shropshire and Varner (1972) have demonstrated a reduction of sympathetic nerve traffic following the administration of methyldopa to renal hypertensive rats.

Alpha-methyldopa is metabolised to α-methylnoradrenaline in the brain. This stimulates the central α-adrenergic receptors, and it is blocked by α-adrenoceptor blocking drugs (Heise and Kroneberg, 1972). The prevention of the metabolism of methyldopa and thus the formation of α-methylnoradrenaline by the administration of a centrally active dopa-decarboxylase inhibitor abolishes the antihypertensive effect of α-methyldopa, but this does not occur when a dopa-decarboxylase inhibitor which does not penetrate the brain is given (Henning and Rubenson, 1971). Likewise the prevention of α-methylnoradrenaline synthesis by the destruction of central adrenergic neurones by intraventricular 6-hydroxydopamine also prevented the hypotensive effect of α-methyldopa, whereas intravenous 6-hydroxydopamine reduced, but did not prevent the hypotensive effect (Finch and Haeusler, 1973). Finally it was also found that hypotensive doses of α-methyldopa failed to reduce the pressor response that is seen when the entire sympathetic outflow is stimulated (Finch and Haeusler, 1973).

Cardiovascular Effects of Methyldopa

Intravenously, α-methyldopa lowers blood pressure principally by reduction in peripheral resistance and the small average reduction in cardiac output for both supine and erect position is not significant (Onesti et al, 1964, Cohen et al, 1967). Chamberlain and Howard (1964) after short-term oral administration of α-methyldopa, 0.75 to 3 g daily, also did not observe any reduction in cardiac output, and the fall in blood pressure in the supine position was associated with a reduction in peripheral resistance. The increased fall in blood pressure on standing was associated with a failure of the peripheral resistance to rise as it did before the administration of α-methyldopa. As the reduction of cardiac output on adopting the erect position was not greater after α-methyldopa, there is no evidence to suggest venous pooling. Many of the blood pressures in these patients were relatively high even after α-methyldopa treatment and these results may not be fully applicable to patients when blood pressure is adequately controlled, although all except one patient showed at least some postural hypotension. Venous pooling may play a part with more adequate control of the blood pressure in some patients with α-methyldopa as a venodepressor effect has been demonstrated after oral administration of α-methyldopa (2 to 5 g daily) over periods between 21 and 49 days (Mason and Braunwald, 1964). However, Lund-Johansen (1972) studied a series of 13 mild hypertensives before and after a year's treatment with α-methyldopa (500 to 1500 mg/day, average 896 mg/day), and it was found that the fall in blood pressure at rest, standing and on exercise was associated with a fall in cardiac output, and no change was seen in peripheral resistance. The patients did not show any postural drop in blood pressure, the supine and standing blood pressures after α-methyldopa were 139/84, and 150/93 mmHg.

There is no doubt that larger doses of α-methyldopa when used in the treatment of hypertension are associated with postural and exercise hypotension, although less than that seen with sympathetic inhibiting drugs, bethanidine, or guanethidine (Oates et al, 1965, Prichard et al, 1968).

Clinical Use

Oates et al (1960) first reported the antihypertensive effect of a α-methyldopa. If a level of a standing diastolic pressure of 100 mmHg is taken as reasonable control, α-methyldopa has been found by various investigators to control about half the hypertensive patients to this level (Prichard et al, 1968). Johnson et al (1966) found that the fall in blood pressure in 37 patients on α-methyldopa was similar to that seen in 66 patients of similar severity on guanethidine. This confirmed a previous within patient study in 19 patients of Oates et al (1965) who found α-methyldopa, guanethidine and pargyline produced similar blood pressure control. Likewise Prichard et al (1968) in a within patient study in 30 patients found α-methyldopa produced similar control to bethanidine and guanethidine.

Differences between α-methyldopa and other antihypertensive drugs reside in the effect on cardiovascular response and the nature of side effects. As has been discussed above, control of the blood pressure with methyldopa is associated with less postural and exercise fall in blood pressure than that seen with adrenergic neurone inhibitory drugs.

The usual starting dose is 250 mg two or three times daily, occasionally half this dose. Increments of 250 mg/dose may be made. Some physicians only use up to 2 g/day, others have used higher doses, e.g. 6 g/day (Hamilton and Kopelman, 1963). A diuretic should be used in addition if any side effects occur, such as sedation, and most usually would be added in any case if a daily dose of 2 g is reached. Tolerance is not uncommon, but can usually be overcome by increasing the dose.

Side Effects

Tiredness occurs in about half the patients treated with methyldopa and is the most common factor limiting dose. Other central nervous system side effects occur such as dreams and depression (Johnson et al, 1966; Prichard et al, 1968). Weight gain is another common side effect, and has been reported in as many as 64 per cent of cases (Johnson et al, 1966). Diarrhoea is unusual as are symptoms of postural or exertional hypotension (Johnson et al, 1966; Prichard et al, 1968). Skin rashes have been reported, urticaria and eczema, particularly in patients with previous skin disorders (Church, 1974).

A positive Coombs' test is frequent, about 20 per cent, but an autoimmune haemolytic anaemia only develops in about 0.02 per cent of patients receiving α-methyldopa (Worlledge, Carstairs and Dacie, 1966). Rarely, reversible leucopenia or thrombocytopenia may occur (Benraad and Schoenaker, 1965). Antinuclear factor has been reported in just under 15 per cent of patients on α-methyldopa (Breckenridge et al, 1967).

Alpha-methyldopa may rarely cause a number of other untoward effects, hepatotoxicity, most often an hepatic syndrome (Toghill et al, 1974), hyper-pyrexia (Glontz and Saslaw, 1968), lactation and Parkinsonism. Finally, a paradoxical pressor response has been reported with methyldopa (Levine and Strauch, 1966).

CLONIDINE

Mode of Action

Clonidine was introduced as treatment for hypertension 1966. It was soon evident that the mechanism of action of the drug was unique and this stimulated a large number of basic investigations and renewed interest in the role of the central nervous system in hypertension.

The drug does not block sympathetic ganglia, inhibit release of noradrena-line from postganglionic nerves, deplete noradrenergic neurones of the trans-mitter, nor does it block α- or β-receptors of the cardiovascular system. However, clonidine directly stimulates peripheral α-adrenoceptors and this produces an initial pressor response after i.v. administration.

The antihypertensive effect is primarily due to the drug's stimulation of α-receptors in the hindbrain (Haeusler, 1975; Henning, 1975). Clonidine direct-ly stimulates central α-receptors, and unlike α-methyldopa this action is not dependent on the interposition of noradrenergic neurones (Haeusler, 1974; Kobinger and Pichler, 1974). When given orally or intravenously, or if administered at much smaller doses into a vertebral artery, the ventricular system of the hindbrain, or applied to the 'vasomotor centres' of the medulla oblongata, the consequent reductions of heart rate and blood pressure are associated with diminished neuroelectrical activity of the sympathetic nerves. Administration of these smaller amounts to the brain does not cause the initial pressor action which is produced by larger intravenous doses because there is no stimulation of the peripheral α-receptors. Clonidine does not produce the above mentioned responses if the brain is pretreated with α-receptor blocking drugs.

Clonidine not only reduces spontaneous (resting) sympathetic and increases vagal activity but it also facilitates the evoked autonomic changes caused by stimulation of the carotid sinus and aortic arch baroreceptors (Robson and

Antonaccio, 1975). It also reduces, in animals, the evoked increases of sympathetic nervous system activity which are caused by hypoxia, common carotid artery occlusion, and stimulation of pressor areas of the hypothalamus. These last observations are difficult to extrapolate to man because a major advantage of the drug in treatment is that it rarely produces significant postural hypotension. Therefore, it is assumed that clonidine permits, in man, the necessary evoked increase of sympathetic tone that is induced by decreased carotid sinus stimulation during changes in posture (Tuckman et al, 1968).

Haemodynamic and Renal Effects

There have been but few studies of the haemodynamic effects of clonidine in man and they concerned acute administration of the drug. In the supine position the antihypertensive action was associated with reductions of cardiac output of approximately 20 per cent and insignificant changes in peripheral resistance (Brod et al, 1972; Onesti et al, 1969). Therefore, clonidine prevented the compensatory increase in resistance which would have occurred in untreated subjects with this fall in cardiac output. In upright positions the lowering of blood pressure was accompanied by a diminution of peripheral resistance of about 20 to 25 per cent and more modest decreases in cardiac output (Davidov, Kakaviators and Finnerty, 1967b; Onesti et al, 1969). There is evidence that the reduction in cardiac output caused by clonidine is secondary to the action of the drug on the veins which increases venous distensibility and decreases cardiac filling pressure (Brod et al, 1972).

Haemodynamic investigations of the effect of i.v. clonidine on responses during exercise showed that it did not alter the increases in mean arterial pressure or cardiac output (Muir, Burton and Lawrie, 1969). As expected, this high level of evoked sympathetic stimulation 'broke through' the drug's central inhibitory action and caused normal vasoconstriction in the non-exercising parts of the body. One of the advantages of clonidine in the treatment of hypertension is that it does not produce exertional hypotension.

The antihypertensive action of clonidine does not cause conspicuous elevations of serum creatinine even in patients with poor renal function (Hoobler and Sagastume, 1971; Onesti et al, 1971a). These observations are consistent with the results of several investigations that showed that both acute and chronic administrations of the agent did not lower renal blood flow or glomerular filtration rate (Davidov et al, 1967b; Onesti et al, 1969, 1971a; Brod et al, 1972). Thus, the use of clonidine in antihypertensive treatment, similar to the use of α-methyldopa, tends to preserve renal function.

Clinical Use

Some investigators have suggested that clonidine is a more effective antihypertensive agent in chronic treatment than α-methyldopa (Amery et al, 1970; Onesti et al, 1971b). However, unlike α-methyldopa (Prichard et al,

1968), clonidine rarely controls blood pressure unless it is used with a diuretic (Davidov et al, 1967b); Onesti et al, 1971b). When used with a diuretic it is an effective antihypertensive drug in as many as 80 per cent of patients (Onesti et al, 1971b). After oral administration it begins to lower blood pressure within 30 to 60 min, reaches its peak action within 2 to 4 h and has a significant effect for approximately 6 to 12 h (Davidov et al, 1967b; Onesti et al, 1969). Therefore, the drug has to be given in divided daily doses, usually tds. The range of patients' sensitivities to the antihypertensive effect is large and it has been used in doses between 75 μg and 6 mg/day (Davidov et al, 1967b; Amery et al, 1970; Onesti et al, 1971a).

Side Effects

It was previously emphasised that clonidine rarely causes clinically signicant postural or exercise hypotension and this contrasts with treatment which uses α-methyldopa or the adrenergic inhibiting drugs (Prichard et al, 1968).

Clonidine produces sedation, dryness of the mouth and constipation in a majority of patients. Since these effects are dose dependent and diminish with time (Davidov, et al, 1967b; Hoobler and Sagastume, 1971; Onesti et al, 1971b) it is best to increase the dose gradually at intervals of one or two weeks whenever possible. Sedation is the most serious untoward reaction and often prevents administration of adequately high doses for control of blood pressure. Dryness of the mouth can be alleviated by measures which increase salivary secretion, such as drops of lemon juice, sucking citrus sweets, etc. Constipation is usually of minor severity; however, one instance of paralytic ileus has been reported (Davidov et al, 1967b). The condition was promptly corrected within 24 h after the drug was stopped.

Clonidine is associated with another important and unique side effect. When the drug is abruptly stopped the patient may experience within 8 to 24 h an exaggerated elevation of blood pressure, tachycardia, palpitations, sweating and a feeling of anxiety (Hunyor et al, 1973). This withdrawal syndrome is associated with increases of plasma and urinary catecholamines (Hunyor et al, 1973). It has been treated with i.v. phentolamine and propranolol (Hunyor et al, 1973) but more effective treatment is probably provided by i.v. clonidine, 300 μg (Tuckman, unpublished observations). Oral clonidine, 300 to 600 μg, also is effective, but the onset of action is slower. The incidence of the withdrawal syndrome appears low (Hunyor et al, 1973) and it does not occur if the drug is gradually discontinued during a week. Severe vomiting has occurred following abrupt withdrawal of clonidine and it was relieved by parenteral administration of the drug (Hopkirk, Simpson and Fitzgerald, 1975).

Rarer side effects include rashes, parotid pain, shivering, sleep reversal, exceptionally gynecomastia (Onesti et al, 1971a), Raynaud's phenomenon (Raftos et al, 1973), and visual blurring (Ng et al, 1967). The drug has rarely been associated with de novo episodes or exacerbations of pre-existing psychological disturbances in hypertensive patients (Ng et al, 1967; Raftos et al, 1973). The combined use of large doses of propranolol and clonidine in patients with very poor renal function caused semicoma in five patients. Recovery was rapid when clonidine was withdrawn (Kincaid-Smith et al, 1975).

The role of clonidine today is probably best considered as a substitute for α-methyldopa or the adrenergic neurone inhibiting drugs (ANID) in patients in whom the last two agents cannot be stopped in favour of β-blockers alone or some combination of diuretic, β-blocker and a vasodilating drug. When clonidine, α-methyldopa and/or ANID provide equally effective blood pressure control, the drug of choice will necessarily be the one which causes the fewest side effects.

BETA-ADRENOCEPTOR BLOCKING DRUGS

The use of pronethalol in the treatment of hypertension, was reported in 1964 (Prichard, 1964), and the first report of the antihypertensive effect of propranolol appeared later that year (Prichard and Gillam, 1964). Initially there was a slow start to the acceptance of propranolol as an antihypertensive drug but subsequently its value and that of other beta-adrenoceptor blocking drugs in hypertension has been established (Simpson, 1974).

Haemodynamic Effects of β-Blocking Drugs

Acute effects

The acute administration of propranolol produces a reduction in heart rate and cardiac output, while blood pressure remains unchanged. The overall resistance rises (Shinebourne, Fleming and Hamer, 1967; Tarazi and Dustan, 1972; Gibson, 1974). All β-blocking drugs reduce cardiac output at high levels of sympathetic activity seen on exercise, although at rest those which possess an intrinsic sympathomimetic effect produce less of a reduction in cardiac output.

The reduction in cardiac output is principally rate dependent although other factors play a part as a fall in cardiac output is seen when β-blocking drugs are given to patients with paced hearts (Gibson, 1974). This rate independent fall in cardiac output may in part be due to the fall in plasma volume seen after intravenous propranolol (Julius et al, 1972). The cardio-selective practolol is exceptional in that studies have demonstrated a lesser reduction in cardiac output per unit change in heart rate, although a fall in cardiac output is seen with larger doses of practolol in patients with impaired left ventricular function. (Gibson, 1974).

The haemodynamic effects of β-blocking drugs is a function of the β-receptor inhibition and is not due to any non-specific membrane effect as the D-isomer of propranolol (Bennet et al, 1970) is without significant effect.

Chronic effects

Intravenous administration of propranolol and chronic oral administration of propranolol in doses that produce a similar reduction in cardiac output are markedly different in their effect on blood pressure. Whereas acutely blood pressure is unchanged, with chronic administration there is a fall in blood pressure (Tarazi and Dustan, 1972; Hansson, 1973).

Propranolol added to a diuretic produces similar haemodynamic effects. There is no fall in blood pressure after acute administration but cardiac output falls, as does renin, and thus there is a rise in peripheral resistance, while one month later blood pressure was reduced with a decline of peripheral resistance (Niarchos, Tarazi and Bravo, unpublished; cited by Tarazi, Dustan and Bravo, 1976). Lowering of cardiac output per se does not usually appear to be the reason for the hypotensive effect of β-adrenergic blocking drugs; however, an exception is the addition of a β-receptor blocking drug to a patient receiving a vasodilator. The addition of propranolol to minoxidil led to a further fall in blood pressure, and a fall in cardiac output, with no change in peripheral resistance (Tarazi et al, 1976).

Response of blood pressure to physiological stimuli

Numerous trials have demonstrated that once blood pressure has been lowered by β-blocking agents there is no postural or exercise hypotension (Simpson, 1974) in contrast to the effect seen with sympathetic inhibitory drugs (Prichard and Gillam, 1969; Prichard, Boakes and Graham, 1977). Likewise prolonged oral propranolol does not inhibit the vasoconstriction from obstruction of venous return by Valsalva's manoeuvre unlike sympathetic inhibitory drugs (Prichard, Gillam and Graham, 1970). Finally increasing environmental temperature (from 7 to 30°C) resulted in an increase postural fall in blood pressure on bethanidine or guanethidine, that was not seen on propranolol (Prichard et al, 1970). *In summary* β-adrenergic blocking drugs do not prevent vasoconstriction occurring under various physiological stresses which may lead to an excessive fall in blood pressure with hypotensive drugs that interfere with innervation of the alpha adrenergic receptor.

On the other hand β-adrenergic blocking drugs do reduce the rise in blood pressure to a number of stimuli: exercise (Shinebourne et al, 1967), the stress of sorting ball bearings (Lorimer et al, 1976), coitus (Fox, 1970), but possibly not to painful stimuli (Nicotero et al, 1968).

Mode of Action

The precise mechanism of the antihypertensive effect of β-adrenoceptor blocking drugs is unknown; however, it seems to be a function of their β-receptor inhibitory action not one of the associated properties. Regardless of the presence or absence of membrane stabilising or sympathomimetic action, β-adrenoceptor blocking drugs exert an antihypertensive effect. Moreover, the D-isomer of propranolol has no hypotensive effect in contrast to the usual DL, racemic (i.e. ordinary) propranolol (Simpson, 1974). A number of suggestions have been made to explain the hypotensive effect of β-adrenergic blocking drugs: an antirenin effect, an effect on the central nervous system, an effect on plasma volume, an adrenergic neurone blocking effect, a mechanism consequent on resetting the baroreceptors, and an action secondary to a chronic reduction in cardiac output.

Effect of β-blocking drugs on plasma renin

There is no doubt that plasma renin is lowered by β-adrenergic blocking drugs. Bulher et al (1972) divided their patients into high, intermediate and low renin groups. They found patients with a high pretreatment renin responded well to propranolol unlike those with a low renin. More recently the same pattern has been found with a variety of β-blocking drugs (Buhler et al, 1975). On the other hand many investigators have not found any correlation with the fall in blood pressure and pretreatment levels of plasma renin: for propranolol (Hansson, 1973; Stokes, Weber and Thornell, 1974; Leonetti et al, 1975; Morgan et al, 1975), pindolol (Morgan et al, 1975), sotalol (Verniory et al, 1974), or atenolol (Amery et al, 1976). Bravo, Tarazi and Dustan (1975) found no correlation between the fall in blood pressure and change in renin when propranolol was added to patients on diuretics for their hyptertension, in some renin even increased. An increase in renin with no elevation in blood pressure has been observed when pindolol (Stokes et al, 1974) or atenolol (Amery et al, 1976) was substituted for propranolol. The observation that intravenous propranolol lowers plasma renin without lowering blood pressure (Bravo et al, 1975; Morgan et al, 1975) provides further evidence of the dissociation of renin and antihypertensive effect although it could be argued that the fall in blood pressure, although delayed, was secondary to antirenin effect.

Effect on the central nervous system

There is some animal work to support a central site of action for the antihypertensive effect of β-blocking drugs. The injection of seven β antagonists, with various combinations of the associated properties of membrane activity, intrinsic sympathomimetic activity and cardioselectivity, into the cerebral ventricles of conscious cats result in a hypotensive effect, whereas the D-isomer of propranolol and alprenolol was without effect (Day and Roach, 1974). A similar effect was seen in conscious rabbits from propranolol (Myers et al, 1975).

Recently Lewis and Hauesler (1975) noted that racemic propranolol, but not the (+) isomer, infused into the conscious rabbit resulted in a fall of blood pressure and splanchnic efferent nerve activity. Practolol on the contrary failed to reduce sympathetic nerve activity and when pressure fell

9

following large doses there was a rise in sympathetic nerve activity (Lewis and Haeusler, cited by Dollery and Lewis, 1976).

There are other considerations that mitigate against depression of central sympathetic activity being regarded as the explanation for the antihypertensive action of β-blocking drugs in man. Those that fail to penetrate into the central nervous system, such as practolol (Scales and Cosgrove, 1970) or sotalol (Garvey and Ram, 1975a) are effective antihypertensive drugs. Lastly with the exception of some observations of Garvey and Ram (1975b), the effects reported in animals are of acute onset, unlike the response seen in man (Prichard and Gillam, 1969; Prichard and Boakes, 1974).

Plasma volume

Oral propranolol appears to reduce plasma volume although the cardio-pulmonary volume is unchanged suggesting systemic vasoconstriction (Tarazi et al, 1974). The fall in blood volume does not correlate with the antihypertensive effect of β-adrenoceptor blocking drugs. A fall in plasma volume occurs after intravenous administration without any change in blood pressure. Also diuretics reduce plasma volume, and in a group of patients already on a diuretic, propranolol was found to increase plasma volume almost to pre-diuretic control levels even though the addition of propranolol produced a further fall in blood pressure (Bravo et al, 1975).

Adrenergic neurone blocking effects

An adrenergic neurone inhibition from propranolol has been observed in rats and rabbits, but this action is also seen with the ($+$) isomer (Barrett and Nunn, 1970) which is devoid of antihypertensive effect in man. However, in cats an inhibition of nerve stimulation was seen with racemic propranolol but not the ($+$) isomer (Ablad et al, 1970). The fact that β-adrenergic blocking drugs control the blood pressure without producing postural hypotension characteristic of the adrenergic neurone inhibitory drugs indicates that any effect from this action is not important in man.

Resetting the baroreceptors

An explanation for the antihypertensive action of propranolol and other β-blocking drugs has to explain why, though marked haemodynamic changes occur after intravenous injection, no change in blood pressure is seen.

The hypotensive effect in mild hypertension appears rapidly, while in more severely affected patients some delay in the antihypertensive effect is often seen although the greater part takes place in the first two weeks. When the blood pressure in groups of patients observed under standardised clinic conditions was analysed, those patients receiving propranolol showed a significant fall in blood pressure from the visit to outpatients after stabilisation of the dosage of propranolol and one month subsequent to this (Prichard and Gillam, 1969). The visit to outpatients after stabilisation of dosage was on average three weeks after final adjustment of the dosage of propranolol. Following one month after stabilisation of dosage, a further fall in pressure was seen. The average heart rate was unchanged throughout. When groups of patients treated with bethanidine, methyldopa and guanethidine were assessed there was no such fall after stabilisation of dosage at up to three months. A similar delay in full hypotensive effect has been observed under double blind conditions with sotalol (Prichard and Boakes, 1974).

Arterial pressure is a function of cardiac output and peripheral resistance; and whereas propranolol reduces cardiac output after intravenous propranolol there is little effect on arterial pressure (Shinebourne et al, 1967). The reduction in cardiac output is therefore associated with a rise in peripheral resistance. Inhibition of the cardiac sympathetic activity would, however, be expected to reduce the cardiac contribution to any pressor event, thus attenuating it. As discussed above there is a reduced rise in blood pressure on exercise, the pressor overshoot of Valsalva's manoeuvre is reduced, and although the response to painful stimuli may not be reduced, the pressor effect of some stresses is inhibited.

To explain the difference between acute and chronic administration it has been suggested (Prichard and Gillam, 1964, 1969) that an attenuation of the pressor response to various stimuli leads to the baroreceptors generating their inhibitory impulses at a lower level of blood pressure and mean pressure falls, with prolonged oral use peripheral resistance is reduced (Tarazi and Dustan, 1972). When a hypertensive patient is put to bed a similar state of affairs results. In this case there is a reduction in sensory input, thus pressor events, and the baroreceptors over a period of a few days lower blood pressure by a variable amount.

Observations in dogs have demonstrated that pressor response to carotid occlusion is blunted by chronic propranolol therapy (Dunlop and Shanks, 1969) while short-term administration produces no effect. If chronic propranolol administration increased baroreceptor sensitivity an acute fall in carotid sinus pressure (from carotid occlusion) would result in more inhibitory impulses remaining, than in the absence of chronic propranolol administration, and thus with the greater afferent inhibitory traffic an occlusion would then result in a reduced rise in blood pressure. Baroreceptor reflexes in response to pressor effects appear blunted in hypertension, and this reflex is enhanced modestly by propranolol in normals (Pickering et al, 1972).

Hypertension is a multifactorial disease and it may be that an agent with such wide actions as a β-receptor inhibitory drug may act to lower the blood pressure by more than one mechanism. In some cases one of the effects of a β-receptor blocking drug may be of particular importance, e.g. lowering plasma renin in patients with a high renin, in other instances one of its other effects may assume dominance.

Blood Pressure Control with β-Blocking Drugs

The value of β-blocking drugs although originally observed with pronethalol has been established with propranolol. Most work has been done with this latter drug, although it appears that all β-adrenergic blocking drugs lower the blood pressure (Simpson, 1974). There is at present no good evidence as to the comparative merit of the various agents.

The degree of blood pressure control obtained with propranolol appeared similar to that obtained with bethanidine, guanethidine or methyldopa (Prichard and Gillam, 1969; Zacharias et al, 1972). Prichard et al (1977) in a formal within-patient comparison of the design previously used (Prichard et al, 1968) have confirmed these earier results.

As other β-blocking drugs have become available they have been found effective antihypertensive drugs (Simpson, 1974), oxprenolol (Leishman et al, 1970; Tuckman, Messerli and Hodler, 1973), alprenolol (Furberg and Michaelson, 1969), pindolol (Waal-Manning, 1970; Laver, Fang and Kincaid-Smith, 1974; Waal-Manning and Simpson, 1974), sotalol (Prichard and Boakes, 1974), timolol (Brogden, Speight and Avery, 1975) and drugs of the cardioselective group practolol (Prichard, Boakes and Day, 1971), atenolol (Hansson et al, 1975), metoprolol (Bengtsson, Johnsson and Regardh, 1975) and acebutolol (Letac, Fillastoe and Wolf, 1974).

Beta-adrenergic Receptor Blocking Drugs in Combination with Other Drugs

Diuretics

Beta-adrenergic blocking drugs have been used in combination with diuretics since the earliest studies (Prichard and Gillam, 1969; Zacharias et al, 1972). Approximately equal numbers of patients require the addition of a diuretic as on other potent drugs (Prichard and Gillam, 1969; Prichard et al, 1976).

Blockade of α-Receptor Mediated Vasoconstriction

Beta-receptor blocking drugs and drugs inhibiting the action of vasoconstrictor nerves, either at the nerve endings or α-adrenoceptor site may be combined. The combination of propranolol with either methyldopa or the sympathetic inhibitory agent bethanidine showed at least an additive effect or possibly even a potentiating action. However, this was at the expense of some postural and exercise hypotension, absent on propranolol alone (Prichard, 1976). Phenoxybenzamine the α-adrenoceptor blocking drug combined with propranolol also resulted in a considerable postural fall of blood pressure (Beilin and Juel-Jensen, 1972). Labetalol is a β-adrenoceptor blocking drug which in addition possesses some α-receptor blocking activity, but less than a quarter that of its β-blocking action. Our studies with this drug in the long-term treatment of hypertension indicate many patients can be controlled without postural or exercise hypotension although this may be seen at large doses (Prichard et al, 1975).

Vasodilators

Recently interest has been directed toward using β-receptor blocking drugs with agents that are direct vascular smooth muscle relaxants, hydrallazine and the closely related dihydrallazine, guancydine and minoxidil. Guancydine was discontinued as it resulted in an increased incidence of carcinoma in rats when given with propranolol (personal communication from American Cyanamid Company, USA). Minoxidil is reserved for the treatment of severe refractory hypertension, as it causes serious sodium and fluid retention, inexplicable hypertrichosis (Gottlieb, Kutz and Chidsey, 1972; Dormois, Young and Nies, 1975), and in dogs in large doses it may produce right atrial lesions (Du Charme et al, 1973). Suspicious cardiac lesions have also been reported in man (Gifford, 1975).

The vasodilators produce reflex increases in heart rate and cardiac output. When used alone to treat hypertension they have to be given in such large doses that unacceptable levels of tachycardia may result which could be dangerous in patients with ischaemic heart disease. Sodium and fluid retention and other side effects such as headaches, nervousness and gastrointestinal disturbances also occur (Kincaid-Smith, 1975). They can, however, be used at lower doses and also with a marked reduction of untoward reactions if they are administered with a diuretic and drugs which inhibit reflex sympathetic activity. The adrenergic blocking agents also inhibit the vasodilator-induced increase of plasma renin activity and this may be important in the combined antihypertensive regime (Pettinger and Keeton, 1975).

Beta-adrenergic blocking drugs may be given in doses just large enough to inhibit reflex sympathetic activity from vasodilators (Zacest, Gilmore and Koch-Weser, 1972). Another approach is to use larger amounts of the β-blockers than is necessary to inhibit the side effects due to the vasodilators (Hansson et al, 1971).

Prazosin hydrochloride is a peripheral vasodilator that probably acts distal to the vascular α-receptors (Constantine, 1974). In contrast to the vasodilators discussed it does not produce a marked tachycardia or an increase in cardiac output (Lund-Johansen, 1974). Prazosin lowers blood pressure when used alone and the antihypertensive effect is increased when it is administered with propranolol (Stokes and Weber, 1974).

Selection of Patients for Treatment with β-Adrenergic Blocking Drugs

Efforts to identify factors of predictive value in forecasting the hypotensive response of a given patient to a β-adrenergic blocking drug have not been very successful. The possible relevance of renin has been discussed above. The suggestion has also been made that old patients respond less favourably to β-adrenergic blocking drugs, perhaps because renin levels fall with age (Buhler et al, 1975). No correlation has been found between cardiac output and response to β-blocking drugs (Birkenhäger et al, 1971; Tarazi and Dustan, 1972; Hansson et al, 1974). Birkenhager et al (1971) also found no prediction could be made from age, blood volume and renin, while Hansson et al (1974) found age, blood volume, peripheral resistance, urinary adrenaline and noradrenaline aldosterone levels and heart rate response to isoprenaline were likewise of no predictive value.

Side Effects

Zacharias et al (1972), in his series of 311 patients, found that 55 patients experienced 'tolerable' side effects from propranolol, in 7 patients they were dose limiting and in 26 patients sufficient for the drug to be stopped. The overall incidence of side effects is probably at least no more than other potent antihypertensive drugs (Prichard and Gillam, 1969; Zacharias et al, 1972; Prichard et al, 1976).

Two *important untoward effects* from β-adrenergic blocking drugs can be avoided by careful patient selection: *heart failure and asthma*. Patients in overt heart failure, or even patients who have a history suggestive of left ventricular insufficiency (not necessarily with signs of heart failure on physical examination or chest x-ray), are critically dependent on cardiac sympathetic activity in order to maintain the cardiac output. In these patients consideration should only be given to treatment with a β-receptor blocking drug after prior administration of digitalis and diuretics. If these measures alleviate the dyspnoea it is possible, with extra caution, to commence a β-blocking drug. There have been reports of patients who have been put into failure by propranolol and were subsequently able to tolerate the drug after the administration of digoxin and a diuretic (Gillam and Prichard, 1965; Amsterdam, Gorlin and Wolfson, 1969). Uncontrolled heart failure is a contraindication to β-adrenergic blocking drugs. β-Adrenergic inhibitory drugs with intrinsic sympathomimetic stimulating action may also precipitate heart failure; and neither is there evidence that the direct membrane effect of some β-blocking drugs is of relevance in the possible precipitation of heart failure. Prichard (1974) has pointed out the most dramatic change in the sympathetic environment of the heart takes place when treatment is commenced with a β-adrenergic receptor blocking drug, i.e. the small starting dose.

The effects of β-adrenergic blocking drugs on respiratory function has been reviewed by Beumer (1974). Inhibition of sympathetic tone in bronchial smooth muscle is likely to produce a significant increase in airways resistance. The cardioselective agents show only modest selectivity; a serious increase in airways resistance has been reported with practolol (Waal-Manning and Simpson, 1971).

The occurrence of cold extremities is a common side effect from β-adrenergic blocking drugs. This probably results from peripheral vasoconstriction from the reduced cardiac output and peripheral β-adrenergic blockade. It was reported in 25 of the series of Zacharias et al (1972), leading to the drug being stopped in three patients.

The rise of blood sugar by glycogenolysis is in part controlled by β-receptors and therefore theoretically β-blockade would interfere with this mechanism. However, hypoglycaemia is very rare but diabetics receiving propranolol may have the hypoglycaemic response to insulin increased. This has also been reported after anaesthesia in children, and in partial gastrectomy patients (Dollery, Patterson and Conolly, 1969).

Central nervous system side effects occur as most β-adrenergic blocking drugs cross the blood-barrier. They include lack of concentration, loss of ambition, depression, disturbance of sleep patterns, and troublesome dreams (Zacharias et al, 1972). Dreams and insomnia can usually be reduced or abolished by taking the last dose no later than say early evening, and also reducing that dose if necessary.

Indigestion, often with some nausea, is a not an uncommon side effect which can often be avoided by taking the drug with meals (Prichard and Gillam, 1969). Diarrhoea is unusual (Zacharias et al, 1972).

Impotence failed to occur in any of the series of Zacharias et al (1972). While in eight patients who had impotence on previous therapy, in four it disappeared, in two it was improved, and in the other two it was unchanged.

A number of severe sensitivity reactions have been recently reported with practolol, and this drug can no longer be used in long-term therapy.

Important adverse reactions to β-adrenergic blocking drugs are uncommon except with practolol (which is no longer used as long-term treatment). Rare severe adverse reactions such as heart failure from errors in patient selection tend to occur soon after initiation of therapy, even with small doses, but once treatment has been started gradual increments in dosage are most unlikely to be associated with sudden adverse reactions.

The importance of β-Blocking Drugs

Beta-adrenoceptor blocking drugs represent a useful new group of drugs in the treatment of hypertension. Although their mode of action is unknown other than it appears to be a function of β-adrenoceptor blockade, they offer certain advantages as they do not inhibit the innervation of the α-adrenoceptor.

The blood pressure control they produce is not influenced by posture, and exercise hypotension is not seen, nor does increasing environmental temperature lead to postural or exercise hypotension. There is in addition the possibility that β-receptor blocking drugs, unlike other hypotensive drugs, reduce mortality from myocardial infarction. There is some suggestive evidence in mild hypertensives with angina pectoris, that this is so (Lambert, 1976).

CONCLUSIONS

Hypertensive emergencies are now relatively rare and occur mostly in patients with advanced renal impairment. Although the indications for particular drugs under these circumstances are straightforward, treatment is frequently complicated because some of the agents are not always available.

The choice of drugs in chronic treatment is based on the ability of a given medication to lower pressure in relation to the side effects that it produces. The reduction of blood pressure seems to be the basis for the therapeutic benefit. There are three factors which often influence the responses obtained with antihypertensive drugs. First, many physicians use an inadequate dose of a drug. Secondly, too rapid an increase in dosage may result in severe side effects and this is likely to jeopardise patient confidence and compliance. Thirdly, the chronic treatment of hypertension is usually more successful if patients are properly motivated and they understand the long-term preventative object of therapy.

When hypertension is severe it is best to start treatment with a combined regime of a diuretic and ANID, the dose of the latter being increased until the hypertension is controlled. The ANID frequently produce untoward reactions and/or poor control of the supine pressure. If this occurs, once blood pressure is stabilised, an attempt can be made to phase them out gradually and to introduce a β-adrenergic blocking agent with or without a vasodilator, α-methyldopa and clonidine being alternatives. If the newer combination achieves good regulation of pressure for a prolonged period it is sometimes possible to discontinue the diuretic. Further, some patients require a multiple regime of diuretic, ANID and, in addition, one or rarely even more of the other agents. Many multiple regimes could be avoided if the dosages of drugs were raised to maximal levels.

In less serious cases of hypertension two different approaches can be used. Some physicians give a diuretic as initial and perhaps sole therapy, and if the pressure is not sufficiently lowered they add one of the other drugs. Others prefer to use first the more 'potent' antihypertensive drugs alone or in combination and to add a diuretic only when required.

ACKNOWLEDGMENTS

We are grateful to Mrs J. Cant, Miss A. Crowe, Miss J. C. Owens, Mr B. R. Graham and Mr W. Lim for help in the preparation of this paper.

REFERENCES

Ablad, B., Ek, L., Johansson, B. & Waldeck, B. (1970) Inhibitory effect of propranolol on the vasoconstrictor response to sympathetic nerve stimulation. *Journal of Pharmacy and Pharmacology*, **22**, 627–628.

Abrams, W. B., Pocelinko, R., Klausner, M., Hanauer, L. & Whitman, E. N. (1964) Clinical pharmacological studies with debrisoquin sulphate, a new antihypertensive agent. *Journal of New Drugs*, **4**, 268–283.

Adi, F. C., Eze, C. J. & Anwunah, A. (1975) Comparison of debrisoquine and guanethidine in the treatment of hypertension. *British Medical Journal*, **1**, 482–485.

AMA Committee on Hypertension (1974) The treatment of malignant hypertension and hypertensive emergencies. *Journal of the American Medical Association*, **228**, 1673–1679.

Amery, A. & Deloof, W. (1970) Letter: Cheese reaction during debrisoquine treatment. *Lancet*, **2**, 613.

Amery, A., De Plaen, J. F., Fagard, R., Lijnen, P. & Reybrouck, T. (1976) The relationship between beta-blockade, hyporeninaemic and hypotensive effect of two beta-blocking agents. *Postgraduate Medical Journal*, **52**, Suppl. 4, 102–108.

Amery, A., Verstraete, M., Bossaert, H. & Verstreken, G. (1970) Hypotensive action and side effects of clonidine-chlorthalidone and methyldopa-chlorthalidone in treatment of hypertension. *British Medical Journal*, **4**, 392–395.

Aminu, J., D'Mello, A. & Vere, D. W. (1970) Interaction between debrisoquine and phenylephrine. *Lancet*, **2**, 935–936.

Amsterdam, E. A., Gorlin, R. & Wolfson, S. (1969) Evaluation of long-term use of propranolol in angina pectoris. *Journal of the American Medical Association*, **210**, 103–106.

Anderton, J. L. & Kincaid-Smith, P. (1971) Diuretics. I. Physiological and pharmacological considerations. *Drugs*, **1**, 54–81.

Baker, D. R., Schrader, W. H. & Hitchcock, C. R. (1964) Small bowel ulceration apparently associated with thiazide and potassium therapy. *Journal of the American Medical Association*, **190**, 586–590.

Barrett, A. M. & Nunn, B. (1970) Adrenergic neuron blocking properties of ($\pm$)-propranolol and (+)-propranolol. *Journal of Pharmacy and Pharmacology*, **22**, 806–810.

Bauer, G. E., Hull, R. D., Stokes, C. S. & Raftos, J. (1973) The reversibility of side effects of guanethidine therapy. *Medical Journal of Australia*, **1**, 930–933.

Baum, T., Shropshire, A. T. & Varner, L. L. (1972) Contribution of the central nervous system to the action of several antihypertensive agents (methyldopa, hydralazine and guanethidine). *Journal of Pharmacology and Experimental Therapeutics*, **182**, 135–144.

Beilin, L. J. & Juel-Jensen, B. E. (1972) Alpha- and beta-adrenergic blockade in hypertension. *Lancet*, **1**, 979–982.

Bengtsson, C., Johnsson, G. & Regardh, C.-G. (1975) Plasma levels and effects of metopolol on blood pressure and heart rate in hypertensive patients after acute dose and between two doses during long-term treatment. *Clinical Pharmacology and Therapeutics*, **17**, 400–408.

Bengtsson, C., Johnsson, G., Sannerstedt, R. & Werko, L. (1975) Effect of different doses of chlorthalidone on blood pressure, serum potassium and serum urate. *British Medical Journal*, **1**, 197–199.

Bennet, D., Balcon, R., Hoy, J. & Sowton, E. (1970) Haemodynamic effects of dextropranolol in acute myocardial infarction. *Thorax*, **25**, 86–88.

Benraad, A. H. & Schoenaker, A. H. (1965) Thrombopenia after use of methyldopa. *Lancet*, **2**, 292.

Beumer, H. M. (1974) Adverse effects of β-adrenergic receptor blocking drugs on respiratory function. *Drugs*, **7**, 130–138.

Birkenhäger, W. H., Krauss, X. H., Schalekamp, M. A. D. H., Kolsters, G. & Kroon, B. J. M. (1971) Antihypertensive effects of propranolol. Observations on predictability. *Folia medica neerlanda*, **14**, 67–71.

Boura, A. L. A. & Green, A. F. (1965) Adrenergic neurone blocking agents. *Annual Review of Pharmacology*, **5**, 183–212.

Bravo, E. H., Tarazi, R. C. & Dustan, H. P. (1975) β-Adrenergic blockade in diuretic-treated patients with essential hypertension. *New England Journal of Medicine*, **292**, 66–70.

Breckenridge, A., Dollery, C. T., Worlledge, S. M., Holborn, E. J. & Johnson, G. D. (1967) Positive direct Coombs tests and antinuclear factor in patients treated with methyldopa. *Lancet*, **2**, 1265–1268.

Brod, J., Horback, L., Just, H., Rosenthal, J. & Nicolescu, R. (1972) Acute effects of clonidine on central and peripheral haemodynamics and plasma renin activity. *European Journal of Clinical Pharmacology*, **4**, 107–114.

Brogden, R. N., Speight, T. M. & Avery, G. S. (1975) Timolol: a preliminary report of its pharmacological properties and therapeutic efficacy in angina and hypertension. *Drugs*, **9**, 164–177.

Buhler, F. R., Burkart, F., Lutold, B. E., Kung, M., Marbet, G. & Pfisterer, M. (1975) Antihypertensive beta-blocking action as related to renin and age: a pharmacologic tool to identify pathogenic mechanisms in essential hypertension. *American Journal of Cardiology*, **36**, 653–669.

Buhler, F. R., Laragh, J. H., Baer, L., Vaughan, E. D. & Brunner, H. R. (1972) Propranolol inhibition of renin secretion. A specific approach to diagnosis and treatment of renin-dependent hypertensive diseases. *New England Journal of Medicine*, **287**, 1209–1214.

Chamberlain, D. A. & Howard, J. (1964) Guanethidine and methyldopa: a haemodynamic study. *British Heart Journal*, **26**, 528–536.

Church, R. (1974) Eczema provoked by methyldopa. *British Journal of Dermatology*, **91**, 373–378.

Cohen, A., Maxmen, J. S., Ragheb, M., Baleiron, H., Zaleski, E. J. & Bing, R. J. (1967) Effects of alpha-methyldopa on the myocardial blood flow, utilising the coincidence counting method. *Journal of Clinical Pharmacology*, **7**, 77–83.

Cohn, J. N. (1973) Vasodilator therapy for heart failure. *Circulation*, **48**, 5–8.

Cohn, J. N., Liptak, T. E. & Freis, E. D. (1963) Hemodynamic effects of guanethidine in man. *Circulation Research*, **12**, 298–307.

Constantine, J. W. (1974) Analysis of the hypotensive action of prazosin. In *Prazosin: Evaluation of a New Antihypertensive Agent*, pp. 16–86. Amsterdam: Excerpta Medica.

Cranston, W. I., Juel-Jensen, B. E., Semmence, A. M., Handfield, R. P. C., Forbes, J. A. & Mutch, L. M. M. (1963) Effects of oral diuretics on raised arterial pressure. *Lancet*, **2**, 966–970.

Dargie, H. J., Boddy, K., Kennedy, A. C., King, P. C., Read, P. R. & Ward, D. M. (1974) Total body potassium in long-term frusemide therapy: is potassium supplementation necessary? *British Medical Journal*, **4**, 316–319.

Davidov, M., Kakaviatos, N. & Finnerty, F. A., Jr (1967a) Antihypertensive properties of furosemide. *Circulation*, **36**, 125–135.

Davidov, M., Kakaviatos, N. & Finnerty, F. A., Jr (1967b) The antihypertensive effects of an imidazoline compound. *Clinical Pharmacology and Therapeutics*, **8**, 810–816.

Davies, D. L. & Wilson, G. M. (1975) Diuretics: mechanism of action and clinical application. *Drugs*, **9**, 178–226.

Day, M. D. & Rand, M. J. (1963) A hypothesis for the mode of action of α-methyldopa in relieving hypertension. *Journal of Pharmacy and Pharmacology*, **15**, 221–224.

Day, M. D. & Roach, A. G. (1974) Cardiovascular effects of β-adrenoceptor blocking agents after intracerebroventricular administration on conscious normotensive cats. *Clinical and Experimental Pharmacology and Physiology*, **1**, 333–339.

Degnbol, N., Dorph, S. & Marner, T. (1973) The effect of different diuretics on elevated blood pressure and serum potassium. *Acta medica scandinavica*, **193**, 407–410.

Dollery, C. T., Emslie-Smith, D. & Shillingford, J. P. (1961) Haemodynamic effects of guanethidine. *Lancet*, **2**, 331–334.

Dollery, C. T. & Lewis, P. J. (1976) Central hypotensive effect of propranolol. *Postgraduate Medical Journal*, **52**, Suppl. 4, 116–120.

Dollery, C. T., Paterson, J. W. & Conolly, M. E. (1969) Clinical pharmacology of β-receptor blocking drugs. *Clinical Pharmacology and Therapeutics*, **10**, 765–799.

Dormois, J. C., Young, J. L. & Nies, A. S. (1975) Minoxidil in severe hypertension: value when conventional drugs have failed. *American Heart Journal*, **90**, 360–368.

Du Charme, D. W., Freyburger, W. A., Graham, B. E. & Carlson, R. G. (1973) Pharmacologic properties of minoxidil, a new hypotensive agent. *Journal of Pharmacology and Experimental Therapeutics*, **184**, 662–670.

Dunlop, D. & Shanks, R. G. (1969) Inhibition of the carotid sinus reflex by the chronic administration of propranolol. *British Journal of Pharmacology*, **36**, 132–143.

Dustan, H. P., Tarazi, R. C. & Bravo, E. L. (1974) Diuretic and diet treatment of hypertension. *Archives of Internal Medicine*, **133**, 1007–1013.

Edmonds, C. J. & Jasani, B. (1972) Total body potassium in hypertensive patients during prolonged diuretic therapy. *Lancet*, **2**, 8–12.

Fewings, J. D., Hodge, R. L., Scroop, G. C. & Whelan, R. F. (1964) The effect of bethanidine on the peripheral circulation in man. *British Journal of Pharmacology*, **23**, 115–122.

Finch, L. & Haeusler, G. (1973) Further evidence for a central hypotensive action of α-methyldopa in both the rat and cat. *British Journal of Pharmacology*, **47**, 217–228.

Finnerty, F. A., Jr (1974) Malignant hypertension. *American Heart Journal*, **88**, 265–268.

Fox, C. A. (1970) Reduction in the rise of systolic blood pressure during human coitus by the β-adrenergic blocking agent, propranolol. *Journal of Reproduction and Fertility*, **22**, 587–590.

Furberg, C. & Michaelson, G. (1969) Effect of aptin, a β-adrenergic blocking agent, in arterial hypertension. *Acta medica scandinavica*, **186**, 447–450.

Furst, C. I. (1967) The biochemistry of guanethidine. *Advances in Drug Research*, **4**, 133–161.

Garvey, H. L. & Ram, N. (1975a) Comparative antihypertensive effects and tissue distribution of beta-adrenergic blocking drugs. *Journal of Pharmacology and Experimental Therapeutics*, **194**, 220–233.

Garvey, H. L. & Ram, N. (1975b) Centrally induced hypotensive effect of β-adrenergic blocking drugs. *European Journal of Pharmacology*, **33**, 283–294.

Gibson, D. G. (1974) Pharmacodynamic properties of β-adrenergic blocking drugs in man. *Drugs*, **7**, 8–23.

Gifford, R. W. (1975) Clinical applications of new antihypertensive drugs. *Cleveland Clinic Quarterly*, **42**, 255–262.

Gillam, P. M. S. & Prichard, B. N. C. (1965) Use of propranolol in angina pectoris. *British Medical Journal*, **2**, 337–339.

Glontz, G. E. & Saslaw, S. (1968) Methyldopa fever. *Archives of Internal Medicine*, **122**, 445–447.

Gottlieb, T. B., Katz, F. H. & Chidsey, C. A. (1972) Combined therapy with vasodilator drugs and beta-adrenergic blockade in hypertension. A comparative study of minoxidil and hydralazine. *Circulation*, **45**, 571–582.

Haefely, W., Hürlimann, A. & Thoenen, H. (1967) Adrenergic transmitter changes and response to sympathetic nerve stimulation after differing pretreatment with α-methyldopa. *British Journal of Pharmacology and Chemotherapy*, **31**, 105–109.

Haeusler, G. (1974) Clonidine-induced inhibition of sympathetic nerve activity: no indication for a central presynaptic or an indirect sympathomimetic mode of action. *Naunyn-Schmiedebergs Archiv fur experimentelle Pathologie u. Pharmakologia*, **286**, 97–111.

Haeusler, G. (1975) Cardiovascular regulation by central adrenergic mechanisms and its alteration of hypotensive drugs. *Circulation Research*, **36**, Suppl. I, 223–232.

Hamilton, M. & Kopelman, H. (1963) The treatment of severe hypertension with methyldopa. *British Medical Journal*, **1**, 151–155.

Hansen, J. (1968) Hydrochlorothiazide in the treatment of hypertension. The effects on blood volume, exchangeable sodium and blood pressure. *Acta medica scandinavica*, **183**, 317–321.

Hansson, L. (1973) Beta-adrenergic blockade in essential hypertension. Effects of propranolol on haemodynamic parameters and plasma renin activity. *Acta medica scandinavica*, Suppl. **55**, 1–40.

Hansson, L., Aberg, H., Karlberg, B. E. & Westerlund, A. (1975) Controlled study of atenolol in treatment of hypertension. *British Medical Journal*, **1**, 367–370.

Hansson, L., Olander, R., Aberg, H., Malmcrona, R. & Westerlund, A. (1971) Treatment of hypertension with propranolol and hydralazine. *Acta medica scandinavica*, **190**, 531–534.

Hansson, L., Zweifler, A. J., Julius, S. & Ellis, C. N. (1974) Propranolol therapy in essential hypertension. Observations on predictability of therapeutic response. *International Journal of Clinical Pharmacology*, **10**, 79–89.

Heise, A. & Kroneberg, G. (1972) α-Sympathetic receptor stimulation in the brain and hypotensive activity of α-methyldopa. *European Journal of Pharmacology*, **17**, 315–317.

Henning, M. (1975) Central sympathetic transmitters and hypertension. *Clinical Science and Molecular Medicine*, **48**, 195s–203s.

Henning, M. & Rubenson, A. (1971) Evidence that the hypotensive action of methyldopa is mediated by the central actions of methylnoradrenaline. *Journal of Pharmacy and Pharmacology*, **23**, 407–411.

Hoobler, S. W. & Sagastume, E. (1971) Clonidine hydrochloride in the treatment of hypertension. *American Journal of Cardiology*, **28**, 67–73.

Hopkirk, J. A. C., Simpson, N. B. & Fitzgerald, W. R. (1975) Letter: Vomiting with clonidine withdrawal. *British Medical Journal*, **3**, 435.

Howie, A. O. & Strachan, R. W. (1975) Case report: Slow release potassium chloride treatment. *British Medical Journal*, 2, 176.

Hunyor, S. N., Hansson, L., Harrison, T. S. & Hoobler, S. W. (1973) Effects of clonidine withdrawal: possible mechanisms and suggestions for management. *British Medical Journal*, 2, 209–211.

Iversen, L. L. (1973) Catecholamine uptake processes. *British Medical Bulletin*, 29, 130–135.

Johnson, P., Kitchin, A. H., Lowther, C. P. & Turner, R. W. D. (1966) Treatment of hypertension with methyldopa. *British Medical Journal*, 1, 133–137.

Johnston, A. W., Prichard, B. N. C. & Rosenheim, M. L. (1964) The use of bethanidine in the treatment of hypertension. *Lancet*, 2, 659–661.

Julius, S., Pascual, A. V., Abbrecht, P. H. & London, R. (1972) Effect of beta-adrenergic blockade on plasma volume in human subjects. *Proceedings of the Society of Experimental Biology and Medicine*, 140, 982–985.

Kakaviatos, N., Tuckman, J., Chupkovich, V. & Finnerty, F. A., Jr (1964) Pressor and depressor effects of Ro5-3307/1 (Declinex). *American Journal of Cardiology*, 13, 111–112.

Khatri, I. M. & Cohn, J. N. (1970) Mechanism of exercise hypotension after sympathetic blockade. *American Journal of Cardiology*, 25, 329–338.

Kincaid-Smith, P. (1975) Vasodilators in the treatment of hypertension. *Medical Journal of Australia*, Special Suppl. 1, 7–9.

Kincaid-Smith, P., Macdonald, I. M., Hua, A., Laver, M. C. & Fang, P. (1975) Changing concepts in the management of hypertension. *Medical Journal of Australia*, 1, 327–332.

Kitchen, A. H. & Turner, R. W. D. (1966) Studies on debrisoquine sulphate. *British Medical Journal*, 2, 728–731.

Kobinger, W. & Pichler, L. (1974) Evidence for direct alpha-adrenoceptor stimulation of effector neurons in cardiovascular centres by clonidine. *European Journal of Pharmacology*, 27, 151–154.

Lambert, D. M. D. (1976) Effect of propranolol on mortality in patients with angina. *Postgraduate Medical Journal*, 52, Suppl. 4, 57–60.

Laver, M. C., Fang, P. & Kincaid-Smith, Priscilla (1974) Double blind comparison of two beta-blocking drugs with previous therapy in the treatment of hypertension. *Medical Journal of Australia*, 1, 174–176.

Laverty, R. (1973) The mechanisms of action of some antihypertensive drugs. *British Medical Bulletin*, 29, 152–157.

Lee, R. E. (1966) Management of hypertensive crisis. In *Antihypertensive Therapy*, ed. Gross, F., pp. 313–319. Berlin: Springer-Verlag.

Leishman, A. W. D., Thirkettle, J. L., Allen, B. R. & Dixon, R. A. (1970) Controlled trial of oxprenolol and practolol in hypertension. *British Medical Journal*, 4, 342–344.

Leonetti, G., Mayer, Genevieve, Morganti, A., Terzoli, Laura, Zanchetti, A., Bianchetti, G., DiSalle, E., Morselli, P. L. & Chidsey, C. A. (1975) Hypotensive and renin-suppressing activities of propranolol in hypertensive patients. *Clinical Science and Molecular Medicine*, 48, 491–499.

Letac, B., Fillastre, J. P. & Wolf, L. M. (1974) The treatment of essential hypertension with acebutolol (sectral). *Clinical Trials Journal*, 11, Suppl. 3, 92–95.

Leth, A. (1970) Changes in plasma and extracellular fluid volumes, in patients with essential hypertension during long-term treatment with hydrochlorothiazide. *Circulation*, 42, 479–485.

Levine, R. J. & Strauch, B. S. (1966) Hypertensive responses to methyldopa. *New England Journal of Medicine*, 275, 946–948.

Lewis, P. J. & Haeusler, G. (1975) Reduction in sympathetic nervous activity as a mechanism for hypotensive effect of propranolol. *Nature*, 256, 440.

Lorimer, A. R., Dunn, F. G., Jones, J. V., Clark, B. & Lawrie, T. D. V. (1976) Indications for beta-adrenoceptor blocking drugs in hypertension. *Postgraduate Medical Journal*, 52, Suppl. 4, 81–86.

Lund-Johansen, P. (1970) Haemodynamic changes in long-term diuretic therapy of essential hypertension. A comparative study of chlorthalidone polythiazide and hydrochlorothiazide. *Acta medica scandinavica*, 187, 509–518.

Lund-Johansen, P. (1972) Haemodynamic changes in long term α-methyldopa therapy of essential hypertension. *Acta medica scandinavica*, 192, 221–226.

Lund-Johnasen, P. (1974) Haemodynamic changes at rest and during exercise in long-term prazosin therapy of essential hypertension. In *Prazosin: Evaluation of a New Antihypertensive Agent*, pp. 43–53. Amsterdam: Excerpta Medica.

Luria, M. H. & Freis, E. D. (1965) Treatment of hypertension with debrisoquin sulphate (declinax). *Current Therapeutic Research*, **7**, 289–296.

Mason, D. T. & Braunwald, E. (1964) Effects of guanethidine, reserpine and methyldopa on reflex venous and arterial constriction in man. *Journal of Clinical Investigation*, **43**, 1449–1463.

Mitchell, J. R., Cavanaugh, J. H., Arias, L. & Oates, J. A. (1970) Guanethidine and related agents, 3. Antagonism of drugs which inhibit the norepinephrine pump in man. *Journal of Clinical Investigation*, **49**, 1596–1604.

Montuschi, E. & Pickens, P. T. (1962) A clinical trial of two related adrenergic-neurone-blocking agents—BW 392C60 and BW 467C60. *Lancet*, **2**, 897–901.

Morgan, T. O., Roberts, R., Carney, S. L., Louis, W. J. & Doyle, A. E. (1975) Beta-adrenergic receptor blocking drugs, hypertension and plasma renin. *British Journal of Clinical Pharmacology*, **2**, 159–164.

Muir, A. L., Burton, J. L. & Lawrie, D. M. (1969) Cirulatory effects at rest and exercise of clonidine, an imidazoline derivative with hypotensive properties. *Lancet*, **2**, 181–185.

Myers, M. G., Lewis, P. J., Reid, J. L. & Dollery, C. T. (1975) Brain concentration of propanolol in relation to hypotensive effect in the rabbit with observations on brain propranolol levels in man. *Journal of Pharmacology and Experimental Therapeutics*, **192**, 327–335.

Ng, J., Phelan, E. L., McGregor, D. D., Laverty, R., Taylor, K. M. & Smirk, H. (1967) Properties of catapres, a new hypotensive drug: a preliminary report. *New Zealand Medical Journal*, **66**, 864–870.

Nicotero, J. A., Beamer, Virginia, Moutsos, S. E. & Shapiro, A. P. (1968) Effects of propranolol on pressor responses to noxious stimuli in hypertensive patients. *American Journal of Cardiology*, **22**, 657–666.

Novack, P. (1961) The effect of guanethidine on renal, cerebral and cardiac hemodynamics. *Hypertension, Recent Advances*. The Second Hahnemann Symposium on Hypertensive Diseases, pp. 444–448. Philadelphia: Lea & Febiger.

Oates, J. A., Gillespie, L., Udenfriend, S. & Sjoerdsma, A. (1960) Decarboxylase inhibition and blood pressure reduction by α-methyl-3,4-dihydroxy-DL-phenylalamine. *Science*, **131**, 1890–1891.

Oates, J. A., Seligmann, A. W., Clark, M. A., Rousseau, P. & Lee, R. E. (1965) The relative efficacy of guanethidine, methyldopa and pargyline as antihypertensive agents. *New England Journal of Medicine*, **273**, 729–734.

Onesti, G., Brest, A. N., Novack, P., Kasparin, J. & Moyer, J. H. (1964) Pharmacodynamic effects of α-methyldopa in hypertensive subjects. *American Heart Journal*, **67**, 32–38.

Onesti, G., La Schiazza, D., Brest, A. N. & Moyer, J. H. (1966) Cardiac and renal haemodynamic effects of debrisoquin sulphate in hypertensive patients. *Clinical Pharmacology and Therapeutics*, **7**, 17–20.

Onesti, G., Schwartz, A. B., Kim, K. E., Swartz, C. & Brest, A. N. (1969) Pharmacodynamic effects of a new antihypertensive drug, catapres (ST-155). *Circulation*, **39**, 219–228.

Onesti, G., Bock, K. D., Heimsoth, V., Kim, K. E. & Merguet, P. (1971a) Clonidine a new antihypertensive agent. *American Journal of Cardiology*, **28**, 74–83.

Onesti, G., Schwartz, A. B., Kim, K. E., Paz-Martinez, V. & Swartz, C. (1971b) Antihypertensive effect of clonidine. *Circulation Research*, **28**, Suppl. 2, 53–69.

Page, I. H., Corcoran, A. C., Dustan, H. P. D. & Koppanyi, T. (1955) Cardiovascular actions of sodium nitroprusside in animals and hypertensive patients. *Circulation*, **11**, 188–198.

Palmer, R. F. & Lasseter, K. C. (1975a) Sodium nitroprusside. *New England Journal of Medicine*, **292**, 294–297.

Palmer, R. F. & Lasseter, K. C. (1975b) Use and toxicity of nitroprusside. *New England Journal of Medicine*, **292**, 1081–1082.

Pickering, T. G., Gribbin, B., Petersen, E. S., Cunningham, D. J. C. & Sleight, P. (1972) Effects of autonomic blockade on the baroreflex in man at rest and during exercise. *Circulation Research*, **30**, 177–185.

Pettinger, W. A. & Keeton, K. (1975) Altered renin release and propranolol potentiation of vasodilatory drug hypotension. *Journal of Clinical Investigation*, **55**, 236–243.

Pettinger, W. A., Korn, A., Spiegel, H., Solomon, H. M., Pocelinko, R. & Abrams, W. B. (1969) Debrisoquin: a selective inhibitor of intraneuronal monoamine oxidase in man. *Clinical Pharmacology and Therapeutics*, **10**, 667–674.

Prichard, B. N. C. (1964) Hypotensive action of pronethalol. *British Medical Journal*, **1**, 1227–1228.

Prichard, B. N. C. (1976) The combined effect of propranolol with bethanidine or methyldopa in hypertension. *International Journal of Clinical Pharmacology*. Suppl. Advances in Clinical Pharmacology, **11**, 107–113.

Prichard, B. N. C. & Boakes, A. J. (1974) The use of sotalol in the treatment of hypertension. In *Clinical Advances in Beta adrenergic Blocking Therapy. Sotalol*, ed. Smart, A. G., Vol. IV, pp. 7–24. Amsterdam: Excerpta Medica.

Prichard, B. N. C., Boakes, A. J. & Day, Gillian M. (1971) Practolol in the treatment of hypertension. *Postgraduate Medical Journal*, **47**, Suppl., 84–91.

Prichard, B. N. C., Boakes, A. J. & Graham, B. R. (1977) A within-patient comparison of bethanidine, methyldopa and propranolol in the treatment of hypertension. *Clinical Science and Molecular Medicine* (in press).

Prichard, B. N. C. & Gillam, P. M. S. (1964) Use of propranolol (inderal) in the treatment of hypertension. *British Medical Journal*, **2**, 725–727.

Prichard, B. N. C. & Gillam, P. M. S. (1969) Treatment of hypertension with propranolol. *British Medical Journal*, **1**, 7–16.

Prichard, B. N. C., Gillam, P. M. S. & Graham, B. R. (1970) Beta-receptor antagonism in hypertension; comparison with the effect of adrenergic neurone inhibition on cardiovascular responses. *International Journal of Clinical Pharmacology*, **4**, 131–140.

Prichard, B. N. C., Johnston, A. W., Hill, I. D. & Rosenheim, M. L. (1968) Bethanidine, guanethidine and methyldopa in the treatment of hypertension; a within-patient comparison. *British Medical Journal*, **1**, 135–144.

Prichard, B. N. C., Thompson, F. O., Boakes, A. J. & Joekes, A. M. (1975) Some haemodynamic effects of compound AH 5158 compared with propranolol, propranolol plus hydrallazine and diazoxide; the use of AH 5158 in the treatment of hypertension. *Clinical Science and Molecular Medicine*, **48**, 97–100s.

Raftos, J., Bauer, G. E., Lewis, R. G., Stokes, G. S., Mitchell, A. S., Young, A. A. & Machlachlan, I. (1973) Clonidine in the treatment of severe hypertension trial carried out in 1968–1972. *Medical Journal of Australia*, **1**, 786–793.

Relman, A. S. & Schwartz, W. B. (1958) The kidney in potassium depletion. *American Journal of Medicine*, **24**, 764–773.

Richardson, D. W., Wysso, E. M., Magee, J. H. & Cavell, G. C. (1960) Circulatory effects of guanethidine–clinical, renal and cardiac responses to treatment with a novel antihypertensive agent. *Circulation*, **22**, 184–190.

Robson, R. D. & Antonaccio, M. J. (1975) Modification of baroreceptor function by clonidine: evidence for an opposing action on baroreceptors of different location. *Recent Advances in Hypertension*, ed. Milliez, P. & Safar, M. Vol. 2, pp. 37–47. Reims, France: Société Alina.

Rosei, E. A., Trust, P. M., Brown, J. J., Lever, A. F. & Robertson, J. I. S. (1975) Intravenous labetalol in severe hypertension. *Lancet*, **2**, 1093–1094.

Scales, B. & Cosgrove, M. B. (1970) The metabolism and distribution of the selective betablocking agent practolol. *Journal of Pharmacology and Experimental Therapeutics*, **175**, 338–347.

Sellers, E. M. & Koch-Weser, J. (1973) Influence of intravenous injection rate on protein binding and vascular activity of diazoxide. *Annals of the New York Academy of Sciences*, **226**, 319–332.

Shinebourne, E., Fleming, J. & Hamer, J. (1967) Effects of beta-adrenergic blockade during exercise in hypertensive and ischaemic heart disease. *Lancet*, **2**, 1217–1220.

Simpson, F. O. (1974) Beta-adrenergic blocking drugs in hypertension. *Drugs*, **7**, 85–105.

Stokes, G. S. & Weber, M. A. (1974) Prazosin: preliminary report and comparative studies with other antihypertensive agents. *British Medical Journal*, **2**, 298–300.

Stokes, G. S., Weber, M. A. & Thornell, I. R. (1974) Beta-blockers and plasma renin activity in hypertension. *British Medical Journal*, **1**, 60–62.

Tarazi, R. C. & Dustan, Harriet, P. (1972) Beta-adrenergic blockade in hypertension. Practical and theoretical implications of long-term haemodynamic variations. *American Journal of Cardiology*, **29**, 633–640.

Tarazi, R. C., Dustan, Harriet, P. & Bravo, E. L. (1976) Haemodynamic effects of propranolol in hypertension. *Postgraduate Medical Journal*, **52**, Suppl. 4, 92–101.

Tarazi, R. C., Dustan, Harriet, P. & Frolich, E. D. (1970) Long-term thiazide therapy in essential hypertension. Evidence for persistent alteration in plasma volume and renin activity. *Circulation*, **41**, 709–717.

Tarazi, R. C. & Gifford, R. W. (1975) Drug treatment of hypertension. *Current Cardiovascular Topics*, Vol. 1, Part 2. In *Drugs in Cardiology*, ed. Donoso, E. Stuttgart: George Thieme.

Tarazi, R. C., Ibrahim, M. M., Dustan, Harriet, P. & Ferrario, C. M. (1974) Cardiac factors in hypertension. *Circulation Research*, **34**, Suppl. 1, 213–221.

Taylor, S. H., Sutherland, G. R., Hutchison, D. C., Langford-Kidd, B. S., Robertson, P. C., Kennelly, B. M. & Donald, K. W. (1962) The effects of intravenous guanethidine on the systemic and pulmonary circulation in man. *American Heart Journal*, **63**, 239–264.

Toghill, P. J., Smith, P. G., Benton, P., Brown, R. C. & Matthews, H. L. (1974) Methyldopa liver damage. *British Medical Journal*, **3**, 545–548.

Tuckman, J., Messerli, F. & Hodler, J. (1973) Treatment of hypertension with large doses of the β-adrenergic blocking drug oxprenolol, alone and in combination with the vasodilatator dihydralazine. *Clinical Science and Molecular Medicine*, **45**, 159–161s.

Tuckman, J., Reich, T., Lyon, A. F., Goodman, B., Mendlowitz, M. & Jacobson, J. H. (1968) Electrical stimulation of the sinus nerves in hypertensive patients. *Hypertension*, **16** 23–38.

Verniory, A., Staroukine, M., Telerman, M. & Delwiche, F. (1974) Effect of sotalol on arterial pressure and renin–angiotensin system in hypertensive patients. In *Clinical Advances in Beta-Blocking Therapy. Sotalol*, ed. Smart, A. G. Vol. IV, pp. 36–45. Amsterdam: Excerpta Medica.

Villarreal, H., Exaire, J. E., Rubio, V. & Davila, H. (1964) Effect of guanethidine and bretylium tosylate on systemic and renal hemodynamics in essential hypertension. *American Journal of Cardiology*, **14**, 633–640.

Waal-Manning, H. J. (1970) Comparative studies on the hypotensive effects of beta-adrenergic receptor blockade. In *Symposium on Beta-adrenergic Receptor Blocking Drugs*, ed. Simpson, F. O., p. 64. Auckland: CIBA.

Waal-Manning, H. J. & Simpson, F. O. (1971) Practolol treatment in asthmatics. *Lancet*, **2**, 1264–1265.

Waal-Manning, H. J. & Simpson, F. O. (1974) Pindolol: a comparison with other antihypertensive drugs and a double-blind placebo trial. *New Zealand Medical Journal*, **80**, 151–157.

Wilkinson, P. R., Issler, H., Hesp, R. & Raftery, E. B. (1975) Total body and serum potassium during prolonged thiazide therapy for essential hypertension. *Lancet*, **1**, 759–762.

Winer, B. M. (1961) The antihypertensive actions of benzothiadiazines. *Circulation*, **23**, 211–218.

Worlledge, Sheila M., Carstairs, K. C. & Dacie, J. V. (1966) Autoimmune haemolytic anaemia associated with α-methyldopa therapy. *Lancet*, **2**, 135–139.

Zacest, R., Gilmore, E. & Koch-Weser, J. (1972) Treatment of essential hypertension with combined vasodilation and beta-adrenergic blockade. *New England Journal of Medicine*, **286**, 617–622.

Zacharias, F. J., Cowan, K. J., Vickers, Jean & Wall, B. G. (1972) Propranolol in hypertension. A study of long-term therapy 1964–1970. *American Heart Journal*, **83**, 755–761.

10

CARDIAC METABOLISM

M. R. Stephens   J. R. Muir

Since the first review of this series (Muir, 1973), there has been a continued advance in our knowledge of cardiac metabolism both at a basic and an applied level. Particular areas of relevance to the cardiologist and the physician are now more clearly understood in biochemical and physiological terms. This article will concentrate on these aspects, and most especially on those most pertinent to human disease. Furthermore, an attempt will be made to correlate information from ultrastructural, biochemical and physiological studies, as such an approach should be useful in the more meaningful interpretation of many models of human heart disease.

As space does not permit a detailed discussion of all aspects of cardiac metabolism, those subjects which have been previously reviewed in detail will be treated here in brief. The reader is again referred to previous reviews (Olson, 1962; Weber, 1966; Opie, 1968).

THE STRUCTURE AND METABOLISM OF THE NORMAL MYOCARDIUM

Ultrastructure

The contractile units of cardiac muscle are the myofibrils and these are composed of many sarcomeres separated from each other by Z-lines (Fig. 10.1). The striated appearance of each sarcomere is due to the overlapping of two different types of myofilament (Huxley, 1951, 1953a, b). The thick centrally placed filament is composed of myosin, while the thin filaments projecting from the Z-line are made up essentially of actin. Thus, the central A-band (anisotropic) contains a dark area of overlapping thick and thin filaments and a central light area, the H-zone, consisting of only thick filaments. The areas of the sarcomere adjacent to the Z-lines, which contain only thin actin filaments, are called the I-bands (isotropic).

Mitochondria are arranged in densely packed rows between the bundles of myofibrils (Fig. 10.1). These organelles are the main site of energy production by oxidative phosphorylation, which leads to the formation of adenosine triphosphate (ATP). It is of interest that mitochondria are more abundant in the more active types of muscle, and in particular the heart, which has a high metabolic activity, contains a very large number of mitochondria.

Sarcolemma. The cardiac muscle cells are surrounded by the sarcolemmal membrane, which is responsible for the control of the action potential and the maintenance of the ionic 'milieu' of the sarcoplasm. Unlike skeletal muscle where individual fibres are innervated by their own motor end plates, the heart must be activated as a whole. This is made possible by the existence of connecting gap junctions between adjacent cells (Sommer and Johnson, 1970). Following the action potential there is an increase in the intracellular calcium ion concentration, which in turn activates the contractile units. Therefore there must be an efficient mechanism for the rapid distribution of

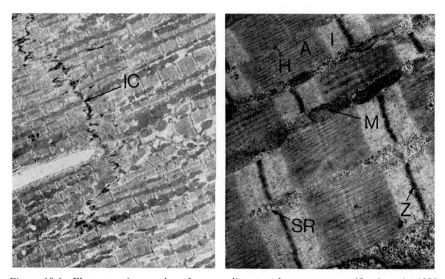

Figure 10.1 Electron micrographs of rat cardiac muscle at two magnifications (×4300, ×20 000). Mitochondria (M) are seen between the myofibrils. The structure of the sarcomeres, between the Z-bands, is shown to be composed of I-bands (thin filaments), A-bands (overlapping thick and thin filaments), and the central H-bands (thick filaments) in the centre of which is a darker line, M-line, which is due to interconnections between the thick filaments. Elements of the sarcoplasmic reticulum (SR) and the intercallated discs (IC) are also seen

calcium throughout the sarcoplasm. It is now thought that two different membrane systems, the sarcolemma and the sarcoplasmic reticulum, play important roles in the release of calcium in the sarcoplasm. Firstly, calcium ions may penetrate or be displaced from the sarcolemma, whose surface area is greatly increased by invaginations that penetrate into the sarcoplasm as a transverse tubular system in close proximity to the Z-lines. Secondly, there exists a separate internal membrane system, the *sarocplasmic reticulum*, which is capable of accumulating and releasing calcium ions. It is thought that this second system may play a role in the beat to beat regulation of calcium ion concentration within the cell. This membrane surrounds the sarcomeres and terminates in cisternal swellings, which lie in close proximity to the transverse tubules of the sarcolemma (Fig. 10.1).

Energy Metabolism

The division of myocardial metabolism into three phases (energy liberation, energy conservation, and energy utilisation), proposed by Olson (1962) remains a useful working hypothesis.

Energy liberation. Energy is liberated from the substrates available to the heart by a number of mechanisms including the Embden–Meyerhoff glycolytic pathway, the pentose shunt, the oxidation of fatty acids, and the Krebs citric acid cycle. The free energy of the 'nascent' hydrogen thus produced is transported through the electron transport chain of the mitochondria, and is finally combined with oxygen to form water. During this process electrons are transferred enzymatically from a donor to a series of acceptors, releasing energy which is conserved by phosphorylation of adenosine diphosphate (ADP) to form ATP. The myocardium, with its need to regulate performance rapidly in accordance with work demand, needs an efficient method for the storage of energy. This is achieved by the transfer of the terminal high energy phosphate bond of ATP to creatine by creatine phosphotransferase to form creatine phosphate (CP). This provides a store for the rapid regeneration of ATP to meet immediate increases in demand.

High-energy phosphates. The direct source of energy for contraction is ATP which is hydrolysed by an enzyme adenosine triphosphatase (ATP-ase) located on the myosin molecule. This enzyme liberates the large amount of energy in the terminal phosphate bond of ATP. Energy is also required for other processes in the cardiac muscle cell, and in particular for the control of the movement of calcium ions and other ions which play a key role in excitation–contraction coupling in the cell.

Excitation–Contraction Coupling

The resting potential across the sarcolemmal membrane is about -80 mV but this polarity is reversed by the depolarisation of the membrane by the passage of the action potential. This is brought about by the inward movement of positively charged cations due to a voltage-dependent selective increase in membrane permeability to sodium and calcium ions. It is associated with some outward movement of potassium ions. There is an initial rapid and short-lived influx of sodium ions, the fast sodium current. This is followed by a more prolonged influx of calcium ions, the slow calcium current, which is mainly responsible for the maintenance of the plateau of the action potential (Fig. 10.2). In this respect heart muscle differs from skeletal muscle, in which the action potential is very short and contractile activity is relatively independent of external calcium ion concentration. The long duration of the action potential in the heart may be related to the importance of inward calcium movements in modulating contraction. It is also probably important in terms of the physiological role of the heart which is fulfilled by regular twitch contractions rather than the occasional tetanic contraction, and where the presence of a long refractory period is important. During repolarisation the ionic movements are reversed, sodium being pumped out of the cell in exchange for potassium by an energy dependent pump (Na-K ATP-ase), which is inhibited by the cardiac glycosides. This also appears to be linked to sodium/calcium transport across the membrane which is not energy dependent.

Ca ion action

The influx of extracellular calcium across the sarcolemma during the plateau of the action potential does provide some calcium ions for the activation of the contractile proteins. However, it seems unlikely that this mechan-

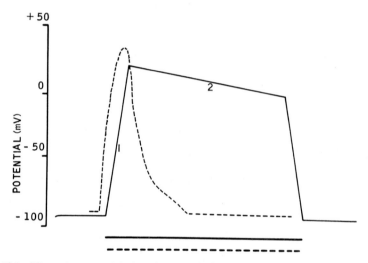

Figure 10.2   The action potential of cardiac ventricular muscle (solid line) and skeletal muscle (broken line). (1) The fast sodium current, (2) the slow calcium current. The duration of contraction is represented by the corresponding horizontal lines below

ism by itself is capable of increasing the sarcoplasmic calcium ion concentration to a sufficient level with sufficient rapidity. Heart muscle contains a significant amount of sarcoplasmic reticulum, the actual amount varying in different animal species. This membrane system is almost certainly responsible for the removal of calcium ions from the sarcoplasm. The resulting fall in sarcoplasmic calcium ion concentration causes mechanical relaxation. It is structurally suited for this role being in close proximity to the sarcomeres and hence the myosin enzyme sites. It is therefore also suitably placed to provide a source of calcium for internal release following excitation. Although the sarcoplasmic reticulum is not in direct communication with the sarcolemma, the two systems are anatomically in close apposition at functional processes which appear as dimples between them (Sommer and Johnson, 1970). Furthermore, in the mammalian heart a specialised area of the sarcoplasmic reticulum has been described in the immediate subsarcolemmal space. This observation provides further suggestive evidence that there may be a close interrelationship between the functions of the two possible sources of calcium (Hirakow, 1970). In addition there is now a considerable amount of direct experimental evidence that calcium ions can be released to the contractile proteins from the sarcoplasmic reticulum. Therefore there is potentially a dual source of calcium ions in the cardiac muscle cell; influx from the extracellular space during the action potential and release from internal stores. This dual mechanism may provide a sensitive method for modulating the calcium ion concentration in the sarcoplasm from beat to beat. Variations in the amount of calcium supplied to the contractile sites are ultimately responsible for the variations in inotropic state, which is an integral physiological control mechanism in the heart.

Contractile Proteins and Control of Myosin ATP-ase

The myofibrils are composed of myofilaments which are arranged in a highly organised fashion. The protein components of myofibrils can be separated by electrophoresis on polyacrylamide gels. Myofibrils are initially incubated with a dissociating agent such as sodium docedyl sulphate (SDS) which allows separation of the proteins on the gel according to their molecular weight (Fig. 10.3). The thick filament of the sarcomere is composed essentially of *myosin*. In the presence of SDS this protein is split into a heavy chain and two light chain components. Myosin is an unusual protein in that it consists of both fibrous (structural) and globular (enzymic) components which are covalently linked. The subunit structure of myosin has been identified by studying the effect of the action of different proteases (protein splitting enzymes) on the molecule (Fig. 10.4). Trypsin digests the molecule into two parts, light meromyosin (LMM) and heavy meromysin (HMM). The latter component is further split by papain into S1 and S2 subunits (Lowey et al, 1969). The S1 subunit contains globular heads which are the site of the enzyme, ATP-ase. In the sarcomere these globular heads project out from the thick filaments and lie in close proximity to the thin filaments.

Actin

The thin filament is composed of the protein, actin, which can be extracted with solutions of high ionic strength at an alkline pH. Actin extracted in this way is a globular protein of molecular weight 68 000 (G-actin). In the presence of ATP, potassium chloride, and magnesium chloride, G-actin polymerises into two long threads which microscopically show a rigid helical structure (F-actin). Actin in vivo is probably a polymer of these two strands wrapped around each other.

Associated with the thin actin filaments, and occurring at regular intervals, are the two regulatory proteins tropomyosin (Tm) and troponin (Tn). The interaction between these two proteins, actin, and calcium ions, is the basis of the regulatory mechanism involved in modulation of myosin ATP-ase. Although the exact nature of this important interaction remains uncertain, some aspects now appear to be established.

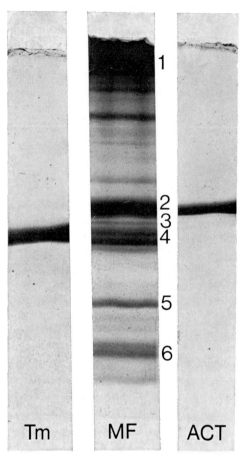

Figure 10.3   The protein components of rat cardiac myofibrils separated by polyacrylamide gel electrophoresis after dissociation with SDS. Myofibrils (MF) are flanked by tropomyosin (Tm) and actin (ACT) as markers. Key: (1) Myosin heavy chain, (2) actin, (3) 37 000 troponin component, (4) tropomyosin, (5, 6) light chains of myosin

Regulatory proteins

The two regulatory proteins are closely associated with the thin actin filaments. The arrangement of these proteins on the actin filament is exact, troponin recurring at regular intervals with tropomyosin situated in the groove of the actin filament between the troponin complexes (Fig. 10.5). The project-ing enzyme heads of myosin lie in close proximity to the sites of troponin on the actin filament and these areas form the potential crossbridges. The function of these interacting sites is to affect binding of the two filaments and to control sliding of the one relative to the other. Troponin is known to be a complex of three protein components (Perry, 1973), which can be separated on

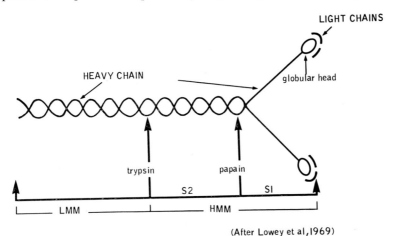

(After Lowey et al,1969)

Figure 10.4 Schematic representation of the myosin molecule

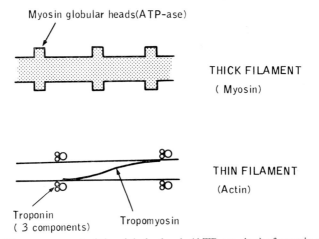

Figure 10.5 The arrangement of the globular heads (ATP-ase sites) of myosin on the thick filament, and tropomyosin and troponin on the actin thin filament (after Perry, 1973)

polyacrylamide gels. While one of these components can be seen in the electrophoretic separation illustrated in Figure 10.3 (p. 268), the other two migrate close to the light chains of myosin and are thus not clearly visible. The three troponin components are: (1) a calcium binding protein (Tn-C, molecular weight 18 000) (2) an inhibitory protein (Tn-I, molecular weight 23 000), and (3) a third component known as the 37 000 component after its molecular weight. Tn-I acts as a strong and specific inhibitor of the magnesium stimulated ATP-ase activity of reconstituted pure actin and myosin (actomyosin) but has no effect on the calcium stimulated ATP-ase (Perry et al, 1973). Furthermore, this inhibitory action is greatly enhanced by tropomyosin. Tn-C possesses a strong affinity for binding calcium ions and this binding neutralises the action of the inhibitory protein. The role of the 37 000 component remains unclear, but it may be related to the attachment of troponin to tropomyosin (Greaser and Gergely, 1971).

The properties of the regulatory proteins have been defined by in vitro experiments using purified components. The nature of the mechanism in vivo is of course more difficult to identify. However, the regular arrangement of the contractile proteins, and in particular of the globular myosin heads, has important implications. Thus at any one sarcomere length the number of globular myosin heads in proximity to the actin filament and the attached regulatory proteins is fixed, and therefore the number of potential ATP-ase sites is also fixed. The increased ATP hydrolysis necessary to augment the speed of fibre shortening that occurs with an increase in the inotropic state must therefore be obtained from the same quantity of enzyme. The regulatory system may thus be more than a simple 'on–off' trigger mechanism. It may also be able to induce a change in the enzyme itself which would result in a higher rate of enzyme activity. Such a change might be induced by minor conformational alterations resulting in reversion to an isoenzyme form possessing a greater capacity for ATP hydrolysis (Trayer and Perry, 1966; Perry, 1973).

These observations have led to some tentative hypotheses concerning the mode of action of the regulatory system in muscles. It is suggested that in resting muscle Tn-I is the controlling component, its inhibitory effect being extended by tropomyosin to several adjacent actin monomers. While it is known that Tn-C will neutralise the inhibitory effect of Tn-I independent of tropomyosin, the exact mechanism by which the binding of calcium to TN-C effects the interaction of the crossbridges, enabling the thick and thin filaments to slide one on another, remains to be clarified.

A further problem remaining to be solved is that of the biological role of the light chain subunits of myosin. In this context species differences are of interest. In the mollusc for example, in which species neither troponin nor tropomyosin are present, the myosin light chains will bind calcium and inhibit myosin ATP-ase activity (Kendrick-Jones, 1974). Perry (1973) has therefore suggested that a troponin–tropomyosin system has evolved in the higher animals. The light chain components of myosin in vertebrate cardiac muscle from a variety of species show differences in both their number and molecular weight, and these differences correlate with the differences in maximal speed of unloaded fibre shortening (V_{max}) in these species (Delcayre and Swynghedauw, 1975; Henderson et al, 1970). Despite these observations, the role of the light chains remains unclear. At the present time there is considerable interest in the light chain components of myosin particularly in relation to the alterations in myosin ATP-ase activity which have been found in association with chronic cardiac hypertrophy (see below).

SOME BIOCHEMICAL–MECHANICAL CORRELATES

The simplest measure of overall cardiac performance is the stroke output. This function is determined by the change in length of the muscle fibres. The main determinants of muscle fibre shortening are:

1. *The load sensed by the fibre.* In the intact heart, this will be controlled by three factors; the pressure against which the heart must eject (the afterload); the wall thickness or the number of contractile units having to share this load; and Laplace's law. As a muscle can either shorten or develop force, these two functions will be inversely related.

2. *Initial fibre length.* The influence of this factor is enunciated in Starling's law. Implicit in this relationship is the fact that, all other things being equal, muscle always shortens to the same end-systolic length. Therefore the degree of fibre shortening will be determined by the initial stretch of the fibre as set by the resting force (the preload). Cardiac muscle, unlike skeletal muscle, is very resistant to stretch at rest, it being very difficult to exceed a sarcomere length of about 2.3 μm. This high resting stiffness of heart muscle implies that as the maximal sarcomere length is approached resting wall tension rises steeply. In the intact heart this is manifested as a steeply rising end diastolic pressure. However, an advantage of this resting stiffness is that it prevents cardiac myofilaments being pulled apart which would result in a reduction or even abolition in the number of possible crossbridge sites between the two filaments.

3. *Contractility (inotropic state, or mechanical capability).* Mechanical activity is manifest as shortening and/or force development. The ability of a muscle to shorten or develop force is dependent on the concentration of calcium ions around the myofilaments, and the contractile state is therefore intimately related to calcium availability.

Inotropic Mechanisms

A positive inotropic effect such as that induced by cardiac glycosides or catecholamines, is associated with a decreased duration of contraction and an increase in the rate of isovolumic tension development (maximal dP/dt). In the case of cardiac glycosides such a change is associated with an increase of intracellular calcium and sodium, and a decrease of intracellular potassium. These changes are similar to those seen with the positive staircase response to increasing frequency of contraction (Langer and Serena, 1970; Langer, 1968). The primary action of the cardiac glycosides is to inhibit the sarcolemmal Na-K, ATP-ase, so leading directly to an accumulation of intracellular sodium ions. The increase in available calcium appears to be secondary to this, perhaps related to calcium/sodium ion competition at membrane binding sites. If, as has been suggested, it is true that sodium competes with calcium for binding to internal storage sites such as the sarcoplasmic reticulum, then the cardiac glycosides might act to increase the free calcium available to the myofilaments.

Sympathetic stimulation

The inotropic effect of adrenaline involves a different process, although the net result is similar in that available internal calcium increases. It now seems probable that adrenaline operates through an intracellular 'messenger'

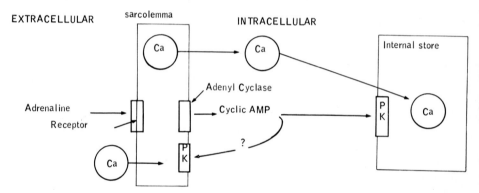

Figure 10.6 Schematic representation of the possible role of cyclic AMP in mediating the changes in calcium ion concentration associated with the positive inotropic response to adrenaline. Adrenaline acts on the sarcolemmal membrane to stimulate adenyl cyclase to produce cyclic AMP which activates the sarcoplasmic reticulum (one of the possible internal stores) and possibly the sarcolemmal protein kinase (PK). This has the effect of phosphorylating the membrane site regulating calcium transport and leads to an increased calcium uptake

substance 3′:5′-cyclic adenosine monophosphate (cyclic AMP). Changes in the intracellular cyclic AMP concentration correlate with the inotropic response to catecholamines (Kukovetz, Poch and Wurm, 1973). The basic mechanism is depicted in Figure 10.6. It is suggested that adrenaline activates a membrane-bound enzyme, adenyl cyclase, the increased activity of which leads to a rise in intracellular cyclic AMP. Cyclic AMP then acts as a second 'messenger' (Sutherland, Oye and Butcher, 1965), stimulating specific membrane enzymes, the protein kinases. The effect of these enzymes is to phosphorylate proteins using ATP as substrate. Protein kinases are thought to occur on cardiac sarcoplasmic reticulum (LaRaia and Morkin, 1974) and cyclic AMP increases the calcium accumulation by this membrane (Morkin and LaRaia, 1974). It is also probable that phosphorylation of the sarcolemma enhances calcium transport across this membrane and thus increases calcium influx into the cell (Wollenberger, 1975). Therefore we can postulate that adrenaline acting through cyclic AMP increases both calcium influx across the sarcolemma, and the accumulation of calcium by internal stores (sarcoplasmic reticulum and possibly others). This would result in an increase both in the calcium immediately available to the myofilaments and in the calcium in the sarcoplasmic reticulum stores, thereby increasing the calcium available for future release to the myofilament crossbridge sites.

NORMAL AND ABNORMAL CARDIAC GROWTH

One of the most intriguing properties of the heart is its ability to vary its mass in response to alterations in its work load. This property is well illustrated by comparisons between different animal species, and even between different animals within the same species; for example, the cardiac mass of the wild rat is greater than that of its domestic brother (Zak, 1974). In considering the factors involved in the growth of heart muscle we shall concern ourselves with three aspects: (1) Is normal and abnormal growth accompanied by cell division (hyperplasia), or cell enlargement (hypertrophy)? (2) What is the mechanism of activation of protein synthesis? and (3) What abnormalities underlie pathological hypertrophy progressing to heart failure?

Hypertrophy or Hyperplasia

The basic question whether the heart increases its muscle mass by hypertrophy or hyperplasia of cells, has now been clarified to some extent by studies of normal and exaggerated growth in the experimental animal. During the early postnatal period, when rapid growth is normal, the nuclei of heart muscle cells still retain the ability to divide by mitosis. On the other hand this is not the case for skeletal muscle cells, which show total absence of nuclear division after birth (Zak, 1973). However, the detailed studies of Bishop (1974) using the neonatal puppy suggest that this ability of the cardiac myocyte to divide persists for only a few weeks after birth. In this respect the muscle cell is fundamentally different from the other cells in the heart, which retain the ability to divide by mitosis throughout their normal life span. It is interesting that in the heart these other cells have a different developmental origin from the myocyte (Grove et al, 1969).

The response of heart cells to an increased work load varies according to the age at which the load is applied. Early observations in the adult animal suggested that the increase in mass that followed aortic constriction was due to both hyperplasia and hypertrophy of cells (Grimm, Kubato and Whitehorn, 1966; Nowy and Frings, 1960). However, more recent studies using autoradiography have shown that the hyperplastic response is confined to cells other than muscle cells and that the muscle cell mass enlarges by hypertrophy alone (Morkin and Ashford, 1968). In contrast, certain experiments have suggested that in the weanling rat anaemia causes hypertrophy and hyperplasia of both muscle and other cells in the myocardium (Neffgen and Korecky, 1972). Observations such as these have been based on the demonstration of increased labelling of nuclei by ^{3}H-thymidine using autoradiographic techniques. However, the finding of increased labelling in the muscle nuclei does not necessarily indicate normal mitotic division, as it may follow increased deoxyribonucleic acid (DNA) synthesis without nuclear division (polyploid nuclei) or nuclear division without cytoplasmic division (multinucleated cells). The observations of Adler and Hueck (1971) that in severe human cardiac hypertrophy up to 75 per cent of all nuclear components may show increased polyploidy are of considerable interest in this context. Finally, Linzbach (1973) has found that in severe cardiac hypertrophy in man mitotic division of muscle cells does not occur, but that the ventricular muscle cells appear to divide by an unusual type of longitudinal splitting involving the apparent cleavage of polyploid nuclei.

In summary, it is probable that soon after birth hyperplasia of muscle cells ceases to occur, whereas mitotic division continues in the other cells in the heart. Under the influence of stimulated growth, the cells other than the muscle cells show a significant increase in mitosis, whereas the response of the muscle cells is less clear cut. It seems likely that in severe cardiac hypertrophy in man an increase in DNA can result from the production of polyploid or even multinucleate cells.

Protein Synthesis in Cardiac Hypertrophy

Protein synthesis in the normal heart

The contractile proteins in heart muscle are in a continuous state of flux, and their mass can be rapidly increased in response to an increased work demand. It is therefore clear that an efficient mechanism for the synthesis of these proteins must be present.

The templates for protein synthesis are contained in the nucleic acid, deoxyribonucleic acid (DNA). The transcription of the code contained in DNA is mediated by messenger ribonucleic acid (m-RNA) under the control of the enzyme RNA polymerase (Fig. 10.7). The m-RNA, synthesised in the nucleoplasm, then passes through the cytoplasm to attach to the ribosomes, which are large ribonucleoprotein particles. It is on the ribosomes, which are found both free and bound to the rough endoplasmic reticulum, that proteins are assembled by the process of translation of amino acids. The amino acids are 'activated' by reacting with ATP under the influence of their own specific activating enzymes (amino acyl-t-RNA synthetases). The ATP–amino acid complex then reacts with a further specific RNA, transfer RNA (t-RNA), to produce amino acyl t-RNA which migrates to the polyribosomes to take part in protein synthesis. The assembly of amino acids on the polyribosomes (translation) involves the binding of the amino acyl t-RNA molecules to the ribosomes, those bound being determined by the arrangement of the specific m-RNA on the ribosomes. The synthesis of protein then occurs by peptide bond formation between the amino acyl t-RNA molecules with subsequent release of t-RNA.

The RNA concentration of any tissue appears to be directly proportional to its protein synthetic activity, and in this respect the heart has a higher RNA concentration than any other muscle (Zak, 1962). Most RNA in muscle tissue is found in the ribosomes, 1 per cent being in the form of m-RNA, and about 14 per cent t-RNA (Gilbert, 1963).

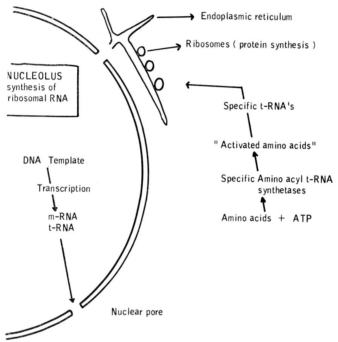

Figure 10.7 Diagram to illustrate the major components of the protein-synthesising mechanism in the cell (see text for discussion)

Protein synthesis in cardiac hypertrophy

The changes that occur in protein synthesis in response to an increased work load have been studied both in the isolated perfused heart and in the intact animal following aortic constriction. One of the earliest responses to an increased work load is an increase in RNA concentration, which is proportional to the increase in heart weight (Nair et al, 1968). This increase affects both ribosomal and transfer RNA but no preferential synthesis of messenger RNA has been found (Koide and Rabinowitz, 1969). At this stage protein synthesis can be blocked by actinomycin D (Morkin, Garrett and Fishman, 1968).

Associated with this early increase in RNA is an increased amino acid incorporation into protein, which is also proportional to the increase in heart weight (Zak and Fischman, 1971). The findings of Fanburg and Posner (1968) that RNA polymerase activity is increased within 12 h following aortic constriction, suggest that m-RNA is involved in the early stages of activation of protein synthesis.

The role of amino acids in the control of protein synthesis in the hypertrophying heart is controversial. Experimental results are difficult to interpret as the quantity of amino acids released by protein degradation, which are reutilised, is difficult to measure, and as the degree of compartmentalisation of the amino acids within the cell is uncertain. The various pools involved are either not measurable or quite possibly not even known. In the isolated perfused heart, subjected to an increased afterload, where the *known* amino acid pools are to some extent controllable, increased transport of lysine could not be demonstrated (Schreiber, Oratz and Rothschild, 1971). This observation is consistent with those of Morgan et al (1971) who showed that intracellular amino acid concentrations remained constant in spite of increased protein synthesis. However, using an artificial amino acid (amino isobutyric acid), which employs the same transport system as lysine but which is not reutilised, an increased uptake of this amino acid was found in the perfused overloaded heart (Ahren, Hjalmarson and Isaksson, 1972). Whatever these results indicate it remains uncertain whether amino acids themselves have any regulatory function to play in the development of cardiac hypertrophy.

The final result of activation of the RNA ribosomal system is a net increase in the amount of contractile protein. The term 'net increase' is specifically chosen because an increase in muscle mass may be due to changes in either protein synthesis or breakdown. During developing cardiac hypertrophy in the rabbit, following banding of the aorta, the increase in myosin mass follows an accelerated turnover of myosin, which is the result of both an increase in the synthesis and to a lesser extent in the degradation of this protein (Morkin, Kimata and Skillman, 1972). As a consequence of these changes approximately 90 per cent of the original myosin is replaced within 15 days of the operation.

Although much is now known of the biochemical events associated with the development of cardiac hypertrophy, little is known about its regression. It is certainly true that in the experimental animal protein synthesis can be rapidly turned on and off in accordance with varying work demands (Stephens et al, 1974). However, whether this is due to alterations in either protein synthesis or degradation, or both, remains to be established.

Biochemical Defects in Cardiac Hypertrophy

There is now little doubt that in 'compensated' cardiac hypertrophy the mechanical performance of ventricular muscle is abnormal. This abnormality varies with the nature of the stimulus to hypertrophy (Skelton and Sonnenblick, 1974). In the mechanically stressed ventricle it is a mild decrease in force development and a significant reduction in the maximal velocity of isotonic fibre shortening. Although longstanding hypertrophy in the human heart often terminates in cardiac failure, a similar situation is difficult to produce in the experimental animal. Therefore we have relatively little knowledge of the true progression of biochemical or mechanical events underlying this important clinical condition. However, in this section we shall discuss briefly certain aspects of cardiac metabolism that are known to be abnormal in hypertrophy.

Contractile proteins

In 1962, Alpert and Gordon showed that the ATP-ase activity of myofibrils extracted from hypertrophied human hearts was depressed. This important observation has since been confirmed in many different experimental models (reviewed by Alpert, Hamrell and Halpern, 1974). Using purified myofibrils and myosin from hypertrophied hearts, Swynghedauw, Bouveret and Hatt (1973) have shown that this depression of the myofibrillar ATP-ase activity reflects a definite abnormality in the enzyme activity of myosin. These observations could explain some of the mechanical abnormalities known to be associated with cardiac hypertrophy. The relationship between the mechanical properties and the enzyme activity of different muscles can also be established in comparative physiology, for it is known that the maximal speed of unloaded fibre shortening (V_{max}) of the various muscles, and of the same muscle in different species, correlates with the myosin ATP-ase activity (Barany, 1967; Barany et al, 1967). Such a relationship is compatible with the sliding filament hypothesis of musclar contraction in which shortening of the muscle is thought to result from the making and breaking of crossbridges between actin and myosin, a process known to be controlled by the enzymatic hydrolysis of ATP by myosin. The cause of this alteration in the enzyme activity of myosin remains unknown. However, it is known that the development of cardiac hypertrophy is associated with an increased turnover of myosin, and also that a chronological relationship exists between the progressive lowering of the myofibrillar ATP-ase activity that occurs and the protein synthetic activity in hypertrophying myofibrils (Stephens et al, 1977). Such observations are consistent with the view that during the development of cardiac hypertrophy the muscle cell produces an abnormal myosin molecule. However, myosin from hypertrophied hearts has a normal appearance on polyacrylamide gel electrophoresis (Berson and Swynghedauw, 1973), which would indicate normal molecular weights for the different components of this protein. In addition the proportion of light and heavy subunits of myosin, and their molecular weights, have also been found to be normal, and the light chains have a normal amino acid composition (Morkin and LaRaia, 1974). However, further studies of the detailed molecular structure and composition of myosin from hypertrophied hearts are needed to resolve this problem. Alternative explanations for the depressed enzyme activity in hypertrophy, such as the production of an ATP-ase inhibitor or the activation of proteolytic enzymes, have not been investigated in great detail.

Finally the possibility that the protein components of the thin filament may be abnormal has received little attention. Although they are present in normal proportions and have normal molecular weights in hypertrophied cardiac muscle, their structure has not been studied. The functioning of the regulatory protein system also remains to be investigated.

Excitation–contraction coupling

The mechanical impairment demonstrable in isolated preparations of papillary muscles from hypertrophied hearts could be explained, in part at least, by a disturbance of excitation–contraction coupling. Kauffman, Homburger and Wirth (1971), using microelectrode measurements of electrical activity from hypertrophied cat right ventricles, were unable to demonstrate any abnormality of transmembrane potentials. In this model contractility was depressed but could be restored to normal by supramaximal calcium activation. These findings implied a disturbance in excitation–contraction coupling. Furthermore the decrease in contractility was directly related to the increase in cell volume associated with hypertrophy. Thus, if the calcium entering the cell was normal in the face of an increased cell size, the calcium available per unit cell volume would be diminished.

Further evidence of impaired excitation–contraction coupling in cardiac hypertrophy was recently reported by Henry et al (1972). In this study a comparison of ATP-ase activity and isometric tension development was made in both glycerinated fibres (membrane free) and intact papillary muscles from hypertrophied rabbit hearts. They found a depressed length–tension curve in intact papillary muscles but a normal curve in the glycerinated fibres. They therefore suggested that in this model hypertrophy is associated with abnormal membrane function. It is also known (Ito, Suko and Chidsey, 1974) that a progressive decline of in vitro calcium accumulation by isolated sarcoplasmic reticulum occurs in hypertrophied heart muscle, and that the depression becomes even more marked when overt cardiac failure develops.

A further way in which the impaired mechanical performance of hypertrophied muscle could be explained would be in terms of inadequate ATP stores in the myocardium. The evidence at the present time remains inconclusive on this important point. In hypertrophied hearts energy stores appear to be normal (Pool, Spann and Buccino, 1967), but these may not be a true reflection of the ability of the energy liberating processes to maintain them at normal levels under conditions of increased demands.

In summary, there is good evidence that in severe cardiac hypertrophy several different aspects of cardiac metabolism are disturbed. These include an intrinsic defect in the contractile proteins, and defective control of the ionic 'milieu' of the cell. It thus seems likely that the depressed mechanical performance in cardiac hypertrophy is not due to one single defect in function but rather to an orchestra of events.

ISCHAEMIA

The normal extraction of oxygen from the blood by the resting myocardium is very efficient and therefore the oxygen content of the coronary venous blood is low. As the arteriovenous oxygen difference across the myocardium is already wide, any increased oxygen delivery to the myocardium is critically dependent on an increase in coronary blood flow, which may be limited in ischaemic heart disease. A situation may thus develop in which energy demands exceed supply. The duration of this negative energy balance will determine whether there is permanent tissue damage with necrosis or reversible ischaemia resulting in the clinical syndrome of angina pectoris.

Ligation of major coronary vessels in the experimental animal cannot be claimed to mimic accurately the situation of acute myocardial infarction in man, where pre-existing patchy fibrosis and collateral circulation may be important factors (Oliver, 1975). However, such models have demonstrated the profound effects of a limited oxygen supply on subcellular myocardial metabolism and are currently of interest in terms of possible metabolic interventions aimed at limiting infarct size.

Substrate Metabolism in Ischaemia

The heart normally derives its energy supply by the strictly aerobic metabolism of substrates that are extracted from the blood in direct proportion to their arterial concentration. Glucose, pyruvate, lactic acid, ketones and free fatty acids (FFA) are all important sources of fuel for the heart. The aerobic metabolism of glucose involves initial glycolysis to pyruvic acid. This is then converted to acetyl coenzyme A to be metabolised by the tricarboxylic acid cycle in the mitochondria. Glucose metabolised in this fashion will potentially yield 39 mol of ATP for each mole of glucose used. Under conditions of ischaemia, the myocardial uptake of glucose increases and there is an initial stimulation of glycogenolysis which is the result of activation of the enzyme phosphorylase 'a' (Brachfeld, 1969). It should be noted that in myocardial infarction in man, plasma insulin levels are decreased and may diminish the intracellular uptake of glucose (Vetter et al, 1974).

Glycolysis

In ischaemic heart tissue, cellular oxidation of glucose cannot occur although pyruvic acid is formed from glycolysis which is not oxygen dependent. The energy yield from this is, however, low. Pyruvic acid is then converted to lactic acid under the influence of lactic dehydrogenase. The intracellular accumulation of lactic acid which follows leads to intracellular acidosis which

10

is further aggravated by the continuing breakdown of ATP. The degree of this acidosis is important because a major rate-limiting step in glycolysis, the phosphofructokinase reaction, is inhibited by ATP and this inhibition is exaggerated by acidosis (Danforth, 1965). The potential thus exists in the ischaemic myocardium for a vicious circle of events to develop in which anaerobic glycolysis leads to lactic acid accumulation with progressive intracellular acidosis and therefore further inhibition of glycolysis.

Fatty acid metabolism

Ischaemia also effects utilisation of FFA by the myocardium. These substrates cannot be oxidised under conditions of oxygen deprivation and they therefore accumulate within the myocardial cells (Owen et al, 1970; Opie, 1969). Plasma levels of FFA are also increased in severe myocardial infarction (Kurien and Oliver, 1966) and, if plasma albumin binding of FFA is saturated, they may be taken up by the myocardium in greatly increased amounts (Oliver, 1975). Investigations of substrate extraction by the heart in resting man suggest that these high circulating levels of FFA may inhibit glucose uptake (Lassers et al, 1972). There is now a considerable amount of experimental evidence to indicate that excess FFA are harmful to the myocardium. They increase the oxygen cost of mechanical work and thus decrease mechanical performance when the oxygen supply is limited (Kjekshus and Mjos, 1972; Henderson et al, 1970). Elevated levels of FFA increase infarct size in the experimental animal (Kjekshus and Mjos, 1973). Furthermore there is both experimental and clinical evidence to indicate that high levels of circulating FFA are associated with an increased tendency to ventricular arrhythmias (Kurien, Yates and Oliver, 1971; Oliver, Kurien and Greenwood, 1968).

Mitochondrial and Sarcoplasmic Reticulum Function in Ischaemia

The abundance of mitochondria in heart muscle is clearly related to the high metabolic activity of the heart with its constant need for an adequate supply of ATP. Mitochondria are the site of oxidative phosphorylation, the tricarboxylic acid cycle, and fatty acid oxidation, and the enzymes responsible for these reactions are located either within the matrix or on the various sections of the membrane. The functional integrity of the mitochondria is thus a vital factor in the utilisation of substrates available to the heart, and in the production of the ATP essential to the contractile process.

An early feature of ischaemia is a loss of myocardial ATP and CP, and a rise in local concentrations of adenosine and hydrogen ions (Berne et al, 1971). Following occlusion of a coronary artery, changes occur in the function of the mitochondria which indicate a disruption of the respiratory pathways and a loss of phosphorylating efficiency (Schwartz et al, 1973). These include an uncoupling of oxidative phosphorylation, so that the amount of oxygen consumed by mitochondria remains normal in the face of a decreased ATP production (a decline in P/O ratio) (Lochner et al, 1975). The actual mitochondrial content of cytochrome enzymes is also depressed (Schwartz et al, 1973). Associated with these biochemical changes are morphological alterations which include swelling and even disruption of the mitochondria. These latter findings appear to be reversible and this may be related to the synthesis of new organelles. In this respect it is of interest that mitochondria are synthesised from their own DNA complement and contain the necessary mechanism for synthesis independent of cell nuclear control.

An important early effect of ischaemia is a decline in the mechanical performance of the heart. While this could be explained in terms of a decreased energy supply, other factors may be important. One of these could be an impairment of the transport of calcium ion across the cell membranes. It has been shown that isolated sarcoplasmic reticulum from animal models of myocardial infarction have a decreased ability to accumulate calcium, which eventually becomes irreversible (Lee, Ladinski and Stuckey, 1967). Intracellular acidosis can also in itself depress mechanical performance, and this is probably related to disturbances of excitation–contraction coupling mechanisms at a variety of sites (Poole-Wilson and Langer, 1975, Williams et al, 1975).

Clinical correlations

The clinical implications of these metabolic changes are now becoming an important consideration in the management of acute myocardial infarction. Many of the changes which have been discussed lead to an early decline in the contractile state of the ischaemic muscle. This will result in a local decrease in energy utilisation which should be beneficial in terms of the eventual survival of the tissue. The overall function of the heart as a pump at this time will of course be related to the extent of the ischaemic area. Severe prolonged ischaemia will result in a central area of irreversible cell death. However, surrounding this area will be a peri-infarction zone, supplied to a variable extent by collaterals, where the ischaemia is potentially reversible. The rational management of this situation in light of the known metabolic disturbances forms the basis of a new approach to acute myocardial infarction which holds exciting possibilities for the future.

REFERENCES

Adler, C. P. & Hueck, C. (1971) Numerical hyperplasia in human heart hypertrophy. *Experimentia*, 27, 1435.

Ahren, K., Hjalmarson, A. & Isaksson, O. (1972) In vitro work load and rat heart metabolism. II. Effect on amino acid transport. *Acta Physiologica Scandinavica*, 86, 257.

Alpert, N. R. & Gordon, M. S. (1962) Myofibrillar adenosine triphosphatase activity in congestive heart failure. *American Journal of Physiology*, 202, 940.

Alpert, N. R., Hamrell, B. B. & Halpern, W. (1974) Mechanical and biochemical correlates of cardiac hypertrophy. *Circulation Research* (Suppl. II), 34–35, 11–71.

Barany, M. (1967) ATP-ase activity of myosin correlated with speed of muscle shortening. *Journal of General Physiology*, 50, 197.

Barany, M., Conover, T. E., Schlisefield, L. H., Gaetjens, E. & Goffard, M. (1967) Relation of properties of isolated myosin to those of intact muscles of the cat and sloth. *European Journal of Biochemistry*, **2**, 156.

Berne, R. M., Rubio, R., Dobson, J. G. & Curnish, R. R. (1971) Adenosine and adenine nucleotides as possible mediators of cardiac and skeletal muscle blood flow regulation. *Circulation Research* (Suppl. I), **28–29**, 115.

Berson, G. & Swynghedauw, B. (1973) Cardiac myofibrillar ATPase and electrophonetic pattern in experimental heart failure produced by a two-step mechanical overloading in the rat. *Cardiovascular Research*, **7**, 464.

Bishop S. (1974) Discussion: Cardiac hypertrophy and cardiomyopathy. *Circulation Research* (Suppl. II), **34–35**, 11–106.

Brachfield, N. (1969) Maintenance of cell viability. *Circulation* (Suppl. IV), **40**, 202.

Danforth, W. H. (1965) In *Control of Energy Metabolism*, ed. Chance, B., Estabrook, R. & Williamson, J. R., p. 287. New York: Academic Press.

Delcayre, C. & Swynghedauw, B. (1975) A comparative study of heart myosin ATPase and light subunits from different species. *Pflügers Archiv.*, **355**, 39–47.

Fanburg, B. L. & Posner, B. I. (1968) Ribonucleic acid synthesis in experimental cardiac hypertrophy in rats. *Circulation Research*, **23**, 123.

Gilbert, W. (1963) Polypeptide synthesis in Escherichia coli. II. The polypeptide chain and s-RNA. *Journal of Molecular Biology*, **6**, 389.

Greaser, M. L. & Gergely, J. (1971) The regulation of rabbit skeletal muscle contraction. *Journal of Biological Chemistry*, **246**, 4866.

Grimm, A. F., Kubato, R. & Whitehorn, W. V. (1966) Ventricular nucleic acid and protein levels with myocardial growth and hypertrophy. *Circulation Research*, **19**, 552.

Grove, D., Zak, R., Nair, K. G. & Aschenbrenner, V. (1969) Biochemical correlates of cardiac hypertrophy. *Circulation Research*, **25**, 473.

Henderson, A. H., Craig, R. J., Gorlin, R. & Sonnenblick, E. H. (1970) Free fatty acids and myocardial function in perfused rat hearts. *Cardiovascular Research*, **4**, 466.

Henderson, A. H., Craig, R. J., Sonnenblick, E. H. & Urschel, C. W. (1970) Species differences in intrinsic myocardial contractility. *Proceedings of the Society of Experimental Biology* (N.Y.), **134**, 930.

Henry, P. D., Ahumada, G. G., Friedman, W. F. & Sobel, B. E. (1972) Simultaneously measured isometric tension and ATP hydrolysis in glycerinated fibers from normal and hypertrophied rabbit heart. *Circulation Research*, **31**, 740.

Hirakow, R. (1970) Ultrastructural characteristics of the mammalian and sauropsidon heart. *American Journal of Cardiology*, **25**, 195.

Huxley, H. E. (1951) Discussions. *Faraday Society*, **11**, 148.

Huxley, H. E. (1953a) *Proceedings of the Royal Society, London*, **64**, 67.

Huxley, H. E. (1953b) Electron microscopic studies of the organisation of filament in striated muscles. *Biochemica et Biophysica Acta*, **12**, 387.

Ito, Y., Suko, J., Chidsey, C. A. (1974) Intracellular calcium and myocardial contractility. V. Calcium uptake of sarcoplasmic reticulum fractions in hypertrophied and failing rabbit hearts. *Journal of Molecular and Cellular Cardiology*, **6**, 237.

Kauffman, R. L., Homburger, H. & Wirth, H. (1971) Disorder in excitation–contraction coupling of cardiac muscle from cats with experimentally produced right ventricular hypertrophy. *Circulation Research*, **28**, 346.

Kendrick-Jones, J. (1974) Role of myosin light chains in calcium regulation. *Nature*, **249**, 631.

Kjekshus, J. K. & Mjos, O. D. (1972) Effect of free fatty acids on myocardial function and metabolism in the ischaemic dog heart. *Journal of Clinical Investigation*, **51**, 1767.

Kjekshus, J. K. & Mjos, O. D. (1973) Effect of inhibition of lipolysis on infarct size after experimental coronary artery occlusion. *Journal of Clinical Investigation*, **52**, 1770.

Koide, T. & Ribinowitz, M. (1969) Biochemical correlates of cardiac hypertrophy. *Circulation Research*, **24**, 9.

Kukovetz, W. R., Poch, G. & Wurm, A. (1973) Effect of catecholamines, histamine and oxyfedrine on isotonic contraction and cyclic AMP in the guinea pig heart. *Naunyn Schmeideberg's Archiv für experimentelle Pathologie und Pharmakologie*, **278**, 403.

Kurien, V. A. & Oliver, M. F. (1966) Serum free fatty acids after acute myocardial infarction and cerebral vascular occlusion. *Lancet*, **2**, 122.

Kurien, V. A., Yates, P. A. & Oliver, M. F. (1971) The role of free fatty acids in the production of ventricular arrhythmias after coronary artery ligation. *European Journal of Clinical Investigation*, **1**, 225.

Langer, G. A. (1968) Ion fluxes in cardiac excitation and contraction and their relation to myocardial contractility. *Physiological Review*, **48**, 708.

Langer, G. A. & Serena, S. D. (1970) Effects of straphonthidin upon contraction and ionic exchange in rabbit ventricular myocardial relation to control of active state. *Journal of Molecular and Cellular Cardiology*, **1**, 65.

LaRaia, P. J. & Morkin, E. (1974) Phosphorylation–dephosphorylation of cardiac microsomes —a possible mechanism for control of calcium uptake by cyclic AMP. In *Myocardial Biology*, ed. Dhalla, N. S., p. 417. Baltimore: University Park Press.

Lassers, B. W., Carlson, L. A., Kaijser, L. & Wahlqvist, M. (1972) In *Effect of Acute Ischaemia on Myocardial Function*, ed. Oliver, M. F., Julian, D. G. & Donald, K. W., p. 200. Edinburgh: Churchill Livingstone.

Lee, K. S., Ladinski, H. & Stuckey, J. H. (1967) Decreased Ca^{2+} uptake by sarcoplasmic reticulum after coronary artery occlusion for 60 and 90 minutes. *Circulation Research*, **21**, 439.

Linzbach, A. J. (1973) Hypertrophy, structural dilation and chronic failure of the human heart. *Folia Facultatis Medicæ Universitatis Comenianae Bratislaviensis* (Suppl. 10), 75.

Lochner, A., Opie, L. H., Owen, P., Kotzi, J. C. N., Bruyneel, K. & Gevers, W. (1975) Oxidative phosphorylation in infarcting baboon and dog myocardium: Effects of mitochondrial isolation and incubation media. *Journal of Molecular and Cellular Cardiology*, **1**, 204.

Lowey, S., Slayter, H. S., Weeds, A. G. & Baker, H. (1969) Structure of the myosin molecule. *Journal of Molecular Biology*, **42**, 1.

Morgan, H. E., Earl, D. C. N., Broadus, A., Wolpert, E. B., Giger, K. E. & Jefferson, L. S. (1971) Regulation of protein synthesis in heart muscle. *Journal of Biological Chemistry*, **246**, 2152.

Morkin, E. & Ashford, T. P. (1968) Myocardial DNA synthesis in experimental cardiac hypertrophy. *American Journal of Physiology*, **215**, 1409.

Morkin, E., Garrett, J. C. & Fishman, A. P. (1968) Effects of actinomycin D and hypophysectomy on development of myocardial hypertrophy in the rat. *American Journal of Physiology*, **214**, 6.

Morkin, E., Kimata, S. & Skillman, J. J. (1972) Myosin synthesis and degradation during development of cardiac hypertrophy in the rabbit. *Circulation Research*, **30**, 690.

Morkin, E. & LaRaia, P. J. (1974) Biochemical studies on the regulation of myocardial contractility. *New England Journal of Medicine*, **290**, 445.

Muir, J. R. (1973) Myocardial metabolism. In *Recent Advances in Cardiology*, (6), ed. Hamer, J., p. 132. Edinburgh: Churchill Livingstone.

Nair, K. G., Cutilletta, A. F., Zak, R., Koide, T. & Rabinowitz, M. (1968) Biochemical correlates of cardiac hypertrophy. *Circulation Research*, **23**, 451.

Neffgen, J. F. & Korecky, B. (1972) Cellular hyperplasia and hypertrophy in cardiomegalies induced by anaemia in young and adult rats. *Circulation Research*, **30**, 104.

Nowy, H. & Frings, H. D. (1960) Nuclein sauren im hypertrophischen Herzmuskel. *Zeitschrift für die gesamte experimentelle Medizin*, **132**, 538.

Oliver, M. F. (1975) Vulnerable ischaemic myocardium and its metabolism. In *Modern Trends in Cardiology* (3), ed. Oliver, M. F., p. 280. London: Butterworths.

Oliver, M. F., Kurien, V. A. & Greenwood, T. W. (1968) Relation between serum free-fatty-acids and arrhythmias and death after acute myocardial infarction. *Lancet*, **1**, 710.

Olson, R. E. (1962) Physiology of cardiac muscle. In *Handbook of Physiology. Circulation* 1, ed. Hamilton, W. F., p. 199. Washington, D.C.: American Physiological Society.

Opie, L. H. (1968) Metabolism of the heart in health and disease. Part 1. *American Heart Journal*, **76**, 685.

Opie, L. H. (1969) Metabolism of the heart in health and disease. Part II. *American Heart Journal*, **77**, 100.

Owen, P., Thomas, M., Young, V. & Opie, L. H. (1970) Comparison between metabolic changes in local venous and coronary sinus blood after acute experimental coronary arterial occlusion. *American Journal of Cardiology*, **25**, 562.

Perry, S. V. (1973) The control of muscular contraction. *Symposium for the Society of Experimental Biology*, **27**, 531–550.

Perry, S. V., Cole, H. A., Head, J. F. & Wilson, F. (1973) Localisation and mode of action of the inhibitory protein component of the troponin complex. *Coldspring Harbour Symposia on Quantitative Biology*, **37**, 251.

Pool, P. E., Spann, J. F. & Buccino, R. A. (1967) Myocardial high energy phosphate stores in cardiac hypertrophy and heart failure. *Circulation Research*, **21**, 365.

Poole-Wilson, P. A. & Langer, G. A. (1975) Effect of pH on ionic exchange and function in rat and rabbit myocardium. *American Journal of Physiology*, **229**, 570.

Schreiber, S. F., Oratz, M. & Rothschild, M. A. (1971) In *Cardiac Hypertrophy*, ed. Alpert, N. A., p. 215. New York: Academic Press.

Schwartz, A., Wood, J. N., Allen, J. C., Burnett, E. P., Entam, M. L., Goldstein, M. A., Sordahl, L. A. & Suzuki, M. (1973) Biochemical and morphologic correlates of cardiac ischaemia. *American Journal of Cardiology*, **32**, 46.

Skelton, L. & Sonnenblick, E. H. (1974) Heterogeneity of contractile function in cardiac hypertrophy. *Circulation Research* (Suppl. II), **34–35**, 11–83.

Sommer, J. R. & Johnson, E. A. (1970) Comparative ultrastructure of cardiac cell membrane specialisations. A review. *American Journal of Cardiology*, **25**, 184.

Stephens, M. R., Leger, J. J., Preteseille, M. & Swynghedauw, B. (1974) The incorporation of ^{3}H-lysine into cardiac myofibrils in cardiac hypertrophy in the rat. *Clinical Science and Molecular Biology*, **47**, 17p.

Sutherland, E. W., Oye, I. & Butcher, R. W. (1965) The action of epinephrine and the rate of the adenyl cyclase system in hormone action. *Recent Progress in Hormone Research*, **21**, 623.

Swynghedauw, B., Bouveret, P. & Hatt, P. Y. (1973) New fractionation scheme for preparation of heart particle. ATPase activity of purified myofibrils in chronic aortic insufficiency in the rabbit. *Journal of Molecular and Cellular Cardiology*, **5**, 44.

Trayer, J. P. & Perry, S. V. (1966) The myosin of developing skeletal muscle. *Biochemische Zietschrift*, **345**, 87.

Vetter, N., Strange, R. C., Adams, W. & Oliver, M. F. (1974) Initial metabolic and hormonal response to acute myocardial infarction. *Lancet*, **1**, 284.

Weber, A. (1966). *Current Topics of Bioenergetics*, **1**, 203.

Williams, G. J., Collins, S., Muir, J. R. & Stephens, M. R. (1975) In *Basic Functions of Cations in Myocardial Activity*, ed. Fleckenstein, A. & Dhalla, N. S., p. 273. Baltimore: University Park Press.

Wollenberger, A. (1975) *Myocardial Membranes and Calcium Myocardial Cell Damage*, ed. Fleckenstein, A. Baltimore: University Park Press.

Zak, R. (1962) Activity and RNA content of muscle. *Federation Proceedings, Federation of American Societies for Experimental Biology*, **21**, (2), 319.

Zak, R. (1973) Cell proliferation during cardiac growth. *American Journal of Cardiology*, **31**, 211.

Zak, R. (1974) Development and proliferative capacity of cardiac muscle cells. *Circulation Research* (Suppl. II), **34–35**, 11–17.

Zak, R. & Fischman, D. A. (1971). In *Cardiac Hypertrophy*, ed. Alpert, N. A., p. 247. New York: Academic Press.

11
MYOCARDIAL PERFORMANCE
M. I. M. Noble

Recent efforts to widen knowledge of basic mechanisms in heart disease have continued to be directed towards an understanding of the myocardium.

In most patients the behaviour of the myocardium is central to understanding of the response of the heart in disease, although in some situations, such as pericardial tamponade or constrictive pericarditis, or mitral or tricuspid stenosis, mechanical factors are important. The increased load placed on the ventricle by systemic or pulmonary hypertension, or by aortic or mitral valve disease, produces changes in myocardial performance which lead eventually to an inadequate cardiac output, increased stiffness of the ventricular muscle and excessive fluid retention. Intrinsic myocardial diseases, such as infarction or cardiomyopathy, have similar effects. Useful description of the behaviour of the heart muscle under these circumstances must involve consideration of the mechanical alterations produced by dilatation, hypertrophy or local damage, as well as changes in the physical properties of the myocardium in diastole and variations in the process of contraction (Hamer, 1973).

Assessment in Heart Disease

Attempts to measure the disturbances found in patients with heart disease have improved our understanding of the mechanisms involved. Reliance on a single estimate of cardiac performance, such as filling pressure, as an estimate of failure is clearly inadequate as this measurement will assess only one aspect of the underlying myocardial disturbances. The relation between the filling pressure and the work done by the ventricle gives more useful information. Attempts to measure the energy used by the myocardium have indicated a distinction between the response to an increase in ventricular work from a greater pressure load and from a greater volume load. The measurement of ventricular volume needed to assess these factors has allowed more complex calculations of myocardial behaviour. The distinction between the force and velocity of contraction originally established in skeletal muscle has been applied to the myocardium in spite of considerable differences in the behaviour of the two types of muscle. However, even at this more sophisticated level attempts to measure isolated aspects of contraction, such as ventricular wall force, ejection fraction or maximal velocity of contraction, although useful, still give inadequate descriptions of the response of the myocardium to stress. In spite of these difficulties, objective description of the disturbances in myocardial function in heart disease must be encouraged, as detailed analysis must, in the long run, prove helpful in improving our understanding of the fundamental changes involved.

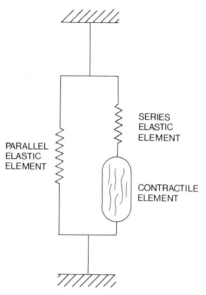

Figure 11.1   Model of a muscle as contractile and elastic elements. If the part of the muscle responsible for active contraction could be separated as the 'contractile element', the parts of the tissue responsible for the passive physical properties of the muscle may be considered as 'elastic elements' arranged either in series or in parallel with the contractile element. The parallel elastic element is responsible for any resting tension, and contraction must stretch the series elastic element before it can become effective

PHYSICAL PROPERTIES OF THE MYOCARDIUM

A useful model of the structure of a muscle is obtained by regarding it as a contractile element linked with elastic elements both in series and in parallel (Fig. 11.1) (Hamer, 1973). The series elastic elements must be stretched before contraction can become effective, and are responsible for the restoration of resting conditions at the end of contraction. The elastic elements are also responsible for the steep rise in tension when the whole muscle is stretched. The series and parallel elastic elements cannot be identified with specific structures in the muscle; these terms refer only to special aspects of the physical properties of the tissue. Cardiac muscle becomes stiff more easily than skeletal muscle when stretched (Spiro and Sonnenblick, 1964); as the properties of the contractile proteins are similar in the two types of muscle and the differences probably arise in the connective tissue (Katz, 1965).

In recent years it has become possible to measure sarcomere length directly in living muscle at rest and during contraction (Ciba Symposium, 1974). Such studies have now been applied to cardiac muscle and have demonstrated that considerable shortening of sarcomeres takes place during a contraction in which the overall length of the muscle is kept constant (isometric). This sarcomere shortening has a magnitude of about 10 per cent of optimum length according to Pollack and Krueger (1975). There is therefore an elastic element in series with the sarcomere as shown in Figure 11.2. The importance of this development is that it may now be possible to stretch heart muscle as it

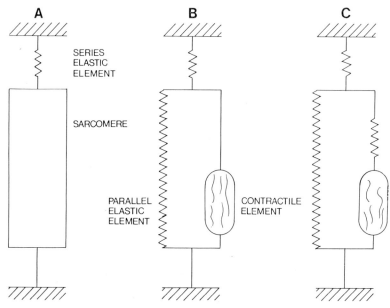

Figure 11.2 *A* Arrangement demonstrated experimentally. *B* and *C* Alternative full models depending on arrangement of elastic elements at sarcomere level

contracts in such a way that sarcomere length is controlled; this has already been done in skeletal muscle (Gordon, Huxley and Julian, 1966; Cleworth and Edman, 1972). By extending methods adopted in skeletal muscle it may then be possible to determine the distribution of elastic properties within the sarcomere. If heart muscle is shown in the future to be similar in this respect to skeletal muscle (Huxley and Simmons, 1971), the full model would become similar to Figure 11.2B; this is suggested by the results of Noble and Else (1972) and Pollack, Huntsman and Verdugo (1972). Further series elastic behaviour within the sarcomere would result in model C in Figure 11.2.

During diastole, the contractile element in Figure 11.2 is assumed to be freely distensible. However, there is no definite evidence to show that all interaction between filaments is zero at this time. The physical properties of the myocardium during diastole are mainly elastic, i.e. related to the length of the tissue components, but viscous and inertial factors, related to the velocity and acceleration of ventricular wall movement, are also found (Noble et al, 1969a).

The force (or pressure) recorded as one increases heart muscle length (or ventricular volume) during diastole increases more and more steeply; this is characteristic of an alinear spring which gets stiffer as it is stretched. This property fulfils the physiological function of preventing overstretch of heart muscle which is not protected from this hazard, as is skeletal muscle, by skeletal structures. When skeletal muscle is stretched so that sarcomere length exceeds 2.2μm, contractile force declines with increasing sarcomere length (Gordon et al, 1966). Similar behaviour on the part of cardiac muscle would be disadvantageous and does not occur because of the high diastolic stiffness. This high diastolic stiffness has, however, made it very difficult to determine the relationship between sarcomere length and active contractile force. Previous estimates (Hamer, 1973) have recently been shown to be erroneous for two reasons. The sarcomere lengths were measured in diastole. As has already been described, it has now been shown that considerable sarcomere shortening occurs even if the muscle is kept at constant length. The sarcomere length at the moment when peak contractile tension was measured was therefore less, as was the contribution to that tension of the parallel elastic element (Fig. 11.2). Failure to allow for this led to an error in the estimate of both sarcomere length and active tension (i.e. tension over and above that contributed by the passive stretched components). The other source of error was the shrinkage artefacts which took place during fixation and histological preparation of specimens for measurement of sarcomere length (Ciba Symposium, 1974).

Both these sources of error can be overcome by an exciting development of 1974 to 1975 which has been the direct measurement of sarcomere length in living contracting muscle by new optical techniques. The most recent data to my knowledge are unpublished results of Pollack and Krueger (1975). Figure 11.3 is a diagram derived from their data which is approximate and subject to a further error. The data was obtained from isometric contractions in which sarcomere shortening occurred, and in which the force was reduced because of the inverse relationship between force and velocity (Hamer, 1973). More reliable data will become available when sarcomere shortening is prevented by stretching the muscle appropriately during contraction (Cleworth and Edman, 1972). This, however, is the best estimate available at the present time and already enables one to realise that the heart has a Frank–Starling mechanism (increasing force with increasing sarcomere length and muscle length) over the range of sarcomere lengths 2.0 to 2.18μm of optimum overlap of thin and thick filaments. In skeletal muscle, contractile force is constant over this range of sarcomere lengths (Huxley, 1974). The difference is likely to be due to the fact that skeletal muscle is studied when fully activated and tetanised into steady state prolonged contraction, whereas heart muscle is studied during incompletely activated twitch contractions similar to physiological cardiac systoles. Inspection of Figure 11.3 shows that over the range of sarcomere length being discussed (2.0–2.18 μm) diastolic force is low, suggesting that this is the physiological range in life; and that over this range there is a near doubling of active force.

From the mixture of new data and uncertainty which has emerged and has been described above, it is possible to conclude that the Frank–Starling mechanism is not due to decreasing double overlap of actin filaments (actin

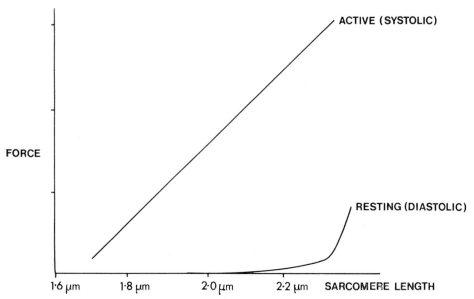

Figure 11.3 Relationship between the force developed by resting heart muscle (diastole) when stretched to increasing sarcomere lengths, and the active contractile force (systole) developed at different sarcomere lengths. Sarcomere lengths measured directly by optical methods

filaments are 1.0 μm long). Several other possible explanations have been preferred (Ciba Symposium, 1974).

Changes in Physical Properties in Diseases

The majority of the well-documented examples of change in the physical properties of the myocardium in disease are confined to the diastolic behaviour. Attempts to detect changes in series elastic and contractile element properties are of considerable interest but have been unsound in theory and unreliable in practice up to the present time.

There are a number of problems associated with measurements of diastolic ventricular compliance. The relationship between pressure and volume is alinear (Fig. 11.4). A number of simultaneous measurements of pressure and volume are therefore required to construct the curve. Routine cardiac catheterisation studies often yield only one or two measures of volume (which are often subject to systematic errors), and give ventricular pressure relative to atmospheric pressure rather than transmural pressure. To infer compliance or 'indices of compliance' from such data is therefore theoretically unsound. An obvious problem when comparing different patients is the dependence of volume on the size of the individual (children have smaller hearts than adults); normalisation of volume with respect to body size is required in this case. However, it is often possible to come to clear conclusions about the direction of a change, e.g. 'the ventricle is stiffer in situation A than in situation B' by showing a clear-cut change in volume at a given pressure or vice versa. If the ventricle is filling rapidly at the time of measurement, the results may be

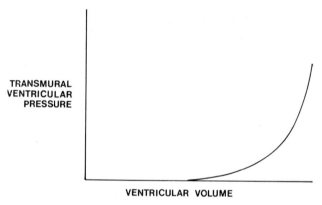

TRANSMURAL
VENTRICULAR
PRESSURE

VENTRICULAR VOLUME

Figure 11.4   Relationship between pressure across the wall of the left ventricle and its internal volume. Note that the slope is not constant, i.e. compliance is a function of volume

affected by viscous or other factors not strictly related to compliance. A radiographic or ultrasonic measure of volume in mid-diastole (diastasis) combined with simultaneous left ventricular transmural pressure, are therefore the measurements of choice for these comparisons.

It has been clearly shown that the pressure–volume relationship of a ventricle can be influenced by a change (e.g. increased systolic pressure) in the other ventricle. This applies both to the adult heart (Elzinga, 1972) and to the neonatal heart, in which the interaction betweeen ventricles changes with age (Harwick, 1974). A further non-ventricular cause of a change in ventricular pressure–volume relationships (apparent change of compliance) is constriction by the pericardium. These factors should be borne in mind when interpreting a raised end-diastolic pressure (see below).

The thicker left ventricle is normally stiffer and more resistant to filling than the right ventricle, and in the intact normal circulation where the degree of filling of each ventricle is similar the left atrial pressure is considerably higher than the right. The difference in the physical properties of the two ventricles leads to a large left-to-right shunt when an atrial septal defect is present, as the two atria then form a common venous reservoir and the less stiff right ventricle fills much more easily than the left ventricle. Left ventricular disease in these patients tends to make the left ventricle even stiffer and may increase the size of the left-to-right shunt.

The ventricular wall may become stiffer either because it is thicker or because it is truly stiffer for a given thickness. Thus an increased stiffness has been demonstrated in most conditions involving hypertrophy, e.g. outflow obstruction, pulmonary or systemic hypertension, hypertrophic cardio-myopathy.

An increase in true stiffness of a given thickness of ventricular wall is easy to demonstrate in experimental preparations (Hamer, 1973), but much more difficult to show in patients. Experimental ischaemia certainly produces increased diastolic stiffness, and this probably also occurs in clinical ischaemia including episodes of angina (Oliver, Julian and Donald, 1972). Obvious increase in true stiffness occurs in constrictive cardiomyopathy and amyloid disease (Hamer, 1973).

Decreased stiffness (increased compliance) occurs when the ventricle is chronically dilated. Such ventricles are found to have much increased end-systolic and end-diastolic volumes without grossly raised diastolic pressures. It is likely that this change occurs as a result of stress relaxation rather than to a direct effect of the disease on myocardial compliance. Chronic distension is thus another complicating factor in the study of diastolic physical properties.

One cause of ventricular distension is fluid retention accompanied by an increase in intrathoracic blood volume. In the acute phase in ventricles of normal compliance, this pushes the ventricle along its pressure volume curve (to the right in Fig. 11.4) where the curve is steeper. This results in clinical features similar to those associated with increased stiffness i.e. increased end-diastolic pressure and larger 'a' waves (Hamer, 1973), but is solely due to the increased volume together with the alinearity of the pressure–volume relation-ship. In the normal heart the greater stiffness of the left ventricle compared to the right leads to a greater effect on left atrial and pulmonary venous pressures, than on right atrial and systemic venous pressures; this is simple to demonstrate by infusing fluid into an animal and following left and right atrial pressures. This pattern is disturbed when fluid retention occurs in the presence of disease and increased stiffness of one ventricle relative to the other; this leads to a disproportionately larger rise in pulmonary venous pressure in left ventricular disease and to a greater increase in systemic venous than in pulmonary venous pressure in right ventricular disease.

From the considerations described above, it will be clear that an increase in end-diastolic pressure occurs (1) with increased end-diastolic volume and no change in compliance (e.g. ischaemia), (2) from pericardial constriction, (3) from hypertrophy of the ventricular wall, (4) from increased stiffness of the ventricular muscle. All these factors are brought together and understood if the pressure–volume relationship (Fig. 11.4) can be determined in each situation.

Frank–Starling Mechanism

The relationship between sarcomere length and force illustrated in Figure 11.3 is the basis of the dependence of force production on initial muscle length (Frank, 1895). This concept was elaborated by Starling (Patterson, Piper and Starling, 1914) from studies of the isolated canine heart–lung preparation. Much discussion has centred on whether the length of the muscle fibres or their tension at the onset of systole determined the ventricular response. Although fibre length is the fundamental factor, length and tension are of course closely related in the resting ventricular wall. In a distensible ventricle

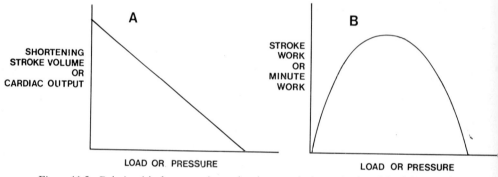

Figure 11.5   Relationship between shortening (or ventricular output) and load (pressure)

large changes in fibre length can occur with little alteration in pressure (Fig. 11.4), but if the pressure changes can be measured accurately they provide a useful index of variations in fibre length, although the relationship is not linear. The use of such an index of fibre length results in ambiguity if there is a change in diastolic compliance (see above). Measurements of cardiac dimensions are theoretically preferable, but radiographic and ultrasonic techniques for this are not yet perfected.

In addition to the difficulty of gauging the stretch of the fibres, a problem arises in an intact situation in measuring the response. This should be measured as an isometric force or isovolumic pressure; this can be done in animals (Ciba Symposium, 1974), but not in patients. When the fibres are allowed to shorten, or the ventricle to eject, the mechanical output is determined by the opposing load (Fig. 11.5). The higher the load the less the shortening or volume ejected (Fig. 11.5A). However, if the aortic pressure is held constant, these variables can be shown to be dependent on the stretch of the fibres. Work is equal to shortening times load, and therefore the relationship between work and load is as shown in Figure 11.5B. This is also true for work rate or power. Again, if the aortic pressure is held constant these variables can be shown to be dependent on the initial fibre length (heart size). This was the approach used to confirm the Frank–Starling hypothesis in sophisticated animal work (Sarnoff and Berglund, 1954). Braunwald (1965) has been responsible for a series of studies in patients using similar principles to confirm the operation of the Frank–Starling mechanism in the intact human heart.

In isolated heart–lung preparations a progressive increase in presystolic ventricular volume leads eventually to a reduction in the force of contraction, giving a descending limb to the response curve. This finding seemed to provide an explanation of the situation in heart failure in which a distended ventricle produces an inadequate response. However, the evidence of a reduction in ventricular response at high filling pressures in animal work has been explained as a shift to a lower curve as the condition of the preparation deteriorated. Case, Berglund and Sarnoff (1954) could not demonstrate a descending limb of the response curve unless left ventricular function was impaired by reducing coronary blood flow. Tricuspid or mitral incompetence due to gross ventricular dilatation or subendocardial ischaemia may be responsible for a fall in cardiac output in animal preparations. It seems unlikely that the 'descending limb' of the ventricular function curve is due to a descending limb of the length–force curve of the cardiac muscle.

Studies of diastolic sarcomere length without correction for shrinkage (see above) have yielded a figure of $2.2\ \mu$m for maximum force development.The normal ventricle appears to operate at an end-diastolic sarcomere length of 2.0 to $2.1\ \mu$m, but the experimental production of filling pressures above 12 to 15 mmHg in the left ventricle, or 7 to 8 mmHg in the right ventricle, leads to a sarcomere length of $2.2\ \mu$m, and the force developed begins to fall with excessive stretch (Sonnenblick et al, 1967). However, the sarcomeres are not as stretched as might be expected in the chronically dilated heart as the fibres slide over one another (Linzbach, 1960). Direct measurements of myocardial specimens from patients with dilated left ventricles showed average sarcomere lengths from 1.9 to $2.3\ \mu$m, and there was no relation between sarcomere length and ventricular filling pressure or volume. In chronic heart disease ventricular dilatation is always associated with hypertrophy, and the consequent increase in thickness of the ventricular wall will also tend to reduce the effect of dilatation on the individual sarcomeres. On the basis of this evidence it seems unlikely that sufficient stretching of the sarcomeres occurs for a descending limb of the response curve to be responsible for the reduced ventricular performance in heart failure.

In the intact heart atrial contraction plays an important part in the regulation of ventricular function. Atrial systole produces an increase in ventricular end-diastolic pressure and volume at the critical time in the cardiac cycle to lead to a greater ventricular response by the Frank–Starling mechanism. As the atria are influenced by both sympathetic and vagal tone, changes in atrial contraction under autonomic control can produce major alterations in ventricular response. The effect of atrial systole is well seen when there are variations in the timing of atrial and ventricular contraction, as in complete heart block. If a diseased ventricle requires a considerable elevation of end-diastolic pressure for satisfactory performance, an increase in the force of atrial systole produces the required effect without a serious rise in mean atrial pressure or the consequent effects of venous congestion. However, the great increases in atrial systolic pressure seen in severe ventricular hypertrophy are largely due to the increased stiffness of the ventricular wall and are mainly needed to maintain a normal end-diastolic tension in the individual muscle fibres rather than to augment the ventricular response through the Frank–Starling mechanism.

The atria have other important functions, including acting as a reservoir for the rapid filling phase of the ventricles during diastole (Grant, Bunnell and Greene, 1964). During ventricular systole atrial relaxation assists the flow of blood from the venous systems, and the systolic pulsatile nature of venous blood flow helps to refill the atria. The left atrium forms, with the pulmonary veins, a closed compartment in which changes in volume and pressure are related by the physical properties of the atrial wall. A steep rise in pressure occurs as the volume increases. There are great variations in left atrial properties in disease states which have a considerable effect on the interpretation of left atrial pressure records (Hamer, Roy and Dow, 1959). The right atrium on the other hand is effectively open to the systemic venous system which fills progressively as the pressure rises, and large volume changes are accommodated more easily than in the left atrium. Atrial contraction plays an important, but probably not an essential, part in atrioventricular valve closure. In atrial fibrillation effective atrial contraction is lost, and tricuspid valve incompetence frequently follows, but the mitral valve is less easily made regurgitant. The loss of atrial systole in atrial fibrillation has a profound effect on ventricular function as the end-diastolic pressure cannot be maintained without a considerable increase in mean atrial pressure.

Force–Velocity Relationships

While the Frank–Starling mechanism controls the overall performance of cardiac muscle as a function of its length, the measured variables of mechanical performance at any given length are a function of the load. In isolated skeletal and cardiac muscle this dependence can be defined in prolonged steady state ('tetanic') contractions by the relationship between velocity of shortening and force (load) (Fig. 11.6). Much work has been done to define this force–velocity relation during simple twitch contractions in isolated papillary muscles. Most of the results so derived are inaccurate because of the interaction of one or other complicating factor (Noble, 1973). However, it is possible to show that in such contractions the inverse force–velocity relation is present. It is also possible to predict with considerable confidence that valid measurement of the force–velocity relation in patients is not possible.

In recent years such attempts have been mainly based on equations for deriving the force–velocity curve from left ventricular pressure records alone. These have now been shown to be erroneous (van den Bos et al, 1973). The crux of the problem is to calculate from measurable variables such as ventricular dimensions (radiographic, ultrasonic), left ventricular pressure and instantaneous left ventricular outflow velocity, the velocity of shortening and force acting on a representative part of the ventricular wall. This was realised initially by Fry, Griggs and Greenfield (1964) whose early attempt is probably still the most reasonable.

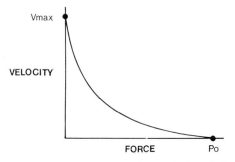

Figure 11.6 Diagrammatic representation of the force/velocity relationship in a muscle. An inverse relation between the force and the velocity of contraction produces a hyperbolic curve. Maximum force (P_0) is obtained when there is no movement and velocity is zero. Maximum velocity (V_{max}) is reached in the absence of load when force is zero. These ideal measurements are useful indices of the behaviour of a muscle, but can only be obtained from extrapolation of data obtained for other points on the curve

Simple geometrical principles, regarding the ventricle as a spherical chamber, can be used to estimate ventricular wall force if the pressure and volume are known (Burton, 1957). The relation between the force per unit circumference (f) in the wall of a sphere and the internal pressure (P) is given by the law of Laplace as $f = \frac{1}{2}Pr$, where r is the radius of the sphere. From this relation, an increase in ventricular volume that doubles the radius must be accompanied by a similar increase in force to maintain the ventricular pressure. The total wall force (F) is the product of this force (f) and ventricular circumference ($2\pi r$) ($F = 2\pi r \times \frac{1}{2}Pr = \pi Pr^2$), and as circumference also doubles with the radius the total wall force increases four-fold as the radius is doubled (Fig. 11.7). This analysis is clearly an over-simplification as it takes no account of the complex shape of the ventricle or of variations in the thickness of the ventricular wall. The left ventricle is approximately ellipsoidal in shape (Arvidsson, 1961), and becomes more spherical during systole (Hawthorne, 1961), but as areas of greater curvature are compensated by regions of lesser curvature the spherical approximation does not produce a large error (Gorlin et al, 1964). Another similar approach is to consider the force (F) tending to pull the part of the ventricle illustrated in Figure 11.7 away from the upper part (not illustrated). This can be shown to be equal to the pressure in the ventricle (P) times the cross-sectional area of the cavity, (A) = πr^2, giving the same result, $F = \pi r^2 P$, as the previous calculation. Hefner et al (1962) sampled this force using a force gauge and showed that this relationship held true experimentally.

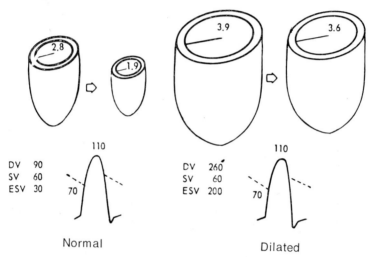

Figure 11.7   The effect of dilatation on ventricular wall force (from Gorlin, 1962). The end-diastolic and end-systolic situation is shown for a normal and a dilated ventricle assuming identical ventricular pressures and stroke volumes. The mean wall force in systole is $2\frac{1}{2}$ times greater in the dilated ventricle. Although the radius must shorten by 0.9 cm in the normal ventricle, the stroke volume is maintained by only 0.3 cm shortening after dilatation. DV = diastolic volume; SV = stroke volume; ESV = end-systolic volume. Volumes in ml, radii in cm, pressures in mmHg

When the wall force so derived is plotted against time during contraction, one finds that it attains a peak in early systole and then declines. It will be apparent from inspection of Figure 11.2 that when the force on the muscle changes, the length of the series elastic element (SE) also changes as it is stretched and relaxed, and that therefore the changes in length of the muscle do not reflect active contraction only. Thus it is not possible to measure a meaningful velocity of shortening in an intact heart with the possible exception of: (1) making the measurement at peak wall force when the SE has just reached maximum length and is just about to start shortening; and (2) making corrections for SE length changes. The second approach has been adopted on a large scale, even though it involves making arbitrary assumptions about the physical properties of the SE in patients. When it is also understood that contractile activity (the entire force–velocity relationship) waxes and wanes with time during contraction, the extreme difficulty of the problem becomes apparent.

Myocardial Contractility

It will be apparent from the previous two sections that the mechanical performance of myocardium is (1) a function of length and (2) at a given length can be determined by the force–velocity relation. If for a given length the isometric force or the force–velocity relation changes, this indicates a fundamental change in the contractile properties—a change in 'myocardial contractility'. The three variables describing a state of contractility can be plotted on three-dimensional diagrams (Fry, 1962), leading to the concept of a force–velocity–length plane describing contractility. Unfortunately, contractility waxes and wanes with time so that in order to describe a cardiac contraction in these terms it is necessary to conceive of a three-dimensional force–velocity–length plane which moves up and down with time during the beat! This complexity demands much of the practical cardiologist and makes it difficult to come to terms with the concept.

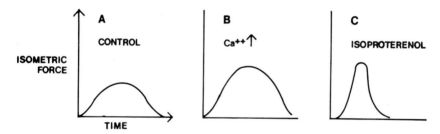

Figure 11.8 *A* Isometric force during contraction of a papillary muscle. *B* Effect of increasing calcium ion concentration. *C* Effect of adding isoproterenol.

If depolarisation of heart muscle is not followed by any mechanical response, the muscle can be said to have no contractility. If a mechanical response is obtained, contractility is present. When contractility is present the mechanical response increases with increase in muscle fibre length. This is the length–tension relationship, i.e. the Frank–Starling mechanism, Starling's law of the heart (see above; Ciba Symposium, 1974). Such changes in mechanical response are not considered to be changes in contractility. A change in mechanical response at a constant muscle length represents a change in contractility.

The measurement of contractility can be considered to be unambiguous only when it is carried out in isolated strips of cardiac muscle contracting isometrically (i.e. no shortening allowed). In this case a change in isometric force development at the same initial muscle length denotes a change in contractility (Fig. 11.8A, B). However, ambiguity can still arise when there is a change in time course of contractions. Figure 11.8B shows a clear-cut increase in contractility with an increase in isometric force and no change in time course, but in Figure 11.8C there has been an increase in peak force with a marked shortening in the contraction period. When measurement is attempted in any system more complex than this, ambiguities increase. When the muscle is allowed to shorten all variables are a function of the load, e.g. velocity of shortening (see above). For this reason many cardiologists have focused on the isovolumic contraction period. A variable such as the maximum rate of rise of left ventricular pressure ($LVdP/dt_{max}$) has been found to reflect changes in contractility provided all measurements are made at the same heart size. In comparison, other indices derived from the isovolumic contraction period ($dP/dt/P$, 'V_{max}', etc.), have severe disadvantages (van den Bos et al, 1973).

In view of the difficulties in measuring force–velocity curves (see above), other ways of defining mechanical performance as a function of load are gaining popularity. A relationship such as that in Figure 11.5A is easier to use in practice than that in Figure 11.5B because of the shape of the latter. What are the most appropriate and useful variables to plot in Figure 11.5A? The answer which appears to be emerging from recent work (Ciba Symposium, 1974) is the mean left ventricular pressure on the y-axis against the mean ventricular outflow on the x-axis. This conforms to standard engineering methods for defining the performance of a pump. The intercept of this line on the y-axis is called the 'hydromotive pressure' and the slope of the line the 'source resistance' (Elzinga and Westerhof, 1973). If one thinks of the heart as analogous to an electrical generator supply current ($\equiv$ flow) to an external circuit ($\equiv$ systemic arterial system), the hydromotive pressure is equivalent to the electromotive force (voltage) of the generator (Ciba Symposium, 1974). In terms of muscle mechanics, the hydromotive pressure is the average active state; the source 'resistance' is less easy to equate but it seems possible that its value depends partly on series elastic properties, but that it has dimensions of resistance because of the presence of the mitral and aortic valves.

The practical usefulness of this approach will depend on how linear this relationship turns out to be. Early results are promising (Ciba Symposium, 1974). A consistently linear relationship allows easy extrapolation to zero flow to obtain the hydromotive pressure which describes the mean level of mechanical activity of the heart. This variable is increased by an increase in initial fibre length (heart size) and by an increase of contractility (e.g. by infusing catecholamine). In order to obtain sufficient data to construct the line and extrapolate, it is necessary to measure mean left ventricular pressure and outflow over a range of different left ventricular pressures. Clearly there are a number of practical difficulties in achieving this; the problem of control of initial muscle length remains.

The desire to avoid control of initial (end-diastolic) muscle length has led a number of investigators to look at variables of mechanical performance to see whether any show independence of end-diastolic dimensions. This empirical approach led to the introduction of maximum acceleration of blood from the left ventricle as such an index (Noble, Trenchard and Guz, 1966a). Comparison of a number of such indices shows that none of them is insensitive to changes in heart size and load (aortic pressure) under all circumstances (van den Bos et al, 1973; Parmley et al, 1973; Patterson, Kent and Peirce, 1972), although LV dP/dt_{max} (see above) and maximum acceleration may reasonably be used in certain circumstances.

There has been considerable effort in recent years to assess myocardial contractility in patients. These efforts have been largely frustrated by theoretical objections (Noble, 1972a) coupled with the fact that many of the patients

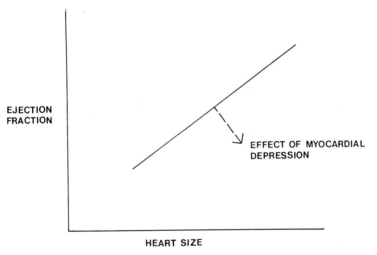

Figure 11.9 Relationship between ejection fraction and heart size. Arrow indicates that myocardial depression usually produces a fall of ejection fraction and cardiac dilatation

of interest have regional disease affecting different parts of the ventricle to different degrees. However, if one admits that one is not measuring 'contractility' as strictly defined by the physiologist one can still assess the effectiveness of cardiac contraction in a general sense, and make reasonable deductions. If, for instance, one chooses a variable which is certainly not an index of contractility but is a function of heart size, namely ejection fraction (stroke volume/ end-diastolic volume) (Fig. 11.9) one can show that the reduction in this variable in disease or with myocardial depression or regional ischaemia is accompanied by ventricular dilatation. Since the effect of increasing ventricular size per se is to increase ejection fraction, the decrease in ejection fraction in the first case reflects worsening of myocardial contraction in an unambiguous manner. In comparison, 'indices of contractility' are relatively insensitive (Kreulen et al, 1975).

Similar reasoning applies to other indices of ejection such as maximum acceleration and peak velocity of left ventricular outflow (Bennett et al, 1974) which are now being introduced into cardiac catheterisation procedures to give continuous assessment not requiring the contrast medium injection needed for ejection fraction. The introduction of non-invasive cardiac imaging with ultrasound brings forward the exciting prospect of obtaining similar information without catheterisation. Unfortunately, the use of a single beam is too liable to error and complex and expensive equipment (Bom et al, 1971) is required at present to make valid measurements.

Dependence of Contraction on Frequency of Stimulation (Heart Rate)

Changes in contractility associated with alterations in both force and velocity of contraction are found after sudden changes in heart rate (Bowditch, 1871). This was referred to by Sarnoff and colleagues (1960) as one aspect of 'homeometric autoregulation'. The original description of the Bowditch effect showed a force 'staircase' but studies on isolated cardiac muscle including human (Sonnenblick, Morrow and Williams, 1966) show that the entire force–velocity curve is affected. Animal work suggests that the net effect is small over the physiological range (Furnival, Linden and Snow, 1970; Noble et al, 1969b).

Koch-Weser and Blinks (1963) showed that the response was complex, with three components. Two of these are seen during a sudden increase in heart rate in an intact animal (Noble et al, 1969b). There is an immediate fall of contractility (the negative effect of Koch-Weser and Blinks, 1963) followed by a slower exponential increase in contractility (the positive effect of Koch-Weser and Blinks (1963), the true Bowditch effect). These effects persist after total denervations of the heart (Noble et al, 1972). Recent work by Edman and Johannsson (1976) in isolated rabbit cardiac muscle has provided an elegant explanation for these effects. The strength of a contraction depends upon the amount of calcium ion available for immediate release during depolarisation. This can be located in a releasable store (probably the lateral cisternae of the sarcoplasmic reticulum, situated near the ends of the myosin filaments (Legato and Langer, 1969). Relaxation is achieved by uptake of calcium ion by a separate 'compartment' (probably the sarcoplasmic reticulum). Time is required for the calcium so taken up to be transferred to the releasable store. At a given time after contraction the amount in the releasable store reaches a maximum. In rabbit myocardium this time is 0.8 s. If the next contraction occurs before this time, the contraction is weaker and becomes progressively less forceful when the interval is made shorter. Once a new, faster frequency of contraction has been established, the total time per minute during which the cell membrane is depolarised is greater, i.e. there is a greater total time per minute during which the calcium inward current (accompanying the plateaux of the action potentials) is flowing (Reuter, 1974). Consequently the amount of intracellular calcium builds up, including the amount in the releasable store on which strength of contraction depends. An increase in intracellular calcium ion concentration compatible with such a mechanism has been detected by radio-active tracer techniques (Langer, 1968). The dependence of such releasable calcium ion on the duration of depolarisation is supported by the effect of postectopic potentiation and paired pulse stimulation which doubles the duration of depolarisation per beat and greatly strengthens the mechanical response (Hoffman, Bindler and Suckling, 1956; Cranefield, 1965).

Interrelationship of Contractility and Intracellular Calcium Ion

The hypothesis presented by Edman and Johannsson (1976) to explain the frequency effect (above) is in tune with current ideas concerning the central role of calcium ion in excitation–contraction coupling and control of

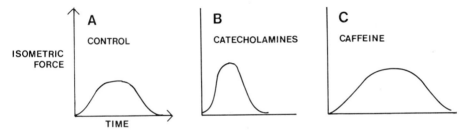

Figure 11.10 *A* Isometric force during contraction of a papillary muscle. *B* A typical effect of catecholamine. *C* Effect sometimes obtained with caffeine

contractility (Tanz, Kavaler and Roberts, 1967; Wood, Hepner and Weidmann, 1969; Trautwein, 1973). The concept of separate 'uptake' and 'release' compartments also fits with the effects of catecholamines and caffeine on cardiac contraction (Fig. 11.10). One would expect that the time course of the contraction/relaxation cycle would depend upon the relative timings and rates of activity of the two compartments. In particular, acceleration of the activity of the uptake compartment will cause earlier and more rapid relaxation with overall shortening of the contraction (Fig. 11.10B). This is precisely what happens with catecholamine and (since noradrenaline is the neuro-transmitter) with sympathetic stimulation, calcium ion uptake by sarcoplasmic reticulum is accelerated by catecholamines (Shinebourne et al, 1969).

Conversely, a reduction in the ability of the uptake compartment to sequester Ca^{2+} leads to the opposite effects, namely later and slower relaxation with overall lengthening of contraction (Fig. 11.10C). This is the effect of caffeine (Blinks et al, 1972). Caffeine impairs sequestration of Ca^{2+} by sarcoplasmic reticulum (Weber and Herz, 1968; Fuchs, 1969). By using this effect it has been possible to release more Ca^{2+} by applying further stimuli before relaxation is complete and to fuse contractions into a tetanic contracture (Henderson et al, 1971; Forman, Ford and Sonnenblick, 1972).

Load-dependent Changes in Contractility

Increases in contractility were found after sudden increases in aortic pressure by Anrep (1912). This was the other aspect of Sarnoff's 'homeometric autoregulation'. It has not been possible to demonstrate this effect in isolated strips of heart muscle, suggesting that this is not a direct intrinsic effect of increased load on muscle. Some evidence (Monroe et al, 1972; Ciba Symposium, 1974) suggests that subendocardial ischaemia (see below) may be involved. This would fit with the lack of an Anrep effect in intact dogs with denervated hearts. However, such a mechanism does not explain why the effect can be observed in the right ventricle.

It has been clearly shown in papillary muscles (Parmley, Brutsaert and Sonnenblick, 1969; Jewell and Rovell, 1973) that a decrease in load increases

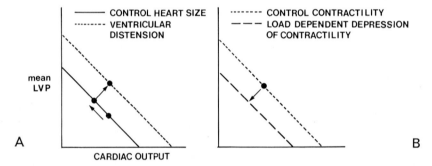

Figure 11.11 Effect of raising aortic pressure described in terms of relationship between mean left ventricular pressure and cardiac output. Cardiac output falls by moving along the control curve to the left (*A*). Cardiac dilatation then causes a shift of the line to the right due to the Frank–Starling mechanism. A shift backwards to the left may occur due to the effect of Parmley et al, and due to the baroreflex (*B*)

contractility while an increase in load decreases contractility. This effect is opposite in sign to the Anrep effect and appears to be a direct intrinsic effect of change in load on muscle. An increase in load is associated with a decrease in the duration of the action potential (Kaufman et al, 1971) from which one would expect a decrease in the amount of Ca^{2+} carried with the cell (decreased duration of calcium current inflow). This may be the reason why contractility subsequently declines.

This effect also appears to be present in the intact dog with denervated heart. The effect of raising aortic pressure (e.g. by aortic occlusion) in an intact animal is not only related to such a mechanism. The output declines (along the source resistance line) but since inflow transiently continues at the same level there is an increase in ventricular end-diastolic dimensions and pressure. This results in an increased forcefulness of contraction according to the Frank–Starling mechanism. (Fig. 11.11A). At the same time contractility declines according to the effect of Parmley et al (1969) (Fig. 11.11B). When the heart is innervated there is a further decline of output due to baroreflex bradycardia. Even if heart rate is held constant by pacing there is parasympathetic stimulation of ventricular muscle which has a slight negative inotropic effect. The net effect of all these influences is not easy to sort out. However, it does appear that diseased hearts show a net response which is negative with respect to normal hearts. This is a useful observation for clinical assessment since it is quite feasible to measure the effect of an acute hypertensive stress on some index of contraction, e.g. LV dP/dt_{max}; such a stress can be obtained by asking the patient to perform isometric handgrip contractions (Krayenbuehl, 1974).

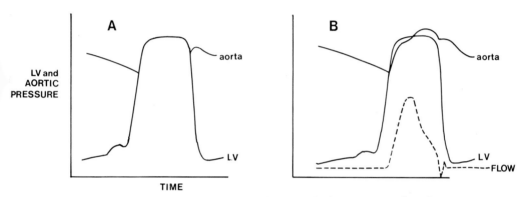

Figure 11.12   A Wiggers' textbook diagram of left ventricular pressure and aortic pressure. *B* Relationship demonstrated by modern manometry. The instantaneous aortic outflow is also shown

THE INTEGRATION OF CARDIAC PERFORMANCE

The Cardiac Cycle

Since the time of Wiggers (1928), textbooks have depicted the cardiac cycle according to his idea of the pressure changes in left atrium, ventricle and aorta. Figure 11.12A shows left ventricular and aortic pressure as equal during ejection. Spencer and Greiss (1962) measured the pressure difference from left ventricle to aorta during systole and found it to be positive in early ejection and negative in the second two-thirds of systole. The presence of a negative pressure difference was denied by Driscol and Eckstein (1965). Noble (1968) investigated this problem using the new high-fidelity micromanometers; these can now be used inside heart chambers directly without the use of fluid-filled catheter–manometer systems (which are liable to waveform distortion). The results (Fig. 11.12B) confirmed that aortic pressure was higher than left ventricular pressure in late systole. The ability with modern flowmeters to measure left ventricular outflow simultaneously adds another basic dimension to the cardiac cycle diagram (Fig. 11.12B) and shows that the reversed pressure gradient in late systole is related to deceleration. Such a relationship would be expected from modern concepts of pulsatile haemodynamics (McDonald, 1974).

Relationship of Cardiac Output to Contractile State

One extraordinary fact that has never been adequately explained is that when the contractility of a normal heart is increased, the stroke volume (at constant heart rate), remains constant (Noble et al, 1966b, 1972; Braunwald, 1971). By contrast, stroke volume and cardiac output are markedly affected by changes in end-diastolic volume (Frank–Starling mechanism) which may in turn be controlled to a certain extent by the peripheral circulation in which blood may pool or be shunted centrally according to the tone of peripheral capacitance vessels. In addition stroke volume and cardiac output are markedly affected by the load imposed by systemic arterial impedance (Fig. 11.5A). This again places control of cardiac output with the peripheral circulation. This contrasts markedly with the situation in disease where cardiac output is depressed due to weak contraction of the muscle. Under these circumstances stroke volume and cardiac output are increased (back toward normal) by a positive inotropic intervention (e.g. digitalis).

Relationship of Myocardial Oxygen Consumption to Mechanical Aspects of Contraction

The major determinant of oxygen consumption in an isolated strip of heart muscle is the force developed (McDonald, 1966) (Fig. 11.13C). As oxygen consumption increases with the force opposing shortening, shortening decreases and external work rises to a maximum and then falls. Thus the most economical way for the heart to contract in terms of energy requirements is to eject a maximum amount of blood against a very low aortic pressure. A more efficient contraction in terms of work occurs against a moderate load where work is at a maximum (Fig. 11.13B). This is where the normal heart appears to operate (Wilcken et al, 1964). However, the force which determines oxygen consumption is the force in the wall of the ventricle. This depends not only on pressure but ventricular size (see above and Fig. 11.7). Thus in the dilated diseased heart, the wall force (and therefore oxygen demand) is higher than would be the case for a normal heart at the same pressure. This is why the volume of the ventricle must be taken into consideration in the estimation of the energy used by the myocardium in disease states associated with ventricular dilatation or a reduction in stroke output (Hamer, 1973). It is also a limitation to use of the tension–time index for estimating myocardial oxygen demand (Sarnoff et al, 1958).

Vigorous contractions produced by sympathetic stimulation have been found to produce a greater myocardial oxygen consumption than expected on the basis of force measurements (Britman and Levine, 1964). If one increases the contractility of myocardium so that the force–velocity curve is shifted upwards, it follows that more energy is required to generate a higher velocity of contraction at the same level of force (Sonnenblick, 1965). This increased oxygen demand consequent upon the administration of positive inotropic agents (digoxin, catecholamines) is a disadvantage when impaired oxygen supply is present (see below).

Relationship of Myocardial Ischaemia to the Balance of Oxygen Supply and Demand

The reduction/oxidation (redox) state of myocardial metabolism at a given site in the myocardium depends on the amount coming in (supply) and the amount being consumed (demand). Either a reduction in supply or an increase in demand results in a shift in the direction of ischaemia. In coronary artery disease the supply is limited by the obstructions to blood flow. Any of the

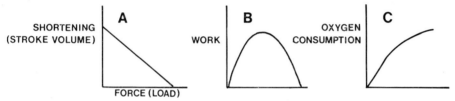

Figure 11.13 Relationship of contractile performance and oxygen consumption to load as demonstrated by isolated papillary muscle experiment. *A* Shortening (equivalent to stroke volume in the intact heart). *B* Work. *C* Oxygen consumption

factors mentioned in the previous section which increase demand; a rise of the aortic pressure, increase in heart size, positive inotropic effects such as sympathetic activation or an increase in the 'number of demands', i.e. in heart rate, therefore causes a shift in the direction of ischaemia.

The same principles may be applied to different sites across the wall of the left ventricle. In this case the demand is probably the same in the subendo-cardium and subepicardium. However, supply is much more precarious in the subendocardium because contraction results in much greater systolic compression forces on subendocardial blood vessels (van der Meer et al, 1970; Kirk and Honig, 1964; Brandi and McGregor, 1969). This effect stops subendo-cardial flow during systole so that perfusion of this region depends on the difference between coronary perfusion pressure and left ventricular pressure in diastole. This explains the greater susceptibility of the subendocardium to ischaemia (Noble, 1972b). In the absence of coronary arteries, this increased susceptibility can be predicted from the ratio of an index of diastolic perfusion to an index of myocardial oxygen consumption, e.g. diastolic pressure time index/tension time index (Buckberg et al, 1972). An intriguing consequence of this interplay of factors is that whereas in most circumstances tachycardia increases the tendency to subendocardial ischaemia by reducing diastolic time relative to systolic time, tachycardia reduces the tendency to subendo-cardial ischaemia in the presence of severe aortic incompetence by cutting short long diastoles when late diastolic aortic (coronary perfusion) pressure is very low (Lewis et al, 1974; Hoffman et al, 1972).

Another useful way of estimating the adequacy of supply in relation to demand is to measure the reactive hyperaemia that follows coronary artery occlusion. Normally coronary blood flow increases so that the time integrated flow 'lost' during the period of occlusion is overpaid during the period of hyperaemia. This function is impaired when ischaemia lurks, e.g. when the blood flow in the subendocardium becomes less than that in the subepicar-dium (Buckberg et al, 1972). A practical example of the use of the reactive hyperaemic response was the study of Reneman and Spencer (1972) who measured it after coronary saphenous vein bypass surgery. A poor response indicated poor anastomosis, and further coronary stenosis peripheral to the site of bypass and the likelihood that the operation would be of no benefit to the patient.

Myocardial Hypertrophy

The need for an increase in the force of contraction in disease seems to act as a stimulus to myocardial hypertrophy. Grant, Green and Bunnell (1965) noted a constant relation between ventricular wall thickness and radius in patients with an increased stroke volume. The hypertrophy of the wall was sufficient to prevent any increase in the systolic force in the individual fibres. Similarly, in patients with hypertension or outflow obstruction the thickening of the wall allows a higher systolic pressure without increasing the load on each myofibril. However, the structural changes associated with hypertrophy seem eventually to produce a reduction in the performance of the ventricle, leading to cardiac failure. The increased stiffness of the hypertrophied ventricle requires an increased end-diastolic pressure for adequate filling, and disturb-ances of contractility reduce the stroke volume. The process is accompanied by an increase in ventricular volume which produces further deterioration in the effectiveness of contraction, and often increases the load on the ventricle by producing mitral or tricuspid incompetence.

The myocardial changes in hypertrophy and failure have been studied in experimental models in animals. Meerson and his colleagues (1968) describe three stages in the response to aortic obstruction. Activation of protein and nucleic acid synthesis in the first stage leads to a second stage of compensating hypertrophy, followed by a final stage in which the metabolic response is inadequate and progressive destructive changes in the myocardium lead to failure. A similar sequence of events is found in the natural inherited cardio-myopathy of the hamster (Bajusz, 1969), leading to changes in distensibility and contractility of the heart muscle (Brink and Lochner, 1969).

The ultrastructural changes associated with hypertrophy involve the sarco-lemma which becomes highly vesiculated, with many mitochondria and pinocytic vesicles, suggesting an increase in active transport mechanisms at the cell surface. The transverse tubules enlarge, and the longitudinal sarcoplasmic reticulum becomes dilated. The myofibrils increase in number, but the individual filaments are normal in form, and the hexagonal pattern in cross-section is not disturbed (Leyton and Sonnenblick, 1969). Focal widening of the Z-bands suggests that new contractile units arise at this site in the cell (Legato, 1970). Changes in the mitochondria and the nuclei are less extensive than might be expected and this disproportion has suggested that functional disturbances may appear. Only a small increase in the number of mitochon-dria occurs, and the cristae are widened and reduced in number, so energy supply for the greater number of myofibrils may be inadequate. The nuclei are a little larger and have more nucleoli, suggesting increased production of nucleotides leading to greater protein synthesis, but the apparent increase in nucleotide content may be due to reduplication of the chromosomes (poly-ploidy) and the functional effect is uncertain (Meessen, 1968). Failure of these processes to keep pace with the increase in cell size may eventually lead to the disturbance of contraction responsible for failure (Meerson et al, 1968). There is also an increase in connective tissue.

In primary myocardial disease there is greater structural disturbance at an early stage. Myocardial ischaemia produces serious disorganisation, with disruption of the sarcolemmal membrane, and of the transverse tubules and the longitudinal sarcoplasmic reticulum. Mitochondria become swollen and granular with shrinkage or disappearance of the cristae and disintegration of the mitochondrial membrane. These changes are related to serious disturb-ance of the mitochondrial enzyme systems. Zones of supercontracted and of relaxed sarcomeres are found, possibly secondary to disturbances of calcium transport. The filaments may be disarranged and ruptured in the Z-band region, or eventually lost. The nuclei degenerate and glycogen granules are reduced in number. Alcoholic cardiomyopathy, on the other hand, does not affect the transverse tubules or sarcoplasmic reticulum until a late stage. Many mitochondria become swollen and dense with deformed cristae, and eventu-ally degenerate; this is probably the primary change. The myofibrils are first affected in the region of the Z-line, but progressive deterioration finally leaves a finely granular mass. The nuclei are often degenerate and lipid globules appear (Leyton and Sonnenblick, 1969).

It has been suggested that local hypoxia is responsible for the impaired performance of the hypertrophied myocardium. However, the coronary blood flow is well adapted to the oxygen requirements of the tissue, and the cardiac venous oxygen saturation remains little changed by exercise or other stress in normal subjects. In most situations the increase in arterial pressure and the vasodilating effect of local hypoxia are sufficient to maintain the myocardial oxygen supply. The major coronary arteries are usually larger than normal in the hypertrophied heart (Harrison and Wood, 1949), and there is a compensatory increase in the capillary bed. The absence of angina in many patients with ventricular hypertrophy confirms that there is no general myocardial ischaemia, and the ST and T wave changes in the electrocardiogram are secondary to the alterations in the QRS complex, and must be regarded as part of the pattern of hypertrophy rather than as evidence of ischaemia. However, the enlargement of the sarcomeres in hypertrophy will tend to increase the diffusion distance for oxygen from the capillaries to the myofibrils, and may

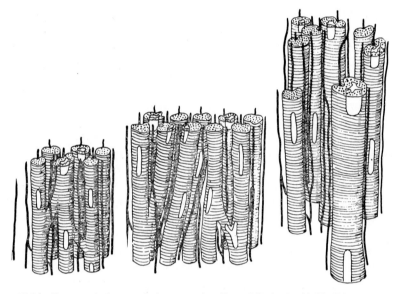

Figure 11.14 Structural changes in hypertrophy (from Linzbach, 1960). Diagram to show the disorganisation of the myocardial fibres in severe hypertrophy (right), compared to the simple increase in the size and number of the fibres in less severe hypertrophy (centre). Normal myocardium is shown on the left. Irregular hypertrophy and scattered loss of fibres in severe hypertrophy may disturb the relation between the contractile tissue and the capillary bed

lead to functional disturbances from relative ischaemia within the myocardial cells.

The impaired performance of the hypertrophied heart that leads to failure has been attributed to the structural disorganisation that eventually occurs. Local unevenness of blood supply may lead to loss of some cells and excessive hypertrophy of others (Linzbach, 1960) (Fig. 11.14). Structural disorganisation may reduce the effectiveness of contraction of the remaining adequately functioning sarcomeres as non-contracting areas must be tensed before effective systole can begin. Asynergic contraction in different parts of the ventricle may have a further deleterious effect, particularly in relation to atrioventricular valve closure (Harrison, 1965), and probably plays a major part in ischaemic heart disease. In coronary artery disease the effects of local ischaemia on myocardial performance are very striking.

During spontaneous angina the myocardial oxygen consumption is increased for a given amount of external work (Messer et al, 1963) and the rate of ejection from the left ventricle is decreased (Cohen et al, 1965). A transient rise in left ventricular end-diastolic pressure is usually found during angina, and Sharma and Taylor (1970) have suggested that an increase in myocardial oxygen consumption may accentuate the myocardial ischaemia. The transient increase in left ventricular stiffness that accompanies the ischaemia may be a more fundamental disturbance.

Impairment of myocardial performance in cardiac failure has been demonstrated in experimental animal models. Ross et al (1966) induced failure by barbiturates or β-sympathetic blockade in a dog left ventricular preparation. When end-diastolic pressure was held constant, failure reduced the extent of shortening of the circumference, and there was a fall in both maximal velocity (by 30 per cent) and maximal tension (by 23 per cent) in isometric contractions produced by sudden balloon occlusion of the aortic root. The duration of contraction was always increased, and peak velocity and peak tension delayed. A digitalis preparation tended to reverse these changes. When end-diastolic volume was allowed to increase at a constant stroke volume, circumferential shortening was reduced (by 47 per cent), and velocity was reduced at tensions comparable to control; maximal velocity was also reduced. Work expended on stretching the series elastic component was nearly doubled, so although external work diminished there was little change in total contractile element work. The extent of shortening was reduced in spite of the prolongation of contraction.

Study of cardiac muscle from animals with experimental hypertrophy induced by constriction of the pulmonary artery showed evidence of depressed contractility even when there was no evidence of failure (Spann et al, 1967). Active tension was reduced a little in the hypertrophied muscle, and very greatly reduced in the muscle from failing hearts. The rate of force development (peak dF/dt) was considerably reduced, but the time taken to reach peak force was normal. If the series elastic tissue is not abnormal in the failing heart (Parmley et al, 1968) these changes must indicate reduced contractility, and although the duration of the active state is unchanged the maximum force produced is much less than in normal muscle. The force–velocity curve is depressed, with a great reduction in the maximum velocity of shortening (V_{max}). The depressed contractility of the failing muscle was not fully restored by paired pacing, increased rate, or digitalis glycosides.

The findings with regard to contractility were confirmed in the intact ventricle by Spann and his colleagues (1967). The maximum velocity of shortening (V_{max}) was 40 per cent below normal in both hypertrophied and failing hearts. At normal end-diastolic volumes the active tension in the hypertrophied and failing hearts was reduced to half the normal value, but the spontaneous end-diastolic volume was increased with an end-diastolic tension twice the normal, allowing a normal peak force during isometric contraction through the Frank–Starling mechanism. The production of thyrotoxicosis in dogs increased contractility, and induced hypothyroidism has the reverse effect (Taylor, Covell and Ross, 1969). In contrast, animals put into apparent gross heart failure by the creation of a large arteriovenous anastomosis retained normal myocardial function (Taylor, Covell and Ross, 1968), showing that fluid retention may occur without myocardial disturbance.

The mechanism of the dilatation of the ventricle that frequently accompanies failure is obscure. As the layers of fibres in the ventricular wall slide over one another there is less stretching of the myofibril than might be expected and the extent of any beneficial effect from the Frank–Starling mechanism is difficult to assess. The increase in volume will require a greater total wall force to maintain the systolic pressure, and will consequently lead to an increase in myocardial oxygen consumption (Gorlin, 1962) (Fig. 11.7). However, dilatation does offer some mechanical advantages in that stroke volume can be maintained with very little shortening of the myofibrils, and consequently with relatively low velocities of contraction. Dilatation may be a compensatory response to an impaired velocity of contraction, allowing an effective stroke volume in spite of this disadvantage at the expense of a greater total wall force. If a reduced velocity of contraction uses less oxygen, the net effect on oxygen consumption may not be as serious as expected from the changes in the force of contraction. However, Levine and his colleagues (1963) found a disproportionate increase in myocardial oxygen consumption on effort in patients with left ventricular failure, suggesting that the increase in volume was in fact a disadvantage from this point of view.

REFERENCES

Anrep, G. von (1912) On the part played by the suprarenals in the normal vascular reactions of the body. *Journal of Physiology (London)*, **45**, 307.

Arvidsson, H. (1961) Angiocardiographic determination of left ventricular volume. *Acta radiologica (Stockholm)*, **56**, 321.

Bajusz, E. (1969) Hereditary cardiomyopathy: a new disease model. *American Heart Journal*, **77**, 686.

Bennett, E. D., Else, W., Miller, G. A. H., Sutton, G. C., Miller, H. C. & Noble, M. I. M. (1974) Maximum acceleration of blood from the left ventricle in patients with ischaemic heart disease. *Clinical Science and Molecular Medicine*, **46**, 49.

Blinks, J. R., Olsen, C. B., Jewell, B. R. & Braveny, P. (1972) Influence of caffeine and other methylxanthines on mechanical properties of isolated mammalian heart muscle: evidence for a dual mechanism of action. *Circulation Research*, **30**, 367.

Bom, M., Lancée, C. T., Honkoop, J. & Hugenholtz, P. G. (1971) Ultrasonic viewer for cross-sectional analyses of moving cardiac structures. *Bio-medical Engineering*, **6**, 500.

Bos, G. C. van den, Elzinga, G., Westerhof, N. & Noble, M. I. M. (1973) Problems in the use of indices of myocardial contractility. *Cardiovascular Research*, **7**, 834.

Bowditch, H. P. (1871) Uber die Eigenthümlichkeiten der Reizbarkeit, welche die Müskel-fasern des Herzens zeigen. *Arbeit Physiologie (Leipzit)*, **6**, 139.

Brandi, G. & McGregor, M. (1969) Intramural pressure in the left ventricle of the dog. *Cardiovascular Research*, **3**, 472.

Braunwald, E. (1965) The control of ventricular function in man. *British Heart Journal*, **27**, 1.

Braunwald, E. (1971) Editorial: On the difference between the heart's output and its contractile state. *Circulation*, **43**, 171.

Brink, A. J. & Lochner, A. (1969) Contractility and tension development of the myopathic hamster (BIO 14.6) heart. *Cardiovascular Research*, **3**, 453.

Britman, N. A. & Levine, H. J. (1964) Contractile element work: a major determinant of myocardial oxygen consumption. *Journal of Clinical Investigation*, **43**, 1397.

Buckberg, G. D., Fixler, D. E., Archie, J. P. & Hoffman, J. I. E. (1972) Experimental subendocardial ischaemia in dogs with normal coronary arteries. *Circulation Research*, **30**, 67.

Burton, A. C. (1957) Editorial: The importance of the shape and size of the heart. *American Heart Journal*, **54**, 801.

Case, R. B., Berglund, E. & Sarnoff, S. J. (1954) Ventricular function: II. Quantitative relationship between coronary flow and ventricular function with observations on unilateral failure. *Circulation Research*, **2**, 319.

Ciba Foundation Symposium 24 (new series) (1974) *The Physiological Basis of Starling's Law of the Heart*, ed. Porter R. & Fitzsimons, D. W. Amsterdam: Elsevier.

Cleworth, D. R. & Edman, K. A. P. (1972) Changes in sarcomere length during isometric tension development in frog skeletal muscle. *Journal of Physiology (London)*, **227**, 1.

Cohen, L. S., Elliott, W. C., Rolett, E. L. & Gorlin, R. (1965) Haemodynamic studies during angina pectoris. *Circulation*, **31**, 409.

Cranefield, P. F. (Conference chairman) (1965) Conference on paired pulse stimulation and post-extrasystolic potentiation in the heart. *Bulletin of the New York Academy of Medicine*, **41**, 417.

Driscol, T. E. & Eckstein, R. W. (1965) Systolic pressure gradients across the aortic valve and in the ascending aorta. *American Journal of Physiology*, **209**, 557.

Edman, K. A. P. & Johannson, M. (1976) The contractile state of rabbit papillary muscle in relation to stimulation frequency. *Journal of Physiology (London)*, **254**, 565.

Elzinga G. (1972) Crosstalk between right and left heart. Ph.D. thesis. Free University of Amsterdam.

Elzinga, G. & Westerhof, N. (1973) Pressure and flow generated by the left ventricle against different impedances. *Circulation Research*, **32**, 178.

Forman, R., Ford, L. E. & Sonnenblick, E. H. (1972) Effect of muscle length on the force–velocity relationship of tetanised cardiac muscle. *Circulation Research*, **31**, 195.

Frank, O. (1895) Zur Dynamik des Herzmuskels. *Zeitschrift fur Biologie*, **32**, 370.

Fry, D. L. (1962) Implications of muscle mechanics in the heart. *Federation Proceedings. Federation of American Societies for Experimental Biology*, **21**, 991.

Fry, D. L., Griggs, D. M., Jr & Greenfield, J. C., Jr (1964) Myocardial mechanics: tension–velocity–length relationships of heart muscle. *Circulation Research*, **14**, 73.

Fuchs, F. (1969) Inhibition of sarcotubular calcium transport by caffeine: species and temperature dependence. *Biochimica et biophysica acta*, **172**, 566.

Furnival, C. M., Linden, R. J. & Snow, H. M. (1970) Inotropic changes in the left ventricle: the effect of changes in heart rate, aortic pressure and end-diastolic pressure. *Journal of Physiology (London)*, **211**, 359.

Gordon, A. M., Huxley, A. F. & Julian, F. J. (1966) The variation in isometric tension with sarcomere length in vertebrate muscle fibres. *Journal of Physiology (London)*, **184**, 170.

Gorlin, R. (1962) Recent conceptual advances in congestive heart failure. *Journal of the American Medical Association*, **179**, 441.

Gorlin, R., Rolett, E. L., Yurchak, P. M. & Elliott, W. C. (1964) Left ventricular volume in man measured by thermodilution. *Journal of Clinical Investigation*, **43**, 1203.

Grant, C., Bunnell, I. L. & Greene, D. G. (1964) The reservoir function of the left atrium during ventricular systole: an angiocardiographic study of atrial stroke volume and work. *American Journal of Medicine*, **37**, 36.

Grant, C., Green, D. G. & Bunnell, I. L. (1965) Left ventricular enlargement and hypertrophy: a clinical and angiocardiographic study. *American Journal of Medicine*, **39**, 895.

Hamer, J. (1973) Fundamental aspects of myocardial performance. In *Recent Advances in Cardiology*, 6th edn, ed. Hamer, J., p. 156. Edinburgh & London: Churchill Livingstone.

Hamer, N. A. J., Roy, S. B. & Dow, J. W. (1959) Determinants of the left atrial pressure pulse in mitral valve disease. *Circulation*, **19**, 257.

Harrison, C. V. & Wood, P. (1949) Hypertensive and ischaemic heart disease: a comparative clinical and pathological study. *British Heart Journal*, **11**, 205.

Harrison, T. R. (1965) Some unanswered questions concerning enlargement and failure of the heart. *American Heart Journal*, **69**, 100.

Harwick, E. (1974) Wederzijdse beinvloeding can be beide hartshelften en veranderingen hiervan na de geboorts. Thesis, University Leiden.

Hawthorne, E. W. (1961) Instantaneous dimensional changes of the left ventricle in dogs. *Circulation Research*, **9**, 110.

Hefner, L. L., Sheffield, L. T., Cobbs, G. C. & Klip, W. (1962) Relation between mural force and pressure in the left ventricle of the dog. *Circulation Research*, **11**, 654.

Henderson, A. H., Forman, R., Brutsaert, D. L. & Sonnenblick, E. H. (1971) Tetanic contraction in mammalian cardiac muscle. *Cardiovascular Research*, **5** Suppl. 1, 96.

Hoffman, B. F., Bindler, E. & Suckling, E. E. (1956) Post-extrasystolic potentiation of contraction in cardiac muscle. *American Journal of Physiology*, **185**, 95.

Hoffman, J. I. E., Buckberg, G. D., Fixler, D. E. & Archie, J. P. (1972) In *Myocardial Blood Flow in Man: Methods and Significance in Coronary Disease*, proceedings of an international symposium held in Pisa, Italy, 10th–12th June, 1971, ed. Maseri, A. Minerva Medica.

Huxley, A. F. (1974) Review lecture: Muscular contraction. *Journal of Physiology (London)*, **243**, 1.

Huxley, A. F. & Simmons, R. M. (1971) Proposed mechanism of force generation in striated muscle. *Nature (London)*, **233**, 533.

Jewell, B. R. & Rovell, J. M. (1973) Influence of previous mechanical events on the contractility of isolated cat papillary muscle. *Journal of Physiology (London)*, **235**, 715.

Katz, A. M. (1965) Editorial: The descending limb of the Starling curve and the failing heart. *Circulation*, **32**, 871.

Kaufmann, R. L., Lab, M. J., Hennekes, R. & Krause, H. (1971) Feedback interaction of mechanical and electrical events in the isolated mammalian ventricular myocardium (cat papillary muscle). *Pflugers Archiv. fur die Gesante Physiologie des Menschen und der Tiere*, **324**, 100.

Kirk, E. S. & Honig, C. R. (1964) An experimental and theoretical analysis of myocardial tissue pressure. *American Journal of Physiology*, **207**, 361.

Koch-Weser, J. & Blinks, J. R. (1963) The influence of the interval between beats on myocardial contractility. *Pharmacological Review*, **15**, 601.

Krayenbuehl, H. P. (1974) Evluation of left ventricular function by handgrip. *European Journal of Cardiology*, **1**, 283.

Kreulen, T. H., Bove, A. A., McDonough, M. T., Sands, M. J. & Spann, J. F. (1975) The evaluation of left ventricular function in man: a comparison of methods. *Circulation*, **51**, 677.

Langer, G. A. (1968) Ion fluxes in cardiac excitation and contraction and their relation to myocardial contractility. *Physiological Reviews*, **48**, 708.

Legato, M. J. (1970) Sarcomerogenesis in human myocardium. *Journal of Molecular and Cellular Cardiology*, **1**, 425.

Legato, M. J. & Langer, G. A. (1969) The subcellular localisation of calcium ion in mammalian myocardium. *Journal of Cellular Biology*, **41**, 401.

Levine, H. J., Messer, J. V., Neill, W. A. & Gorlin, R. (1963) The effect of exercise on cardiac performance in human subjects with congestive heart failure. *American Heart Journal*, **66**, 731.

Lewis, A. B., Heymann, M. A., Stanger, P., Hoffman, J. I. E. & Rudolph, A. M. (1974) Evaluation of subendocardial ischaemia in valvar aortic stenosis in children. *Circulation*, **49**, 978.

Leyton, R. A. & Sonnenblick, E. H. (1969) The ultrastructure of the failing heart. *American Journal of Medical Science*, **258**, 304.

Linzbach, A. J. (1960) Heart failure from the point of view of quantitative anatomy. *American Journal of Cardiology*, **5**, 370.

McDonald, D. A. (1974) *Blood Flow in Arteries*, 2nd edn. London: Edward Arnold.

McDonald, R. H., Jr (1966) Developed tension: a major determinant of myocardial oxygen consumption. *American Journal of Physiology*, **210**, 351.

Meerson, F. Z., Alekhina, G. M., Akeksandrov, P. N. & Bazardjan, A. G. (1968) Dynamics of nucleic acid and protein synthesis of the myocardium in compensatory hyperfunction and hypertrophy of the heart. *American Journal of Cardiology*, **22**, 337.

Meer, J. J. van der, Reneman, R. S., Schneider, H. & Wiederdink, J. (1970) A technique for estimation of intramyocardial pressure in acute and chronic experiments. *Cardiovascular Research*, **4**, 132.

Meessen, H. (1968) Ultrastructure of the myocardium: its significance in myocardial disease. *American Journal of Cardiology*, **22**, 319.

Messer, J. V., Levine, H. J., Wagman, R. J. & Gorlin, R. (1963) Effect of exercise on cardiac performance in human subjects with coronary artery disease. *Circulation*, **28**, 404.

Monroe, R. G., Gamble, W. J., LaFarge, C. G., Kumar, A. E., Stark, J., Sanders, G. L., Phornphutkul, C. & Davis, M. (1972) The Anrep effect reconsidered. *Journal of Clinical Investigation*, **51**, 2573.

Noble, M. I. M. (1968) The contribution of blood momentum to left ventricular ejection in the dog. *Circulation Research*, **23**, 663.

Noble, M. I. M. (1972a) Problems concerning the application of concepts of muscle mechanics to the determination of the contractile state of the heart. *Circulation*, **45**, 252.

Noble, M. I. M. (1972b) Relationship of ischaemia to local myocardial oxygen requirements. In *Effect of Acute Ischaemia on Myocardial Function*, ed. Oliver M. F., Julian, D. G. & Donald, K. W., p. 277. Edinburgh: Churchill Livingstone.

Noble, M. I. M. (1973) Problems in the definition of contractility in terms of myocardial mechanics. *European Journal of Cardiology*, **1**, 209.

Noble, M. I. M. & Else, W. (1972) Re-examination of the applicability of the Hill model of muscle to cat myocardium. *Circulation Research*, **31**, 580.

Noble, M. I. M., Milne, E. N. C., Goerke, R. J., Carlsson, E., Domench, R. J., Saunders, K. B. & Hoffman, J. I. E. (1969a) Left ventricular filling and diastolic pressure–volume relations in the conscious dog. *Circulation Research*, **24**, 269.

Noble, M. I. M., Wyler, J., Milne, E. N. C., Trenchard, D. & Guz, A. (1969b) Effect of changes in heart rate on left ventricular performance in conscious dogs. *Circulation Research*, **24**, 285.

Noble, M. I. M., Stubbs, J., Trenchard, D., Else, W., Eisele, J. H. & Guz, A. (1972) Left ventricular performance in the conscious dog with chronically denervated heart. *Cardiovascular Research*, **6**, 457.

Noble, M. I. M., Trenchard, D. & Guz, A. (1966a) Left ventricular ejection in conscious dogs. I. Measurement and significance of the maximum acceleration of blood from the left ventricle. *Circulation Research*, **19**, 139.

Noble, M. I. M., Trenchard, D. & Guz, A. (1966b) Left ventricular ejection in conscious dogs. II. Determinants of stroke volume. *Circulation Research*, **19**, 148.

Oliver, M. F., Julian, D. G. & Donald, K. W. (ed.) (1972) *Effect of Acute Ischaemia on Myocardial Function*. Edinburgh: Churchill Livingstone.

Parmley, W. W., Brutsaert, D. L. & Sonnenblick, E. H. (1969) Effects of altered loading on contractile events in isolated cat papillary muscle. *Circulation Research*, **24**, 521.

Parmley, W., Chuck, L., Yeatman, L. & Sonnenblick, E. H. (1973) Comparative evaluation of the specificity and sensitivity of isometric indices of contractility. *American Journal of Cardiology*, **31**, 151.

Parmley, W. W., Spann, J. F., Taylor, R. R. & Sonnenblick, E. H. (1968) The series elasticity of cardiac muscle in hyperthyroidism, ventricular hypertrophy and heart failure. *Proceedings of the Society for Experimental Biology and Medicine*, **127**, 606.

Patterson, R. E., Kent, B. B. & Pierce, E. C. (1972) A comparison of empiric contractile indices in intact dogs. *Cardiology*, **57**, 277.

Patterson, S. W., Piper, H. & Starling, E. H. (1914) The regulation of the heart beat. *Journal of Physiology* (*London*), **48**, 465.

Pollack, G. H., Huntsman, L. L. & Verdugo, P. (1972) Cardiac muscle models: an over-extension of series elasticity? *Circulation Research*, **31**, 569.

Pollack, G. H. & Krueger, J. W. (1975) Effect of controlled changes of muscle length on sarcomere dynamics in mammalian heart muscle. *Federation Proceedings. Federation of American Socieites for Experimental Biology*, **34**, 412.

Reneman, R. S. & Spencer, M. P. (1972) The use of diastolic reactive hyperemia to evaluate the coronary vascular system. *Annals of Thoracic Surgery*, **13**, 477.

Reuter, H. (1974) Exchange of calcium ions in the mammalian myocardium: mechanisms and physiological significance. *Circulation Research*, **34**, 599.

Ross, J., Covell, J. W., Sonnenblick, E. H. & Braunwald, E. (1966) Contractile state of the heart characterised by force–velocity relations in variably afterloaded and isovolumic beats. *Circulation Research*, **18**, 149.

Sarnoff, S. J. & Berglund, E. (1954) Ventricular function. I. Starling's law of the heart studied by means of simultaneous right and left ventricular function curves in the dog. *Circulation*, **9**, 706.

Sarnoff, S. J., Mitchell, J. H., Gilmore, J. P. & Remensnyde, J. P. (1960) Homeometric autoregulation of the heart. *Circulation Research*, **8**, 1077.

Sarnoff, S. J., Braunwald, E., Welch, G. H., Case, R. B., Stainsby, W. N. & Macruz, R. (1958) Haemodynamic determinants of oxygen consumption of the heart with special reference to the tension–time index. *American Journal of Physiology*, **192**, 148.

Sharma, B. & Taylor, S. H. (1970) Reversible left-ventricular failure in angina pectoris. *Lancet*, **2**, 902.

Shinebourne, E. A., Hess, M. L., White, R. J. & Hamer, J. (1969) The effect of noradrenaline on the calcium uptake of the sarcoplasmic reticulum. *Cardiovascular Research*, **3**, 113.

Sonnenblick, E. H. (1965) Instantaneous force–velocity–length determinants in the contraction of heart muscle. *Circulation Research*, **16**, 441.

Sonnenblick, E. H., Morrow, A. G. & Williams, J. F. (1966) Effects of heart rate on the dynamics of force development in the intact human ventricle. *Circulation*, **33**, 945.

Sonnenblick, E. H., Ross, J., Jr, Covell, J. W., Spotnitz, H. M. & Spiro, D. (1967) The ultrastructure of the heart in systole and diastole. *Circulation Research*, **21**, 423.

Spann, J. F., Covell, J. W., Eckberg, D. L., Sonnenblick, E. H., Ross, J. & Braunwald, E. (1967) Myocardial contractile state in hypertrophy and congestive failure: studies in the intact heart and the isolated muscle. *Circulation*, **36**, Suppl. 2, 241.

Spencer, M. P. & Greiss, F. C. (1962) Dynamics of ventricular ejection. *Circulation Research*, **10**, 274.

Spiro, D. & Sonnenblick, E. H. (1964) Comparison of the ultrastructural basis of the contractile process in heart and skeletal muscle. *Circulation Research*, **15**, Suppl. 2, 14.

Tanz, R. D., Kavaler, F. & Roberts, J. (eds) (1967) *Factors Influencing Myocardial Contractility*. New York: Academic Press.

Taylor, R. R., Covell, J. W. & Ross, J. (1968) Left ventricular function in experimental aorto-caval fistulae with circulatory congestion and fluid retention. *Journal of Clinical Investigation*, **47**, 1333.

Taylor, R. R., Covell, J. W. & Ross, J. (1969) Influence of the thyroid state on left ventricular tension–velocity relations in the intact sedated dog. *Journal of Clinical Investigation*, **65**, 775.

Trautwein, W. (1973) Membrane currents in cardiac muscle fibres. *Physiological Reviews*, **53**, 793.

Weber, A. & Herz, R. (1968) The relationship between caffeine contracture of intact muscle and the effect of caffeine on reticulum. *Journal of General Physiology*, **52**, 750.

Wiggers, C. J. (1928) *The Pressure Pulses in the Cardiovascular System*. New York: Longmans.

Wilcken, D. E. L., Charlier, A. A., Hoffman, J. I. E. & Guz, A. (1964) Effects of alterations in aortic impedance on the performance of the ventricles. *Circulation Research*, **14**, 283.

Wood, E. H., Heppner, R. L. & Weidmann, S. (1969) Inotropic effects of electric currents. I. Positive and negative effects of constant electric currents or current pulses applied during cardiac action potentials. II. Hypotheses: calcium movements, excitation–contraction coupling and inotropic effects. *Circulation Research*, **24**, 409.

12
CLINICAL ASSESSMENT OF LEFT VENTRICULAR FUNCTION

D. G. Gibson

Understanding the function of the left ventricle remains a central problem in cardiology, and over the past few years significant progress has been made in describing events during filling and ejection in normal subjects and in elucidating abnormalities that may occur in patients with heart disease. In general, these studies have been along two lines. The first has been purely descriptive and has attempted to give as complete an account as possible of the normal structure and contraction pattern of the left ventricle in man. On this basis, abnormalities occurring in patients with heart disease can be characterised and their variation defined with respect to position in the left ventricle, or time during the cardiac cycle. The second approach assumes that left ventricular disease can be described as a failure of 'contractility' and seeks to define 'indices' or 'parameters' which will allow this to be uniquely quantified. These quantities may be empirical or may be based on the properties of isolated heart muscle, but all assume that the function of the left ventricle can be described as a single number. These two approaches are not necessarily compatible.

In the present review an account will be given of recent developments in primary methods used to study the behaviour of the left ventricle in man. This will be followed by a description of the normal contraction pattern, and of abnormalities that may occur in patients with heart disease. Finally, an account will be given of methods used to quantify left ventricular function in clinical practice, although no attempt has been made to discuss the effects of acute interventions on left ventricular behaviour. It does not appear that any of these questions have been finally settled, but the objective of this review is to give a description of current problems.

METHODS

Determination of left ventricular cavity size and the position of its walls throughout the cardiac cycle remains fundamental to a study of its function. Although a number of techniques have been developed, angiography remains the most widely used and forms the basis of comparison for other methods. There has been no fundamental change in technique over the past few years, but introduction of caesium iodide screens with superior resolution, widespread use of biplane cine-angiographic equipment, and optimisation of radiographic and other methods allowing reduction in the quantity of dye injected, has led to a very significant improvement in the quality of the angiographic images from which measurements are made in comparison with those available five years ago (Sandler and Alderman, 1974).

Angiography

A primary objective of angiographic methods has been the determination of the volume of left ventricular cavity (Dodge et al, 1966). If manual techniques of measurement are to be used it is necessary to assume that the cavity can be represented as a simple geometrical figure, such as ellipsoid, and thus that its projection in any plane is an ellipse. Measurement of the area of the projection can be performed either by measuring its axes directly (Arvidsson, 1961) or by deriving the minor axis from direct measurement of long axis and estimation of area by planimetry without simplifying assumptions (Dodge et al, 1960). Correction must be made for magnification resulting from variation in distances between the tube, the intensifier and the patient, and also for distortion of the field. Comparison of left ventricular volume calculated in this way with values derived from plaster casts of postmortem specimens shows consistent over-estimation of volume by angiographic estimates of stroke volume are compared with direct measurements. Calculated values must therefore be corrected by appropriate regression equations based on postmortem specimens (Davila and San Marco, 1966). Although ventricular volume was initially estimated from biplane angiograms, very close correlation has been demonstrated with values derived from single plane images with PA or RAO projections (Greene et al, 1967; Sandler and Dodge, 1968).

Angiographic estimates of left ventricular volume are subject to a number of limitations. The results do not take the volume of the papillary muscles into account, and there is difficulty in defining the boundary of the ventricle in the region of the mitral valve during diastole. Experimental studies have shown that the outer border of angiographic dye may be separated from metal markers on the endocardium itself, particularly at end-systole, with consequent underestimation of volume (Mitchell, Wildenthal and Mullins, 1969). In patients in whom left ventricular cavity shape is normal, the error produced by the assumption of ellipsoidal geometry is probably not a very significant one at end-diastole, but in the presence of left ventricular disease, shape may depart widely from any simple geometrical figure. Angiographic methods require cardiac catheterisation and injection of radiopaque contrast medium which has significant effects on the circulation, both by increasing blood volume and by depressing left ventricular function, although these are small for the first two to three beats after injection (Rahimtoola, Duffy and Swan, 1967; Carleton, 1971; Karliner, Bouchard and Gault, 1972). Finally, measurement of left ventricular volume from angiograms is tedious to perform manually, so that these methods are normally applicable only on a research basis. In spite of these limitations, however, the picture of left ventricular wall movement given by technically satisfactory biplane angiograms is so comprehensive that it has become apparent that a major problem exists in extracting and handling the large amount of information that such records contain. It is not surprising, therefore, that considerable effort has been devoted to the use of computing techniques in processing angiographic data, and it is likely that such methods will make major contributions in the future.

Initial efforts were directed towards facilitating calculations required for manual methods, so that relatively simple resources were required (Nelson and Lipchik, 1966; Rackley et al, 1968). More complex techniques make use of semiautomated methods involving the cardiologist tracing the outline of the left ventricular cavity with a light pen or pencil follower (Alderman et al, 1973; Marcus et al, 1972; Covvey et al, 1972), thus generating a set of points whose coordinates are stored by the computer. From this information a variety of calculations can be performed, including derivation of cavity area by numerical integration, measurement of long axis, and estimation of volumes using appropriate regression equations.

These semiautomated methods have considerably increased the scope of angiographic techniques. They make it possible to study successive cine frames exposed at a rate of 50 to 100/s, and also to make calculations more elaborate than simple volume estimates. They are relatively simple and the computer resources that they require are small compared with those that appear to be necessary if complete automation is undertaken. In addition, the programming is very much less complex than that required to distinguish, for example, between a cavity outline on the one hand and mitral valve, a stream of undyed blood or even a rib on the other. In spite of the obvious subjective element, the results are remarkably consistent provided that angiograms of adequate technical quality are available.

Further development towards complete automation has proceeded in two directions. The first involves the use of more sophisticated boundary following techniques, involving complex operator interaction to mask out other interfering shadows (Chow and Kaneko, 1972). The second uses the technique of videodensitometry, which is based on estimating the density of contrast over the whole area of the cavity projection as well as recognition of the boundary (Heintzen, 1971; Johnson et al, 1974). If uniform mixing of due is assumed to take place it is possible to estimate the path length through which the x-rays must have passed, and combining information from two orthogonal planes it is possible, in many circumstances, to derive a three dimensional model of the left ventricular cavity. These methods allow concave as well as convex regions to be defined from biplane angiograms provided that they are not extensive. Although these techniques are not currently available for use in patients with heart disease, they have considerable potential in displaying complex data (Greenleaf et al, 1972), it seems likely that they will provide the basis for significant contributions in the future.

Echocardiography

Since the first description of measurement of cavity diameter by echocardiography in 1969 (Chapelle and Mensch, 1969; Feigenbaum et al, 1969), there has been increasing interest in the use of this technique for the study of left ventricular function. The method depends on recording echoes from the left side of the interventricular septum as well as from the endocardial surface of the posterior wall, so that only a single dimension is measured. Since echoes can be recorded from both sides of the septum as well as from epicardial and endocardial surfaces of the posterior wall; both septal and myocardial thickness can also be estimated. The transverse dimension measured is not unique, and an additional requirement for a reproducible record is that it should include part of the anterior cusp echo and also the posterior papillary muscle (Feigenbaum, 1973; Fortuin, Hood and Craige, 1972; Gibson, 1973). Such measurements of transverse diameter correlate closely with angiographic minor axis. Early empirical observations suggested that the cube of this dimension approximated to ventricular volume, and initial comparisons showed agreement to be remarkably close. However, more extended comparison has demonstrated that this is only the case when cavity shape and contraction pattern are normal (Gibson, 1973; Teicholtz, Herman and Gorlin, 1973). When the cavity is dilated, this relation no longer applies, while if local contraction abnormalities are present, the echo dimension is no longer representative of the cavity as a whole, and serious errors may result. In retrospect, it appears that such volume estimates should be treated as semiquantitative at best, although they undoubtedly have some value in the clinical context. Measurements of dimension, however, appear to give reliable information about the region of the left ventricle studied.

The echocardiogram of the left ventricular cavity lends itself to semi-automatic digitisation in the same manner as the cineangiogram (Gibson and Brown, 1973; Griffith and Henry, 1973). Using a pencil follower, strings of coordinates can be generated for the positions of the posterior wall and septal echoes, and left ventricular dimension derived continuously by subtraction, so that peak rates of wall movement can also be estimated, allowing ventricular ejection and filling to be investigated in more detail than is possible by simply measuring end-systolic and end-diastolic dimensions. Similar methods can be used to measure posterior wall and septal thicknesses continuously and such data, when combined with cavity pressure measurements made by micromanometer, allow a variety of mechanical determinants of left ventricular function to be calculated continuously throughout the cardiac cycle (Gibson and Brown, 1974, 1976).

The value of echocardiography in studying left ventricular function can be extended in other ways. The extent of the left ventricular cavity explored can be increased by scanning manually from the aortic root towards the apex, using a strip chart recorder, so that regions of increased or abnormal contraction pattern can be localised (Jacobs et al, 1973). Alternatively, mechanical sector scanning has been employed, using a transducer oscillating over an arc of 30 or 60 degrees at a frequency of 12/s (Griffith and Henry, 1974). Other approaches which have shown some promise have been the use of a multi-element transducer, which allows two-dimensional scanning at a frequency of 80/s, and also standard B-scanning methods (King, 1973; Bom et al, 1973; Kloster et al, 1974). Unfortunately, resolution of the endocardium is rather unsatisfactory with these, and estimates of left ventricular cavity size made with it show no improvement over single beam methods when compared with angiograms. A more promising approach has been the development of phased array systems in which the ultrasound beam is steered and focused electronically from a linear array of transducers (von Ramm and Thurstone, 1976; Kisslo, von Ramm and Thurstone, 1976). This provides a frame rate of 20/s, with high lateral resolution and an $80°$ field of view. Preliminary clinical results have been encouraging.

Estimation of Left Ventricular Wall Stress

The myocardium of the left ventricle does work on the circulation by the development of force during systole, so that estimation of the magnitude of such forces is fundamental to any description of cardiac performance in mechanical terms. A stress is a force per unit cross-sectional area; if the force is perpendicular to the cross-section it is spoken of as a normal stress, and if parallel, as a shear stress. Stresses need not be uniformly distributed in the left ventricular wall, and such non-uniformity may be dependent on the structure of the myocardium, or position between its inner and outer surfaces, and may vary in different regions of the ventricle.

Left ventricular wall stress has most frequently been estimated using Laplace's law:

$$p = t \left(\frac{1}{r} + \frac{1}{R} \right)$$

where p = cavity pressure, t = wall tension and r and R are the principal radii of curvature (Love, 1888). This formulation was originally applied to surface tension, and thus a significant number of important assumptions are made in its application to the left ventricle. The myocardium is assumed to be linearly elastic (Hooke's law), isotropic and homogenous (i.e. that its properties are uniform with respect to direction and position). Myocardial distortion is assumed to occur in a purely radial direction and all other wall forces, such as bending moments or shear stresses, are neglected. The heart wall is taken as being in a state of static equilibrium, so that dynamic components are ignored.

Although apparently taking wall thickness into account, formulations based on this, Love's first approximation to Laplace's law are, in fact, only applicable to thin shells. Here, stress is considered constant across the wall, and the normal stress zero, in addition to the other assumptions enumerated above. In general, this can only be taken as applying to a shell whose wall thickness is less than one-tenth of the radius of curvature of the reference surface, and it will be noted that the normal thickness of the left ventricular wall falls well outside this range. If these assumptions are granted, then values for circumferential and longitudinal stress can be calculated from measurements of left ventricular long and minor axes, and wall thickness and cavity pressure, using one of several formulations that have been proposed (Sandler and Dodge, 1963; Falsetti et al, 1970).

In practice, these assumptions are limiting. In the normal subject left ventricular shape may depart significantly from an ellipsoid, particularly at end-systole, and these changes may be pronounced in the presence of heart disease (Rackley et al, 1970a; Gibson and Brown, 1975b). The necessity to assume that the wall is isotropic and homogeneous, and therefore to consider only average stresses, has directed attention away from regional abnormalities of fibre orientation or of abnormalities in different parts of the ventricle in disease states (Streeter and Bassett, 1966; Streeter and Hanna, 1973). The possibility of variation in wall stress across the wall is clearly of importance when myocardial force–velocity relations are extrapolated to the intact heart. In addition, the possibility exists that shear stresses may be developed, which might modify left ventricular behaviour in early diastole, but which cannot be studied using methods based on the Laplace relation (Rushmer and Crystal, 1951). It is clear, therefore, that more comprehensive descriptions might be of value in the investigation of left ventricular function.

Two alternative approaches have been described. The first is based on a true thick-walled model (Ghista and Sandler, 1969; Wong and Rautaharju, 1968; Mirsky, 1969). This allows for a thick-walled left ventricle and variation of stress across it, but it is still restricted by requiring an idealised left ventricular shape based on an ellipsoid. Although the mathematics of such a model are more complex, it is of interest that when used to calculate average stresses, these are of the same order of magnitude as those derived from the Laplace relation, significant differences occurring only at the apex. The second approach is to make use of finite element methods, an engineering method of stress analysis for structures of irregular and complex shape. In this method the whole structure is broken down into small elements of a simpler geometry (Zienkiewicz, 1967). The elements can then be reconstructed to form the complex shape whilst being able to define the material to the degree of complexity required. The left ventricular model itself may be based on the rotation of a two-dimensional structure or be defined in three dimensions, the latter being considerably more complex. Successful use of finite element methods requires sophisticated computing facilities, but they have the advantage that structures of completely irregular shape and anisotropic, non-linear materials can be studied, with regional variation in properties (Janz and Grimm, 1972; Ghista et al, 1973).

NORMAL LEFT VENTRICULAR CONTRACTION PATTERN

Information is now available from a variety of sources from which a picture of the normal left ventricular contraction pattern in man can be built up. This includes data from normal subjects, patients with atypical chest pain found at cardiac catheter to have no haemodynamic or angiographic abnormality and, in some cases, patients with operable heart disease but with no lesion likely to put a pressure or volume load on the left ventricle or to be associated with disease of the myocardium itself.

Wall movement during the pre-ejection period has been studied by angiography which gives information about the endocardium (Karliner et al, 1971), or by radiographic studies of metal clips sutured to the epicardium at the time of corrective surgery for lesions such as mitral stenosis or atrial septal defect (McDonald, 1970). In all normal subjects, the onset of left ventricular contraction is associated with a reduction in transverse left ventricular dimension and downward movement of the base of the heart, but with no significant change in long axis, so that there is a reduction in cavity area of around 5 per cent. At the same time there is an increase in wall thickness associated with a slight increase in epicardial diameter (Rushmer, Crystal and Wagner, 1953). Observations of epicardial markers have also demonstrated slight counter-clockwise rotation, together with a small upward thrust of the apex (McDonald, 1970), the last corresponding with the onset of outward wall movement recorded by apexcardiography.

During the period of ejection, inward left ventricular wall movement is uniform in the normal subject (Hood and Rolett, 1969; Gault, Ross and Braunwald, 1968). The main change is in transverse diameter, but downward movement of the aortic ring also occurs as well as some upward movement of the apex (Harvey, 1628). All parts of the cavity move in phase with one another, as can be demonstrated by superimposition of chords from different regions of the ventricle. The predominance of transverse rather than longitudinal shortening results in the cavity becoming less spherical, or its projection less circular during ejection. These changes in shape can be expressed either in terms of eccentricity, assuming that the cavity is ellipsoidal, which is defined as:

$$\sqrt{\frac{L^2 - D^2}{L}}$$

where L=long axis, D=minor axis; or, in more general terms as a shape index, such as:

$$\frac{4\pi(\text{area})}{(\text{perimeter})^2}$$

which is a measure of cavity area enclosed by unit perimeter, and which does not assume that the cavity projection can be represented by any specific geometrical figure (Gibson and Brown, 1975b). Shape changes proceed concomitantly with those in cavity volume during ejection.

Along with the reduction in cavity size, there is an increase in wall thickness which may be estimated by echocardiography (Feigenbaum et al, 1968; Sjogren, Hytonen and Frick, 1970; Troy, Pombo and Rackley, 1972), or angiography (Rackley et al, 1964; Kennedy et al, 1967; Gault et al, 1968; Eber et al, 1969; Falsetti et al, 1970). Mean end-diastolic wall thickness estimated by either method is approximately 10.9 ± 2.0 mm increasing by approximately 100 per cent at end-systole (Hood, Rackley and Rolett, 1968). Continuous estimates of wall thickness of left ventricular free wall have been made by videodensitometry, and this has demonstrated a small presystolic dip in thickness (Dumesnil et al, 1974). The peak rate of increase of wall thickness in normal subjects was 7 cm/s, with a mean value of 4 cm/s.

Septal movement can be studied most satisfactorily by echocardiography (Popp et al, 1969; McDonald, Feigenbaum and Chang, 1972). In normal subjects the dominant deflection during systole is usually in a posterior direction, but for a variable period at end-ejection both septum and posterior wall may move in the same direction. Increases in septal thickness during systole are less than those occurring in the posterior wall, the difference being possibly related to the altered pattern of septal contraction (Keith, 1918).

Overall movement of the left ventricle can most satisfactorily be investigated by angiography. When referred to an external system of coordinates, Leighton, Wilt and Lewis (1974) found a systolic rotation of the long axis of 1.9 degrees, while movement of the centroid is usually undetectable for the initial part of ejection, but during the last third it moves downwards and to the right. The parallel movement of septum and posterior wall demonstrated by echocardiography suggests an additional posterior movement at this time in the cardiac cycle (McDonald et al, 1972).

Ventricular volume changes have been studied in normal subjects by a number of authors using angiographic techniques (Kennedy et al, 1966; Dodge et al, 1966). Values of end-diastolic volume between 70 and 88 ml/m² and of end-systolic volume of 24 to 34 ml/m² have been reported, resulting in an ejection fraction (stroke volume/end-diastolic volume) of 0.64 to 0.67. Peak systolic ejection rate, determined by cineangiography, has been given by Hammermeister, Brooks and Warbasse (1974) as 430 ± 130 ml/s. Rates of left ventricular wall movement have also been extensively studied in normal subjects, since these form a basis for comparison with values derived from patients with heart disease, both echocardiographic and angiographic techniques having been used. The transverse diameter has been most frequently studied and values in normal subjects are in the range 25 to 40 cm/s, expressed as peak rate of change of mid-wall circumference (Wilcken, 1965; Gault et al, 1968; Karliner Bouchard, and Gault, 1971). These values may be normalised by division by end-diastolic or instantaneous circumference, resulting in a normal range of 1.28 to 2.53 s^{-1}. Mean rates of wall movement are more readily measured than peak ones using simple techniques. To derive mean shortening rate angiographically, measurement of only two cine frames is required, that simultaneous with end-diastole being identified from the Q-wave of a simultaneous ECG, and that corresponding with end-systole as the one with the smallest cavity area (Karliner et al, 1971). Total shortening is given by the difference in minor axis on the two frames, and ejection time as the interval between the two frames less 50 ms in all patients but those with mitral regurgitation. Similar measurements can be derived from left ventricular echocardiograms as systolic reduction in circumference divided by ejection time measured from an indirect carotid pulse (Paraskos et al, 1971; Cooper et al, 1972a). Normal values are in the range 18 to 60 cm/s or 1.3 to 2.3 s^{-1} when normalised to end-diastolic circumference.

Normal left ventricular pressures measured with a micromanometer show characteristic patterns. The onset of pressure rise is synchronous with the first appearance of mechanical activity. Peak rate of rise of pressure occurs during the pre-ejection period, or at the time of aortic valve opening (Gleason and Braunwald, 1962). Peak rate of rise of pressure is affected by a number of variables including end-diastolic volume, the time of aortic valve opening, heart rate and by drugs or other manoeuvres which may have direct myocardial effects or lead to secondary reflex changes in the level of sympathetic activity (Mason, 1969).

With a knowledge of left ventricular cavity size, wall thickness and cavity pressure, wall stress can be calculated subject to the limitations enumerated above. In normal subjects, peak values of circumferential wall tension are in the range 190 to 400 g cm^{-3} or 300 to 400 g cm^{-2} expressed as wall stress, allowing for wall thickness (Sandler and Dodge, 1963; Gault et al, 1968; Hood et al, 1968). Peak wall stress is reached early in systole, later values being appreciably lower, reflecting the substantial relative reduction in left ventricular cavity dimensions occurring during ejection in normal subjects.

ABNORMALITIES OF LEFT VENTRICULAR SYSTOLIC FUNCTION

A number of potentially separable processes can be defined which may lead to impairment of left ventricular systolic function in patients with heart disease. These include abnormalities of left ventricular cavity architecture, local disturbances of wall movement leading to incoordinate contraction and, finally, a reduction in the peak rate of wall movement or stress development. Although more than one of these may be present in individual patients they will be considered separately, since they form the physiological basis for any discussion of methods used for evaluating left ventricular function in clinical practice.

Abnormal Left Ventricular Architecture

The abnormal left ventricle is frequently larger than normal. This increase in size may be expressed in terms of absolute volume, corrected for body surface area, or in terms of a single dimension, usually the transverse one (Dodge and Sandler, 1974). Neither of these forms a satisfactory definition of left ventricular disease, since left ventricular size may also be increased as the result of a large stroke volume due to valvular regurgitation or a shunt with no evidence of myocardial disease. In order to separate these two groups of patients, ejection fraction, the ratio of stroke volume to end-diastolic volume, can be used (Bristow et al, 1964; Miller and Swan, 1964), low values representing an inappropriate increase in end-diastolic volume with respect to the stroke volume. It has proved a very satisfactory method of identifying patients with left ventricular disease illustrating the importance of a large cavity size in the definition of impaired myocardial function.

An increase in cavity size has a number of implications affecting the pattern of left ventricular contraction (Burton, 1957). At constant stroke volume, the overall amplitude of wall movement is reduced in inverse ratio to the square of the radius of the cavity as its size increases. Since ejection time is not greatly different from normal, rates of wall movement, both mean and peak, are also correspondingly reduced as the dimension increases (Paley, McDonald and Weissler, 1964; Gault et al, 1968; Karliner et al, 1971). Since cavity pressure is also not significantly different from normal during systole, the increased radius of curvature of the wall, by the law of Laplace, is associated with a corresponding increase in wall tension. In these circumstances, wall stresses depend on associated changes in wall thickness, which may not be compensatory in patients with increased cavity size, so that high values of wall stress result (Hood et al, 1968; Gault et al, 1968). In the isolated papillary muscle there is an inverse relation between applied force and velocity of contraction but in patients in whom the left ventricle is dilated the reduction in shortening velocity is greater than would be predicted from the increase in wall stress. The implications of this altered pattern of contraction are not clear, although it has been suggested that it may result from a reduction in myocardial contractility (Gault et al, 1968). The reduced amplitude of wall movement also has functional significance, in that high values of wall stress are maintained throughout ejection. This is in sharp contrast to the normal heart where the relatively greater reduction in left ventricular dimension leads to a progressive drop in wall stress as ejection proceeds.

The mechanism by which left ventricular cavity dilatation occurs has not been studied in detail. In general, wall thickness is normal or increased so that, with an increase in cavity size, there is a corresponding increase in left ventricular muscle mass (Rackley et al, 1964), indicating that hypertrophy has occurred (Dodge et al, 1960). The relation between end-diastolic pressure and volume has been studied in a number of patients with left ventricular disease (Jones et al, 1964; Rackley et al, 1970b; Grant, 1965), who demon-strated no clear relation between the two and that patients with a considerable increase in cavity size could have a normal end-diastolic pressure. It is possible that the underlying mechanism is of slippage and reorientation of myocardial fibres associated with hypertrophy, although there is little direct information available at present (Linzbach, 1960; Jean, Streeter and Reichenbach, 1972). Nevertheless, it can be concluded that a large left ventricle cannot be regarded simply as a small one distended and it is inappropriate to apply ideas based on acute changes in filling pressure or end-diastolic volume directly to patients in whom the left ventricular cavity is dilated.

The cavity of the dilated left ventricle is also more circular than normal. This has been documented in several ways—as the ratio of long to short axis, as eccentricity, or in terms of shape index (Hood and Rolett, 1969; Frimer et al, 1969; McDonald, 1970; Teicholtz et al, 1972; Vokonas et al, 1973; Gould et al, 1974; Gibson and Brown, 1975b). These methods indicate that, in damaged hearts, the cavity becomes more spherical at end-diastole and, more important, these departures from normality are greater at end-systole. This failure of shape change correlates closely with the presence of reduced ejection fraction and has several consequences. The similarity of major and minor axes results in an increase in the calculated value of longitudinal stress, while circumferential stress does not alter significantly. This change may have as its basis an alteration in myocardial fibre orientation, and pre-liminary evidence for this has been reported. The normal shape change during systole means that the reduction in cavity volume is brought about with relatively less myocardial shortening than would have been necessary had the end-diastolic configuration beeen maintained throughout ejection. This effect is lost in patients in whom shape changes do not occur, and might be expected to be associated with a reduction in the functional capacity of the ventricle as a whole.

Specific abnormalities of left ventricular structure in disease do not appear to have been studied in the detail that they merit. Grant (1953, 1965) des-cribed a number of disturbances of left ventricular architectonics, finding that ventricular dilatation was eccentric, involving primarily the part of the chamber anterior to the mitral valve and apex. This resulted in posterior displacement of the origins of the papillary muscles and lengthening of all components of the mitral valve apparatus, and also in a change in the orienta-tion of the mitral ring. In the presence of left ventricular hypertrophy, circum-ferential thickening of the wall and septum was observed, together with elongation of the chamber. The most striking change occurred in the posterior and superior walls, the anterior left ventricular wall being embraced by the right ventricular outflow tract, and the inferior surface being constrained by the diaphragm. It seems that description of such abnormalities in greater detail may contribute significantly to a greater understanding of impaired function.

Incoordinate Contraction

Localised abnormalities of wall movement play an important role in interfering with left ventricular contraction, particularly in patients with ischaemic heart disease. Initial analyses of these disturbances have been based on left ventricular angiograms, and four types of abnormal systolic behaviour described (Herman and Gorlin, 1969) which refer to departures from the normal pattern of concentric inward movement.

1. Akinesis, in which there is no inward movement of the affected area.
2. Asyneresis, in which the overall amplitude of movement is reduced, although its direction and timing are normal.
3. Dyskinesis, in which the direction of movement is abnormal, i.e. there is systolic outward movement in the affected area.
4. Asynchrony, in which the time relations of local wall movement differ from those of the rest of the ventricle, although overall amplitude and direction of movement may be normal.

Although these abnormalities are clearly defined, their recognition in individual patients may present difficulties. One of the most important of these is in the definition of a reference point relative to which position can be assessed, so that local abnormalities of movement can be distinguished from overall movement of the heart within the thorax. Such overall movement would cause apparent abnormalities of wall movement in a normally contracting ventricle, so that the impression of localised akinesis or even outward systolic bulging might be produced. There is, however, little agreement as to what frame of reference should be used when comparing cavity outlines at different phases of systole. There are three possibilities for movement of the left ventricle relative to the x-ray tube; thoracic cage motion, downward movement of the aortic root, and systolic rotation of the left ventricle. A number of methods have been proposed. The simplest is to use a system of external landmarks, fixed with respect to the x-ray tube (Chaitman, Bristow and Rahimtoola, 1973), and a second is to assume that the point of intersection of the long axis and its bisecting perpendicular remains fixed, implying that contraction is always concentric (Hamilton, Murray and Kennedy, 1972; Chatterjee et al, 1973). A third method assumes that the point of intersection of the long axis and the aortic valve is fixed, so that any shortening of the long axis must be due to upward movement of the apex, and downward movement of the aortic ring cannot by definition occur: this is clearly incompatible with the previous method (Helfant, Herman and Gorlin, 1973; Rees et al, 1971). More complex methods have also been described, such as that of Leighton et al (1974), in which the cavity projection is divided into two halves of equal area by a line from the apex to a point on the aortic valve ring. This line is defined by trial and error for each cine frame to be studied, and these lines are superimposed when movement is to be assessed. It is apparent, therefore,

that methods should be sought for defining local abnormalities of wall movement. One of the most promising of these is based on the observation of
Dumesnil et al (1974) that normal local contraction is associated with a
predictable increase in wall thickness. If this fails to occur it may indicate
impaired local contraction, while with paradoxical movement a reduction in
thickness may be observed. The method is only available for the free wall of
the ventricle where measurements of thickness can be made, but nevertheless
appears to provide a means of describing local function without the need for
an external reference point. A less rigorous approach is to assume that in
ischaemic heart disease affected areas of myocardium are likely to be those
supplied by diseased arteries, and therefore a method of examination which
gives close correlation between the two is likely to be more physiologically
valid than one that does not. This does not allow for the fact that normal left
ventricular contraction may occur in the presence of severe ischaemic heart
disease, so that the relation between arterial lesions and wall movement is not
clear-cut. The problem of defining a suitable reference point for the analysis
of wall movement is stressed because it is fundamental when regional function
or local wall properties are derived from measures of displacement and cavity
pressure.

Echocardiography may also be used to study abnormalities of the movement
of the septum or posterior wall. These may consist of a reduction in amplitude
or a reversal of the normal direction of wall movement (Inoue et al, 1971;
Fogelman et al, 1972; Jacobs et al, 1973; Heikkila and Nieminen, 1975).
Disease of the anterior descending coronary artery is frequently associated
with reversed or reduced septal movement (Brown, Popp and Harrison, 1973)
while reduced amplitude of posterior wall movement may occur in the presence
of inferior ischaemia (Inoue et al, 1971). Unfortunately, abnormalities of
local movement cannot be taken as evidence of local disease, since reversed
septal movement also occurs in patients with large right ventricular stroke
volume, due, for example, to atrial septal defect (Diamond et al, 1971). In
these circumstances, reversed septal movement may well represent overall
movement of the left ventricle relative to the transducer on the anterior chest
wall, again stressing the necessity for defining the point of reference for
measurements of position. Localised abnormalities of ventricular function
have also been studied by observation of epicardial clips, and include reduced
fractional shortening, premature cessation of shortening, lack of movement or
even lengthening during the pre-ejection period or ejection itself (McDonald,
1972).

Incoordinate contraction has a number of physiological consequences
beyond those due to loss of regional function (Herman and Gorlin, 1969). In
the presence of dyskinesia, abnormal bulging may impose a volume load on
the left ventricle, comparable to that associated with mitral regurgitation, whose
magnitude depends on the properties of the affected region (Herman and
Gorlin, 1969). In addition, such regions cannot support local tension, so that

local increase in wall curvature develops. Localised asyneresis requires a compensatory increase in myocardial shortening elsewhere in the left ventricle if stroke volume is to be maintained. and if the abnormal region involves more than 20 to 25 per cent of the myocardium, cavity dilatation occurs, with a corresponding increase in wall stresses. Abnormalities in the time relations of local contraction lead to more complex disturbances of function. These can be studied by relating local function to that of the ventricle as a whole, as reflected in the pressure pulse (Gibson and Brown, 1976). Distortion of pressure–dimension loops constructed in such circumstances can be used to demonstrate a striking loss of mechanical efficiency resulting from these processes.

Although localised abnormalities of wall movement have been recognised for longest in patients with ischaemic heart disease, they are also present in patients in whom ventricular activation is abnormal, particularly in ventricular ectopic beats, and in left bundle branch block, where echocardiography has demonstrated reversed septal movement (Gibson, 1972) sometimes preceded by a small early systolic posterior displacement. More recently, localised disturbances of wall movement have been documented in patients with valvular heart disease, cardiomyopathy, and in missed beats in atrial fibrillation, although the pattern of ventricular activation is normal (McDonald, 1972; Kreulen, Gorlin and Herman, 1973; Gibson and Brown, 1976). Characteristic disturbances of wall movement have also been associated with the presence of mitral valve prolapse (Gooch et al, 1972). It seems reasonable to suppose, therefore, that incoordinate contraction may be associated with any form of left ventricular disease. It is likely to result in impairment of all time-related measurements of contraction, in particular with the peak rate of rise of pressure and derived quantities, and also of peak aortic flow rate and acceleration. It is clear that any method seeking to give a comprehensive description of impaired left ventricular function must allow for this mechanism.

Rate of Contraction

Disturbances of time-related functions of left ventricular contraction may occur in patients with heart disease. These have received considerable attention, since it seemed possible that their measurement might form the basis of an absolute definition of impairment of left ventricular function.

Rate of rise of pressure. Peak rate of rise of left ventricular pressure may be abnormal in patients with heart disease, and a number of mechanisms have been identified which contribute to this (Gleason and Braunwald, 1962; Mason, 1969). Peak rate of rise of pressure usually occurs at the time of aortic valve opening, so that delay in the onset of ejection, as occurs for instance in aortic stenosis or systemic hypertension, is associated with an increase in the peak value. A reduction in aortic impedance in aortic or mitral regurgitation has the reverse effect. Peak dP/dt is also reduced by abnormalities of activation, including ventricular ectopic beats, left bundle branch block, right ventricular pacing, and to a lesser extent by left anterior hemiblock. In the absence of any of these factors, a reduction in peak dP/dt is usually taken as evidence of severe left ventricular disease, although the normal range is so wide that it cannot be regarded as a specific or sensitive index.

Rates of wall movement. Rates of left ventricular wall movement have been measured by angiography or by echocardiography, and both peak and mean rates studied (Paley et al, 1964; Gault et al, 1968; Karliner et al, 1971; Paraskos et al, 1971; Gibson and Brown, 1975a). The results may be expressed in a number of ways, the commonest being as rates of shortening of left ventricular minor axis, or of mid-wall circumference in the equatorial region of the ventricle. In order to study local function, the long axis quadrasection method has been used in which shortening of three transverse chords, equally spaced along and perpendicular to the major axis, is measured (Herman and Gorlin, 1969).

In patients with heart disease, peak rates of circumferential shortening are reduced from normal values of 30 to 35 cm/s to mean values in the range of 15 to 20 cm/s. However, considerable overlap is present between normal and abnormal groups even when the latter consists of patients with severe cardiomyopathy. Separation is even less clear-cut when patients with moderately severe or compensated left ventricular disease are studied, and a more effective means of identifying these patients has been to use normalised shortening rates. These are derived by dividing peak rates of shortening by the dimension at end diastole, a manipulation adopted to give a figure equivalent to the rate of shortening of unit length of dimension. This manoeuvre is justified by analogy with cardiac muscle mechanics to provide a means whereby values from different patients can be compared. Peak normalised shortening rate (V_{CF}) in normal subjects is in the range 1.3 to 2.5 s^{-1}, while in patients with severe heart disease values are very much lower with a mean of 0.6 to 0.9 s^{-1} depending on the patient population studied. V_{CF} is particularly effective in detecting left ventricular abnormalities associated with increased cavity size, but may be normal in hypertrophic cardiomyopathy, although severe left ventricular disease is present.

Derivation of peak shortening rates requires data handling facilities or involves tedious manual calculations. Mean V_{CF} can be calculated very much more easily and so is more suitable for routine evaluation of patients. Normal values are in the range 18 to 60 cm/s, while appreciably lower values may be recorded in patients with left ventricular disease (2–30 cm/s). As with peak values, separation between normal and abnormal groups is increased when values are normalised, patients with normal left ventricular function having values in the range 1.3 to 2.3 s^{-1}, while in those in whom it is depressed, values lie between 0.15 and 1.3 s^{-1}.

Values of V_{CF} are increased by administration of drugs with a positive inotropic effect, and also by exercise. However, both peak and mean V_{CF} are affected by acute alterations in arterial pressure, being increased by amyl nitrate inhalation and reduced by angiotensin administration (Quinones et al, 1975). In addition, abnormally high values may be observed in patients with mitral regurgitation, ventricular septal defect with high pulmonary flow, and particularly in those with transposition of the great arteries when the left ventricle ejects into a normal pulmonary vascular bed. V_{CF} cannot therefore be taken as an unambiguous measure of left ventricular function unless the effects of ejection pressure and impedance are taken into account.

The rate of change of left ventricular volume can also be measured from left ventricular angiograms (Hammermeister et al, 1974). Unlike the velocity of wall movement, the rate of ejection appears little affected by the presence of left ventricular disease; peak rates of 430 ± 130 ml/s being recorded in normal subjects and 495 ± 85 ml/s in those with cardiomyopathy. The only group of patients in whom peak rate of change of volume was different significantly from normal was those with mitral regurgitation, in whom it was increased to 650 ± 290 ml/s. It appears that, in the presence of left ventricular disease, peak rates of change of ventricular volume remain virtually constant so that with increasing cavity size, peak rates of wall movement are reduced. There is no doubt that normalised rates of wall movement are sensitive methods of detecting patients with impaired left ventricular function, but it is difficult to avoid the conclusion that they do so because they reflect an increase in cavity size rather than any abnormality of contraction pattern.

Rates of left ventricular ejection may also be assessed by measurement of peak rates of aortic blood velocity and acceleration. Maximum acceleration in three normal subjects was recorded by Bennett et al (1974) as being greater than 1500 cm^{-2} and peak velocity as greater than 60 cm s^{-1}. In a group of patients with coronary artery disease, lower values were recorded with a positive correlation between peak velocity or acceleration, and ejection fraction measured by angiography.

Isovolumic Contraction and Relaxation

Dimensional changes in the pre-ejection period have been studied in detail using angiographic methods by Karliner et al (1971). In the presence of left ventricular disease, the normal pattern of uniform inward wall movement causing a reduction of equatorial diameter by approximately 1 mm, was replaced by appreciably greater changes in cavity configuration. In mitral regurgitation, a mean reduction of equatorial diameter of 2.8 mm occurred, accounting for 8 per cent of the end-diastolic volume. In patients with wall motion abnormalities due to ischaemic heart disease, equatorial diameter was reduced by a mean value of 1.7 mm, while in patients with cardiomyopathy, non-homogeneous involvement was suggested by an increase in transverse diameter in the equatorial region and a reduction towards the apex.

Events during isovolumic relaxation have also been studied by angiographic methods. The start of this period can usually be identified as the time of aortic valve closure or of minimum cavity area, while the onset of mitral valve opening is taken as the time of first appearance of unopacified blood in the ventricle. Although there have been a number of descriptions of left ventricular wall movement during this period, there is still no general agreement as to their significance. Most frequently reported is outward wall movement involving the anterior and apical regions which has been observed in normal subjects (Ruttley et al, 1974) in patients with ischaemic heart disease, and in patients with prolapsing mitral valve cusps (Gooch et al, 1971). This outward wall movement is associated with an apparent increase in left ventricular volume of 10 to 20 per cent which has been explained as being due to downward movement of the mitral valve ring, herniation of valve cusps into the cavity, or by aortic regurgitation due to the presence of a retrograde catheter entering the left ventricle. These characteristic wall movements are not always present, having been identified in 50 out of 305 patients by Wilson et al (1975), while Hamby et al (1974) found them in all of 21 patients with angina and Altieri, Wilt and Leighton (1973) in 83 out of 100 successive patients with coronary artery disease. Left ventricular iso-volumic wall movements appear to be accentuated in patients with ischaemic heart disease in whom outward movement occurs in those regions showing normal systolic function. Inward movement may occur in regions that contract poorly during systole and considerable variation in timing of maxi-mum rates of wall movement may be demonstrable in different parts of the cavity. Such asynchronous wall movement may be responsible for the decrease in peak negative dP/dt observed in ischaemic heart disease (McLaurin, Rolett and Grossman, 1973). More comprehensive methods of display indicate that, in patients with ischaemic heart disease, regions showing normal and abnormal behaviour may be quite sharply demarcated (Gibson, Prewitt and Brown, 1976).

Left ventricular shape changes occurring during isovolumic relaxation can also be studied by echocardiography. Mitral valve movement can be recorded directly and changes in left ventricular dimension correlated with it (Upton, Gibson and Brown, 1976). In normal subjects, there is little change in dimension before mitral valve opening, but in patients with ischaemic heart disease, up to 60 per cent of total diastolic wall movement may occur before the onset of filling, representing the effect of an isovolumic shape change. These changes correlated strongly with the presence of localised systolic abnormalities of contraction, demonstrated by angiography.

The overall significance of these changes is not clear. It seems probable that a small symmetrical increase in left ventricular cavity size is a normal finding in the isovolumic relaxation period. In the presence of ischaemic heart disease, these changes seem to be much more complex, and to represent a transient disequilibrium in the wall at this stage of the cardiac cycle. This may reflect the presence of stored energy in the wall or the asynchronous termination of the active state apparently related to the local severity of the ischaemic lesions.

The effect of isovolumic shape changes on overall left ventricular performance can be considered from two points of view. Outward wall movement, when pressure is still raised, must be associated with dissipation of mechanical energy and corresponding loss of mechanical efficiency of the contractile process as a whole. This can be demonstrated by constructing pressure–dimension loops, which allow this loss to be quantified for the region studied (Gibson and Brown, 1976). Ischaemic shape changes may also be considered in terms of their effect on the succeeding diastole, since they appear to be associated with abnormalities of the early rapid phase of ventricular filling.

ABNORMALITIES OF LEFT VENTRICULAR DIASTOLIC FUNCTION

Early Diastolic Filling

The early diastolic filling period may be taken as starting with opening of the mitral valve. This often occurs before minimum ventricular pressure is reached, so that early diastolic filling is associated with a reduction rather than an increase in left ventricular pressure (Dodge, Hay and Sandler, 1962). There is still no general agreement as to the implications of this, although it is clear that left ventricular pressure–volume relations at this stage of the cardiac cycle cannot be described in terms of a passive model. Katz (1930) concluded that it reflected a sucking effect of the left ventricle, drawing blood into its chamber, and more recently Brecher (1958) and Horwitz and Bishop (1972) have produced further evidence for such diastolic suction. The relative importance of filling during this period increases with heart rate, and with the tachycardia associated with maximum exercise tolerance almost all ventricular filling occurs as pressure is falling. It seems likely that further study of events at this stage in the cardiac cycle will prove very fruitful in understanding the limitations of ventricular performance at the extremes of exercise tolerance.

Mid-diastole

After the minimum left ventricular pressure has been reached, both pressure and volume increase together, as might be expected if the ventricle was behaving passively. Pressure–volume relations of the isolated canine left ventricle have been studied by a number of authors (Diamond et al, 1971; Gaasch et al, 1972), and shown to be curvilinear, an empirical relation of the form

$$\mathrm{Log_e}\ P = kV + b$$

applying, where P = transmural left ventricular pressure, V = volume, b is an intercept representing pressure at zero volume and k the slope of the ln P–V relation, frequently termed the stiffness constant. This exponential relation does not apply when the transmural pressure is below 3 mmHg.

In order to study left ventricular pressure–volume relations in man, it is clearly desirable to make multiple measurements of both throughout diastole. However, in order to avoid associated technical difficulties, Gaasch et al (1972) have measured the stiffness constant from single determinations of pressure and volume at end-diastole by assuming that an exponential relation of the type described above applied, and that b, the intercept corresponding to pressure at zero volume, was constant, with a value of 0.43 mmHg, derived from experiments in dogs. With a knowledge of the stiffness constant calculated in this way, an index of distensibility, dP/dV and compliance $1/V.dP/dV$ were derived. Compliance, thus defined, was found to be significantly reduced in idiopathic left ventricular hypertrophy, aortic stenosis and congestive cardiomyopathy.

A limited number of studies have been performed in man in which multiple determinations of pressure and volume have been made. These show that the relation between the two is curvilinear, but cannot be said to demonstrate unequivocally that it is exponential rather than some other continuous monotonically increasing function. If an exponential relation is assumed, then k is a measure of the rate of change of ln P with volume. High values have been observed in patients with hypertrophic cardiomyopathy and lower than normal ones in patients with large dilated hearts (Gaasch et al, 1975). The intercept b, also taken as representing diastolic 'tone', is not fixed but has been shown to rise considerably during attacks of pacing-induced angina (Barry et al, 1974) and to fall after propranolol administration in patients with severe ischaemic heart disease (Coltart et al, 1975). Gaasch et al (1975) also found b to vary from less than 1 to more than 30 mmHg in different patients. The assumption that b is fixed, therefore, is not a realistic one since values have been reported over the entire range of physiological and pathological diastolic pressures and large variations have been documented in individual patients. In addition, left ventricular diastolic pressure–volume relations may vary in individual patients. Sodium nitroprusside or propranolol administration may cause a reduction in diastolic pressure without a corresponding change in volume, and thus displace the pressure–volume curve, while angiotensin has the reverse effect (Coltart et al, 1975; Grossman et al, 1975; Alderman and Glantz, 1976).

Left ventricular pressure–volume relations do not give any information about the properties of the left ventricular wall itself. In order to do this, Mirsky and Parmley (1973) have derived myocardial stress–strain curves of the form

$$\frac{d\sigma}{d\varepsilon} = k\sigma + c$$

where σ = wall stress, ε = wall strain, $d\sigma/d\varepsilon$ = elastic stiffness, k a stiffness constant, and c an intercept. Wall stresses were calculated from cavity pressure and cavity and wall volumes, assuming that the ventricle remained spherical throughout diastole. An exponential relation between left ventricular pressure and volume was also assumed, and the intercept b was taken as constant at 0.43 mmHg. The highest values of elastic stiffness occurred in patients with congestive cardiomyopathy while, in normal subjects and those with hypertrophic cardiomyopathy, values were lower and not significantly different in the two groups. However, the stiffness constant k was found to be significantly higher in the patients with hypertrophic cardiomyopathy. These ideas are developed in greater detail by Mirsky (1976) in a comprehensive review.

In an attempt to avoid some of these assumptions, an alternative approach has been used in which simultaneous echocardiograms and left ventricular pressure have been recorded (Gibson and Brown, 1974). Wall thickness and cavity diameter were derived continuously from the echocardiogram by digitisation, and wall stress calculated on the basis of an ellipsoid of finite wall thickness. Measurements of wall stress and strain could thus be recorded directly throughout diastole. Using this method it was possible to demonstrate an early diastolic period when diameter increased as pressure fell, and a late diastolic period when the stress–strain curve had a finite slope which cor-related with cardiographic evidence of left ventricular hypertrophy. In addition, there was a mid-diastolic period when negligible change in calculated stress occurred in spite of an increase in circumference, due possibly to shape changes or to failure of myocardium to develop passive stress at fibre lengths reached at end-systole (Grimm et al, 1970).

Such methods have a number of limitations. Some are dependent on the assumption of an exponential relation between pressure and volume which has not been shown to apply in man. Measurements of cavity pressure, particularly when expressed on a logarithmic scale, are critically dependent on the zero used, and if the properties of the myocardium are to be studied, then the transmural gradient must be known. Very few measurements of pericardial pressure have been made in man, so it cannot be taken as proved that it is equal to the pressure at mid-thorax, or even that it remains constant throughout the cardiac cycle. Measurements of pericardial pressure in experi-mental animals (Holt, Rhode and Kines, 1960), and limited studies in a patient with malignant disease (Sharp et al, 1960), or in man after open heart surgery (Sutton and Gibson, 1975), suggest that this is not the case, and that considerable errors may result if transmural gradients are estimated from cavity pressure. Measurement of myocardial stress–strain relations is further complicated by the fact that, if cavity shape departs from a sphere, then at constant cavity pressure, local myocardial tension depends on local curvature. Similarly, when a thick-walled ventricle is considered, differences in myo-cardial stress are present across the wall. In these circumstances, a series of overlapping stress–strain curves are being measured in a single ventricle, and it would indeed be surprising if the overall resultant approximated to any simple mathematical relation.

An additional problem is that measured pressure–volume relations may include dynamic components, and could thus be affected by the rate of ventricular filling (Noble et al, 1969; Gibson and Brown, 1974; Gaasch et al, 1975). Inertial forces, due to outward acceleration of the wall, lead to cavity pressure being lower than in the static situation. Viscous forces are proportional to the rate of distension of myocardium, and would result in wall stiffness being greater at the same cavity size than in the static situation. Inertial forces are probably negligible since the greatest outward acceleration of left ventricular wall observed in adult man occurs in patients with non-rheumatic mitral regurgitation, and is of the order of $0.35\,g$, corresponding to a reduction in pressure of less than 1 mmHg. The presence of viscous forces is still uncertain. An increase in wall stiffness during atrial systole when filling rates increase has been taken as evidence for their presence, but this conclusion assumes that the mechanism of ventricular filling at this time is identical to that earlier in diastole. It is also necessary that there is no significant change in pericardial pressure at this stage in the cardiac cycle, since the conclusion that the wall shows increased stiffness depends on the presence of a greater slope of the $\log_e P$–volume curve during atrial systole.

Yet another difficulty in determining left ventricular stress–strain relations is that significant changes in shape may occur during filling, the cavity being less spherical at end-systole than end-diastole, so that there is no fixed relation between volume changes and distension of the wall (Gibson and Brown, 1975b). The shape change during systole, as has been pointed out, is considerably less in patients with low ejection fraction, and also in those with local abnormalities of contraction. In these patients the ventricle may show increased stiffness when expressed in terms of pressure–volume relations because a greater part of the diastolic inflow has to be accommodated by distension of myocardium rather than by a change to a more spherical configuration. In these circumstances reduced compliance may be measured, although the properties of the ventricular myocardium itself could be normal.

In view of these difficulties it is not surprising that a number of other methods have been described in order to define the diastolic properties in intact man. The simplest of these is to measure the ratio $\Delta P/\Delta V$. ΔP is the difference between minimum and end-diastolic pressure, and ΔV is taken as stroke volume (Diamond and Forrester, 1972). Passive elastic modulus has been defined as the relation between this ratio and the mean diastolic pressure. Normal values of $\Delta P/\Delta V$ are in the range 0.015 to 0.12 mmHg/ml, while in patients with low stroke volume and high end-diastolic pressure after myocardial infarction, values of 0.28 to 1.3 mmHg/ml have been observed. Although this approach is a simple one, the entry of a significant amount of blood into the left ventricle before minimum pressure casts doubt on its validity, since stroke volume is not a measure of ΔV. This effect becomes progressively more significant as heart rate increases, with a relative reduction in filling period.

A second method, devised by Grossman et al (1973), measures the change in left ventricular pressure by micromanometer, and the change in cavity diameter by echocardiography during left atrial systole. Late diastolic stiffness, defined as the ratio between the two, was greater in patients with aortic stenosis (8.9 mmHg/mm increase in dimension), and low in mitral stenosis (1.5 mmHg/mm), its magnitude correlating with cardiographic evidence of left ventricular hypertrophy.

It is apparent from this discussion that diastolic filling of the left ventricle is a complex process and poorly understood. All current methods of study have severe limitations, and a more comprehensive description must await measurement of true transmural pressure gradients, more adequate methods of stress analysis in the wall, a greater understanding of changes in shape and fibre orientation with increase in cavity volume, and an adequate understanding of events during the early diastolic filling period.

ASSESSMENT OF CONTRACTILITY IN MAN

Much effort has been devoted to the determination of what is described as 'myocardial contractility', or the 'contractile state of the left ventricle' in man. This is based on the assumption that the extent of shortening of mammalian heart muscle, and therefore the stroke volume of the intact left ventricle is, in the final analysis, determined by three influences: the length of the muscle at the onset of contraction (the preload), the tension that the muscle is called upon to develop (the afterload), and the contractile state of the muscle (that is, the position on the force–velocity length curve) (Braunwald, Ross and Sonnenblick, 1967). In congestive heart failure, the fundamental abnormality is assumed to reside in depression of the myocardial length–active tension curve and the force–velocity relation, reflecting reductions in the contractile state of the myocardium. The objective of determination of contractility in man is thus to define the force–velocity curve and, in particular, to estimate V_{max}, the maximum velocity of shortening of contractile elements when the load against which they act is zero. This quantity is held to be independent of initial fibre length, and to be a unique measure of contractile state. It has the units s^{-1}, and thus the characteristics of a normalised velocity. In terms of V_{max}, therefore, impaired left ventricular function can, by definition, be due only to a reduction in the peak rate of shortening of the myocardial contractile elements.

In clinical practice, V_{max} is usually determined from the left ventricular pressure recorded during isovolumic systole, with a micromanometer (Mason, Spann and Zelis, 1970; Grossman et al, 1971). It is assumed that during this period, contractile element shortening causes corresponding lengthening of the series elastic component, with consequent development of tension within the wall (Taylor, 1970). The rate of development of tension can be used to estimate the rate of lengthening of the series elastic elements if their length–tension relation is known. As left ventricular pressure rises, values for the rate of increase of wall stress can be calculated from dP/dt with a knowledge of wall thickness and cavity dimensions, so that the rate of shortening of the contractile elements estimated at any left ventricular pressure, and a force–velocity curve constructed. V_{max} is estimated by extrapolation to the rate of shortening at zero wall stress, which corresponds to zero cavity pressure, regardless of cavity dimensions or wall thickness. It is possible thus to estimate V_{max} from pressure measurements alone, using the relation:

$$V_{max} = \frac{dP/dt}{kP + c}$$

where k is described as a stiffness constant, being dimensionless, while the intercept c is small, and usually neglected. P may be taken as cavity pressure, or 'developed' pressure, which represents cavity pressure minus end-diastolic pressure (Grossman et al, 1972).

This method may be considered from two points of view: whether it provides a valid measure of V_{max}, and whether it is of clinical value in separating patients with chronic impairment of myocardial function from those without.

From the first point of view, these measurements have been criticised on a number of grounds, referable to the definition of V_{max} in terms of heart muscle mechanics (Pollack, 1970; Noble, 1972). These will not be reviewed in detail, but in brief, there is no general agreement as to whether changes in contractile state are separable from those in preload, and the resulting measurements of maximum velocity are critically dependent on the muscle model employed. In the intact heart, it is assumed that no change in left ventricular dimension occurs between the onset of mechanical activity and the time of peak $dP/dt/P$. As has been stated above (Karliner et al, 1971), definite outward wall movement occurs during this period in normal subjects, and changes are accentuated in patients with left ventricular disease or mitral regurgitation. Secondly, determination of V_{max} involves extrapolation to zero pressure, but since the form of the force–velocity curve has not been defined in physical terms, there is no predetermined method as to how this extrapolation should be performed. Accordingly, linear, exponential, hyperbolic, polynomial, or simple manual methods have all been used, with corresponding loss of definition of the value of V_{max} itself (Peterson et al, 1974; Kreulen et al, 1975; Mirsky et al, 1974). A third factor is that k, the stiffness constant, is not measured directly, but instead, an arbitrary value is employed, frequently derived from animal data. Since abnormalities in the elastic properties of the ventricle might be anticipated in disease, this is clearly an unsatisfactory expedient. Reduced values of peak dP/dt and thus of calculated V_{max}, can clearly be due to causes other than impaired contractile element velocity:

incoordinate contraction or abnormal activation are obvious ones, and a single measurement of V_{max} cannot give any information about regional abnormalities of left ventricular function which have been shown to occur in all types of heart disease. Further, V_{max} takes no account of variation in fibre angle, or differences in either stress or shortening velocity across the thickness of the wall.

The use of V_{max} as an indicator of myocardial performance in man has been examined by a number of authors, in groups of patients with abnormal left ventricular function defined in terms of ejection fraction, raised end-diastolic pressure, and evidence of regional contractional abnormalities on angiography (Peterson et al, 1974; Kreulen et al, 1975). In these circumstances V_{max} appeared an insensitive method of separating patients with normal left ventricular function from those in whom it was depressed on these other criteria. This insensitivity was associated with a very wide range of values recorded in subjects with apparently normal left ventricular function, and was not reduced by performing studies at a fixed atrial pacing rate of 100/min. Since many of these patients had advanced and unequivocal left ventricular disease, it must be concluded that the use of V_{max} as an index of myocardial function cannot be supported on pragmatic, any more than on theoretical, grounds.

A second method of investigating left ventricular function depends on measurements of rates of wall movement during ejection, particularly those along the minor axis. As has been stated above, such measurements distinguish poorly between patients with normal and abnormal left ventricular function when expressed directly as cm/s. Their sensitivity, however, is greatly increased when they are normalised in terms of end-diastolic or instantaneous fibre length, and their performance in detecting left ventricular disease defined in terms of ejection fraction, raised end-diastolic pressure and local abnormalities of wall movement, is considerably superior to that of V_{max}. However, it must be pointed out that a normalised shortening velocity and a measurement of ejection fraction are both reduced by a low amplitude of wall movement and a large end-diastolic cavity size (Lewis and Sandler, 1971). It is not surprising, therefore, that there is good agreement between these two variables, since the features of impaired ventricular function that they reflect are so similar.

Ejection Fraction

Since ejection fraction is the single most widely used index of left ventricular function, it is difficult to obtain independent evidence as to its sensitivity, particularly as there is still no unequivocal basis on which an absolute measure of myocardial function can be defined. A number of lines of evidence have been used, however. Measurements of ejection fraction are closely related to prognosis in cardiomyopathy (Field et al, 1973) and valvular heart disease, and to survival after coronary artery surgery (Chatterjee et al, 1971; Collins et al, 1973; Bruschke, Proudfit and Sones, 1973). The range of normal values is clearly defined and remarkably constant between different studies. Reduced ejection fraction occurs in patients with specific types of myocardial disease, and forms the functional definition of congestive cardiomyopathy; however, it may be normal or even increased in the presence of severe heart muscle disease due to hypertrophic cardiomyopathy. It also gives no indication of the presence of incoordinate contraction and in such patients values derived from angiograms exposed in orthogonal planes may show considerable discrepancies between one another.

The reason for the sensitivity of ejection fraction is not clear. It is not a measure of contractility, as defined in acute experiments (Krayenbuehl et al, 1968). It is dimensionless, unlike measurements of contractility which have the dimensions of s^{-1}. Ejection fraction is affected variably by propranolol administration, while it is very sensitive to arterial pressure, volume loading (Liedtke et al, 1972), and a very wide beat-to-beat variation may occur in atrial fibrillation (Vogel and Adams, 1974). The most probable determinant of ejection fraction appears to be the size and architecture of the left ventricular cavity, although it clearly gives no information about regional abnormalities of contraction.

Left Ventricular End-diastolic Pressure

Left ventricular end-diastolic pressure is widely used as a non-specific index of left ventricular function (Rahimtoola, 1973). Initially, such elevation was explained in terms of the Frank–Starling law, a high end-diastolic pressure being held to reflect the presence of a high end-diastolic volume, and by analogy, with acute experiments in the heart–lung preparation; this in turn was associated with increased energy released at the subsequent contraction of the heart. This view is no longer tenable. There is no correlation in chronic heart disease between end-diastolic pressure and end-diastolic volume (Jones et al, 1964; Grant, Bunnell and Greene, 1965). Rackley et al (1970b) have demonstrated further that end-diastolic pressure is also independent of left ventricular mass, peak systolic pressure, stroke volume and ejection fraction. A raised end-diastolic pressure does not, therefore, give information about the systolic function of the ventricle.

It is possible that end-diastolic pressure might reflect diastolic abnormalities of the left ventricle. This question was considered by Braunwald and Ross (1963), who concluded that such information was, at best, indirect. As has been pointed out, it cannot be used to predict volume, even in individual patients, since large changes in volume may occur early in diastole with no change in pressure. Fluid overload may cause considerable increase in end-diastolic pressure in patients with normal left ventricular function (Eichna, 1960). End-diastolic pressure may also be affected by pericardial tamponade or constriction, infiltration of the myocardium, or thickening of the endo-cardium. Finally, end-diastolic pressure is heart-rate dependent and may be reduced by tachycardia induced by atrial pacing. It must therefore be concluded that end-diastolic pressure is not a measure of end-diastolic volume, and still less of end-diastolic fibre length. Although a raised value usually implies some abnormality of the left ventricle, it may also occur with fluid overload or pericardial disease, while normal values may be present with severe impairment of ventricular function.

CONCLUSION

Assessment of left ventricular function in clinical practice is complex. The most constant feature of the diseased left ventricle is an increase in cavity size out of proportion to the stroke volume, and a reduction in the amplitude of wall movement. This abnormality can be quantified by measurement of either ejection fraction or normalised rates of wall movement. A second process, which can be clearly distinguished from an increase in cavity size, is the presence of local abnormalities of contraction leading to incoordinate contraction, which is best assessed by angiography. It is possible that a reduced rate of contraction also occurs in patients with left ventricular disease, but this has not yet been established as occurring independently of structural abnormalities and incoordinate contraction.

It is probably premature to attempt to summarise the position with respect to diastolic abnormalities of the left ventricle. An increase in left ventricular stiffness, associated with abnormal filling, seems very likely, while disturbances in early diastole when filling is not passive are an additional possibility.

It seems likely that further progress will come from investigation of the many mechanisms involved in coordinate ventricular filling and ejection, which are unobtrusive when function is normal, but which may become apparent in the presence of disease. This approach seems more fruitful than one which attempts to impose a number of simplistic ideas on the understanding of what is a most highly organised and complex process.

REFERENCES

Alderman, E. L. & Glantz, S. A. (1976) Acute hemodynamic interventions shift the diastolic pressure–volume curve in man. *Circulation*, **54**, 662.

Alderman, E. L., Sandler, H., Brooker, J. Z., Sanders, W. J., Simpson, C. & Harrison, D. C. (1973) Light pen computer processing of video image for the determination of left ventricular volume. *Circulation*, **47**, 309.

Altieri, P. I., Wilt, S. M. & Leighton, R. F. (1973) Left ventricular wall motion during the isovolumic relaxation period. *Circulation*, **48**, 499.

Arvidsson, H. (1961) Angiographic determination of left ventricular volume. *Acta radiologica*, **56**, 321.

Barry, W. H., Brooker, J. Z., Alderman, E. L. & Harrison, D. C. (1974) Changes in diastolic stiffness and tone of the left ventricle during angina pectoris. *Circulation*, **49**, 255.

Bennett, E. D., Else, W., Miller, G. A. H., Sutton, G. C., Miller, H. C. & Noble, M. I. M. (1974) Maximum acceleration of blood from the left ventricle in patients with ischaemic heart disease. *Clinical Science and Molecular Medicine.* **46**, 49.

Bom, N., Lancée, C. T., van Zweiten, G., Kloster, F. E. & Roelandt, J. (1973) Multiscan echocardiography. I. Technical description. *Circulation,* **48**, 1066.

Braunwald, E. & Ross, J., Jr (1963) The ventricular end-diastolic pressure; appraisal of its value in the recognition of ventricular failure in man. *American Journal of Medicine,* **34**, 147.

Braunwald, E., Ross, J., Jr & Sonnenblick, E. H. (1967) Mechanisms of contraction in the normal and failing heart. *New England Journal of Medicine,* **277**, 1012.

Brecher, G. A. (1958) Critical review of recent work on ventricular diastolic suction. *Circulation Research,* **6**, 554.

Bristow, J. D., Crislip, R. L., Farreh, I., Harris, W. E., Lewis, R. P., Sutherland, D. W. & Griswold, H. E. (1964) Left ventricular volume measurements in man by thermodilution. *Journal of Clinical Investigation,* **43**, 1015.

Brown, O. R., Popp, R. L. & Harrison, D. C. (1973) Abnormal interventricular septal motion in patients with significant disease of the left anterior descending coronary artery (Abs). *American Journal of Cardiology,* **31**, 123.

Bruschke, A. V. G., Proudfit, W. L. & Sones, F. M., Jr (1973) Progress study of 590 consecutive non-surgical cases of coronary artery disease, followed 5–9 years. III. Ventriculographic and other correlates. *Circulation,* **47**, 1154.

Burton, A. C. (1957) The importance of the shape and size of the heart. *American Heart Journal,* **54**, 801.

Carleton, R. A. (1971) Changes in left ventricular volume during angiocardiography. *American Journal of Cardiology,* **27**, 460.

Chaitman, B. R., Bristow, J. D. & Rahimtoola, S. H. (1973) Left ventricular wall motion assessed by using fixed external reference systems. *Circulation,* **48**, 1043.

Chapelle, M. & Mensch, B. (1969) Etude des variations du diamètre ventriculaire gauche chez l'homme par échocardiographie transthoracique. *Archives des maladies du coeur et des vaissaux,* **62**, 1505.

Chatterjee, K., Sacoor, M., Sutton, G. C. & Miller, G. A. H. (1971) Angiographic assessment of left ventricular function in patients with ischaemic heart disease without clinical heart failure. *British Heart Journal,* **33**, 559.

Chatterjee, K., Swan, H. J. C., Parmley, W. W., Sustaita, H., Marcus, H. S. & Matloff, J. (1973) Influence of direct myocardial revascularisation on left ventricular asynergy and function in patients with coronary artery disease. *Circulation,* **47**, 276.

Chow, C. K. & Kaneko, T. (1972) Automatic boundary detection of the left ventricle from cineangiograms. *Computers and Biomedical Research,* **5**, 388.

Cohn, P. F., Gorlin, R., Adams, D. F., Chahine, R. A., Vokonas, P. S. & Herman, M. L. (1974) Comparison of biplane and single plane left ventriculograms in patients with coronary artery disease. *American Journal of Cardiology,* **33**, 331.

Collins, J. J., Jr, Cohn, L. H., Sonnenblick, E. H., Herman, M. V., Cohn, P. F. & Gorlin, R. (1973) Determinants of survival after coronary artery bypass surgery (abstract). *Circulation,* **48**, III-132.

Cooper, R. H., O'Rourke, R. A., Karliner, J. S., Peterson, K. L. & Leopold, G. R. (1972a) Comparison of ultrasound and cineangiographic measurements of the mean rate of circumferential fibre shortening in man. *Circulation,* **46**, 914.

Cooper, R., Karliner, J. S., O'Rourke, R. A., Peterson, K. L. & Leopold, G. R. (1972b) Ultrasound determinations of mean fiber shortening rate in man. *American Journal of Cardiology,* **29**, 251.

Coltart, D. J., Alderman, E. L., Robison, S. C. & Harrison, D. C. (1975) Effect of propranolol on left ventricular function, segmental wall motion and diastolic pressure–volume relation in man. *British Heart Journal,* **37**, 357.

Covvey, H. D. J., Adelman, A. G., Felderhof, C. H., Taylor, K. W. & Wigle, E. D. (1972) Television/computer dimensional analysis interface with special reference to left ventricular cineangiograms. *Computers in Biology and Medicine,* **2**, 221.

Davila, J. C. & San Marco, M. E. (1966) Analysis of the fit of mathematical models applicable to the measurement of left ventricular volume. *American Journal of Cardiology,* **18**, 31.

Diamond, G., Forrester, J. S., Hargis, J., Parmley, W. W., Danzig, R. & Swan, H. J. C. (1971) Diastolic pressure–volume relationship in canine left ventricle. *Circulation Research*, **39**, 267.

Diamond, G. & Forrester, J. S. (1972) Effect of coronary artery disease and acute myocardial infarction on left ventricular compliance in man. *Circulation*, **40**, 11.

Diamond, M. A., Dillon, J. C., Haine, C. L., Chang, S. & Feigenbaum, H. (1971) Echo-cardiographic features of atrial septal defect. *Circulation*, **43**, 129.

Dodge, H. T., Hay, R. E. & Sandler, H. (1962) Pressure–volume characteristics of the dia-stolic left ventricle of man with heart disease. *American Heart Journal*, **64**, 503.

Dodge, H. T., Sandler, H., Baxley, W. A. & Hawley, R. R. (1966) Usefulness and limitations of radiographic methods for determining left ventricular volumes. *American Journal of Cardiology*, **18**, 10.

Dodge, H. T., Sandler, H., Ballew, D. W. & Lord, J. D. (1960) The use of biplane angiography for measurement of left ventricular volume in man. *American Heart Journal*, **60**, 762.

Dodge, H. T. & Sandler, H. (1974) *Clinical Applications of Angiocardiography* in *Myocardial Mechanics*, ed. Mirsky, I., Ghista, D. N. & Sandler, H. New York: John Wiley.

Dumesnil, J. G., Ritman, E. L., Frye, R. L., Gau, G. T., Rutherford, E. D. & Davis, G. D. (1974) Quantitative determination of regional left ventricular wall dynamics by roentgen videometry. *Circulation*, **50**, 700.

Eber, L. M., Greenberg, H. M., Cooke, J. M. & Gorlin, R. (1969) Dynamic changes in left ventricular free wall thickness in the human heart. *Circulation*, **39**, 455.

Eichna, L. W. (1960) Circulatory congestion or heart failure. *Circulation*, **22**, 864.

Falsetti, H. L., Mates, R. E., Grant, C., Greene, D. G., Bunnell, I. L. (1970) Left ventricular wall stress calculated from one-plane angiography: an approach to force–velocity analysis in man. *Circulation Research*, **26**, 71.

Feigenbaum, H. (1973) *Echocardiography*. New York: Henry Kimpton.

Feigenbaum, H., Popp, R. L., Chip, J. N. & Haine, C. L. (1968) Left ventricular wall thick-ness measured by ultrasound. *Archives of Internal Medicine*, **121**, 391.

Feigenbaum, H., Wolfe, S. B., Popp, R. L., Haine, C. L. & Dodge, H. T. (1969) Correlation of ultrasound and angiocardiography in measuring left ventricular volume (abstract). *American Journal of Cardiology*, **23**, 111.

Field, B. J., Baxley, W. A., Russell, R. O., Hood, W. P., Holt, J. H., Dowling, J. T. & Rackley, C. E. (1973) Left ventricular function and hypertrophy in cardiomyopathy with depressed ejection fraction. *Circulation*, **47**, 1022.

Fogelman, A. M., Abbasi, A. S., Pearce, M. L. & Kattus, A. A. (1972) Echocardiographic study of abnormal motion of the posterior left ventricular wall during angina pectoris. *Circulation*, **46**, 905.

Fortuin, N. J., Hood, W. P. & Craige, E. (1972) Evaluation of left ventricular function by echocardiography. *Circulation*, **46**, 26.

Frimer, M., Porter, C. M. G., Rackley, C. E. & Dodge, H. T. (1969) Left ventricular chamber geometry and function in heart disease. *Circulation*, **46**, Supplement III, 85.

Gaasch, W. H., Battle, W. E., Oboler, A. A., Banas, J. S., Jr & Levine, H. J. (1972) Left ventricular stress and compliance in man: with special reference to normalised ventricular function curves. *Circulation*, **45**, 746.

Gaasch, W. H., Cole, J. S., Quinones, M. A. & Alexander, J. K. (1975) Dynamic determinants of left ventricular pressure–volume relations in man. *Circulation*, **51**, 317.

Gaasch, W. J., Peterson, K. L. & Shabetai, R. (1974) Left ventricular function in chronic constrictive pericarditis. *American Journal of Cardiology*, **34**, 107.

Gault, J. H., Ross, J., Jr & Braunwald, E. (1968) Contractile state of the left ventricle in man: instantaneous tension–velocity–length relations in patients with and without disease of the left ventricular myocardium. *Circulation Research*, **22**, 451.

Ghista, D. N., Patil, K. M., Gould, P. & Woo, K. B. (1973) Computerised left ventricular mechanics and control system analyses models relevant for cardiac diagnosis. *Computers in Biology and Medicine*, **3**, 27.

Ghista, D. N. & Sandler, H. (1969) Analytic model for the shape and forces in the left ventricle. *Journal of Biomechanics*, **2**, 35.

Gibson, D. G. (1972) Disordered left ventricular contraction associated with abnormalities of conduction: an echocardiographic study. *Postgraduate Medical Journal*, **48**, 756.

Gibson, D. G. (1973) Estimation of left ventricular size by echocardiography. *British Heart Journal*, **35**, 128.

Gibson, D. G. & Brown, D. J. (1973) Measurement of instantaneous left ventricular dimension and filling rate in man using echocardiography. *British Heart Journal*, **35**, 1141.

Gibson, D. G. & Brown, D. J. (1974) Relation between diastolic left ventricular wall stress and strain in man. *British Heart Journal*, **36**, 1066.

Gibson, D. G. & Brown, D. J. (1975a) Measurement of peak rates of left ventricular wall movement in man: comparison of echocardiography with angiocardiography. *British Heart Journal*, **37**, 677.

Gibson, D. G. & Brown, D. J. (1975b) Continuous assessment of left ventricular shape in man. *British Heart Journal*, **37**, 904.

Gibson, D. G. & Brown, D. J. (1976) Assessment of left ventricular systolic function in man from simultaneous echocardiographic and pressure measurements. *British Heart Journal*, **38**, 8.

Gibson, D. G., Prewitt, T. A. & Brown, D. J. (1976) Analysis of left ventricular wall movement during isovolumic relaxation and its relation to coronary artery disease. *British Heart Journal*, **38**, 1010.

Gleason, W. L. & Braunwald, E. (1962) Studies on the first derivative of the ventricular pressure pulse in man. *Journal of Clinical Investigation*, **41**, 80.

Gooch, A. S., Vicencio, F., Maranhao, V. & Goldberg, H. (1972) Arrhythmias and left ventricular asynergy in the prolapsing mitral leaflet syndrome. *American Journal of Cardiology*, **29**, 611.

Gould, K. L., Lipscomb, K., Hamilton, G. W. & Kennedy, J. W. (1974) Relation of left ventricular shape, function and wall stress in man. *American Journal of Cardiology*, **34**, 627.

Grant, C., Bunnell, I. L. & Greene, D. (1965) Left ventricular enlargement and hypertrophy. A clinical and angiographic study. *American Journal of Medicine*, **39**, 895.

Grant, R. P. (1953) Architectonics of the heart. *American Heart Journal*, **46**, 405.

Grant, R. P. (1965) Notes on the muscular architecture of the left ventricle. *Circulation*, **32**, 301.

Greene, D. G., Carlisle, R., Grant, C. & Bunnell, I. L. (1967) Estimation of left ventricular volume from one-plane cineangiography. *Circulation*, **35**, 61.

Greenleaf, J. F., Ritman, E. L., Coulam, C. M., Sturm, R. E. & Wood, E. H. (1972) Computer graphic techniques for the study of temporal and spatial relationships of multi-dimensional data derived from biplane roentzen videograms with particular reference to cardioangiography. *Computers and Biomedical Research*, **5**, 368.

Griffith, J. M. & Henry, W. L. (1973) Videoscanner analogue computer system for semi-automatic analysis of routine echocardiograms. *American Journal of Cardiology*, **32**, 961.

Griffith, J. M. & Henry, W. L. (1974) A sector scanner for real time two-dimensional echo-cardiography. *Circulation*, **49**, 1147.

Grimm, A. F., Katele, K. V., Kubota, R. & Whitehorn, W. V. (1970) Relation of sarcomere length and muscle length in resting myocardium. *American Journal of Physiology*, **218**, 1412.

Grossman, W., Brodie, B., Mann, T. & McLaurin, L. (1975) Effects of sodium nitroprusside on left ventricular pressure–volume relations (abstract). *Circulation*, **52**, Supplement II, 35.

Grossman, W., Brooks, H., Meister, S., Sherman, H. & Dexter, L. (1971) A new technique for determining instantaneous myocardial force–velocity relations in the intact heart. *Circulation Research*, **28**, 290.

Grossman, W., Brooks, H., Meister, S., Sherman, H. & Dexter, L. (1972) Alterations in preload and myocardial mechanics in the dog and man. *Circulation Research*, **31**, 83.

Grossman, W., Stefadouros, M. A., McLaurin, L. P., Rolett, E. L. & Young, D. T. (1973) Quantitative assessment of left ventricular diastolic stiffness in man. *Circulation*, **47**, 567.

Hamby, R. I., Aintablian, A., Tabrah, F., Reddy, K. & Wisoff, G. (1974) Late systolic bulging of the left ventricle in patients with angina pectoris. *Chest*, **65**, 169.

Hamilton, G. W., Murray, J. A. & Kennedy, J. W. (1972) Quantitative angiography in ischemic heart disease; spectrum of abnormal left ventricular function and the role of abnormally contracting segments. *Circulation*, **45**, 1065.

Hammermeister, K. E., Brooks, R. C. & Warbasse, J. R. (1974) The rate of change of left ventricular volume in man. I. Validation and peak systolic ejection rate in health and disease. *Circulation*, **49**, 729.

Harvey, W. (1628) *De motu cordis et sanguinis*. Translated Willis (1907) London: Everyman Dent.

Heikkilä, J. & Nieminen, M. (1975) Echoventriculographic detection, localisation and quantification of left ventricular asynergy in acute myocardial infarction: a correlative echo- and electrocardiographic study. *British Heart Journal*, **37**, 46.

Heintzen, P. H. (1971) *Roetgen-, Cine- and Video-densitometry: Fundamentals and Applications for Blood Flow and Heart Volume Determinations*. Stuttgart: Georg Thieme Verlag.

Helfant, R. H., Herman, M. V. & Gorlin, R. (1973) Abnormalities of left ventricular contraction induced by beta-adrenergic blockade. *Circulation*, **63**, 641.

Herman, M. V. & Gorlin, R. (1969) Implications of left ventricular asynergy. *American Journal of Cardiology*, **23**, 538.

Holt, J. P., Rhode, E. A. & Kines, H. (1960) Pericardial and ventricular pressure. *Circulation Research*, **8**, 1171.

Hood, W. P., Rackley, C. E. & Rolett, E. L. (1968) Wall stress in normal and hypertrophied left ventricle. *American Journal of Cardiology*, **22**, 550.

Hood, W. P. & Rolett, E. L. (1969) Patterns of contraction in the human left ventricle (abstract). *Circulation*, **40**, Supplement III, 109.

Horwitz, L. D. & Bishop, V. S. (1972) Left ventricular pressure–dimension relationships in the conscious dog. *Cardiovascular Research*, **6**, 163.

Inoue, K., Smulyan, H., Moukherjee, S. & Eich, R. (1971) Ultrasonic measurement of left ventricular wall motion in acute myocardial infarction. *Circulation*, **43**, 778.

Jacobs, J. J., Feigenbaum, H., Corya, B. C. & Phillips, J. F. (1973) Detection of left ventricular asynergy by echocardiography. *Circulation*, **48**, 263.

Janz, R. F. & Grimm, A. F. (1972) Finite element model for the mechanical behavior of the left ventricle. *Circulation Research*, **30**, 244.

Jean, C. F., Streeter, D. D. & Reichenbach, D. D. (1972) Fiber orientation in the normal and hypertensive cadaver left ventricle (abstract). *Circulation*, **46**, II–44.

Johnson, S. A., Robb, R. A., Greenleaf, J. F., Ritman, E. L., Lee, S. L., Herman, G. T., Sturm, R. E. & Wood, E. H. (1974) The problem of accurate measurement of left ventricular shape and dimension from multiplane roentgenographic data. *European Journal of Cardiology*, **1**, 247.

Jones, J. W., Rackley, C. E., Bruce, R. A., Dodge, H. T. & Sandler, H. (1964) Left ventricular volumes in valvular heart disease. *Circulation*, **29**, 887.

Karliner, J. S., Bouchard, R. J. & Gault, J. H. (1971) Dimensional changes of the human left ventricle prior to aortic valve opening. *Circulation*, **44**, 312.

Karliner, J. S., Bouchard, R. J. & Gault, J. S. (1972) Haemodynamic effects of angiographic contrast material in man: a beat by beat analysis. *British Heart Journal*, **34**, 347.

Karliner, J. S., Gault, J. H., Eckberg, D., Mullins, C. B. & Ross, J., Jr (1971) Mean velocity of fiber shortening: a simplified measure of left ventricular myocardial contractility. *Circulation*, **44**, 323.

Katz, L. N. (1930) The role played by the ventricular relaxation in filling of the ventricle. *American Journal of Physiology*, **95**, 542.

Keith, A. (1918) Functional anatomy of the heart. *British Medical Journal*, **1**, 361.

Kennedy, J. W., Baxley, W. A., Figley, M. M., Dodge, H. T. & Blackmon, J. R. (1966) Quantitative angiocardiography: the normal left ventricle in man. *Circulation*, **34**, 272.

Kennedy, J. W., Reichenbach, D. D., Baxley, W. A. & Dodge, H. T. (1967) Left ventricular mass: a comparison of angiocardiographic measurements with autopsy weight. *American Journal of Cardiology*, **19**, 221.

King, D. L. (1973) Cardiac ultrasonography: cross-sectional imaging of the heart. *Circulation*, **47**, 843.

Kisslo, J., von Ramm, O. T. & Thurstone, F. L. (1976) Cardiac imaging using a phased array ultrasound system. II. Clinical technique and application. *Circulation*, **53**, 262.

Kloster, F. E., Roelandt, J., Cate, F. J., Bom, N. & Hugenholtz, P. (1974) Multiscan echocardiography. II. Technique and initial clinical results. *Circulation*, **48**, 1075.

Krayenbuehl, H. P., Bussman, W. D., Turina, M. & Luthy, E. (1968) Is the ejection fraction an index of myocardial contractility? *Cardiology*, **53**, 1.

Kreulen, T., Bove, A. A., McDonough, M. T., Sands, M. J. & Spann, J. F. (1975) The evaluation of left ventricular function in man: a comparison of methods. *Circulation*, **51**, 677.

Kreulen, T., Gorlin, R. & Herman, M. V. (1973) Ventriculographic patterns and hemo-dynamics in primary myocardial disease. *Circulation*, **47**, 299.

Leighton, R. F., Wilt, S. M. & Lewis, R. P. (1974) Detection of hypokinesis by a quantitative analysis of left ventricular cineangiograms. *Circulation*, **50**, 114.

Lewis, R. P. & Sandler, H. (1971) Relationship between left ventricular dimensions and the ejection fraction in man. *Circulation*, **44**, 548.

Liedtke, A. J., Pasternac, A., Sonnenblick, E. H. & Gorlin, R. (1972) Changes in canine ventricular dimensions with acute changes in preload and afterload. *American Journal of Physiology*, **223**, 820.

Linzbach, A. J. (1960) Heart failure from the point of view of quantitative anatomy. *American Journal of Cardiology*, **5**, 370.

Love, A. E. H. (1888) On the small free vibrations and deformations of thin elastic shells. *Philosophical Transactions of the Royal Society*, **17A**, 491.

Ludbrook, P., Karliner, J. S., Peterson, K., Leopold, G. & O'Rourke, R. A. (1973) Com-parison of ultrasound and cineangiographic measurements of left ventricular performance in patients with and without wall motion abnormalities. *British Heart Journal*, **35**, 1026.

McDonald, I. G. (1970) The shape and movement of the human left ventricle during systole: a study by cineangiography of epicardial markers. *American Journal of Cardiology*, **26**, 221.

McDonald, I. G. (1972) Contraction of the hypertrophied left ventricle in man studied by cineangiography of epicardial markers. *American Journal of Cardiology*, **30**, 587.

McDonald, I. G., Feigenbaum, H. & Chang, S. (1972) Analysis of left ventricular wall motion by reflected ultrasound: application to assessment of myocardial function. *Circulation*, **46**, 14.

McLaurin, L. P., Rolett, E. L. & Grossman, W. (1973) Impaired left ventricular relaxation during pacing-induced ischemia. *American Journal of Cardiology*, **32**, 751.

Marcus, M. L., Schuette, W. H., Whitehouse, W. C., Baxley, J. J. & Glancy, D. L. (1972) Automated method for the measurement of left ventricular volume. *Circulation*, **45**, 65.

Mason, D. T. (1969) Usefulness and limitations of the rate of rise of intraventricular pressure in the evaluation of myocardial contractility in man. *American Journal of Cardiology*, **23**, 516.

Mason, D. T., Spann, J. F. & Zelis, R. (1970) Quantification of the contractile state of the intact human heart. Maximal velocity of contractile element shortening determined by the instantaneous relation between the rate of rise of pressure and pressure in the left ventricle during isovolumic systole. *American Journal of Cardiology*, **26**, 248.

Miller, G. A. H. & Swan, H. J. C. (1964) Effects of chronic pressure and volume overload on left heart volumes in subjects with congenital heart disease. *Circulation*, **30**, 205.

Mirsky, I. (1969) Left ventricular stresses in the intact human heart. *Biophysical Journal*, **9**, 189.

Mirsky, I. (1976) Assessment of passive elastic stiffness of cardiac muscle. Mathematical concepts, physiologic and clinical considerations, directions of future research. *Progress in Cardiovascular Diseases*, **18**, 277.

Mirsky, I. & Parmley, W. W. (1973) Assessment of passive elastic stiffness for isolated heart muscle and the intact heart. *Circulation Research*, **33**, 233.

Mirsky, I., Pasternac, A., Ellison, R. C. & Hugenholtz, P. (1974) Clinical applications of force–velocity parameters and the concept of a 'normalised velocity'. In *Cardiac Mechanics*, ed. Mirsky, I., Ghista, D. & Sandler, H. New York: John Wiley.

Mirsky, I., Cohn, P. F., Levine, J. A., Gorlin, R., Herman, M. V., Kreulen, T. & Sonnenblick, E. H. (1975) Assessment of left ventricular stiffness in primary myocardial disease and coronary artery disease. *Circulation*, **50**, 128.

Mitchell, J. H., Wildenthal, K. & Mullins, C. B. (1969) Geometrical studies of the left ventricle utilizing biplane cineangiography. *Federation Proceedings*, **28**, 1334.

Nelson, C. N. & Lipchik, E. O. (1966) A computer method for calculation of left ventricular volume from biplane angiocardiograms. *Investigative Radiology*, **1**, 139.

Noble, M. I. M. (1972) Editorial: Problems concerning the application of muscle mechanics to the determination of the contractile state of the heart. *Circulation*, **45**, 252.

Noble, M. I. M., Milne, E. N. C., Goerke, R. J., Carlsson, E., Domenech, R., Saunders, K. B. & Hoffman, J. I. E. (1969) Left ventricular diastolic filling and diastolic pressure–volume relation in the conscious dog. *Circulation Research*, **24**, 269.

Paley, H. W., McDonald, I. G. & Weissler, A. M. (1964) The relationship of left ventricular circumferential contraction to left ventricular ejection time as an inotropic index (Abstract). *Clinical Research*, **12**, 191.

Paraskos, J. A., Grossman, W., Saltz, S., Dalen, J. E. & Dexter, L. (1971) A non-invasive technique for the determination of velocity of circumferential shortening in man. *Circulation Research*, **29**, 610.

Peterson, K. L., Skloven, D., Ludbrook, P., Utmer, J. B. & Ross, J., Jr (1974) Comparison of isovolumic and ejection phase indices of myocardial performance in man. *Circulation*, **49**, 1088.

Pollack, G. H. (1970) Maximum velocity as an index of contractility in cardiac muscle—a critical evaluation. *Circulation Research*, **26**, 111.

Popp, R. L., Wolfe, S. B., Hirata, T. & Feigenbaum, H. (1969) Estimation of right and left ventricular size by echocardiography. A study of echoes from the interventricular septum. *American Journal of Cardiology*, **24**, 523.

Quinones, M. A., Gaasch, W. H., Cole, J. S. & Alexander, J. K. (1975) Echocardiographic determination of left ventricular stress–strain relations in man, with reference to the effects of loading and contractility. *Circulation*, **51**, 689.

Rackley, C. E., Dodge, H. T., Coble, Y. D., Jr & Hay, R. E. (1964) A method for determining left ventricular mass in man. *Circulation*, **29**, 666.

Rackley, C. E., Hood, W. P., Jr, Cleveland, L. & Stacy, R. W. (1968) Derivation of cardiac mechanical parameters from serial biplane angiograms. *Journal of Applied Physiology*, **24**, 254.

Rackley, C. E., Frimer, M., Porter, C. M. & Dodge, H. T. (1970a) Left ventricular shape in chronic heart disease (abstract). *Circulation*, **42**, III–67.

Rackley, C. E., Hood, W. P., Jr, Rolett, E. L. & Young, D. T. (1970b) Left ventricular end-diastolic pressure in chronic heart disease. *American Journal of Medicine*, **48**, 310.

Rahimtoola, S. H., Duffy, J. P. & Swan, H. J. C. (1967) Ventricular performance after angiocardiography. *Circulation*, **35**, 70.

Rahimtoola, S. H. (1973) Left ventricular end-diastolic and filling pressures in the assessment of left ventricular function. *Chest*, **63**, 858.

Rees, G., Bristow, J. W., Kremkav, E. L., Green, G. S., Herr, R. H., Griswold, H. L. & Starr, A. (1971) Influence of aortocoronary bypass surgery on left ventricular performance. *New England Journal of Medicine*, **284**, 1116.

Rushmer, R. F. (1956) Initial phase of ventricular systole: asynchronous contraction. *American Journal of Physiology*, **184**, 188.

Rushmer, R. F. & Crystal, D. K. (1951) Changes in the configuration of the ventricular chambers during the cardiac cycle. *Circulation*, **4**, 211.

Rushmer, R. F., Crystal, D. K. & Wagner, C. W. (1953) The functional anatomy of ventricular contraction. *Circulation Research*, **1**, 162.

Ruttley, M. S., Adams, D. F., Cohn, P. F. & Abrams, H. L. (1974) Shape and volume changes during 'isovolumetric relaxation' in normal and asynergic ventricles. *Circulation*, **50**, 306.

Sandler, H. & Alderman, E. L. (1974) Determination of left ventricular size and shape. *Circulation Research*, **34**, 1.

Sandler, H. & Dodge, H. T. (1963) Left ventricular tension and stress in man. *Circulation Research*, **13**, 191.

Sandler, H. & Dodge, H. T. (1968) The use of single plan angiocardiograms for the calculation of left ventricular volume in man. *American Heart Journal*, **75**, 325.

Sharp, J. T., Bunnell, I. L., Holland, J. F., Griffith, G. T. & Greene, D. G. (1960) Hemodynamics of induced cardiac tamponade in man. *American Journal of Medicine*, **29**, 640.

Sjögren, A. L., Hytonen, I. & Frick, M. H. (1970) Ultrasonic measurement of left ventricular wall thickness. *Chest*, **57**, 37.

Streeter, D. D., Jr & Bassett, D. L. (1966) Engineering analysis of myocardial fiber orientation in pig's left ventricle during systole. *Anatomical Record*, **155**, 503.

Streeter, D. D., Jr & Hanna, W. T. (1973) Engineering mechanics for successive states in canine left ventricular myocardium. *Circulation Research*, **33**, 639.

Sutton, M. St J. & Gibson, D. (1975) Measurement of postoperative pericardial pressure in man (abstract). *British Heart Journal*, **37**, 780.

Taylor, R. (1970) Theoretical basis of the isovolumic phase of left ventricular contraction in terms of cardiac muscle mechanics. *Cardiovascular Research*, **4**, 429.

Teicholtz, L. E., Herman, M. V. & Gorlin, R. (1972) Problems in echocardiographic volume determinations: echoangiographic correlation (Abstract). *Circulation*, **46**, II–75.

Troy, B. L., Pombo, J. & Rackley, C. E. (1972) Measurement of left ventricular wall thickness and mass by echocardiography. *Circulation*, **45**, 602.

Upton, M. T., Gibson, D. G. & Brown, D. J. (1976) Echocardiographic assessment of abnormal left ventricular relaxation in man. *British Heart Journal*, **38**, 1001.

Vogel, J. H. K. & Adams, N. (1974) Non-invasive ventricular function curves—instability of systolic ejection fraction (EF) (Abstract). *Clinical Research*, **22**, 113A.

Vokonas, P. S., Gorlin, R., Cohn, P. F., Herman, M. V. & Sonnenblick, E. H. (1973) Dynamic geometry of the left ventricle in mitral regurgitation. *Circulation*, **48**, 787.

von Ramm, O. T. & Thurstone, F. L. (1976) Cardiac imaging using a phased array ultrasound system. I. System design. *Circulation*, **53**, 258.

Wilcken, D. E. (1965) Load, work and velocity of muscle shortening of the left ventricle in normal and abnormal human hearts. *Journal of Clinical Investigation*, **44**, 1295.

Wilson, C. S., Krueger, S., Forker, A. D. & Weaver, W. F. (1975) Correlation between segmental early relaxation at the left ventricle and coronary artery disease. *American Heart Journal*, **89**, 474.

Wong, A. Y. K. & Rautaharju, P. M. (1968) Stress distribution within the left ventricular wall approximated as a thick ellipsoidal shell. *American Heart Journal*, **75**, 649.

Zienkiewicz, O. C. (1967) *Finite Element Method in Structural and Continuum Mechanics*. New York: McGraw-Hill.

13
MYOCARDIAL BIOPSY

E. G. J. Olsen

Examination of fresh biological tissue has become routine practice in many specialised fields of medicine. Open or closed biopsy techniques have been applied to organs or tissue such as liver, kidney, lung, pleura, lymph nodes, gastrointestinal tract and prostate.

As far as the heart is concerned, probably because of its inherent nature and the risk of complications, biopsy investigations have tended to lag behind. Despite sophisticated modern techniques of non-invasive investigations, examination of fresh myocardium together with endocardium or pericardium, is often essential to establish a firm diagnosis.

The indications to undertake such a procedure, and the value such a biopsy can yield diagnostically, include infiltrative, metabolic or degenerative conditions of the heart. The most important disease process where biopsy can yield helpful information is that of cardiomyopathy. Not only will biopsy help to establish a diagnosis, but it may also help us to understand the pathogenesis and the underlying cause or causes of these conditions.

Methods of Obtaining Myocardial Biopsies

Many methods have been devised to achieve recovery of fresh myocardial tissue. They have been reported in the literature on the experimental animal or in combination with patients after preliminary testing with animals. Some workers reported their experience on human material alone.

Requirements. Whatever method might be chosen, Bulloch, Murphy and Pearce (1965) summarised the criteria for routine use of any biopsy technique; this included reliability, ease of performance, low morbidity and essentially no mortality. Casten and Marsh (1953), after 10 days' preparatory partial rib resection and anchoring the apex of the heart, subsequently obtained myocardial specimens from dogs, employing a Vim–Silverman needle. This procedure permitted repeated biopsies. In order to avoid possible complications, such as puncturing coronary arteries, irritation of the myocardium or perforation of the ventricles, Sutton, Sutton and Kent (1956) undertook a preliminary investigation in dogs. Thin-walled, highly flexible modified Vim–Silverman needles of varying diameters were inserted into the myocardium under direct vision. This study was then extended to patients, using a percutaneous approach. A further report on 54 patients, using a Terry needle followed (Sutton and Sutton, 1960). Percutaneous needle puncture methods, using modified Vim–Silverman needles or Menghini needles have also been reported by Bercu et al (1964) (using the technique described by Brock, Milstein and Ross (1956)), Timmis et al (1965) and Hirose and Bailey (1965). More recently, Frantsev et al (1972) employed experimentally a transcutaneous method in dogs, using a Hausser needle. Shirey et al (1972), using a thin-walled Silverman needle, described their experience on 254 percutaneous punch biopsies performed in 198 patients.

Catheter biopsy techniques employing a corkscrew type device have been explored experimentally by Dotter (1964), and a catheter-sheathed curved needle containing a retractable cutting device was developed by Bulloch, Murphy and Pearce (1965), and had been successfully applied to dogs and humans. Bulloch et al (1972) employed a technique to investigate 20 patients with cardiomyopathy; 12 of these suffered from idiopathic and 8 from 'alcoholic cardiomyopathy'. A drill biopsy device, introducing a modified Ross transseptal needle through the superior vena cava or carotid artery, has been developed by Leighton et al (1967).

Direct Approaches

Since the report on the percutaneous technique by Sutton and Sutton (1960), exploratory mediastinotomy was considered more valuable than the percutaneous approach (Weinberg et al, 1963; Sutton et al, 1964). A special thin-walled needle was used to recover the myocardial tissue. This technique was an extension of that used by Weinberg, Fell and Lynfield (1958), employing a partial extrapleural resection method, and excising surgically a small area of heart muscle. Raffensperger et al (1964) summarised the total experience of 108 patients who had undergone myocardial biopsy by a variety of techniques.

At thoracotomy, Braimbridge and Niles (1964) found that biopsy material by Vim–Silverman or Menghini needles yielded unsatisfactory results. Resection of a small piece of myocardial tissue left a ragged hole, and they therefore devised a rotatory drill to recover such tissue. At open heart surgery, before and after perfusion, full thickness drill biopsy was obtained by Björk and Hultquist (1967), and can be used to assess the state of the myocardium (Braimbridge, 1970).

Another manner in which fresh endomyocardial tissue could be obtained was that of open surgical operation, where resection of cardiac muscle formed part of the surgical procedure, as in patients suffering from hypertrophic cardiomyopathy with obstruction (Cleland, 1963; Bentall et al, 1965; Morrow et al, 1968, 1971; Cleland et al, 1969). These larger amounts of tissue had been analysed histologically, histochemically and ultrastructurally (van

Noorden, Olsen and Pearse, 1971; Olsen, 1971, 1972a, b; Ferrans, Morrow and Roberts, 1972).

Endocardial Biopsy by Bioptome

A major advance in obtaining myocardial biopsies was achieved by Sakakibara and Konno (1962) and Konno and Sakakibara (1963) by employing an instrument, the bioptome, which permitted fresh endomyocardial tissue to be obtained by using the usual routes of catheterisation, without serious risk to the patient. This method of investigation is gaining world-wide application. The instrument consists of an intracardiac catheter, 100 or 110 cm in length, an operating handle and a cutting claw at the exploring end. These cutting claws consist of two elliptical cups or spoons, the concave aspects facing each other, and are operated by a double hinge mechanism. Control from the operating end is achieved by a wire which runs within the Teflon-covered catheter shaft. The size of the cups in common use measure $2.5 \times 2 \times 1$ mm; larger cups which measure 3.5 mm in diameter are also available.

Since the original bioptome, clinical experience and preference of individual operators has led to modifications of the original instrument, using or modifying other instruments originally devised for other uses. Ali (1974) has used the GFB gastrointestinal catheter (Olympus), which closely resembles the Konno bioptome, but lacks the Teflon sleeve covering of the shaft and has only one 'knurled knob' to fasten the sliding mechanism controlling the cups. The shaft measures 130 cm in length and is 2 mm in diameter. The spoon measurements are 2.5 mm in diameter and 2 mm in depth.

Richardson (1974a) modified the Olympus fibreoptic bronchoscope biopsy forceps, BF5B2. The shaft measures 105 cm and the jaws in the closed position measure only 1.8 mm. The FBIC model has now been modified and is covered with Teflon. The instrument, the 'King's bioptome', has many advantages, which include easier introduction of the catheter into the vessel, greater flexibility and fewer mechanical problems in the operating of the cups and handle (Richardson, 1975).

Another instrument, a modification of the Konno's bioptome, has been described by Caves et al (1974a). The shaft of the biopsy forceps is shorter than the three previously described instruments, measuring only 50 cm in length. The operating handle has been replaced by surgical forceps, which includes a ratchet, permitting locking of the jaw. The flexible spiral wire of the catheter is covered with shrink tubing. The jaws have a span of 2.5 mm in the open position, and are operated on a single hinge mechanism, one jaw being fixed, the other mobile. Each cup measures 1.5 mm in diameter. Also included are Teflon stoppers preventing seepage of blood beneath the catheter tubing.

Although the percutaneous route to obtain myocardial tissue often yielded sufficient material for pathological assessment, Sutton et al (1964) found the approach via a thoracotomy more valuable. Such an approach has the advantages that inspection of pericardium and palpation of coronary arteries can be undertaken. The risk of anaesthesia and surgical operation, though small, exists.

Complications using the percutaneous approach are rare, but nevertheless significant. These include the postpericardiotomy syndrome (Peter et al, 1966; Shirey et al, 1972). The latter authors also described cardiac tamponade and ventricular fibrillation.

The success rate of recovery using needle biopsy techniques has been 76 per cent (Sutton and Sutton, 1960), and 60 per cent (Timmis et al, 1965), compared to 100 per cent with the Konno bioptome (Sakakibara and Konno, 1966) or its modification (Ali, 1974). Somers et al (1971) reported a success rate of only 80 per cent with the Konno bioptome, and the authors suggested that initial excess caution and inexperience accounted for the high failure rate.

It would therefore appear that the bioptome technique is superior to previous devices that have been used to obtain myocardial biopsies. Whichever bioptome is employed, these instruments have become more widely used. Originally the technique was extensively applied by the Japanese workers (Konno and Sakakibara, 1963; Sekiguchi and Konno, 1969; Konno, Sekiguchi and Sakakibara, 1971). More recently this technique and interpretation of material has been reported from other countries, which include Uganda (Somers et al, 1971), West Germany (Harmjanz et al, 1971), East Germany (Müller, Müller and Richter, 1971), France (Kin et al, 1973), Sweden (Torp, 1973), USA (Ali et al, 1973; Ali, 1974; Caves et al, 1974b), and Great Britain (Richardson, 1974a; Olsen, 1974a, b, 1975a; MacKay, Littler and Sleight, 1974; Brooksby et al, 1975; Peters, Bloomfield and Oakley, 1975).

Indications

Although the technique is safe in experienced hands, this method of investigation should only be applied if serious clinical doubt exists as to the cause for the patient's symptomatology (Olsen, 1975b). No helpful results can be expected if, for example, clinical examination and non-invasive laboratory investigations suggest septal defects, valve disease or systemic hypertension, as in all these instances hypertrophy of myocardial fibres, with or without fibrous tissue increase, will be found. If, however, the patient suffers from heart failure, and other intracardiac disease can be excluded, congestive cardiomyopathy seems a likely diagnosis, but myocarditis or possible small vessel disease cannot be ruled out. Degenerative or infiltrative diseases may also be the underlying cause. It is in these circumstances that biopsy has proved of great value.

Any patient considered well enough for cardiac catheterisation, can undergo the biopsy procedure by means of the bioptome. No special preparation of the patients is necessary; sedatives or local anaesthesia may be used (Somers et al, 1971; Konno et al, 1971; Caves et al, 1975). The use of anticoagulants in cases of left ventricular biopsies has been discontinued (Konno et al, 1971).

Most of the published literature on the results of the bioptome investigation deals with pathological evaluation of predominantly right ventricular samples.

Technique of Biopsy

The routes chosen for entering the cardiac chambers are, in the majority of instances, those of catheterisation, using arm or leg veins (Somers et al, 1971; Torp, 1973; Ali, 1974; Richardson, 1974b, 1975; Harmjanz, 1975). Preferences of the route chosen have been documented by individual operators. In patients where left atrial and left ventricular material is deemed necessary, a transseptal approach is used via the right saphenous vein or retrograde arterial catheterisation via the right femoral, or carotid or brachial arteries. Long sheath techniques for introducing the bioptome into the left ventricle transseptally or by an arterial approach have been described by Konno et al (1971), Brooksby et al (1974) and Richardson (1974b). Caves et al (1974b, 1975) used the right internal jugular vein routinely.

Whichever approach is used, the progress of the tip of the bioptome with the cups in the closed position, is followed fluoroscopically, and is advanced towards a suitable position on the ventricular wall. Once this is reached, the instrument is withdrawn for a short distance to permit unimpeded opening of the cups, and the bioptome is again advanced until the instrument is bent slightly. Once this has been achieved, the jaws are vigorously closed and the instrument is rapidly withdrawn (Richardson, 1975) (Fig. 13.1a–d). The action of the Caves–Schulz bioptome and the King's instrument is diagrammatically shown in Fig. 13.2.

Electrocardiographic monitoring and intracardiac recordings form an important part of the procedure (Ali, 1974; Richardson, 1975; Caves et al, 1975). Injury potential with marked ST elevation indicates contact of the bioptome with the myocardial wall. Absence of this finding indicates that contact with the ventricular wall has not been achieved, and although the bioptome may appear to be in the right ventricle, it may be in the anterior cardiac vein or coronary sinus (Richardson, 1975).

Whichever bioptome technique is employed, each biopsy usually measures 2 to 3 mm in diameter, and wet weights of 3 to 16 mg have been recorded (Torp, 1973). Two to five biopsies are usually taken from each chamber during the procedure.

Examination of Specimen

The methods of preparation for light and electron-microscopic examination are fairly standard. The methods employed in the writer's laboratory will be briefly summarised.

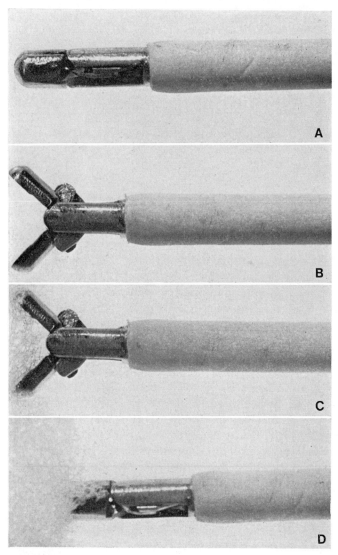

Figure 13.1   Close-up view of the exploring end of the King's bioptome. (a) Cups closed (as during advancement), (b) cups open (in readiness to take biopsy), (c) cups open (pressed against wall (foam rubber)), (d) cups closed (specimen enclosed in cups)

For histological and histochemical evaluation, the biopsies are plunged into melting 'Freon' (BOC), or Arcton (ICI), precooled in liquid nitrogen, and stored at $-70\,^\circ$C. Subsequently, 5 μm thick sections are cut and stained with haematoxylin and eosin and Weigert's elastic van Gieson. Histochemical evaluation includes that for glycogen, succinic dehydrogenase, acid and alkaline phosphatase. For ultrastructural examination fixation in 3 per cent buffered gluteraldehyde solution at 4°C, which is replaced by buffered sucrose washing solution (4°C, pH 7.4) and postfixation with 1 per cent osmium tetroxide, is carried out. The tissue is finally embedded in Epon. Sections 50 nm thick are cut and stained with uranyl acetate and lead citrate.

Variations exist in the scope of parameters examined, strength of fixing fluid and methods of embedding. Björk and Hultquist (1967) for example,

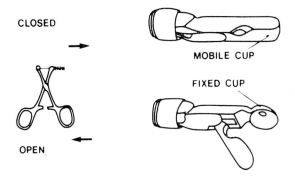

KING'S ENDOMYOCARDIAL BIOPTOME

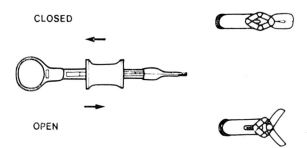

Figure 13.2 Diagrammatic representation of action of the Caves–Schulz bioptome (upper part of the illustration), and the King's instrument. (By kind permission of the author and Editors, Richardson, P. J. (1974) *Biochemical Engineering*, **9**, 353–355)

included phosphotungstic-acid–haematoxylin stain, and histochemical examination included phosphatase, β-hydroxybutarate, glutamate and cytochrome oxidase. Other investigations such as noradrenergic nerve fibre fluorescence, employing the method of Falck and Torp (1961) have also been used (Torp, 1973).

Diagnostic Value of the Biopsy

The samples obtained usually permit patterns of myocardial cell arrangement, the presence of increased connective tissue, small vessels and endocardium, to be assessed. They are also of sufficient size to show specific lesions. A typical biopsy is illustrated in Fig. 13.3.

In most published papers, all, or a considerable number of patients, were suspected of having a form of cardiomyopathy (Sekiguchi and Konno, 1969, 1971; Somers et al, 1971; Torp, 1973; Ali, 1974; Sekiguchi, 1974; Olsen, 1974a, 1975a; MacKay et al, 1974). Confusion in the use of the term 'cardio-myopathy' exists. The definition of 'heart muscle disease of unknown cause or association' (Oakley, 1972, 1975) and restriction of this term to the group previously known as 'primary cardiomyopathy' (Goodwin, 1973), has gained widespread acceptance. (The term 'secondary cardiomyopathy' should be replaced by 'specific heart muscle disease'.) A useful working classification of

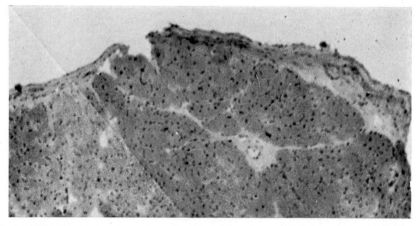

Figure 13.3 Photomicrograph of part of a right ventricular biopsy showing thickened endocardium containing smooth muscle fibres, mildly hypertrophied myocardial fibres and vessels. From a patient suspected to suffer from congestive cardiomyopathy. Haematoxylin and eosin, × 64

cardiomyopathy, according to the myocardial fault and functional distinctions (Goodwin, 1974; Oakley, 1974, 1975) is:

(a) congestive or dilated forms,
(b) hypertrophic obstructive or non-obstructive forms,
(c) restrictive, and
(d) obliterative forms (Löffler's endocarditis parietalis fibroplastica or endomyocardial fibrosis).

Pathological differences for groups (a), (b) and (d) exist, while the rare group (c) is, in pathological terms, less well defined.

The pathological and ultrastructural recognition of these various forms of cardiomyopathy, particularly that of the hypertrophic group, have been previously well established (Teare, 1958; van Noorden et al, 1971; Olsen,

1971, 1972a, b, c; Ferrans et al, 1972; Davies, Pomerance and Teare, 1974) on postmortem or surgically removed tissue.

The pathological criteria previously established have been strictly applied to the material obtained by the bioptome (Olsen, 1974a).

The endomyocardial material has so far largely been utilised for diagnostic purposes (Sekiguchi and Konno, 1969; Somers et al, 1971; Torp, 1973; Olsen, 1974a, b, 1975; MacKay et al, 1974; Richardson et al, 1974; Brooksby et al, 1975) and in the majority of instances the material has come from the right ventricle. It has also enabled Sekiguchi and Konno (1971) to formulate another classification of primary myocardial disease.

The author of this chapter has reported his experience of the material from 121 patients[1] (received principally from five centres in London or Europe), 81 of whom were suspected to suffer from a form of cardiomyopathy (Olsen, 1974b), and has analysed material with emphasis on the useful information that can be obtained on pathological examination. Every patient had a right

Table 13.1 Biopsies from patients with suspected cardiomyopathy

Presumed clinical diagnosis	Total no.	Confirmed	Excluded	Unhelpful pathological results	Failed biopsy
Congestive cardiomyopathy	60	26	14	12	8
Hypertrophic cardiomyopathy	17	5	7	5	0
Obliterative cardiomyopathy	4	2	1	0	1
	81	33	22	17	9
	Per cent	41	27	21	11

ventricular biopsy and in addition, left ventricular sampling was undertaken in 18 cases. The material was examined without knowledge of age, sex, history or suspected clinical diagnosis. After the pathological findings were reported, discussion with the referring physician permitted the results to be tabulated (Olsen, 1974a) under one of the following four headings:

1. Suspected clinical diagnosis confirmed.
2. Suspected clinical diagnosis or diagnoses excluded.
3. Unhelpful result.
4. Failed biopsies.

The findings have been summarised in Tables 13.1 and 13.2; the latter lists the suspected clinical diagnoses other than cardiomyopathy.

The evidence suggests that in nearly 70 per cent of patients, helpful information was obtained. The yield of helpful pathological results would be higher if the suspected disease process is widespread, such as congestive

[1]At the time of writing the total number of patients has increased to over 200.

cardiomyopathy, and frequently in cases of myocarditis, or where the position of the cardiac abnormality can be accurately located as, for example, in hypertrophic cardiomyopathy with obstruction, or intracardiac tumours. Less helpful results will be found if the suspected disease processes are scattered through the myocardium as, for example, in sarcoidosis, but even in this disease, positive results may be obtained.

The failure rate is substantial. Included in the figure of failed biopsy in the above tables are those cases where the diagnostic component was lacking (for example, suspected endomyocardial fibrosis where no endocardium had been included), even though a good myocardial biopsy had been obtained. Excessive

Table 13.2   Other groups

Presumed clinical diagnosis	Total no.	Confirmed	Excluded	Unhelpful pathological results	Failed biopsy
Myocarditis	16	3	13	0	0
Cardiac tumour	4	1	3	0	0
Alcoholic 'cardiomyopathy'	8	1	0	7	0
Rheumatic	3	0	2	0	1
Mitral insufficiency	2	0	0	1	1
Amyloid	2	1	1	0	0
Sarcoid	2	0	2	0	0
Myxoedema	1	1	0	0	0
Atrial septal defect	1	0	0	1	0
Myocardial fibrosis	1	0	1	0	0
	40	7	22	9	2
	Per cent	17.5	55	22.5	5

caution and inexperience may add initially to this failure rate (Somers et al, 1971).

Damage Artefact

A hazard besetting all biopsy material, especially needle biopsies, is that of damage artefact around the edges of the biopsy. In all personally examined biopsies obtained with the bioptome, these artefacts have been minimal. At light microscopic level, pinching of cells has occasionally been observed (Fig. 13.4) and separation of cells involving one or two superficial layers has also been seen occasionally. At electron-microscopic level, contraction bands and occasional disruption of mitochondria near the periphery have also been found (Fig. 13.5). Provided the material is treated as described above, the severe artefacts obtained by using the modified cork borer (Eckner et al, 1967) were not found.

Most of the reported results of bioptome investigation deal with right ventricular samples. Some reports have, however, concentrated on comparing left and right ventricular biopsies, investigating the superiority of one to the other (Richardson et al, 1975; Brooksby et al, 1975). Whether left ventricular biopsy is superior would, of course, depend on the underlying disease process from which the patient is suspected to suffer. In cases of congestive cardiomyopathy, both left and right ventricles are equally affected, and therefore biopsy from either ventricle would be valuable. In cases of hypertrophic

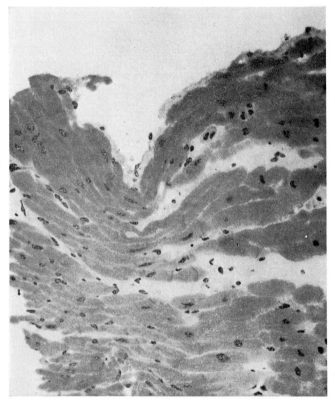

Figure 13.4 Photomicrograph of part of an endomyocardial biopsy showing 'pinch' artefact. Haematoxylin and eosin, ×160

cardiomyopathy, left ventricular sampling might be superior, but the right ventricular biopsy has also yielded positive results (see Table 13.1). In the series of Brooksby et al (1975) patients suffering from aortic valve disease, cardiomyopathy, or rheumatic heart disease, were included in their study of 20 patients in whom left and right ventricular biopsies were compared. Conspicuous histopathological differences existed in 59 per cent of these patients. In an analysis on 15 patients undergoing biventricular biopsy, no major histopathological, histochemical or ultrastructural differences were found between the right and left ventricles (Richardson et al, 1975), but the selection of patients was restricted to those in whom cardiomyopathy was the suspected diagnosis. Left ventricular biopsy is obviously preferable if the cardiac disease is predominantly left sided.

Other Uses of Biopsies

Cardiac transplantation. The use of the bioptome has also been extended to other parameters of clinical diagnosis. Caves et al (1973) had shown in animal

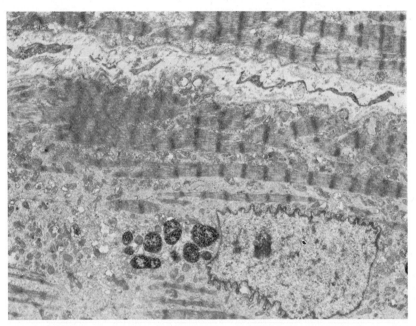

Figure 13.5 Electron micrograph of myocardium obtained by bioptome showing contraction banding. Note the regular arrangement of myofibrils, the patchy increase of mitochondria and lipofuscin granules. From a patient with suspected congestive cardiomyopathy. Lead citrate and uranyl acetate, × 5000

experiments that acute rejection is clinically recognisable by a reduction in the voltages of the electrocardiograph. Similar changes have also been observed in man (Griepp et al, 1971). The technique of serial biopsies has been used on orthotopically transplanted canine hearts, from which it had been learned that histological changes precede significant electrocardiographic changes by 24 to 48 h (Caves et al, 1973). By applying the information gained from these experiments, Caves et al (1974b) have studied 16 patients who had undergone cardiac transplantation. Serial biopsies have been undertaken in 12 of these patients, examining altogether 223 biopsy specimens, and involving a total of 119 biopsy procedures: 37 prerejection episodes were found, 35 of which were successfully reversed by adjusting the dosage of immunosuppressive drugs. Histological studies of biopsies in 11 long-term cardiac transplant survivors have demonstrated, for the first time, that healthy cardiac transplant recipients can have normal histology for up to three years (Caves et al, 1975).

So far the discussion has concentrated on the use of the material for diagnostic purposes. The potential value does not, however, end there.

Assessment of myocardial function. Peters et al (1975) are undertaking biochemical studies on cardiomyopathic tissue, using as controls myocardial tissue obtained at open heart surgery. Ultrasensitive assays have been established for marker enzymes of the main structures of the myocardial cells, such as plasma membrane (5′-nucleotidase, Na^+,K^+-activated ATPase), lysosome (N-acetyl-β-glucosaminidase, cathepsin D,β-glucosidase, acid α-glucosidase), mitochondrion (cytochrome oxidase, malate dehydrogenase, glutamate dehydrogenase, monoamine oxidase), microsome (neutral α-glucosidase), myofibrils (Ca^{2+}-activated ATPase) and cytosol (lactate dehydrogenase). No differences from right and left ventricles in controls or myopathic cardiac tissue have been found as far as assays of microsomal, lysosomal or plasma membrane enzymes are concerned. A reduction in the levels of mitochondrial dehydrogenases and of myofibrillary azide-resistant Ca^{2+}-activated ATPase was found in patients with suspected cardiomyopathy and with poor left ventricular function. Levels of cytosol lactate dehydrogenase were elevated in myopathic heart tissue. Work is in progress to study these changes further.

Virological studies. Another useful approach to utilise fresh endomyocardial tissue is virological investigation in cases of congestive cardiomyopathy, where such a possible aetiology had been suggested (Goodwin, 1964; Gardner et al, 1967). So far serology and tissue culture for viruses have been negative (MacKay et al, 1974; Waterson, 1975).

Effects of drugs. This method of investigation can also be employed to study the effect of drugs on the myocardium, without increased risk to the patient. Klein and Harmjanz (1975) have studied the influence of a moderate dose of ethanol on the ultrastructure of the myocardium in six patients with myocardial and valvular disease. Samples of endomyocardial tissue were obtained with the Konno bioptome before and after infusion. Following infusion, mitochondrial swelling, less dense mitochondrial matrix and dilatation of the sarcoplasmic reticulum were found. Lipid droplets were also seen in two out of the six patients who had suffered from chronic alcoholism.

Reliability of Biopsy Findings

In other fields, such as renal and hepatic disease, biopsies from these organs have shown that representative areas are often obtained, and the question arises whether the small amounts of tissue which are recovered by the bioptome technique reflect the changes that may be present in the heart.

The ultimate confirmation can only be found at necropsy, but only a small number of cases has been reported. None of the described cases died as a result of the bioptome investigation.

Sekiguchi and Konno (1971) reported 15 necropsy cases. Good correlation was found between the diagnosis by biopsy and the postmortem examination. The author has personal experience of one patient, and reports on two other patients who subsequently died elsewhere. The necropsy result confirmed the previously suggested diagnosis made on biopsy material.

The site of the biopsy is usually not found (Somers et al, 1971). Caves et al (1974b) were also not able to locate the site from which the biopsy had been obtained in four out of five patients.

Confirmation on biopsy material has also been obtained at surgical operation in a few cases of hypertrophic obstructive cardiomyopathy and intracardiac tumour (Olsen, 1975, personal observations). Although the number of cases in whom the diagnosis could be confirmed is small, the reported information available suggests that good correlation is obtained.

Complications

It has already been mentioned in this chapter that the investigation with the bioptome is a safe procedure. This also applies to the catheter approach employed by Bulloch et al (1972) where 50 patients were biopsied with the catheter sheathed needle bearing a retractable cutting device. No significant morbidity and no mortality occurred. No complications in 90 patients biopsied with the Konno bioptome have been reported by Harmjanz (1975). Konno et al (1971) and Sekiguchi et al (1972/73) also reported no serious complications in over 500 patients, varying in age between four months and 64 years. During manipulation, no special sensation is experienced by the patient, but in two instances sudden chest pain was felt at the time the myocardium was punched. Premature beats during left ventricular biopsy occasionally occurred just after the instrument had passed through the aortic valve.

Somers et al (1971) also stated that the bioptome procedure is without hazard. One or two ventricular ectopic beats at the time of taking the biopsy may occur, but this is unusual.

No mortality related to the procedure and no serious morbidity was also reported by Caves et al (1974b). Small right-sided pneumothoraces occurred after biopsy in three patients, using the approach via the right internal jugular vein. Isolated premature ventricular contraction usually occurred during the procedure when the biopsy instrument was in contact with the right ventricular endocardium. Persistent atrial flutter was found in one patient.

Richardson (1975) reported in one patient supraventricular tachycardia which produced left ventricular failure, necessitating electroversion. Other complications included short runs of atrial fibrillation, multiple ventricular premature contractions, and chest discomfort of short duration. Very occasionally was pericardial pain experienced, but in two instances was associated with a pericardial rub. (Over 100 patients have now been biopsied.) Brooksby et al (1975) reported on complications in over 100 patients biopsied; these consisted of insignificant haemopericardium in two patients, and ventricular tachycardia requiring electroversion in one patient.

The complications reported above are relatively minor and compare favourably with those experienced by the various forms of needle biopsy techniques.

Conclusions

The evidence suggests that this safe procedure is of value, permitting establishment of a diagnosis where clinical doubt had existed. It has also been clearly established that this method of investigation is of great value in combating acute rejection in transplant patients, permitting early drug adjustment. The analysis of the fresh endomyocardial tissue extends now to biochemical, immunological and viral studies, which will include an immunoperoxidase technique (Waterson, 1975). This line of investigation will offer prospects of information on pathogenesis, treatment, and thus prevention in many fields of cardiology, but particularly those of cardiomyopathy, where the aetiology is often obscure.

The bioptome technique fulfils the criteria of Bulloch et al (1965) which were noted at the beginning of this chapter (p. 349), in that the method is reliable, it is easy to perform, the morbidity is low and there is essentially no mortality. It is hoped that the procedure will continue to be increasingly used throughout the world.

ADDENDUM

At the time of going to press the author's experience of endomyocardial biopsies obtained by bioptome has increased to over 350 patients (355). The evidence suggested that in 70 per cent information helpful to the physician could be obtained on morphological examination, and that this aspect of analysis of the biopsy material is valuable and should continue (Olsen, 1977).

Since writing this chapter, a number of reports on endomyocardial biopsies by bioptome technique have appeared in the literature; for example, from Germany Kuhn et al (1975) reported on 25 patients suspected to suffer from congestive cardiomyopathy. These workers emphasised improvement of the diagnosis of congestive cardiomyopathy after biopsy examination, and clinico-morphological correlation. In six of their patients, changes suspicious of myocarditis or storage disease were encountered. In one patient, Coxsackie virus B3 was isolated from the biopsy material. The authors have also applied a system, awarding points on the electronmicroscopic changes, permitting an assessment of prognosis.

Regarding assessment of prognosis, Bouhour et al (1976) reporting on 38 patients with congestive cardiomyopathy, pointed out that caution should be exercised.

Petitier et al (1976) reported on biopsies from 94 patients, of whom 47 were suffering from congestive cardiomyopathy. These authors did not attempt to establish a morphological diagnosis of congestive cardiomyopathy, but commented on an index of histological and ultrastructural severity of the lesions encountered. They also emphasised the value of biopsy examination in cases of hypertrophic cardiomyopathy and subaortic stenosis.

The value of enzymatic analysis of cardiac biopsy material was reported by Peters and co-workers (1976), investigating patients with valvular heart disease by left ventricular endomyocardial biopsies, and correlating their findings with left ventricular function. In those patients with poor function, myofibrillar calcium dependent adenosine-triphosphatase was strikingly decreased, and lactic dehydrogenase significantly increased.

REFERENCES

Ali, N. (1974) Transvenous endomyocardial biopsy using the gastrointestinal biopsy (Olympus GFB) catheter. *American Heart Journal*, **87**, 294–297.

Ali, N., Ferrans, V. J., Roberts, W. C. & Massumi, R. A. (1973) The clinical evaluation of transvenous catheter technique for endomyocardial biopsy. *Chest*, **63**, 399–402.

Bentall, H. H., Cleland, W. P., Oakley, C. M., Shah, P. M., Steiner, R. E. & Goodwin, J. F. (1965) Surgical treatment and postoperative haemodynamic studies in hypertrophic obstructive cardiomyopathy. *British Heart Journal*, **27**, 585–594.

Bercu, B., Heinz, J., Choudhry, A. & Cabrera, P. (1964) Myocardial biopsy. *American Journal of Cardiology*, **14**, 675–678.

Björk, V. O. & Hultquist, G. (1967) Ultrastructural, enzyme histochemical and light microscopic investigation of the myocardium in cases undergoing open-heart surgery. *Scandinavian Journal of Thoracic and Cardiovascular Surgery*, **1**, 27–41.

Braimbridge, W. V. (1970) Communication at the *VIth International Congress of Cardiology*, London.

Braimbridge, W. V. & Niles, N. R. (1964) Left ventricular drill biopsy. *Journal of Thoracic and Cardiovascular Surgery*, **47**, 685–686.

Brock, R., Milstein, B. B. & Ross, D. N. (1956) Percutaneous left ventricular puncture in the assessment of aortic stenosis. *Thorax*, **11**, 163–171.

Brooksby, I. A. B., Swanton, R. H., Jenkins, B. S. & Webb-Peploe, M. M. (1974) Long sheath technique for introduction of catheter tip manometer or endomyocardial bioptome into left or right heart. *British Heart Journal*, **36**, 908–912.

Brooksby, I., Jenkins, S., Coltart, J., Webb-Peploe, M. & Davies, M. (1975) Myocardial biopsy: description of technique, comparison of right and left ventricular biopsy (Abstract) *British Heart Journal*, **37**, 555.

Bulloch, R. T., Murphy, M. L. & Pearce, M. B. (1965) Intracardiac needle biopsy of the ventricular septum. *American Journal of Cardiology*, **16**, 227–233.

Bulloch, R. T., Pearce, M. B., Murphy, M. L., Jenkins, B. J. & Davis, J. L. (1972) Myocardial lesions in idiopathic and alcoholic cardiomyopathy. Study by ventricular septal biopsy. *American Journal of Cardiology*, **29**, 15–25.

Casten, G. G. & Marsh, J. B. (1953) Metabolic studies on cardiac tissue obtained by needle biopsy in the intact unanesthetised dog. *Circulation Research*, **1**, 226–229.

Caves, P. K., Billingham, M. E., Schulz, W. P., Dong, E., Jr & Shumway, N. E. (1973) Transvenous biopsy from canine orthotopic heart allografts. *American Heart Journal*, **85**, 525–530.

Caves, P. K., Schulz, W. P., Dong, E., Jr, Stinson, E. B. & Shumway, N. E. (1974a) New instrument for transvenous cardiac biopsy. *American Journal of Cardiology*, **33**, 264–267.

Caves, P. K., Stinson, E. B., Billingham, M. E. & Shumway, N. E. (1974b) Serial transvenous biopsy of the transplanted human heart. Improved management of acute rejection episodes. *Lancet*, **1**, 821–826.

Caves, P., Coltart, J., Billingham, M., Rider, A. & Stinson, E. (1975) Transvenous endomyocardial biopsy—application of a method for diagnosing heart disease. *Postgraduate Medical Journal*, **51**, 286–290.

Cleland, W. P. (1963) The surgical management of obstructive cardiomyopathy. *Journal of Cardiovascular Surgery*, **4**, 489–491.

Cleland, W. P., Goodwin, J. F., McDonald, L. & Ross, D. (1969) In *Medical and Surgical Cardiology*, pp. 951–978. Oxford and Edinburgh: Blackwell Scientific Publications.

Davies, M. J., Pomerance, A. & Teare, R. D. (1974) Pathological features of hypertrophic obstructive cardiomyopathy. *Journal of Clinical Pathology*, **27**, 529–535.

Dotter, C. T. (1964) Catheter biopsy. *Radiology*, **82**, 312–314.

Eckner, F. A. O., Thaemert, J. C., Moulder, P. V. & Blackstone, E. H. (1967) Myocardial biopsy in dogs. *Circulation*, **36**, 964–974.

Falck, B. & Torp, A. (1961) A fluorescence method for histochemical demonstration of noradrenalin in the adrenal medulla. *Medicina Experimentalis (Basel)*, **5**, 429–432.

Ferrans, V. J., Morrow, A. G. & Roberts, W. C. (1972) Myocardial ultrastructure in idiopathic hypertrophic stenosis. A study of operatively excised left ventricular outflow tract muscle in 14 patients. *Circulation*, **45**, 769–792.

Frantsev, V. I., Kalikshtein, D. B., Odinokova, V. A., Bogomazov, Yu. I., Bezmenova, E. V., Rybalkina, M. S. & Banina, V. B. (1972) On the transcutaneous puncture biopsy of the myocardium. *Eksperimental 'naya Khirurgiya Anestesial. Moskva*, **17**, 21–24.

Gardner, M. B., Lee, P. V., Norris, J. C., Phillips, E. & Caponegro, P. (1967 Letter): Viruslike particles in cardiac biopsy. *Lancet*, **2**, 95–96.

Goodwin, J. F. (1964) Cardiac function in primary myocardial disorders. *British Medical Journal*, **1**, 1527–1533.

Goodwin, J. F. (1973) Primary myocardial disease. Spectrum of cardiomyopathy and current classification. *Singapore Medical Journal*, **14**, 358–362.

Goodwin, J. F. (1974) Prospects and predictions for the cardiomyopathies. *Circulation*, **50**, 210–219.

Griepp, R. B., Stinson, E. B., Dong, E., Jr, Clark, D. A. & Shumway, N. E. (1971) Acute rejection of the allografted human heart. *Annals of Thoracic Surgery*, **12**, 113–126.

Harmjanz, D. (1975) Problems of myocardial biopsy. *Postgraduate Medical Journal*, **51**, 291–292.

Harmjanz, D., Reale, E., Luciano, L. & Ostertag, P. (1971) Die Endomyokardbiopsie als Hilfsmittel in der Diagnostik von Myokarderkrankungen. Presented at 77 Tagung der Deutschen Gesellschaft für Innere Medizin, April 22. Cited by Sekiguchi, M. (1974) *Journal of Molecular and Cellular Cardiology*, **6**, 111–122.

Hirose, T. & Bailey, C. P. (1965) New myocardial biopsy needle. *Angiology*, **16**, 288–291.

Kin, G., Combes, S., Miray, D. & Grosgogeat, Y. (1973) La biopsie endomyocardique. Technique, résultats et indications. *Nouvelle Presse Médicale*, **2**(46), 3117–3120.

Klein, H. & Harmjanz, D. (1975) Effect of ethanol infusion on the ultrastructure of human myocardium. *Postgraduate Medical Journal*, **51**, 325–329.

Konno, S. & Sakakibara, S. (1963) Endomyocardial biopsy. *Diseases of the Chest*, **44**, 345–350.

Konno, S., Sekiguchi, M. & Sakakibara, S. (1971) Catheter biopsy of the heart. *Radiologic Clinics of North America*, **IX**, 491–510.

Leighton, R. F., Hamlin, R. L., Scarpelli, D. G. & Weissler, A. M. (1967) Drill biopsy of the canine interventricular septum. A new catheterisation technic. *American Journal of Cardiology*, **19**, 365–371.

MacKay, E. H., Littler, W. A. & Sleight, P. (1974) Assessment of value of catheter biopsy of the heart (Abstract). *British Heart Journal*, **36**, 404.

Morrow, A. G., Fogarty, T. J., Hannah, H., III & Braunwald, E. (1968) Operative treatment in idiopathic hypertrophic subaortic stenosis. *Circulation*, **37**, 589–596.

Morrow, A. G., Epstein, S. E., Rodgers, B. M. & Braunwald, E. (1971) Idiopathic, hypertrophic subaortic stenosis: a current assessment of the results of operative treatment in
hypertrophic obstructive cardiomyopathy. *Ciba Foundation Study Group*, No. 37, ed.
Wolstenholme, G. E. W. & O'Connor, M., pp. 140–149. London: J. & A. Churchill.

Müller, S. A., Müller, P. & Richter, G. (1971) Herzbiopsie mit Katheter-Bioptom. *Zeitschrift
fur die Gesamte Innere Medizin*, **36**, 107–113.

Oakley, C. M. (1972) Clinical definition and classification of cardiomyopathies. *Postgraduate
Medical Journal*, **48**, 703–713.

Oakley, C. M. (1974) Clinical recognition of the cardiomyopathies. *Circulation Research*, **35**,
Suppl. 2, 152–167.

Oakley, C. M. (1975) The relation between function and causation in cardiomyopathy.
Postgraduate Medical Journal, **51**, 271–276.

Olsen, E. G. J. (1971) Morbid anatomy and histology. *Ciba Foundation Study Group*, No. 37,
ed. Wolstenholme, G. E. W. & O'Connor, M., pp. 183–191. London: J. & A. Churchill.

Olsen, E. G. J. (1972a) Cardiomyopathies. In Clinical–pathologic correlations, 1. *Cardiovascular Clinics*, ed. Edwards, J. E. & Brest, A. W., Vol. 4, pp. 240–261. Philadelphia:
Davis, Co.

Olsen, E. G. J. (1972b) Pathology of primary cardiomyopathies. *Postgraduate Medical
Journal*, **48**, 732–737.

Olsen, E. G. J. (1972c) Histochemical, ultrastructural and structural changes in primary
cardiomyopathy and in cobalt cardiomyopathy. *Postgraduate Medical Journal*, **48**,
760–762.

Olsen, E. G. J. (1974a) Diagnostic value of the endomyocardial bioptome. *Lancet*, **1**, 658–660.

Olsen, E. G. J. (1974b) Cardiomyopathies. Pathological information from cardiac biopsies.
Presented at the *VIIth World Congress of Cardiology*, Buenos Aires, September 1974.

Olsen, E. G. J. (1975a) Results of endomyocardial biopsy: histological, histochemical and
ultrastructural analysis. *Postgraduate Medical Journal*, **51**, 295–297.

Olsen, E. G. J. (1975b) Diagnostic value of the endomyocardial bioptome (Annotation).
American Heart Journal, **91**, 398–399.

Peter, R. H., Whalen, R. E., Orgain, E. S. & McIntosh, H. D. (1966) Postpericardiotomy
syndrome as a complication of percutaneous left ventricular puncture. *American Journal
of Cardiology*, **17**, 86–90.

Peters, T. J., Bloomfield, F. J. & Oakley, C. M. (1975) Biochemical studies on biopsies from
normal and diseased cardiac tissue (Abstract). *Postgraduate Medical Journal*, **51**, 298.

Raffensperger, J., Driscol, J. F., Sutton, G. C. & Weinberg, M., Jr (1964) Myocardial biopsy.
Archives of Surgery (*Chicago*), **89**, 1021–1023.

Richardson, P. J. (1974a) King's endomyocardial bioptome. *Lancet*, **1**, 660–661.

Richardson, P. J. (1974b) Catheter technique for endomyocardial biopsy. *Journal of Cardiovascular Technology*, **16** (2), 31–37.

Richardson, P. J. (1975) Technique of endomyocardial biopsy—including a description of a
new form of endomyocardial bioptome. *Postgraduate Medical Journal*, **51**, 282–285.

Richardson, P. J., Livesley, B., Oram, S., Olsen, E. G. J. & Armstrong, P. (1974) Angina
pectoris with normal coronary arteries. Transvenous myocardial biopsy in diagnosis.
Lancet, **2**, 667–680.

Richardson, P. J., Olsen, E. G. J., Jewitt, D. E. & Oram, S. (1975) Percutaneous technique
of left ventricular biopsy and comparison between right and left ventricular myocardial
samples (Abstract). *British Heart Journal*, **37**, 556.

Sakakibara, S. & Konno, S. (1962) Endomyocardial biopsy. *Japanese Heart Journal*, **3**,
537–543.

Sakakibara, S. & Konno, S. (1966) Intracardiac heart biopsy. *Japanese Circulation Journal*,
30, 1582–1584.

Sekiguchi, M. (1974) Electron microscopical observation of the myocardium in patients with
idiopathic cardiomyopathy using endomyocardial biopsy. *Journal of Molecular and
Cellular Cardiology*, **6**, 111–122.

Sekiguchi, M. & Konno, S. (1969) Histopathological differentiation employing endomyocardial biopsy in the assessment of primary myocardial disease. *Japanese Heart Journal*,
10, 30–46.

Sekiguchi, M. & Konno, S. (1971) Diagnosis and classification of primary myocardial disease
with the aid of endomyocardial biopsy. *Japanese Circulation Journal*, **35**, 737–754.

Sekiguchi, M., Konno, S., Hasegawa, F. & Hirosawa, K. (1972/73) Some characteristic electron microscopic pictures of diseased myocardium obtained by endomyocardial biopsy. *Bulletin of the Heart Institute Japan*, **14**, 30–52.

Shirey, E. K., Hawk, W. A., Mukerji, D. & Effler, D. B. (1972) Percutaneous myocardial biopsy of the left ventricle. Experience in 198 patients. *Circulation*, **46**, 112–122.

Somers, K., Hutt, M. S. R., Patel, A. K. & D'Arbela, P. G. (1971) Endomyocardial biopsy in diagnosis of cardiomyopathies. *British Heart Journal*, **33**, 822–832.

Sutton, D. C. & Sutton, G. C. (1960) Needle biopsy of the human myocardium: review of 54 consecutive cases. *American Heart Journal*, **60**, 364–370.

Sutton, D. C., Sutton, G. C. & Kent, G. (1956) Needle biopsy of the human ventricular myocardium. *Quarterly Bulletin of Northwestern University Medical School*, **30**, 213–214.

Sutton, G. C., Driscoll, J. F., Gunnar, R. M. & Tobin, J. R., Jr (1964) Exploratory mediastinostomy in primary myocardial disease. *Progress of Cardiovascular Disease*, **7**, 83–97.

Teare, D. (1958) Asymmetrical hypertrophy of the heart in young adults. *British Heart Journal*, **20**, 1–8.

Timmis, G. C., Gordon, S., Baron, R. H. & Brough, A. J. (1965) Percutaneous myocardial biopsy. *American Heart Journal*, **70**, 499–504.

Torp, A. (1973) Endomyocardial biopsy. *Scandinavian Journal of Thoracic and Cardiovascular Surgery*, **7**, 253–261.

Van Noorden, S., Olsen, E. G. J. & Pearse, A. G. E. (1971) Hypertrophic obstructive cardiomyopathy, a histological, histochemical, and ultrastructural study of biopsy material. *Cardiovascular Research*, **5**, 118–131.

Waterson, A. P. (1975) Personal communication.

Weinberg, M., Fell, E. H. & Lynfield, D. J. (1958) Diagnostic biopsy of the pericardium and myocardium. *Archives of Surgery*, **76**, 825–829.

Weinberg, M., Raffensberger, J., Driscoll, J. F., Sutton, G. C. & Tobin, J. R., Jr (1963) Technique for full-thickness myocardial biopsy of the human heart (Abstract). *Circulation*, **28**, 823.

REFERENCES TO ADDENDUM

Bouhour, J. B., Petitier, H., De Lajartre, A. Y., Almazor, M., Nicolas, G. & Horeau, J. (1976) La biopsie myocardique dans les myocardiopathies congestives en apparence primitives. *Archives des Maladies du Coeur et des Vaisseaux*, **69**, 485–494.

Kuhn, H., Breithardt, G., Knieriem, H.-J., Loogen, F., Both, A., Schmidt, W. A. K., Stroobandt, R. & Gleichmann, U. (1975) Die Bedeutung der endomyokardialen Katheterbiopsie für die Diagnostik und die Beurteilung der Prognose der kongestiven Kardiomyopathie. *Deutsche Medizinische Wochenschrift*, **100**, 717–723.

Olsen, E. G. J. (1977) Endomyocardial biopsies; is pathological examination of use? (abstract). Presented at the autumn meeting of the British Cardiac Society. *British Heart Journal*, (in press).

Peters, T. J., Wells, G., Brooksby, I. A. B., Jenkins, B. S., Webb-Peploe, M. M. & Coltart, D. J. (1976) Enzymatic analysis of cardiac biopsy material from patients with valvular heart disease. *Lancet*, **1**, 269–270.

Petitier, H., Bouhour, J. B., de Lajartre, A. Y., Crochet, D., Nicolas, G. & Horeau, J. (1976) La biopsie endomyocardique, innocuité et intérêt clinique. Une expérience de cinq ans. *Archives des Maladies du Coeur et des Vaisseaux*, **69**, 1005–1011.

14
HEART FAILURE—I

S. H. Taylor

The definition of heart failure has long intrigued clinicians, investigators and physiologists. Its clinical basis is relatively easy to define; it is that state in which the heart is unable at a normal filling pressure to pump sufficient blood to meet the current demands of metabolically active tissues. It is an important state to detect as heart failure is the commonest cause of death in Western society today (Klainer, Gibson and White, 1965), and, despite modern methods of treatment, remains amongst the most lethal of disease syndromes (McKee et al, 1971). The spectrum of causes of heart failure in the adult population has radically changed over the past few years; rheumatic disease has now been supplanted by the far more frequent syndromes of hypertensive and coronary heart disease. This has also led to the recognition of another common outcome in advanced coronary heart disease, namely that of unexpected or 'sudden' death. Although all deaths from heart failure are directly due to failure of its pumping activity, dysrhythmias of such severity as to preclude more than token pumping function can be reasonably separately categorised as 'electrical failure'. It is not the purpose of this review to deal with this mode of 'heart failure'; attention will be concentrated on failure of more gradual onset, usually described as 'power' failure of the heart.

Heart failure is a complex subject which can be approached from many directions. A collected review of many aspects of the syndrome, particularly as it relates to coronary heart disease, has recently been presented by Braunwald (1974). Nayler (1975) has also reviewed in detail the biochemical events in the cardiac cell in heart failure, and Henderson (1975) has presented a critical review of the mechanical activity of the failing heart. This review will, therefore, be particularly directed to those clinical and therapeutic aspects of heart failure which have attracted lesser interest.

CLINICAL MANIFESTATIONS OF HEART FAILURE

In the majority of dissertations on heart failure the clinical aspects have usually been avoided. This may have been due in part to the enormous increase in knowledge in other professional fields, e.g. biochemistry, physiology, pharmacology, etc., and, in part, due to the relatively slow progression in the definition of the relevance of methods in practice of the clinical art. This short and possibly controversial review is intended to remedy that situation.

The clinical presentation of heart failure differs substantially in adults and children. This is not surprising when it is considered that heart disease in the child is usually due to congenital causes so that mechanisms of adaptation are gradually deployed in a heart with 'healthy' myocardium. In the adult, particularly the elderly, the myocardium is less able to adapt to the burdens imposed by disease. Although in the terminal phases of heart failure the clinicopathological picture is similar at all ages, in earlier stages the patterns of abnormal circulatory activity and thus clinical presentation often differ widely. The following discussion of the clinical presentation of heart failure will be confined to that in the adult.

Symptoms

Relatively intense effort is expended in teaching the finer details of physical examination, despite the fact that the history yields far more diagnostically useful information in the majority of patients (Hampton et al, 1975). However, this is a statistic that cannot be uncritically applied either to the individual patient or to a particular disease syndrome. Diagnostic predictions from history alone are limited in the case of heart failure by:

1. the priority accorded to various symptoms by the patient,
2. the difficulties of prediction of the severity of the functional impairment of the heart from history alone.

The first point is particularly well illustrated by the simultaneous occurrence of anginal pain and breathlessness during exercise-induced angina pectoris. Pain is perhaps naturally given overriding priority amongst symptoms, even to the exclusion of mention of symptoms which in other circumstances would give rise to severe complaint. Thus, breathlessness was rarely mentioned as a feature of the anginal syndrome until laboratory studies suggested its possibility by describing the reversible left ventricular failure that accompanies the onset of pain (Parker, Di Giorgi and West, 1966; Sharma and Taylor, 1970). For similar reasons haemoptysis is accorded a high priority of complaint, tiredness and fatigue relatively low priorities. Although clinicians are aware of such a natural selection of complaints by the patient it is a fact rarely emphasised to the student of medicine.

The second limiting factor, namely the prediction of the extent of physiological impairment of cardiac function from a patient's account, has conversely received unwarranted and uncritical emphasis in textbooks and teaching alike. Despite the considerable emphasis given by many clinical teachers to the attempted prediction of the severity of heart disease from history alone, this is almost certainly a fruitless exercise. How has this come to pass?

Almost half a century ago it became recognised that the diagnosis of a patient with heart disease could not depend on description of the structural abnormality alone; some estimate of the functional incapacity of the heart was essential for meaningful assessment. On the basis that a patient's symptoms could be expected to be quantitatively related to the extent of his cardiac impairment, a committee of the New York Heart Association eventually recommended a functional classification of heart disease (New York Heart Association Criteria Committee Report, 1942). At a time when there were few other methods of assessment of the functional severity of a patient's cardiac illness, this classification was widely and unquestioningly embraced. The extent to which it pervaded traditional cardiological thinking is illustrated by its uncritical acceptance for more than three decades, despite the enormous advances in physiological knowledge and methods of clinical investigation during this time. It is still widely taught, and is still used extensively in medical literature, particularly in connection with reports of surgical treatment, is still required in some insurance reports and it is still a part of the standard nomenclature in hospital diagnostic coding. Perhaps the fact that the grading was based on such ill-defined expressions as 'slight' or 'marked' limitations in exercise capacity (by breathlessness, fatigue, palpitations or anginal pain), has proved attractive by its very vagueness. Although such a classification demands little or no criticial examination of a patient's historical account of his complaints, its failure to give useful clinical information has now led to its eventual and unqualified demise.

Breathlessness is the commonest symptom of heart failure; it is the prime symptomatic indication of the approaching maximum physical performance of a patient. But its misleading nature as a precise indicator of the extent of pumping failure of the heart has rarely been stressed. Many thousands of words in many textbooks have been devoted to the clinical interpretation and predictive utility of this symptom with none emphasising that its value is at best only qualitative. Although there is a broad association between the symptom of breathlessness and the extent of left heart failure, there is no way of calibrating an individual's complaints that can give certain information about the functional extent of the failure. Many patients who claim to be entirely well are quite unable to meet the ordinary daily requirements of physical activity (Bergy and Bruce, 1955). Neither can the symptom be used to quantitatively evaluate the results of treatment with any precision (Taylor et al, 1975), despite its almost universal use in surgical reports of the results of heart operations. Patients without detectable heart disease may complain of breathlessness indistinguishable from that associated with left ventricular failure; the converse is also true. This is perhaps not surprising when the variable and often varying magnitude of the subjective component of a symptom is considered. It is important to emphasise that symptoms are adjusted by the patient in the light of medical and social circumstances to achieve what he considers the right impact on his physician. Verification is rarely undertaken, despite the fact that it is essential if a complaint such as breathlessness is to be quantitatively interpreted.

As no previous studies could be traced in the literature, an investigation of the problem was recently undertaken in our laboratory in ambulant patients with heart failure. The discrepancy between patients' statements of their exercise incapacity and their measured achievements was so great as to invalidate any evaluation of the severity of cardiac impairment from patients' claims. Many refinements of the New York Heart Association classification have been proposed. Questionnaires based on the distances patients think they are able to walk take no account of a patient's error in judging distance and afford no better indication of their limitation of exercise tolerance than more vague descriptions. The first essential feature of any valid diagnostic classification is that the information should be reproducible, i.e. elicitable by independent observers. The variability of patients' complaints given to different physicians is such that in our recent study radically different conclusions as to their disability were reached by experienced physicians in more than a third of the patients. Any classification of a patient's functional incapacity that allows the entry of guesswork and bias either on the part of the patient or the physician may compound diagnostic difficulties rather than simplify them and therefore rank as 'opinion'. The lack of usefulness of these classifications has probably long been recognised in clinical practice, but has only finally been admitted by the Criteria Committee of the New York Heart Association (1974). Six revisions of its 1953 proposals have been published over the last two decades; the latest rescinds all earlier classifications and abandons any attempt at 'grading' of severity of symptoms of heart failure.

In the context of heart failure, therefore, breathlessness on exertion, cough, undue fatigue and rarely haemoptysis, *may* indicate the presence of impaired pumping function. But they do not *prove* its presence and, importantly, there is no way in which they can be extrapolated to give a reliable estimate of its severity either before or after treatment.

Signs

The clinical value of physical examination of the failing heart varies with the extent of the failure. In early left ventricular failure impairment of pumping function only occurs under such loads as physical exercise; it is irrational therefore to expect that physical examination at rest can yield useful information of the degree of physiological impairment of the heart. In acute severe left ventricular failure, such as that following myocardial infarction, the only abnormal physical sign may be that of a left ventricular gallop rhythm. Although a rapid pulse and small pulse pressure are frequent accompaniments, neither are absolute or accurate correlates of left heart failure. Pulmonary oedema may also be present with few, if any, auscultatory signs of such. When heart failure develops more slowly, secondary mechanisms induce increases in blood volume, which eventually give rise to the clinical features classically described, i.e. pulmonary fine rales, hydrothorax, raised jugular venous pressure, distension of the liver, dependent peripheral oedema and occasionally ascites. Thus, the clinical presentation of left ventricular failure varies more with its *rate* of development than with its *severity*. These observations also indicate that whilst some features of heart failure may be detected clinically, they are of little use as a measure of its severity and, conversely, their absence is of no predictive value. This is not to devalue the correct elicitation of physical signs; only to focus attention on their unreliability as objective indicators of the severity of heart failure.

METHODS OF DETECTION AND MEASUREMENT OF THE SEVERITY OF HEART FAILURE

Laboratory investigations designed to measure the severity of pumping failure of the heart fall into two groups. Those concerned with the anatomical description of the size of the heart and related changes in the lung fields, and those concerned with the measurement of changes in one or more related physiological variables.

Anatomical Description

Chest radiography
The chest radiograph taken standing in full-inspiration, is undoubtedly the most valuable single adjunct to the clinical evaluation of heart failure. Although the size and shape of the x-ray silhouette of the heart may vary with the cause of the heart disease, the associated radiographic changes in the lungs are common to all forms of left heart failure. Signs of pulmonary venous hypertension are reflected in opacification of the veins in the upper lobes and often as peripheral horizontal linear opacities in the basal segments (Kerley B lines). Pulmonary oedema is the invariable end-result of severe left heart failure and, following myocardial infarction, may be detectable *only* by chest x-ray. Similarly, minimal degrees of clinically silent hydrothorax are readily detectable by this method. However, the findings on chest radiography cannot be uncritically extended to the prediction of the severity of the physiological abnormality. There is a broad correlation between the extent of heart failure as judged by elevation of the left heart filling pressure and the radiographic changes in the pulmonary vessels (Moore et al, 1959; Harley, 1961; Milne, 1968; Kostuk et al, 1973). However, the extrapolation of radiographic signs to the prediction of the haemodynamic status of the patient is fraught with hazard; patients with undoubted radiographic signs of pulmonary oedema have been reported who have had normal pulmonary venous pressures (Nixon and Durh, 1968; Lassers et al, 1970). It is possible that these few reported discrepancies may have been due to the radiographic and haemodynamic

measurements not being simultaneous. Until such problems are solved the interpretation of 'anatomical' appearances in terms of physiological derangement will remain open to error. But this apparent absence of absolute agreement must not allow clouding of the undoubted value of the chest radiograph in the clinical detection of heart failure.

Physiological Measurements

Direct intravascular methods

Despite the severe limitations of all techniques used to measure the cardiac output in man, the literature indicates that it is still one of the most used in the attempted evaluation of cardiac function in man. The theoretical limitations of the majority of the techniques in current use have been adequately described in many physiological texts (e.g. *Handbook of Physiology*, Section 2, Vol. I and II). The problems inherent in the application of the two commonest methods in use, namely those dependent upon the Fick principle and those dependent upon the indicator dilution principle have also been published (Taylor, 1966). It can only be concluded that the continuing and uncritical attraction for this measurement by many investigators must depend on factors other than scientific interest or clinical usefulness. Although systematic errors in the measurement of cardiac output are of little consequence, measurement of variability and definition of 'normality' in each laboratory are of vital importance if the results of such studies are to be interpreted. Few of those reported quote these essential prerequisites, despite claims to show 'significant' changes in the measurements made. Moreover, measurement of changes in cardiac output alone without knowledge of ventricular filling pressure cannot be reliably interpreted in terms of cardiac function, particularly as an increase in filling pressure with maintained output is often the initial change in heart failure. This is illustrated by a recent study in our laboratory: in 200 patients with a raised left ventricular filling pressure due to hypertension, aortic stenosis or coronary heart disease, the cardiac output at rest and the increase during bicycle exercise was within 'normal' limits in more than 50 per cent (unpublished observations). Moreover, as filling pressure crudely reflects end-diastolic volume in such patients, at least as regards the left ventricle (Sharma and Taylor, 1975), measurement of left ventricular filling pressure alone is probably the most sensitive and readily available method of detecting *early* left ventricular failure, particularly if a multipoint curve of ventricular activity is obtained by increasing venous return (e.g. by dynamic exercise such as bicycling) or by increasing systemic blood pressure (e.g. by static exercise, such as hand-grip). The clinical applicability of this method is considerably enhanced by the close agreement between left ventricular diastolic, left atrial and pulmonary wedge pressures; the latter measurement can be obtained at the bedside by the use of balloon catheters 'floated' into a peripheral pulmonary artery thus obviating the necessity for radiographic screening facilities. The limitations of this measurement must also be emphasised. It is at its most sensitive in early left ventricular failure when the left ventricular filling pressure is raised only during increased muscular activity. However, it is this state that is most difficult to diagnose by other methods; in advanced heart failure with a raised filling pressure at rest, the significance of further increases in pressure are difficult to interpret and other measurements (e.g. radiographic heart size) are probably of more quantitative utility.

Measurements of cardiac output alone cannot describe the contractile performance of the myocardium (Braunwald, 1971). Attention in recent years has therefore been directed to the development of measurements which describe some of the discrete mechanical accompaniments of left ventricular contraction (see reviews by Hamer, 1973; Dodge, 1974; Henderson, 1975). A knowledge of the behaviour of heart muscle is essential to an understanding of the performance of the heart as a whole, but measurements of integrated cardiac performance cannot be dissected into the constituents of its contractile activity. Considerable advances have been made in elucidating the principles governing the mechanical performance of the heart (Brady, 1968; Edman and Nilsson, 1968; Brutsaert and Sonnenblick, 1969). However, the extrapolation of these principles to the measurement of myocardial mechanical behaviour in the sick patient has not unnaturally posed considerable difficulties, not the least the ethical problems associated with the extensive intravascular cannulation necessary with some methods, e.g. aortic flow probes—and attempted 'short cuts' often lead to invalid results (Taylor, Snow and Linden, 1972). At the present time there is no simple way of measuring the discrete properties of the mechanical behaviour of the myocardium in intact man, and it is irrational to advocate that a measurement of questionable validity should be used because no better exists. Many of the measurements proposed (e.g. maximum dP/dt and its derivations) may indeed reflect changes in inotropic state of the myocardium in an individual in a given set of circumstances, but none have sufficient advantages as diagnostic tools over the simpler methods of measurements of heart size and venous filling pressure to recommend their unqualified clinical acceptance.

Non-invasive methods

The ethical problems associated with intravascular methods and the lack of an easily applicable and physiologically valid method of measurement of myocardial function in intact man have led to the development of interest in non-invasive methods of evaluation of cardiac performance.

The Valsalva manoeuvre was probably the earliest non-invasive (or at least non-cardiac invasive) method specifically suggested as a means of detecting heart failure (Sharpey-Schafer, 1955). There was conspicuous qualitative difference between the response of the systemic blood pressure during expiration against a closed glottis in patients with severe left ventricular failure compared to the response in normal subjects. The principle was later refined to the changes in heart rate thus obviating the need for intra-arterial cannulation. Evidence has been presented that there is a correlation between various components of the heart rate response (longest/shortest RR interval— 'Valsalva ratio') and the pulmonary wedge pressure (Levin, 1966). This report does not appear to have attracted the interest its claims warrant; if confirmed, it would have the potential of furnishing a widely applicable method of detecting left heart failure at the bedside. Unfortunately, detailed examination of the correlation in our laboratory has shown that although there was an overall positive correlation between the Valsalva ratio and left heart filling pressure, the method was insufficiently accurate to detect the most important stage, namely 'early' (exercise-induced) left ventricular insufficiency. Moreover, the method is limited to patients in sinus rhythm. This approach to the detection of heart failure unfortunately appears to lack further diagnostic potential.

A number of other non-invasive methods have been suggested for the clinical measurement of left ventricular function (see Gibson, 1975, for review). These include systolic time intervals derived from simultaneous records of the electrocardiogram, phonocardiogram and carotid pulse (Weissler, Harris and Schoenfeld, 1968), apex cardiography involving measurement of the displacement of the cardiac apex relative to the chest wall (Roberts and Jones, 1963), echocardiography based on the detection of reflected ultrasound pulses, (Edler, 1955) and more recently measurement of changes in cardiac output and thoracic volume by impedance cardiography (Hill and Lowe, 1973; Kubicek et al, 1974). In the hands of skilled investigators each of these methods has been shown to give an estimate of a particular physiologic variable related to left ventricular function. However, their wider application in the routine clinical measurement of cardiac function is severely limited on a number of scores. Repeatable measurements are difficult to obtain, particularly in ill patients. Measurements can only be interpreted in patients in sinus rhythm. The relationship between non-invasive measurements and directly measured variables of cardiac function varies in different disease states and changes with physiologically or therapeutically induced alterations in cardiac performance. The variability of the majority of methods is so wide that the results from grouped statistical analyses are of little or no value in the prediction of changes in the individual patient. It must be concluded therefore that these non-invasive methods are presently of little value in the evaluation of cardiac performance or the routine detection of heart failure in the individual patient. It is possible, however, that with further development they may be usefully amalgamated to give a more complete picture of left ventricular function than is possible at present. It is important that these comments should not be extended to outright condemnation of these methods throughout the whole field of cardiological investigation. Systolic time intervals have proved of value in the measurement of drug effects on the heart and echocardiograms are of proven diagnostic use in locating pericardial effusion and abnormalities of mitral valve movement. The attraction of these methods only wanes when applied to the attempted measurement of discrete aspects of myocardial function.

PHYSIOLOGICAL BASIS OF HEART FAILURE

The circulatory and metabolic accompaniments of heart failure have been reviewed in detail in a previous publication (Taylor, 1973a, b). However, a résumé of the salient points furnishes a useful basis for further discussion.

Failure of the left heart in man may result from many different causes but it is always followed by a similar pattern of circulatory response. Failure to propel the venous return results in a fall in blood pressure and rise in volume in the ventricle and left atrium. These instant sequelae of ventricular failure are rapidly followed by two events, initiation of the Frank–Starling intrinsic adaptive mechanisms and reflex activation of the sympathetic nervous system. The latter results in three main circulatory effects:

1. the heart contracts more frequently, more rapidly and more forcibly,
2. it results in widespread peripheral vasoconstriction thus reducing the capacity of the systemic vascular system,
3. catecholamines are released from sympathetic nerve endings and from the adrenal medulla.

Acute heart failure also results in the immediate activation of other mechanisms. The fall in blood pressure, by reducing renal perfusion pressure, causes renin to be released from the kidney. Renin release is independently facilitated by catecholamine stimulation of β-adrenoceptors in the juxtaglomerular bodies, amines released by catecholamines from sympathetic nerve endings in the kidney or blood borne. Renin subsequently activates the angiotensin pressor system. This has three effects; it results in vasoconstriction by direct action on vascular smooth muscle, it stimulates sympathetic vasomotor centres in the brain and, by stimulating the release of aldosterone from the adrenal cortex, it augments the more rapid pressor effects by the renal retention of sodium. These changes serve to maintain aortic blood pressure, and thus flow, to the vital cerebral and coronary circulations.

Sympathetic Stimulation

The reflex and widespread sympathetic excitation and associated catecholaminaemia also has other effects. Stimulation of β-adrenoceptors in the bronchi results in a reduction in airways resistance, although this may be overwhelmed by the increase in airways resistance due to bronchial mucosal oedema in heart failure. Stimulation of β-adrenoceptors in fat tissue results in the activation of lipolytic enzymes and the release of free-fatty acids and triglycerides into the blood stream. Stimulation of β-adrenoceptors in liver and striated muscle results in the release of glucose. The effects on the pancreas are more complex; stimulation of β-receptors releases insulin but this is opposed by the reduction in pancreatic blood flow and the stimulation of α-receptors; the end result is a suppression of insulin secretion despite the rise in blood glucose. An even more indirect consequence of acute heart failure is the enhancement of the effects of thyroid hormone, the release of growth hormone and stimulation of the release of adrenal corticosteroids. Although these facts are beyond doubt, their consequences and proportionate importance at the various stages of heart failure are far from clear.

This brief summary does little justice to the immense effort that has been involved in unravelling these complex changes. This is illustrated by the fact that a detailed review of any single aspect reveals an immense pool of knowledge. All have a bearing on the mechanisms involved in heart failure, but perhaps the most clinically relevant and therapeutically important are those responsible for the reflex control of cardiac function and those effecting sodium handling by the kidney.

Changes in the Reflex Control of the Failing Heart

Although heart muscle resembles other striated muscle structurally and biochemically, the heart functions as a whole in quite a different way to the discrete behaviour of skeletal muscle: when increased work is demanded of the heart it responds by an increase in energy output of all fibres, not by increasing the number of active muscle fibres as is the case with skeletal muscle. Adaptation to changes in work load on the heart is brought about by two mechanisms. The Frank–Starling mechanism relates the magnitude of the contractile response to the length of the muscle fibre unit at the time of electrical activation; this mechanism is an intrinsic property of all myocardial muscle cells. The autonomic system furnishes the second mechanism controlling cardiac contractile activity by directly altering work output at any given length of cardiac muscle fibre. Together the two mechanisms are not only responsible for the large range of adjustments in work output of the heart in health, but also allow its extended survival in the face of events precipitating its failure.

The fundamental abnormality in myocardial failure is a primary reduction in the intrinsic contractile state of the heart muscle fibres. The secondary support afforded by the sympathetic nerves to the heart appears to decline as failure progresses, and in the terminal state the peripheral metabolic consequences of the reduced output of the heart directly depress myocardial function still further.

In recent years significant advances have been made in our understanding of these processes. Probably the most exciting and that with the most therapeutic potential relates to the changes in autonomic control of the failing heart.

The Efferent Arc

The heart is abundantly supplied with sympathetic nerves; these are distributed throughout the myocardium with local concentrations in the sino-atrial and atrioventricular nodes and the Purkinje system. Stimulation results in the release of noradrenaline from the sympathetic nerve endings which activate 'receptors' in these sites, described in pharmacological terms as β-adrenoceptors. Cardiac sympathetic stimulation by releasing noradrenaline at the sinoatrial node increases the speed of spontaneous diastolic de-polarisation and thus the heart rate (positive chronotropic effect); released at the AV node noradrenaline reduces the period during which the node is refractory to incoming atrial stimuli and also increases the velocity of outgoing impulses thus facilitating transmission of atrial impulses to the ventricle. Released in the myocardium noradrenaline increases the speed and force of contraction developed at a given fibre length (positive inotropic effect). Thus, sympathetic stimulation of the intact heart profoundly increases all aspects of its contractile activity. The integrity of the cardiac sympathetic mechanisms is crucial to the survival of the failing heart; the neurotransmitter nor-adrenaline appears to be the Achilles heel in the system in heart failure.

The heart, like other organs innervated by sympathetic nerves, can so readily extract noradrenaline from the blood that until recently it was as-sumed that this was the source of its neurotransmitter stores. During the past few years, however, it has become increasingly apparent that the predominant source of noradrenaline in the heart is locally synthesised in sympathetic nerve endings from the precursor amino acid tyrosine (Blaschko, 1973).

It is perhaps not surprising therefore to find that in heart failure, the increase in sympathetic nervous activity is associated with an increased urinary excretion of noradrenaline and the increase is broadly correlated with the severity of the heart failure (Chidsey, Braunwald and Morrow, 1965). What is more surprising was the discovery that heart failure was accompanied by depletion of the myocardial stores of noradrenaline both in the experi-mental animal (Chidsey et al, 1964; Spann et al, 1965; Sassa, 1971) and in man (Chidsey et al, 1965; De Quattro et al, 1973). The depletion occurs within days of the onset of failure, is directly correlated with the clinical severity of the failure and inversely with the urinary catecholamine excretion (Gertler, Saluste and Spencer, 1970). Moreover, the depletion of neurotransmitter is unique to the heart; it does not occur in other organs such as the kidney which is also the target for increased sympathetic activity in heart failure.

Three possibilities exist to explain this observation, namely, reduced synthesis, increased breakdown or impaired binding of noradrenaline in sympathetic nerve endings in the heart. The enzyme tyrosine hydroxylase is responsible for the first step in the synthesis of noradrenaline from tyrosine in sympathetic nerve endings and the activity of this enzyme controls the rate of the entire synthetic process. This enzyme is severely depleted in sympathetic nerve endings in the failing heart (Pool et al, 1967; Sassa, 1971; De Quattro et al, 1973). It has also been claimed that the breakdown of catecholamines is increased in the failing heart (Sassa, 1971; De Quattro et al, 1973) although this is disputed (Krakoff et al, 1968). However, there is conclusive evidence that the uptake and binding of noradrenaline by sympathetic nerve terminals is also severely depressed in heart failure (Spann et al, 1965; Oliverio and Wang, 1966). Thus, both biosynthesis of noradrenaline and its uptake and binding are sufficiently impaired in the failing heart to account for its severe myocardial depletion. However, noradrenaline depletion does not appear to alter the contractile activity of myocardium in terms of the Frank–Starling relationship. This suggests that the intrinsic contractile state of the myocardium is not dependent upon its noradrenaline stores, and that the depletion of myocardial noradrenaline does not account for the depressed mechanical behaviour of failing myocardium.

The importance of the depletion in sympathetic neurotransmitter stores in heart failure has been shown by the demonstration in the experimental animal that the normal increases in heart rate and contractile force when the sympathetic nerves to the heart are stimulated were significantly reduced in the presence of heart failure (Braunwald, 1974). The reduced heart rate increments during exercise observed in patients in heart failure may be explained on a similar basis. However, myocardium from the failing heart remains normally responsible to the inotropic action of noradrenaline (Chidsey et al, 1964). Thus, it is reasonable to assume that the depleted neurotransmitter stores are a reflection of a decreased liberation of noradrenaline despite an increase in sympathetic impulses. While myocardial noradrenaline depletion in heart failure does not reduce its intrinsic mechanical performance it does seriously impair the increase in contractile activity afforded by stimulation of the sympathetic nerves to the heart.

These observations may be synthesised into a working hypothesis of the changes in cardiac sympathetic activity that occur in heart failure. The key factor is a reduction in the amount of the rate-limiting enzyme tyrosine hydroxylase in cardiac sympathetic nerve terminals with the result that the amount of noradrenaline available for activation of the β-adrenoceptors in the nodes and muscle of the heart is severely reduced. Depletion of the neurotransmitter stores interferes with transmission of impulses from the cardiac sympathetic nerve endings to the adjacent β-adrenoceptors, reducing still further cardiac performance. This chain of events is retarded to some extent by the fact that the β-receptors in the heart respond to blood-borne as well as locally released catecholamines. The leakage of catecholamines from the increased sympathetic activity in other territories, augmented by those released from the adrenal medulla, result in their increased plasma concentration which thus serves to sustain, at least in part, the contractile function of the failing heart.

This synthesis highlights two significant gaps in knowledge. The cause of the reduction in the key rate-limiting enzyme tyrosine hydroxylase is still unknown; it may be related to the persistent barrage of impulses to which the cardiac sympathetic nerves are subjected as the heart fails, but this affords no real explanation of the observed fact. Neither is it known why this enzyme and noradrenaline stores are *not* reduced in other territories with a high sympathetic representation, such as the kidney. The answer to these questions may have far-reaching therapeutic implications.

These observations may also afford an explanation of the known sensitivity of patients in heart failure to the β-adrenoceptor blocking drugs. Although relatively large amounts of these drugs are necessary to reduce exercise tachycardia in the normal heart, presumably due to the competition afforded by the release of high concentrations of noradrenaline at local receptor sites, the cardiac response to circulating catecholamines is blocked by much smaller amounts (Thadani et al, 1975).

Although recent advances on the role of the autonomic control of cardiac activity have been largely derived from analysis of the sympathetic component, knowledge of the effects of vagal activity on the heart long antedate the elucidation of the role of the sympathoadrenal system. For many years the parasympathetic system was considered to play a minor role in cardiac control and even now is rarely thought of in terms other than its influence on heart rate. This has been due to the lack of clear separation of vagal and sympathetic influences on the heart and the paucity of histological knowledge of the innervation of the ventricles.

The major proportion of the vagal outflow is distributed to the atria and atrioventricular node, but there is a histologically distinct component distributed to the ventricular myocardium and coronary vessels. Functionally the vagal effects are due to the release of acetylcholine from the postganglionic endings. This results in inhibitory effects on the heart by decreasing the duration of the action potential and reducing adenylate cyclase activity and the concentration of cyclic AMP; this latter is essential for myocardial contractile activity. Thus, vagal stimulation not only reduces heart rate but also ventricular performance. However, the picture is confused somewhat by the fact that acetylcholine released from postganglionic vagal nerve endings also stimulates the release of noradrenaline from postganglionic sympathetic nerve endings. The interrelated role of these two activities has recently been clarified. Situations which result in a high level of sympathetic activity are associated with inhibition of the centres in the brain controlling parasympathetic activity, so that the augmentation of heart rate and contractility by the sympathetic component are uninhibited (Levy, 1971). At lower levels of excitation the inhibitory effects of the vagi predominate in the territory of their major anatomical distribution, namely the atria, with a reduction in sinus rate and delayed conduction in the AV node. The direct inhibitory effects of acetylcholine on ventricular myocardium are offset by the stimulatory actions associated with the acetylcholine-induced release of noradrenaline. In addition to these effects of the vagus on heart rate and myocardial contractile function, there is now convincing evidence that vagal stimulation also results in vaso-dilation of the coronary vessels, although the role of this action in the context of cardiac performance is obscure.

The integrity of the efferent vagal component is essential for a number of the cardiovascular reflexes brought into play when the heart fails. One of the most important of these reflexes is the inverse change in heart rate in response to changes in blood pressure. In the normal heart elevation of the blood pressure (except that associated with exercise) results in a reflex reduction in heart rate; a reduction in blood pressure increases heart rate. The sensitivity of this reflex response has been found to be significantly reduced in heart failure and the extent of its reduction was proportional to the extent of the failure. Moreover, vagal influence on the resting heart rate, tested by the administration of atropine after pretreatment with propranolol, has been found to be much less in patients with heart failure than it is in normal subjects (Braunwald, 1974). Together these findings strongly suggest an impairment of vagal activity on the sinus node in the failing heart.

The Afferent Arc

So far this synthesis has dealt only with the efferent arc of the autonomic supply to the heart. However, the functional efficiency of the afferent arc of these reflex responses may also be impaired. Although receptors may exist in the ventricle, stretch receptors in the atria and adjacent large veins appear to be a more numerous source of baroreceptor stimuli regulating cardiac and peripheral mechanisms of circulatory control (see review by Linden, 1973). Stretch of these receptors via an afferent vagal and efferent sympathetic reflex arc operates to maintain a constant heart volume by adjusting heart rate to atrial volume (venous return). This reflex may also operate to maintain heart volume within narrow limits in the face of an increased plasma and extra-cellular volume by stimulation of urine excretion (Ledsome and Linden, 1968), possibly through a specific reduction in sympathetic impulses to the kidney (Karim et al, 1972). Thus, the atrial receptors appear to be a vital first link in a negative feedback mechanism controlling heart volume. Normally, relatively small changes in volume in these sites result in large autonomic adjustments. In heart failure changes in chamber volume far exceed those in the normal heart and yet appear to produce relatively small changes in the behaviour of the heart and circulation. Although part of the impaired response is almost certainly due to partial failure of the efferent arc of the reflex, it has recently been demonstrated that the afferent side of the reflex may also be impaired; stretch of atrial receptors above a certain limit was found to be associated with a reduction in their discharge rate (Greenberg et al, 1973). It is possible that a similar reduction in afferent impulses from other baroreceptor sites in heart failure may also contribute to the reduced efferent activity of the autonomic nerve supply to the heart.

In contrast to the intense effort directed to elucidation of the activity of the autonomic nervous control of the failing heart, it is pertinent to note the relatively small amount of interest taken in the control of the peripheral circulation in these circumstances. Although the changes in cardiac autonomic activity observed in heart failure may possibly be accompanied by similar impairment of sympathetic activity in the peripheral circulation, such a concept does not appear to have concerned investigators to the same extent as the changes in the heart.

SYNOPSIS

The basic mechanisms and biochemical events ultimately responsible for the inadequate function of the autonomic nerves to the failing heart are obscure but the results of such impairment of vital support are easy to see. The ability of the heart to meet the metabolic requirements of the body is dependent upon its ability to pump blood. When the heart cannot pump into the systemic circulation all the blood presented to it, the intrinsic ability of myocardium to respond to increased stretch by increased work output is brought into play. In addition, afferent impulses from stretch receptors in the atria initiate a reflex sympathoadrenal discharge which increases work output of the heart at any given volume. However, if these mechanisms fail to correct the pumping deficiency of the heart within a relatively short time the effectiveness of this support becomes increasingly blunted, possibly due to a relative decrease in afferent impulses, but certainly despite an increased barrage of sympathetic impulses. Some alternative cardiac support is supplied by the increased concentration of catecholamines in the blood, resulting from increased sympathetic discharge to the periphery and adrenal medulla. However, the proportionate importance of this 'exogenous' support is limited, and can be at best only a temporary expedient. The parasympathetic supply to the heart is also impaired in heart failure, reducing the ability to vary the heart rate in response to baroreceptor stimuli. In the failing heart increases in stroke volume are limited and the heart becomes more dependent upon changes in heart rate to increase output. The impairment of vagal activity in these circumstances may contribute to the decline in cardiac performance. Together these events result in the progressive nature of established heart failure.

SALT AND WATER RETENTION IN HEART FAILURE
(see also p. 402)

Many factors operate in heart failure to reduce sodium excretion and retain water; this assists circulatory control by helping to maintain the blood pressure by expansion of the plasma volume, at the potential penalty of oedema. In heart failure changes in sodium handling by the kidney may occur as a result of:

1. reduction in glomerular filtration rate (GFR) consequent upon a reduction in renal blood flow,
2. increase in aldosterone liberation as a result of activation of the renin–angiotensin system,
3. reduction in metabolic breakdown of salt-retaining hormones as a consequence of hepatic impairment due primarily to a low hepatic blood flow.

The reduction of GFR is an immediate result of a reduced renal blood flow which is a direct consequence of the reduced output of the heart and indirectly due to an increase in sympathetic vasoconstrictor activity; it is an effective means of immediately reducing sodium excretion. This mechanism has been known for many years. More recent interest and investigative attention has turned to the changes in renin–angiotensin–aldersterone mechanisms that result from heart failure.

In heart failure renin is liberated from the juxtaglomerular bodies by two independent mechanisms. Reduction of pressure in the renal artery is a potent stimulus for the release of renin which is independent of that due to stimulation of sympathetic β-adrenoceptors in the kidney (Davis, 1971; Johns and Singer, 1974). Renin liberated from the kidney converts angiotensin precursor (α_2-globulin) in the blood into the decapeptide angiotensin I which on passage through the lungs is converted to the octapeptide angiotensin II. This agent has three circulatory actions:

1. it results in direct contraction of vascular smooth muscle (Johnson and Davis, 1972),
2. it stimulates sympathetic vasomotor centres in the brain (Scroop and Whelan, 1966),
3. it results in the release of aldosterone from the zona glomerulosa of the adrenal cortex (Urquhart, Davis and Higgins, 1964).

The increased plasma concentration of renin and aldosterone in heart failure are both directly related to its severity. In the case of aldosterone this is due both to increased liberation from the adrenal cortex and reduced metabolic degradation by the liver. The rate of destruction of aldosterone by the liver is a direct correlate of hepatic blood flow. However, renin degradation by the liver in low output heart failure is within normal limits, indicating that there is some mechanism operative in these circumstances to improve the renin-removing efficiency of the liver despite the reduction in hepatic flow.

If these brief comments appear to furnish a 'closed' account of this important topic it is a fallacy of their presentation. Many factors remain unknown, particularly the quantitative relations of the mechanisms involved. Although a unified concept of the mechanisms involved is still some way off, reduction in glomercular filtration rate and increased aldosterone secretion must be assigned major influences in the retention of salt and water in heart failure.

TREATMENT OF HEART FAILURE

Progress in the treatment of heart failure, particularly chronic heart failure, in clinical practice remains pedestrian. The immense increase in knowledge of the biochemical and contractile functions of the heart and the development of diverse techniques of investigation have so far had little discernible impact on the routine treatment of patients in cardiac failure. Moreover, it is not generally realised how little current clinical practices have influenced the lethal nature of the syndrome. The newer attempts at the treatment of the very sick with vasodilator drugs or in the last resort with mechanical circulatory assistance, originated from considerations which owed little to the tremendous expansion in knowledge of the fundamental workings of the heart. Unfortunately, the evaluation of treatments in heart failure has rarely followed the strict validation required of clinical trials in other situations. This must be borne in mind in evaluating the claims of therapeutic benefit to be reviewed.

The treatment of heart failure is essentially directed to increasing cardiac stroke volume by:

1. increasing myocardial contractility with drugs or procedures that have a positive inotropic action,
2. reducing pressure work load of the left ventricle,
3. improving coronary blood flow by mechanical assistance,
4. improving myocardial performance by correction of adverse metabolic factors.

Inotropic Drugs

Digitalis glycosides (see also p. 413 *et seq.*)

The effects of digitalis in the treatment of patients in heart failure was described by Withering nearly two centuries ago but the use of these compounds in clinical practice continues to remain largely empirical. Tremendous advances have been made in recent years in knowledge of the biochemical and other cellular processes in the myocardium induced by digitalis (see review by Langer, 1974). Unfortunately, this progress has not been reflected in similar advances in the treatment of patients. Beyond the fact that the digitalis glycosides exert positive inotropic effects, particularly in heart failure (Vatner and Braunwald, 1974), that these effects are glucose dependent (Berman, Masuoka and Saunders, 1957), insulin sensitive (Darforth, McKinsey and Stewart, 1962), and reduced by hypoxia and systemic acidaemia, little has been uncovered of clinical application in recent years. A major difficulty has been the choice of a valid measurement of cardiac function that can be used in the ambulant patient to monitor the effects of the drug. This may account in part for the large number of therapeutically important questions that remain unanswered. Why does the clinical effectiveness of the drug vary in different patients with similar degrees of heart failure? Why are the positive inotropic effects of the drug often not translated into clinical improvement? What is the relationship between the degree of heart failure and the degree of clinical response? Can patients who will respond to the drug be predicted? Should digitalis ever be used alone or always combined with diuretics or vasodilator remedies? Despite our extensive knowledge of activity of the drug at a cellular level, this information has yet to supply an answer to these therapeutically vital questions.

Other inotropic drugs
    The limitations of digitalis in many clinical situations has stimulated the search for other agents with positive inotropic activity. The majority of inotropic drugs in clinical use have distinct disadvantages in the treatment of heart failure, particularly that associated with coronary heart disease, due to the induced increase in myocardial energy and oxygen requirements. The sympathomimetic amine isoprenaline is a potent positive inotropic agent by virtue of its stimulation of β-adrenoceptors in the heart, but its clinical use is severely limited by the tachycardia, dysrhythmias and hypotension that often result from its intravenous infusion. Moreover, extension of infarct size, intensification of myocardial ischaemia and even impairment of left ventricular function have been described after its use (Maroko et al, 1971, 1973). Noradrenaline is also a powerful inotropic agent, but has the disadvantage that it causes a marked increase in peripheral resistance as a consequence of its α-adrenoceptor stimulating properties (Vatner, Higgins and Braunwald, 1974a). Dopamine, which has similar inotropic activity but causes less α-receptor stimulation than noradrenaline and less tachycardia than isoprenaline, has also been advocated as a cardiac stimulant in heart failure and shock (Loeb et al, 1971; Goldberg, 1972). However, its vasoconstrictive actions (Higgins et al, 1973) and its tendency to induce dysrhythmias are distinct disadvantages (Gunnar and Loeb, 1972). Dobutamine has recently been introduced as a sympathomimetic amine with the claimed advantage that its positive inotropic actions are accompanied by smaller changes in heart rate and peripheral resistance than the foregoing drugs. Although these claims have been in part substantiated by animal experiments (Vatner, McRitchie and Braunwald, 1974b), intravenous administration of the drug resulted in conspicuous stimulation of both α- and β-adrenoceptors in peripheral vessels. Simultaneous stimulation of both these receptors resulted in a redistribution of the cardiac output favouring the muscle vascular beds at the expense of the renal; the drug also induced significant tachycardia. In man the positive inotropic effects of the drug have been shown to be dose-related and promisingly translated into increases in cardiac output (Jewitt et al, 1974). The drug *may* have therapeutic potential in the treatment of severe heart failure but the

confirmation of these claims must await the results of specific tests in such patients; they cannot be extrapolated from the results so far presented.

Vasodilator Drugs

The rationale for the use of vasodilator drugs and the clinical features limiting their application in man have been discussed in detail previously (Taylor, 1973b). However, in view of the increasing interest in this approach to the alleviation of left ventricular failure and its neglect in traditional therapeutic considerations, the importance of impedance to left ventricular output will be briefly reviewed.

Theoretical basis

Resistance to ejection of blood from the ventricle is due to two factors, the *compliant* impedance of the large arteries (a function of their elasticity or rigidity) and the *resistive* impedance of the peripheral circulation (a function of the length and cross-section of the small arteries and the viscosity of blood as related in the Poiseuilles equation). The resistive component is the most important factor of the two in determining the work of the heart. The generation of energy by the left ventricle takes place largely during the isometric or isovolumic phase of ventricular systole, i.e. before the aortic valve is open. The greater the resistance to run-off of blood from the arterial circulation, the higher the diastolic pressure, the greater the resistive impedance to ejection of blood from the ventricle and the greater its resulting work load. In the 'normal' heart increased impedance to ejection of blood is compensated by the Frank–Starling mechanism which increases work output of the stretched myocardial fibre elements. Although this mechanism operates in the failing heart, increases in impedance are not well tolerated because of differences in left ventricular contraction geometry. To develop a given aortic ejection pressure the work required of the ventricle is a function of its volume (law of La Place), i.e. the larger the ventricle the more energy is required. Moreover, in the normal heart ventricular systole is accompanied by such a large reduction in volume and myocardial fibre shortening that energy expenditure actually lessens as contraction proceeds. The opposite obtains in the failing heart. Not only is energy expenditure increased due to its increased volume, but the increase becomes progressively greater during the isometric phase of contraction due to the impaired fibre shortening. The overall result is that the failing left ventricle delivers a smaller stroke volume at higher energy cost.

As discussed in a previous section, one of the vital adaptive accompaniments of a reduced output of the heart is a reflex vasoconstriction of the majority of peripheral vascular beds due to sympathetic excitation and activation of the renin–angiotensin pressor system. In addition, the stagnation of blood in the peripheral circulation increases its viscosity and further contributes to the increased resistive impedance (Wells, 1964). These increases in resistive impedance are also accompanied by an increase in compliant impedance due to an increase in sodium and water content of vessel walls (Zelis, Delea and Coleman, 1969). This increases vessel wall stiffness sufficiently to counter, in part, the functional sympatholysis that occurs in exercising muscle (Remensnyder, Mitchell and Sarnoff, 1962; Zelis, Mason and Braunwald, 1968). Together, these factors increase overall impedance to left ventricular ejection and increase the work load of the failing heart. The increasing impedance to ventricular ejection and subsequent reduction in output of the heart tends to induce a vicious circle which it is essential to break if the patient is to survive. It is these considerations which first led to the use of the α-adrenoceptor blocking agent phentolamine in this situation (Majid, Sharma and Taylor, 1971). The beneficial effects of this drug in acute heart failure have been confirmed without exception (Kelly et al, 1973; Chatterjee et al, 1973; Walkinsky et al, 1974). Since that time the acute administration of a variety of other vasodilator agents have also been shown to induce significant clinical and haemodynamic reversal of severe heart failure. These include sodium nitroprusside (Franciosa et al, 1972), short-acting sublingual nitroglycerine (Gold, Leinbach and Sanders, 1972), long-acting oral isosorbide dinitrate (Franciosa et al, 1974) and intravenous salbutamol (Lal et al, 1972; Wyse, Gibson and Branthwaite, 1974). Phentolamine produces its effects by vasodilatation which is predominantly concentrated in areas with a high α-adrenoceptor component, e.g. kidney and skin. Sodium nitroprusside, and the nitrates, are non-specific vasodilator agents. Salbutamol produces its effects by stimulation of vasodilator β-adrenoceptors so that its effects are predominantly located in the muscle vascular bed. The major benefit of all these drugs lies unequivocally in their ability to reduce the pressure work load of the left ventricle. However, drugs in which the vasodilator properties are accompanied by α-receptor blocking activity, e.g., phentolamine, have the theoretical advantage that they act proportionately on those parts of the peripheral circulation in which the major resistive element lies, namely the kidney. Drugs which have non-specific vasodilator properties, e.g. sodium nitroprusside, or those in which the vasodilator activity is due to stimulation of β-adrenoceptors, e.g. salbutamol, have the theoretical disadvantage that they may passively divert blood from the non-vasodilated kidney to the non-essential vasodilated muscle vascular beds. Drugs which stimulate both α- and β-receptors, e.g. dobutamine, are theoretically the most disadvantageous due to the potentially active redistribution of available cardiac output from the kidneys to the muscles.

Other beneficial effects

There are other aspects of the action of these drugs in heart failure which are clinically interesting. The improvement in left ventricular performance after vasodilator drugs is not accompanied by increased metabolic cost to the heart (Chatterjee et al, 1973). The increased output of the heart may be a result not only of a reduction in systemic impedance but also to a reduction in preload due to venous dilatation and pooling. It may also be augmented by an increase in contractility due to the secondary release of catecholamines, by a reduction in systemic hypoxaemia and acidaemia, and by an improvement in the metabolic status of the heart due to release of insulin (Taylor 1973b). The administration of vasodilator drugs in normal man is accompanied by a conspicuous increase in heart rate (Taylor et al, 1965). This reflex tachycardia in response to the fall in arterial pressure is much reduced in heart failure, presumably due to the impairment of sympathetic stimulation of the heart for the reasons outlined in the previous section. The reduction in left ventricular pressure and wall tension throughout the cardiac cycle after these drugs can also be expected to favour subendocardial perfusion, particularly during diastole (Moir and Debra, 1967). The proportionate importance of these factors in the spectrum of haemodynamic benefit afforded by these drugs is as yet unclear, but there is little doubt that this group of drugs holds considerable potential in the treatment of heart failure.

These remarks must be tempered with caution. It must be emphasised that as yet no statistically valid trial has confirmed the benefits of vasodilator treatment of heart failure against the more traditional remedy of digitalis and diuretics. Moreover, the continued maintenance of improvement in function of the failing heart by vasodilator agents has yet to be established. This is a field in which further work is urgently required.

Mechanical Circulatory Assistance

The failure of conventional medical treatments to reverse severe uncompensated power failure of the heart ('circulatory shock') following acute myocardial infarction has led to the development of mechanical devices to aid pumping function of the heart. Two contrasting approaches to circulatory assistance have been used. The 'in parallel' pump, analogous to the heart–lung machine, has occasionally been used. The use of mechanical devices implanted into the chest, partial cardiac transplantation and more recently symbiotic support have all been tried. At the present state of knowledge and technology, it is unlikely that this approach will be of value except in certain restricted circumstances. The 'in-series' counterpulsation pump has proved to be the most effective and clinically applicable of the two approaches to date. The object of this method is to improve left ventricular function by decreasing aortic blood pressure during systole and increasing it during diastole, thereby helping to improve the balance between myocardial oxygen supply and demand.

Counterpulsation

The concept of counterpulsation was first put forward by Harken in 1958. As it was originally proposed, it involved the rapid removal of blood from the femoral artery during systole and rapid reinfusion during the diastole.

Although a few reports have described clinical successes with this technique, its clinical application has immense technical drawbacks related to the rapid movement of relatively large amounts of blood. Dormandy and his colleagues (1969) also claim that the method does not increase coronary blood flow. A major advance was the 'blood-less' method of intra-aortic balloon pumping (IABP) suggested by Moulopoulos and his colleagues in 1962. In this method a cylindrical balloon on the end of a catheter, inserted via the femoral artery, is positioned in the descending thoracic aorta. The balloon is inflated during diastole and deflated during systole. This accomplishes the same purpose as counterpulsation by the Harken method, but without its drawbacks. Inflation of the balloon prevents the run-off of blood during diastole so maintaining diastolic pressure and coronary and cerebral perfusion. Deflation of the balloon during systole results in a reduction in impedance to left ventricular ejection by suddenly opening the lower body circulation to aortic run-off. This technique has the immense clinical advantage that only one arteriotomy is required and it can be maintained without vascular detriment for some days. Since Kantrowitz and his colleagues (1968) reported the first successful clinical application of IABP numerous reports have confirmed its efficacy. The benefit of this method in intractable power failure of the left ventricle is probably largely related to the increase induced in coronary blood flow. Coronary blood flow is crucially dependent upon the level of the aortic pressure during diastole, particularly at low diastolic pressures and particularly in the presence of obstructive disease of the coronary arteries. In these circumstances elevation of the aortic pressure during diastole can be expected to result in a conspicuous increase in coronary blood flow (Kralios et al, 1972; Gill et al, 1973). Despite the limitations of the methods of measurements used, IABP has been shown to increase coronary blood flow in circulatory shock (Talpins, Kripke and Goetz, 1968), and reduce the size of myocardial infarcts (Maroko et al, 1972).

More recently the dual-chambered intra-aortic balloon has been introduced (Bregman and Goetz, 1971; Goetz et al, 1972). It is claimed that by inflating the more distal balloon first, the system pumps blood proximally towards the aortic arch more efficiently, thereby avoiding some of the losses of the single-chambered system. However, all balloon techniques require cannulation of the patient with its inherent restrictions on clinical deployment. A recently developed non-invasive method holds great promise in this direction (Soroff and Birtwell, 1974). With the legs encased in rigid metal tubes, water-filled bags are inflated and deflated in diastole and systole respectively. The initial clinical experiences with this external counterpulsation device are encouraging and it possesses the immense clinical advantage that it cannot conceivably harm the patient. Further refinements of these techniques will doubtless follow, but there is no doubt that the technique of counterpulsation has now emerged as the single most promising adjunct in the treatment of refractory power failure of the left ventricle.

In terms of clinical perspective the reader must be reminded that this is a purely *temporary* method of alleviating severe heart failure; it has no place in the treatment of chronic failure of the heart. Even in the acute situation it is not an unqualified success (Dilley, Ross and Bernstein, 1973), and it is unlikely *alone* to contribute to the long-term survival of patients in circulatory shock. Its place is undoubtedly one of circulatory rescue whilst other methods are mobilised to assist the continued survival of the patient.

Correction of Adverse Metabolic Factors

This aspect of the treatment of heart failure has attracted little attention. Since the situation was last reviewed (Taylor, 1973b) little progress has been made in the clinical application of the immense fund of knowledge that exists concerning the biochemical changes that occur both in the failing heart and in the peripheral tissues. At that time prospects were hopeful that metabolic support of the heart would become as rapidly an accepted part of the treatment of severe power failure as vasodilator treatment. Unfortunately, the lag between discovery and clinical application has never been wider than this field. Continuing work in patients in severe chronic heart failure Allison and his colleagues (1972) were able to demonstrate significant increases in urine output, presumably due to improved cardiac function, after infusions of insulin and glucose. We have confirmed this (unpublished observations). Maroko and his colleagues (1971) clearly demonstrated the reduction of myocardial damage after experimental coronary occlusion afforded by glucose–insulin–potassium infusion and also that this combination reduced the depression of myocardial function induced by propranolol. As yet no clinical observations have been reported to substantiate these promising experimental findings.

Natural History of Heart Failure

It is often forgotten that the object of the work described in the foregoing sections is primarily favourably to alter the natural history of heart failure. Yet, despite the incidence of this syndrome in the community and the enormous research and clinical effort directed to the pathogenetic mechanisms involved, its diagnosis and its treatment, relatively little knowledge exists of its natural history. In the past, various isolated accounts have been published directed to the outcome of heart failure in small selected groups with specific disease processes. But there is little data on its rate of occurrence in the community, the relative frequencies of predisposing causes and the prognosis in each. The reported incidence of heart failure in the community has varied by a factor of 40 (Klainer et al, 1965), but all studies of the incidence of heart failure have been hampered by the lack of consistent diagnostic information and comprehensiveness and the period of observation. An interpretative difficulty is the varying nature of the causes of heart failure in different areas of the world. But such studies are important from a number of aspects. The identification of factors that predispose to or influence the course of established disease are vital for a rational approach to prevention. Equally, the influence of treatment in the community is crucially dependent upon the outcome of such studies. A recent report from the Framingham community forms a model for such a study even if its interpretation is limited to Western urban society (McKee et al, 1971). Using uniform critera of diagnosis in a relatively closed community for a period of 16 years, these authors found that clinically serious heart failure developed in 3 per cent of men and 2 per cent of women over this time, i.e. an annual rate of 2.3/1000 for men and 1.4/1000 women. Two factors were prominent as predisposing causes: ageing and hypertension. Heart failure was preceded by hypertension far more frequently than by coronary heart disease: 75 per cent as against 10 per cent (in 40 per cent of patients in heart failure, both were present). This supports numerous less extensive clinical statements in the older literature implicating hypertension as the predominant cause of heart failure in Western man.

Current drug treatments of heart failure are often associated with rapid reversal of heart failure, often giving rise to uncritical optimism on the part of the profession regarding the long-term outlook for these findings. The findings of the Framingham survey are interesting in that they dispel any complacency that may exist regarding the long-term efficacy of current medical treatment of heart failure. Despite earlier recognition and treatment, the clinical course and prognosis remain grim and not much better than those for cancer in general. After the recognition of heart failure in men, more than 50 per cent were dead within five years and less than one in four lived for a decade. It has long been known that the adequate treatment of high blood pressure in hospital clinics significantly reduces the incidence of heart failure and vascular disease. It can only be deduced therefore that hypertension is largely hidden in our society and, when discovered, on the whole is unsatisfactorily treated. The preventative importance of screening of the adult population for hypertension is thus given added impetus; the recent introduction of less unpleasant antihypertensive drugs also gives hope for more successful prophylaxis against heart failure in the future.

CONCLUSIONS

The outstanding impression of present-day cardiology is that the immense increase in our knowledge of the fundamental biochemical and physiological processes of cardiac function has not been accompanied by similar advances in the treatment of patients in heart failure. In fact, the newer therapeutic methods now in use owe little to the background of experimentally derived information; even their conception was largely uninfluenced by traditional physiological thinking. In some instances the 'empirical' methods themselves have stimulated physiological interest and reappraisal of ideas. However, there is no denying that the elucidation of many of the pathophysiological mechanisms brought into play when the heart fails has supplied answers to some of the oustanding clinical questions.

The immense increase in experimental and investigative effort in the modern cardiological scene has unfortunately distracted clinicians from the ideal of their own professional pursuits, i.e. the *application* of knowledge of fundamental processes to the diagnosis and treatment of patients. The increasing dichotomy of real communication between workers in the experimental fields and the clinician in contact with the patient may well explain the increasing aloofness of physicians to experimental information of possible value in the treatment of their patients. These considerations explain two aspects highlighted in this review. The glitter of experimental science has led to the neglect of evaluation of clinical methods of detecting and then monitoring the progress of heart failure. Even the classification of the functional characterisation of heart failure has persisted unchallenged and unchanged for over 30 years—during which time the majority of present-day knowledge of cardiovascular function in health and disease has been accumulated. Even the natural history of heart failure has attracted little attention despite the fact that the incidence and dismal prognosis of the syndrome are self-evident in practice. The unpopularity of heart failure as a clinical topic is also reflected in the low level of clinical therapeutic interest in its correction. Digitalis and diuretics remain incompletely evaluated and uncritically accepted as the agents of choice in treatment—on far less evidence of benefit than is currently demanded of any new drug. It is hoped that such comments may soon be made redundant by the stimulation of clinical interest and perhaps concern for the low level of therapeutic activity in this vital field.

The treatment of the clinically dramatic acute heart failure and shock has attracted far more interest than the care of patients with chronic heart failure. During the past few years a number of significant advances in the treatment of acute severe heart failure have been made. In patients in whom the blood pressure is still maintained, the vasodilator drugs have become a widely accepted and efficacious treatment. In the search for 'different' agents a number of different drugs have been suggested without critical physiological appraisal. Consideration of the pathophysiological events in heart failure underlines the potentially superior value of vasodilator drugs with α-adrenoceptor blocking activity over others. Drugs which act by their positive inotropic activity in heart failure and shock await more adequate proof of their efficacy. This does not now appear to be the case with mechanical circulatory assist devices. During the past two years intra-aortic balloon pumping has become an established, if temporary, expedient for uncompensated hypotension associated with acute heart failure ('shock'). External counterpulsation methods applied to the lower limbs would appear to have even greater potential in their obviously wider application than methods requiring intravascular manipulations. But these mechanical methods cannot be used in isolation. They must only be used as an emergency rescue procedure temporarily improving the circulatory state to a point where the primary cardiac disease is more susceptive to methods of metabolic support or surgical correction.

REFERENCES

Allison, S. P., Morley, C. J. & Burns-Cox, C. J. (1972) Insulin, glucose and potassium in the treatment of congestive heart failure. *British Medical Journal*, **3**, 675.

Bergy, G. G. & Bruce, R. A. (1955) Discrepancies between subjective and objective evaluation of mitral commissurotomy. *New England Journal of Medicine*, **253**, 887.

Berman, D. A., Masuoka, D. T. & Saunders, P. R. (1957) Potentiation by ouabain of contractile response of myocardium to glucose. *Science*, **126**, 746.

Blaschko, H. (1973) Catecholamine biosynthesis. *British Medical Bulletin*, **29**, 105.

Brǝdy, A. J. (1968) Active state in cardiac muscle. *Physiological Reviews*, **48**, 570.

Braunwald, E. (1971) On the difference between the heart's output and its contractile state. *Circulation*, **43**, 171.

Braunwald, E. (1974) The autonomic nervous system in heart failure. In *The Myocardium; Failure and Infarction* ed. Braunwald, E., Ch. 6. New York: HP Publishing Co., Inc.

Braunwald, E. (1974) *The Myocardium: Failure and Infarction*. New York: HP Publishing Co., Inc.

Bregman, D. & Goetz, R. H. (1971) Clinical experience with a new cardiac assist device— the dual-chambered intra-aortic balloon assist. *Journal of Thoracic and Cardiovascular Surgery*, **62**, 577.

Brutsaert, D. L. & Sonnenblick, E. H. (1969) Force–velocity–length–time relations of the contractile elements in heart muscle of the cat. *Circulation Research*, **24**, 137.

Chatterjee, K., Parmley, W. W., Gorg, W., Forrester, J., Walinskij, P., Crexells, C. & Swan, H. J. C. (1973) Haemodynamic and metabolic responses to vasodilator therapy in acute myocardial infarction. *Circulation*, **48**, 1183.

Chidsey, C. A., Kauser, G. A., Sonnenblick, E. H., Spann, J. F. & Braunwald, E. (1964) Cardiac nor-epinephrine stores in experimental heart failure in the dog. *Journal of Clinical Investigation*, **43**, 2386.

Chidsey, C. A., Braunwald, E. & Morrow, A. G. (1965) Catecholamine excretion and cardiac stores of nor-epinephrine in congestive heart failure. *American Journal of Medicine*, **39**, 442.

Darforth, W. H., McKinsey, J. J. & Stewart, J. T. (1962) Transport and phosphorylation of glucose in the dog heart. *Journal of Physiology (London)*, **162**, 367.

Davis, J. O. (1971) What signals the kidney to release renin? *Circulation Research*, **28**, 301.

De Quattro, V., Nagatsu, T., Mendez, A. & Verska, J. (1973) Determinants of cardiac noradrenaline depletion in human congestive failure. *Cardiovascular Research*, **7**, 344.

Dilley, R. B., Ross, J. & Bernstein, E. F. (1973) Serial haemodynamics during intra-aortic balloon counterpulsation for cardiogenic shock. *Circulation*, **7**, Suppl. III, 99.

Dodge, H. T. (1974) Haemodynamic aspects of cardiac failure. In *The Myocardium; Failure and Infarction*, ed. Braunwald, E., Ch. 7. New York: HP Publishing Co., Inc.

Dormandy, J. A., Goetz, R. H. & Kripke, D. C. (1969) Haemodynamics and coronary blood flow with counterpulsation. *Surgery*, **65**, 311.

Edler, I. (1955) The diagnostic use of ultrasound in heart disease. *Acta medica scandinavica*, **152**, Suppl. 308, 32.

Edman, K. A. P. & Nilsson, E. (1968) The mechanical parameters of myocardial contraction studied at constant length of the contractile element. *Acta physiologica scandinavica*, **72**, 205.

Franciosa, J. A., Guiha, N. H., Limas, C. H., Rodriguera, E. & Cohn, J. N. (1972) Improved left ventricular function during nitroprusside infusion in acute myocardial infarction. *Lancet*, **1**, 650.

Franciosa, J. A., Mikulic, E., Cohn, J. N., Jose, E. & Fabie, A. (1974) Hemodynamic effects of orally administered isosorbide dinitrate in patients with congestive heart failure. *Circulation*, **50**, 1020.

Gertler, M. M., Saluste, E. & Spencer, F. (1970) Biochemical analyses of human papillary muscles and guinea-pig ventricles in failure. *Proceedings of the Society for Experimental Biology and Medicine*, **135**, 817.

Gibson, D. G. (1975) Assessment of left ventricular function in man by non-invasive techniques. In *Modern Trends in Cardiology*, 3rd edn, ed. Oliver, M. F., Ch. 9. London: Butterworth.

Gill, C. C., Wechsler, A. S., Newman, G. E. & Oldham, H. N. (1973) Augmentation and redistribution of myocardial blood flow during ischaemia by intra-aortic balloon pumping. *Annals of Thoracic Surgery*, **16**, 445.

Goetz, R. H., Bregman, D., Esrig, B. & Laniado, S. (1972) Unidirectional intra-aortic balloon pumping in cardiogenic shock and intractable left ventricular failure. *American Journal of Cardiology*, **29**, 213.

Gold, H. K., Leinback, R. C. & Sanders, C. A. (1972) Use of sublingual nitroglycerine in congestive failure following acute myocardial infarction. *Circulation*, **46**, 839.

Goldberg, L. I. (1972) Cardiovascular and renal actions of dopamine: potential clinical applications. *Pharmacology Reviews*, **24**, 1.

Greenberg, T. T., Richmond, W. H., Stocking, R. A., Gupta, P. D., Meehan, J. P. & Henry, J. P. (1973) Impaired atrial receptor responses in dogs with heart failure due to tricuspid insufficiency and pulmonary artery stenosis. *Circulation Research*, **32**, 424.

Gunnar, S. F. & Loeb, H. S. (1972) Use of drugs in cardiogenic shock due to acute myocardial infarction. *Circulation*, **45**, 1111.

Gunnar, S. F., McRitchie, R. J. & Braunwald, E. (1974) Effects of dobutamine on left ventricular performance, coronary dynamics and distribution of cardiac output in conscious dogs. *Journal of Clinical Investigation*, **53**, 1265.

Hamer, J. (1973) Fundamental aspects of myocardial performance. In *Recent Advances in Cardiology*, ed Hamer, J., Ch. 8, Edinburgh: Churchill Livingstone.

Hampton, J. R., Harrison, M. J. G., Mitchell, J. R. A., Prichard, J. S. & Seymour, C. (1975) Relative contributions of history taking physical examination and laboratory investigation to diagnosis and management of medical outpatients. *British Medical Journal*, **2**, 486.

Harken, D. E. (1958) Presentation at the International College of Cardiology, Brussels, Belgium.

Harley, H. R. S. (1961) The radiological changes in pulmonary venous hypertension with special reference to the root shadows and lobular pattern. *British Heart Journal*, **23** 75.

Henderson, A. H. (1975) Contractile basis of heart failure. In *Modern Trends in Cardiology*, 3rd edn, ed. Oliver, M. F., Ch. 7. London: Butterworth.

Higgins, C. B., Millard, R. W., Braunwald, E. & Vatner, S. F. (1973) Effects and mechanisms of action of dopamine on regional haemodynamics in the conscious dog. *American Journal of Physiology*, **225**, 432.

Hill, D. W. & Lowe, H. T. (1973) The use of the electrical-impedance technique for the monitoring of cardiac output and limb blood flow during anaesthesia. *Medical and Biological Engineering*, **11**, 534.

Jewitt, D., Birkhead, J., Mitchell, A. & Dollery, C. (1974) Clinical cardiovascular pharmacology of dobutamine. *Lancet*, **2**, 363.

Johns, E. J. & Singer, B. (1974) Specificity of blockade of renal renin release by propranolol in the cat. *Clinical Science and Molecular Medicine*, **47**, 331.

Johnson, J. A. & Davis, J. O. (1972) Effects of an angiotensin II analog on blood pressure and adrenal steroid secretion in dogs with thoracic caval constriction. *Physiologist*, **15**, 184.

Kantrowitz, A., Tjønneland, S., Freed, P. S., Philips, S. H., Butner, A. N. & Sharma, J. L. (1968) Initial clinical experience with intra-aortic balloon pumping in cardiogenic shock. *Journal of the American Heart Association*, **203**, 135.

Karim, F., Kidd, C., Malpus, C. M. & Pinna, P. E. (1972) The effects of stimulation of the left atrial receptors on sympathetic efferent nerve activity. *Journal of Physiology (London)*, **227**, 243.

Kelly, D. T., Delgado, C. E., Taylor, D. R., Pitt, B. & Ross, R. S. (1973) Use of phentolamine in acute myocardial infarction associated with hypertension and left ventricular failure. *Circulation*, **47**, 729.

Klainer, L. M., Gibson, T. C. & White, K. L. (1965) The epidemiology of cardiac failure. *Journal of Chronic Diseases*, **18**, 797.

Kostuk, W., Barr, J. W., Simon, A. L. & Ross, J. (1973) Correlations between the chest film and haemodynamics in acute myocardial infarction. *Circulation*, **48**, 624.

Krakoff, L. R., Buccino, R. A., Spann, J. F. & De Champlain, J. (1968) Cardiac catechol-*o*-methyltransferase and monoamine oxidase activity in congestive heart failure. *American Journal of Physiology*, **215**, 549.

Kralios, A. C., Zwart, H. H. J., Yenching, W., Moulopoulos, S. D. & Kolff, W. J. (1972) Coronary flow supplementation in experimental myocardial infarction with shock. *Chest*, **61**, 365.

Kubicek, W. G., Kottke, F. J., Ramos, M. U., Patterson, R. P., Witso, D. A., Labree, J. W., Remole, W., Layman, T. E., Schoening, H. & Garamela, J. T. (1974) The Minnesota impedance cardiograph—theory and applications. *Biomedical Engineering*, **9**, 410.

Lal, S., Savidge, R. S., Davies, D. M., Ali, M. M. & Soni, V. (1972) Intravenous salbutamol and cardiogenic shock. *Lancet*, **1**, 853.

Langer, G. A. (1974) The mechanism of action of digitalis. In *The Myocardium; Failure and Infarction*, ed. Braunwald, E., Ch. 13, New York: HP Publishing Co., Inc.

Lassers, B. W., George, M., Anderton, J. L., Higgins, M. R. & Philp, T. (1970) Left ventricular failure in acute myocardial infarction. *American Journal of Cardiology*, **25**, 511.

Ledsome, J. R. & Linden, R. J. (1968) The role of the left atrial receptors in the diuretic response to left atrial distension. *Journal of Physiology (London)*, **198**, 487.

Levin, A. B. (1966) A simple test of cardiac function based upon the heart rate changes induced by the Valsalva manoeuvre. *American Journal of Cardiology*, **18**, 90.

Levy, M. N. (1971) Sympathetic–parasympathetic interactions in the heart. *Circulation Research*, **29**, 437.

Linden, R. J. (1973) Function of cardiac receptors. *Circulation*, **48**, 463.

Loeb, H. S., Winslow, B. J. E., Rahimtoola, S. H., Rosen, K. M. & Gunnar, R. M. (1971) Acute haemodynamic effects of dopamine in patients with shock. *Circulation*, **44**, 163.

McKee, P. A., Castelli, W. P., McNamara, P. M. & Kannel, W. B. (1971) The natural history of congestive heart failure; the Framingham study. *New England Journal of Medicine*, **285**, 1441.

Majid, P. A., Sharma, B. & Taylor, S. H. (1971) Phentolamine for vasodilator treatment of severe heart failure. *Lancet*, **2**, 719.

Maroko, P. R., Kjekshus, J. K., Sobel, B. E., Watanabe, T., Covell, J. W., Ross, J. & Braunwald, E. (1971) Factors influencing infarct size following experimental coronary artery occlusion. *Circulation*, **43**, 67.

Maroko, P. R., Bernstein, E. F., Libby, P., Dehamia, G. A., Covell, J. W., Ross, J. & Braunwald, E. (1972) Effects of intra-aortic balloon counterpulsation on the severity of myocardial ischaemia injury following acute coronary occlusion. *Circulation*, **45**, 1150.

Maroko, P. R., Libby, P. & Braunwald, E. (1973) Effect of pharmacologic agents on the function of the ischaemic heart. *American Journal of Cardiology*, **32**, 930.

Milne, E. N. C. (1968) Physiological interpretation of the plain radiograph in mitral stenosis, including a review of criteria for the radiological estimation of pulmonary arterial and venous pressures. *British Journal of Radiology*, **36**, 902.

Moir, T. W. & Debra, D. W. (1967) Effect of left ventricular hypertension, ischaemia and vasoactive drugs on the myocardial distribution of coronary blood flow. *Circulation Research*, **21**, 65.

Moore, C. B., Kraus, W.L., Dock, D. S., Woodward, E. & Dexter, L. (1959) Experimental and laboratory reports. The relationship between pulmonary arterial pressure and roentgenographic appearance in mitral stenosis. *American Heart Journal*, **58**, 576.

Moulopoulos, S. D., Topaz, S. & Kolff, W. J. (1962) Diastolic balloon pumping (with carbon dioxide) in the aorta. A mechanical assistance to the failing circulation. *American Heart Journal*, **63**, 669.

Nayler, W. G. (1975) The ionic basic of contractility, relaxation and cardiac failure. In *Modern Trends in Cardiology*, 3rd edn, ed. Oliver, M. F., Ch. 6. London: Butterworth.

New York Heart Association Criteria Committee Report (1942) *Nomenclature and Criteria for Diagnosis of Diseases of the Heart and Great Vessels*. Boston: Little, Brown.

New York Heart Association Criteria Committee Report (1974) Major changes made by Criteria Committee of the New York Heart Association. *Circulation*, **49**, 390.

Nixon, P. G. F. & Durh, M. B. (1968) Pulmonary oedema with low left ventricular end-diastolic pressure in acute myocardial infarction. *Lancet*, **2**, 146.

Oliverio, A. & Wang, H. L. (1966) Effects of acute heart failure and administration of ouabain on cardiac catecholamine uptake. *Acta physiologica scandinavica*, **66**, 278.

Parker, J. O., Di Giorgi, S. & West, R. O. (1966) A haemodynamic study of acute coronary insufficiency precipitated by exercise. *American Journal of Cardiology*, **17**, 470.

Pool, P. E., Covell, J. W., Levitt, M., Gibb, J. & Braunwald, E. (1967) Reduction of cardiac tyrosine hydroxylase activity in experimental congestive heart failure. *Circulation Research*, **20**, 349.

Remensnyder, J. P., Mitchell, J. H. & Sarnoff, S. J. (1962) Functional sympatholysis during muscular activity. *Circulation Research*, **11**, 370.

Roberts, D. V. & Jones, E. S. (1963) A new system for recording the apex beat. *Lancet*, **1**, 1193.

Sassa, H. (1971) Mechanism of myocardial catecholamine depletion in cardiac hypertrophy and failure in rabbits. *Japanese Circulation Journal*, **35**, 391.

Scroop, G. C. & Whelan, R. F. (1966) A central vasomotor action of angiotensin in man. *Clinical Science*, **30**, 79.

Sharma, B. & Taylor, S. H. (1970) Reversible left ventricular failure in angina pectoris. *Lancet*, **2**, 902.

Sharma, B. & Taylor, S. H. (1975) Localisation of left ventricular ischaemia in angina pectoris by cineangiography during exercise. *British Heart Journal*, **37**, 963.

Sharpey-Schafer, E. P. (1955) Effect of Valsalva's manoeuvre on the normal and failing circulation. *British Medical Journal*, **1**, 693.

Soroff, H. S. & Birtwell, W. C. (1974) Assisted circulation: a progress report. In *The Myocardium; Failure and Infarction*, ed. Braunwald, E., Ch. 33. New York: HP Publishing Co., Inc.

Spann, J. F., Chidsey, C. A., Pool, P. E. & Braunwald, E. (1965) Mechanism of norepinephrine depletion in experimental heart failure produced by aortic constriction in the guinea-pig. *Circulation Research*, **17**, 312.

Talpins, N. L., Kripe, D. C. & Goetz, R. H. (1968) Counterpulsation and intra-aortic balloon pumping in cardiogenic shock. Circulatory dynamics. *Archives of Surgery*, **97**, 991.

Taylor, S. H. (1966) Measurement of the cardiac output in man. *Proceedings of the Royal Society of Medicine*, **59**, Suppl. 'Measurement in therapeutic assessment'.

Taylor, S. H. (1973a) The circulatory consequences of heart failure and shock. In *Recent Advances in Cardiology*, ed. Hamer, J., Ch. 10, Edinburgh: Churchill Livingstone.

Taylor, S. H. (1973b) The metabolic consequences of heart failure and shock. In *Recent Advances in Cardiology*, ed. Hamer, J., Ch. 10. Edinburgh: Churchill Livingstone.

Taylor, S. H. (1975) Beta-receptors and beta-blockers. *Australian Family Physician*, **4**, 9.

Taylor, S. H., Sutherland, G. R., MacKensie, G. J., Staunton, H. P. & Donald, K. W. (1965) The circulatory effects of intravenous phentolamine in man. *Circulation*, **31**, 741.

Taylor, S. H., Snow, H. M. & Linden, R. J. (1972) Relationship between left ventricular and aortic dp/dt (max). *Proceedings of the Royal Society of Medicine*, **65**, 550.

Taylor, S. H., Galvin, M. C., Pakrashi, B. C., Tulpule, A. T., Ionescu, M. I. & Whitaker, W. (1975) Clinical and haemodynamic results of mitral valve replacement with autologous fascia lata grafts; studies in patients with competent prostheses. *Circulation*, **52**, 880.

Urquhart, J., Davis, J. O. & Higgins, J. T. (1964) Simulation of spontaneous secondary hyperaldosteronism by intravenous infusion of angiotensin II in dogs with an arteriovenous fistula. *Journal of Clinical Investigation*, **43**, 1355.

Vatner, S. F. & Braunwald, E. (1974) Effects of chronic heart failure on the inotropic response of the right ventricle of the conscious dog to a cardiac glycoside and to tachycardia. *Circulation*, **50**, 728.

Vatner, S. F., Higgins, C. B. & Braunwald, E. (1974a) Coronary and left ventricular dynamic effects of norepinephrine in conscious dogs. *Circulation Research*, **34**, 812.

Vatner, S. F., McRitchie, R. J. & Braunwald, E. (1974b) Effects of dobutamine on left ventricular performance, coronary dynamics and distribution of cardiac output in conscious dogs. *Journal of Clinical Investigation*, **53**, 1265.

Walinsky, P., Chatterjee, K., Forrester, J., Parmley, W. W. & Swan, H. J. C. (1974) Enhanced left ventricular performance with phentolamine in acute myocardial infarction. *American Journal of Cardiology*, **33**, 37.

Weissler, A. M., Harris, W. S. & Schoenfeld, C. D. (1968) Systolic time intervals in heart failure in man. *Circulation*, **37**, 149.

Wells, R. E. (1964) Rheology of blood in the microvasculature. *New England Journal of Medicine*, **270**, 832.

Wyse, S. D., Gibson, D. G. & Branthwaite, M. A. (1974) Haemodynamic effects of salbutamol in patients needing circulatory support after open-heart surgery. *British Medical Journal*, **3**, 502.

Zelis, R., Mason, D. T. & Braunwald, E. (1968) A comparison of the effects of vasodilator stimuli on peripheral resistance vessels in normal subjects and in patients with congestive heart failure. *Journal of Clinical Investigation*, **47**, 960.

Zelis, R., Delea, C. S. & Coleman, H. M. (1969) Arterial sodium content in experimental congestive heart failure. *American Journal of Cardiology*, **23**, 144.

15
HEART FAILURE—II
John Hamer

THE FUNDAMENTAL DISTURBANCE OF
CONGESTIVE HEART FAILURE

The syndrome of congestive heart failure includes a number of pathological processes which vary in emphasis from one patient to another.

Although fluid retention is the predominant feature, an increase in ventricular filling pressure and a reduction in cardiac output are usual and may play a major part in the production of symptoms.

Filling Pressure

An increase in ventricular filling pressure may be due to operation of the Frank–Starling mechanism, an adaptive process increasing the ventricular response, or to increased ventricular diastolic stiffness from hypertrophy (see p. 289) or disease. Increased stiffness is a dominant feature in constrictive pericarditis in some patients with endomyocardial fibrosis and in some myocardial diseases, such as amyloid of the heart. The fibrotic element in the ischaemic myocardium makes increased stiffness a major factor in the syndrome of congestive heart failure in ischaemic heart disease. In hypertrophic obstructive cardiomyopathy the great increase in diastolic stiffness of the ventricle is associated with the severe hypertrophy of the myocardium. The characteristic feature of these 'stiff' hearts is congestive heart failure with relatively little increase in heart size, for instance on chest x-ray.

Fluid Retention

Fluid retention is generally related to the selective fall in renal blood flow in congestive heart failure (see later, p. 402) although Gibson, Marshall and Lockey (1970), on the basis of studies in patients with atrial septal defect who did not show the usual tendency to increased sodium reabsorption after propranolol, suggest that the underlying mechanism is related not to a disturbance of arterial pressure or flow but to some peripheral aspect of the maintenance of systemic venous return, an effect from changes in left atrial or left ventricular filling was excluded by inconsistencies between patients with mitral stenosis and those with ischaemic heart disease. Changes in the smaller veins where the capacity of the circulation is greatest may play a considerable part in the regulation of the venous return, and consequently in the control of ventricular filling and of cardiac output (Guyton, 1963). An increase in sympathetic tone has a major effect on the peripheral vessels in congestive heart failure and may be triggered by hypoxic effects on skeletal muscle consequent on reduced blood flow (Zelis et al, 1973). The distribution of venous congestion and oedema between the pulmonary and systemic circulation is related to the filling pressures on the two sides of the heart (Guyton, 1963).

Symptoms

Mason (1973) classifies the symptoms of congestive heart failure as those due to adaptive processes, such as dyspnoea from pulmonary congestion, angina from hypertrophy of ventricular muscle in the presence of impaired coronary flow and tachycardia from excessive sympathetic stimulation, and those from frank decompensation with an inadequate cardiac output, such as fatigue at rest and confusional states or other evidence of poor perfusion of vital organs. In most patients with severe heart disease symptoms are related to the increase in circulating blood volume and the collection of oedema fluid in the tissues. Relatively little fluid retention in the small tight left atrial and pulmonary venous compartment is needed to produce serious symptoms from pulmonary congestion in patients with disease of the left side of the heart. In right ventricular failure, as from pulmonary hypertension or tricuspid stenosis, on the other hand, the clinical picture is dominated by systemic oedema associated with the high filling pressure on the right side of the heart where the right atrium is free to expand into the large systemic venous system and the volume of the extracellular fluid may be very greatly increased.

In constrictive pericarditis where the filling pressure is equally raised on both sides of the heart the systemic venous congestion dominates the clinical picture suggesting that a modest elevation of venous pressure is better tolerated in the pulmonary circulation.

Although treatment will produce symptomatic improvement by removing these accumulations of fluid, there are little corresponding changes in the underlying cardiac disturbances after diuresis (Stampfer et al, 1968). In other situations, such as acute cardiac infarction, acute pulmonary embolism or pericardial tamponade, a reduction in cardiac output is the major feature of the condition, presumably as serious effects are evident before compensatory fluid retention can occur. The variations in these components of congestive heart failure make a strict definition difficult but inadequate cardiac performance is involved in each case.

Compensatory Mechanisms

The compensatory mechanisms available to improve the response of the ventricle to the stresses of disease include the Frank–Starling effect (p. 271) augmented by more forceful atrial contraction producing a critical presystolic boost to left ventricular filling pressure but complicated by slippage of myocardial fibres (Linzbach, 1960; Spotnitz and Sonnenblick, 1968), improved myocardial performance by the staircase effect ('treppe') (Sarnoff and Mitchell, 1961), and increased sympathetic stimulation producing tachycardia and improved contraction.

In disease states the compensatory mechanisms are augmented by myocardial hypertrophy which is usually appropriate to restore the stress on the individual fibres to normal (Spotnitz and Sonnenblick, 1973). Digitalis effect may further augment myocardial performance (but see p. 414).

The myocardial response

This differs in different disease states (Mason, 1973). The concentric hypertrophy of pressure load, as in aortic stenosis hypertrophy, allows a great increase in ventricular systolic wall tension at the expense of increased diastolic stiffness and a necessarily raised filling pressure. In contrast, the eccentric hypertrophy of volume load, as in aortic or mitral regurgitation, in which dilatation allows more effective shortening in terms of volume ejected for a given change in length, at the expense of a need for greater wall tension from the Laplace relationship (Fig. 11.7), and diastolic stiffness seems to be diminished (Spotnitz and Sonnenblick, 1973). The reduced outflow impedance in regurgitant valve lesions, particularly mitral regurgitation, tends to reduce the load on the left ventricle in this situation (Mason, 1973); similarly the left ventricle has less load in ventricular septal defect than in persistent ductus arteriosus for an equivalent pulmonary blood flow. In primary myocardial disease both hypertrophy and dilatation are involved in the response (Mason, 1973).

Fluid retention in other situations

Other conditions producing fluid retention may mimic congestive heart failure by producing a raised venous pressure and oedema as in acute glomerulonephritis, nephrotic syndrome or cirrhosis without evidence of impaired myocardial performance. The situation is seen experimentally in animals with arteriovenous fistula (Taylor, Covell and Ross, 1968).

Inadequate Myocardial Performance in Congestive Failure

Local necrosis of fibres is a feature of the hypertrophic myocardium (Linzbach, 1960, Fig. 11.14; Spotnitz and Sonnenblick, 1973) and structural disorganisation on this basis may impair myocardial performance. Chronic excessive sympathetic stimulation (p. 377) is probably not primarily responsible for the impaired myocardial performance but interferes with an important compensatory mechanism (Rutenberg and Spann, 1973), although the response to exogenous catecholamines is increased. In addition to the mechanical problems of the hypertrophic ventricle the intrinsic performance of the muscle fibres seems to be abnormal (Spann et al, 1967).

Although there is no obvious structural change in the myofibrils a variety of biochemical disturbances have been detected in animal models (Schwartz et al, 1973). Phosphorylation in mitochondria is decreased, so energy supply may be disturbed. The ATPase of the actomyosin link may be abnormal, disturbing the contraction process itself. The most likely candidate for the primary disturbance is the process of excitation–contraction coupling involving Ca ions, which may be disturbed by changes in Ca binding or release in the sarcoplasmic reticulum or by interference with binding of Ca ion at the troponin molecule on the myofibril which allows the regulation of contraction by Ca ions. Katz (1973a) suggests that intracellular acidosis releases H ions which compete with Ca ions for the troponin receptor site. Local ischaemia in the hypertrophied myocardium may have such an effect.

SALT AND WATER RETENTION IN HEART FAILURE

Although the concept of fluid retention in the venous system behind a failing ventricle (backward-failure) has a certain attractive naive simplicity, it avoids the problem of the origin of the excess fluid clearly evident as an increase in total exchangeable Na ion; an alternative explanation for the fluid retention of congestive failure on the basis of a disturbance of renal Na excretion secondary to a reduction in cardiac output (forward-failure theory) is more satisfactory (Merrill, 1946) although the mechanisms are not yet fully understood.

The backward-failure theory remains useful to explain the distribution of retained fluid between the left- and right-sided venous systems.

Sodium Retention

Sodium retention in congestive heart failure may be regarded as a disturbance of feed-back control of the circulation, in which a persistent error signal due to inadequate cardiac output leads to an attempt to correct the disturbance by fluid (Na and water) retention, which should increase effective arterial blood volume and improve cardiac output by the Frank–Starling mechanism but which succeeds only in producing venous congestion and oedema. Three factors have been suggested as responsible for renal Na retention but the quantitative role of each component is not clear (Fig. 15.1).

1. Reduction in glomerular filtration rate (GFR).
2. Increased aldosterone activity.
3. A third factor as yet unknown acting on the proximal renal tubule.

Reduction in GFR
Reduction in GFR might be expected as renal blood flow falls as part of

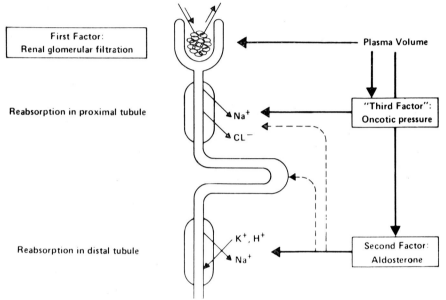

Figure 15.1 Renal sodium regulation. Diagram of the renal tubule to show the three major sites of renal sodium regulation. The first factor, filtration of sodium at the renal glomerulus, is related to renal blood flow and will be reduced by a fall in cardiac output. The second factor (in order of discovery), an increase in aldosterone activity, provoked via the renin–angiotensin–aldosterone mechanism by the reduction in renal blood flow which initiates release of renin from the juxtaglomerular apparatus, leading to the production of angiotensin in the plasma which stimulates the production of aldosterone by the adrenal cortex, producing sodium retention by an exchange mechanism in the distal renal tubule, associated with the loss of potassium and hydrogen ions. A third factor is postulated producing sodium re-absorption in the proximal renal tubule and may be quantitatively important, although the precise mechanism is not yet identified, a 'salt-loosing' hormone active at this site is postulated but physical factors leading to local changes in peritubular oncotic pressure or intrarenal redistribution of blood flow may be responsible. (Reproduced with permission from teaching material distributed by G. D. Searle and Co., High Wycombe)

the reduction in cardiac output. This effect is accentuated by the redistribution of blood flow (Wade and Bishop, 1962) mediated largely by sympathetic stimulation.

The quantitative effect of reduced renal blood flow has been held to be inadequate in itself to account for the Na retention of congestive heart failure, so this cannot be the sole mechanism.

Increased aldosterone activity

Increased aldosterone activity was postulated early (Merrill, 1946) and might be expected from the stimulus to renin secretion produced by reduction in renal perfusion pressure secondary to reduced renal blood flow (Vander, 1967; Davis, 1963, 1974; Johns and Singer, 1974; Brod, 1972).

Renin acts on a plasma precursor to produce the decapeptide angiotensin I, which is converted on passage through the lungs to the octapeptide angiotensin II, which produces the release of aldosterone from the zona glomerulosa of the adrenal cortex (Urquhart, Davis and Higgins, 1964) in addition to its direct action on vascular smooth muscle and its stimulatory effect on cerebral sympathetic vasomotor centres (Scroop and Whelan, 1966).

The importance of increased aldosterone activity is that it operates on an ionic exchange mechanism in the distal renal tubule (Fig. 15.1) so that Na retention is accompanied by loss of K and H ions producing K depletion (White et al, 1969) and metabolic alkalosis.

The influence of diuretic treatment on the aldosterone mechanism in congestive failure has been much clarified by the recent introduction of direct measurement of plasma aldosterone concentration by radioimmunoassay. Parallel changes in plasma renin activity as the aldosterone concentration varies (Nicholls et al, 1974) suggests that impaired hepatic breakdown of aldosterone from hepatic congestion or reduced hepatic arterial blood flow (Genest et al, 1968) plays little part in producing the high plasma aldosterone concentrations.

On the basis of the work of Nicholls et al (1974) three phases can be recognised in the activity of the renin–angiotensin–aldosterone system in congestive cardiac failure:

(a) *In the untreated state at the onset of congestive failure,* a modest increase as outlined above.

(b) *During the diuretic phase,* a paradoxical suppression of the renin–angiotensin–aldosterone system (Genest et al, 1968). Plasma aldosterone concentrations may be undetectable at this stage.

This response may be regarded as paradoxical, as diuretic treatment provokes a brisk increase in plasma aldosterone in normal subjects and in patients with hypertension. The suggestion that the suppression is due to an improved haemodynamic situation as a result of treatment (Genest et al, 1968) based on the hypothesis of a descending limb of the Frank–Starling curve, now discarded, seems unlikely as Stampfer et al (1968) have shown a fall rather than a rise in cardiac output as congestion is lost during diuretic treatment of cardiac failure.

A more likely mechanism is the great increase in Na load reaching the distal renal tubule. Na load to the distal tubule is the other major mechanism controlling renin release (Vander, 1967) and operates through a receptor in the macula densa of the distal tubule which from the convolution of the nephron is adjacent to the source of renin secretion, the juxtaglomerular apparatus on the afferent arteriole. The large Na load produced during diuresis seems capable of reversing other effects stimulating renin release in the situation of congestive heart failure in which some expansion of the circulatory blood volume persists in spite of the diuresis.

The low plasma aldosterone concentrations at this stage in treatment does not nullify the potential value of aldosterone antagonists as the large Na load to the distal tubule may result in extensive Na/K exchange and K loss, even though the plasma aldosterone levels are relatively low. Theoretically, ideal competitive antagonists such as spironolactone may be more effective at this stage, as the effect of lower concentrations of aldosterone is more easily

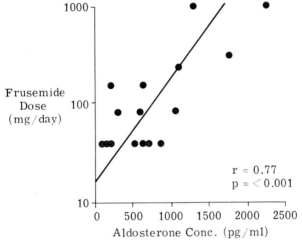

Figure 15.2 Relation of plasma aldosterone concentration to intensity of diuretic therapy. In a series of patients with treated congestive heart failure close to dry weight plasma aldosterone correlates closely ($r = 0.77$) with diuretic therapy expressed as daily dose of frusemide

overcome than that of the higher concentrations found at other stages in the treatment of congestive heart failure.

(c) *As the patient approaches dry weight*, with continued diuretic treatment, plasma aldosterone concentrations rise to very high levels (Nicholls et al, 1974; Hamer et al, 1976). The high plasma aldosterone levels which are related to the intensity of diuretic treatment (Fig. 15.2) are associated with depletion of total exchangeable K (Fig. 15.3) (Hamer et al, 1976). A parallel rise in plasma renin activity in a similar situation (Nicholls et al, 1974) suggests that the stimulus operates through the renin–angiotensin–aldosterone mechanism. A relation between plasma aldosterone and extracellular fluid volume measured as sulphate space (Fig. 15.4) suggests that reduction in effective arterial volume and in renal perfusion pressure is the determinant of the high plasma aldosterone concentrations in these patients (Knight et al,

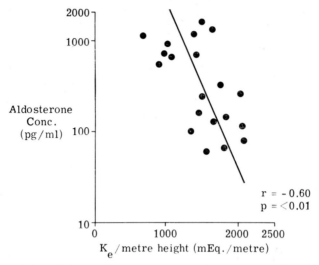

Figure 15.3   Relation of plasma aldosterone concentrations to total exchangeable potassium (K_e). In the same series of patients as Figure 15.2 high plasma aldosterone concentrations were associated with potassium depletion shown as an inverse correlation ($r = -0.60$) with K_e expressed in terms of height to correct for variations in body size in the presence of cachexia

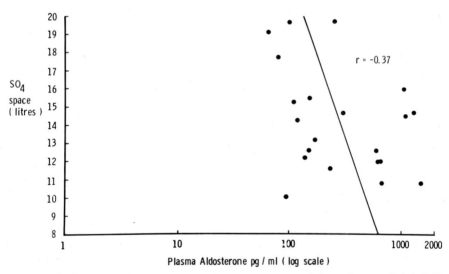

Figure 15.4   Relation between plasma aldosterone concentrations and extracellular fluid volume measured as sulphate space. From the same study as Figures 15.2 and 15.3, sulphate space was measured in some subjects and correlated negatively ($r = -0.37$), with plasma aldosterone, i.e. high plasma aldosterone concentrations were associated with reduced extracellular fluid volume

1975). Na load to the distal tubule will be low at this stage as there is little diuresis and diuretic therapy serves only to maintain dry weight against the stimulus to Na retention produced by the disturbance of cardiac performance.

The complex response makes assessment of data on the renin–angiotensin–aldosterone system in congestive heart failure of little value without further details, and much earlier work on aldosterone in heart failure before the use of radioimmunoassay must probably be discarded (Nicholls et al, 1974).

The third factor

This is a general term to cover unexplained mechanisms of Na retention generally thought to operate at the proximal tubule and perhaps of major importance in congestive heart failure (Gibson et al, 1970).

The existence of an unidentified 'salt-loosing hormone' probably of cerebral origin that can inhibit tubular Na absorption as the extracellular fluid expands has been postulated (Schrier and de Wardener, 1971) and disturbance of such a mechanism could produce the Na retention of congestive heart failure.

Physical factors may operate; for instance, changes in colloid oncotic pressure in peritubular capillaries may favour Na reabsorption as may alterations in the distribution of blood flow within the kidney (Kilcoyne, Schmidt and Cannon, 1971) as a response to the general reduction in renal blood flow; the tendency to medullary rather than cortical blood flow may favour nephrons with more potent Na-retaining properties.

Potassium Depletion in Congestive Heart Failure

Our own studies (White et al, 1969; Hamer et al, 1976) using radioisotope dilution methods have confirmed previous evidence of extensive K depletion in patients living the diuretic life, i.e. with stable severe congestive heart failure being kept relatively well and free of gross oedema by intensive diuretic treatment. Other work using natural ^{40}K (Edmonds and Jasoni, 1972) has confirmed the reduction in total body potassium in hypertensive patients on prolonged diuretic therapy; the changes were more severe in patients with cardiac involvement.

Nagent de Deuxchaisnes and his colleagues (1961, 1974) have analysed the reduced body potassium in heart disease to three components; potassium 'deficiency' which can be corrected by potassium loading, potassium 'depletion' which they suggest may be related to hypoxia and acidosis or to hyper-aldosteronism and cannot be restored by potassium supplements, and 'pseudodepletion' due to muscle wasting which they assessed by comparison with patients having muscular dystrophy; in this situation the intracellular potassium concentration in remaining cells would be unaffected (Fig. 15.5).

There are a number of difficulties in the interpretation of total exchangeable electrolyte data. The concept of lean body mass as a fixed fraction of total body water introduced for the study of obesity is not valid for studies of

14

congestive heart failure where various degrees of oedema and wasting may be present, and the use of body weight as a basis of comparison is excluded on similar grounds. The best index of body size is probably 'ideal weight', expressed in relation to the cube of height, or more simply height itself (as $h^3 \propto h$).

The suspicion that depletion of total exchangeable potassium (TEK) measured by radioisotope dilution was largely related to loss of lean body mass in cardiac cachexia (White et al, 1969) seems to be confirmed by studies of total body potassium (TBK) measuring the natural radioisotope ^{40}K in a

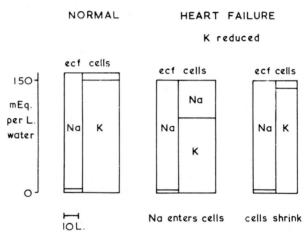

Figure 15.5 Gamble diagrams to show two postulated mechanisms of potassium depletion in heart failure. The normal ECF (extracellular fluid) and cell electrolyte situation is shown on the left. The centre and right-hand diagrams show two possible mechanisms of potassium depletion. In the centre intracellular potassium (K) concentration is reduced but cellular volume and osmolarity are maintained by the entry of sodium (Na) into the cells. At the right a similar reduction in total body potassium is shown but the cell osmotic pressure is maintained by a drastic reduction in cell mass, i.e. a 'pseudodepletion', in that the intracellular potassium concentration of the remaining cells is unaffected

whole body counter (Davidson et al, 1976; Lawson et al, 1976); these workers found no evidence of depletion; their findings were related to the body size of the patients at the time of study. The suggestion (Davidson et al, 1976) that TEK underestimates TBK because of slow equilibration of the isotope in patients with heart disease is countered by Olesen and Valentin (1973) who indicate that the error is unimportant as equilibration is sufficient to give results that are 90 per cent of the true value at 24 hours, the usual time of measurement.

Olesen and Valentin (1973) further confirm the view that loss of potassium is due to reduction in lean body mass by finding that the sodium content of the extracellular fluid volume (extracellular sodium), measured with ^{82}Br was similar to and closely correlated ($r = 0.89$) with total exchangeable sodium;

they suggest this indicates that no sodium has passed from the extracellular fluid to replace potassium lost from the cells, as would be expected to maintain osmotic equilibrium if the intracellular potassium concentration was reduced. Our own data from the study reported by Hamer et al (1976) does not entirely confirm this view. Although potassium depletion correlated to some extent with reduction in body weight ($r = 0.55$) (Fig. 15.6), as in our previous study (White et al, 1969), our calculations of extracellular sodium correlated only poorly ($r = 0.40$) (Fig. 15.7) with total exchangeable sodium and many patients

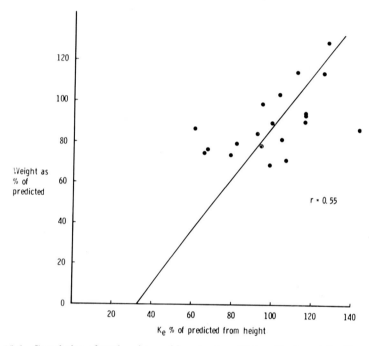

Figure 15.6   Correlation of total exchangeable potassium (K_e) and body weight. Even though K_e is corrected for expected body mass on the basis of height there is a correlation ($r = 0.55$) with body weight as predicted from height, suggesting that depleted K_e is partly due to loss of lean body mass

gave higher values for total exchangeable sodium, indicating some entry of sodium to the cells. These different findings may be in part explained by technical differences as we measured extracellular fluid volume as sulphate space, using an anion which does not enter cells, but Olesen and Valentin (1973) used [82]Br which behaves as an analogue of the chloride ion and may enter cells to some extent; an entry of chloride ions into the cells with sodium ions would obscure a minor reduction of intracellular potassium concentration. Comparison of our findings with plasma aldosterone measurements gave no definite evidence of a greater reduction of intracellular potassium concentration in hyperaldosteronism.

Direct attempts to measure intracellular potassium concentration have been difficult to interpret. A study of myocardial biopsies at operation (Schinert et al, 1966) is difficult to interpret because of drying of the specimens; and a study of leucocyte electrolytes by Edmondson et al (1974) fails to consider the effect of digitalis therapy in patients with heart disease, which may allow unusual entry of sodium into the cells in exchange for potassium.

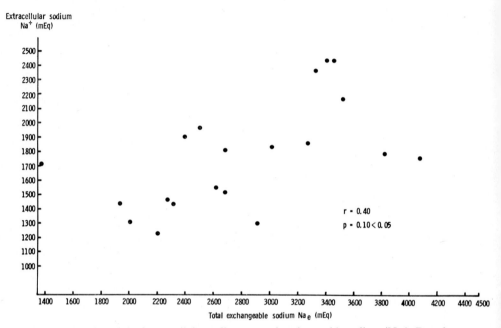

Figure 15.7   Relation of extracellular sodium to total exchangeable sodium (Na_e). Data from the same study as Figures 15.2, 15.3 and 15.4. Extracellular sodium calculated from total body water less sulphate space, and from sodium concentration in plasma water is related to total exchangeable sodium (Na_e). If all the sodium in the body is in the extracellular fluid these values should be the same, and the points should approximate to the line of identity. Although there is some correlation ($r = 0.40$) deviation from the line of identity towards the horizontal axis (Na_e) indicates entry of sodium into the cells so that total exchangeable sodium exceeds extracellular sodium

Although cardiac cachexia seems to play a major part in reducing body potassium due to loss of lean body mass, the 'pseudodepletion' of Nagent de Deuxchaisnes and colleagues (1961, 1974), some reduction of intracellular potassium concentration is difficult to exclude. If reflected in the myocardial cells, any reduction in intracellular potassium concentration would reduce the membrane potential leading to slow intercellular conduction and may possibly initiate late after-potentials, setting the background for serious ventricular ectopic rhythms or ventricular fibrillation. The finding (Lockey et al, 1966) of an increased incidence of arrhythmias after cardiac surgery in the presence of potassium depletion could not be confirmed by Olesen and Valentin (1973).

Therapeutic attention should be mainly directed to the maintenance of a normal plasma potassium concentration to avoid the synergistic effect of hypokalaemia and digitalis therapy. The plasma potassium forms part of a labile pool which is easily repleted by potassium supplements, but the difficulty in replacing lost body potassium after correction of hypokalaemia (Nagent de Deuxchaisnes and colleagues, 1961, 1974; White, 1970) (Fig. 15.8) might be in part related to the inappropriateness of the attempt to restore lean body mass unless the underlying heart disease is corrected, or an indication

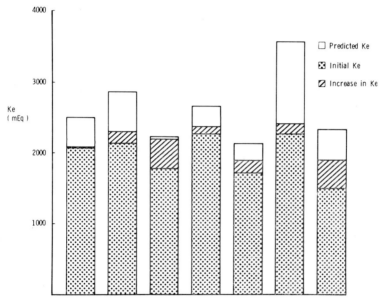

EFFECT OF POTASSIUM SUPPLEMENTS (48 mEq /day) or Ke

Figure 15.8 Effect of potassium supplements on total exchangeable potassium (K_e). Intensive therapy with potassium supplements (48 mEq/day), as Slow-K (Ciba) produced a consistent increase in K_e but the rise did not approach the predicted normal value in these patients with severe potassium depletion following intensive diuretic therapy for severe congestive heart failure. (From White, 1970)

that the potassium depletion is related to hyperaldosteronism which Schwartz and Swartz (1974) suggest may not respond to potassium therapy. In this case aldosterone antagonists may provide a more useful therapeutic approach which maintains the plasma potassium (Croxson, Neutze and John, 1972; Davidson and Gillebrand, 1973) and may in the long-term restore lost intracellular potassium.

It seems unlikely that hyperaldosteronism is directly responsible for the loss of tissue evident as cardiac cachexia, and a hypercatabolic state due to excess sympathetic stimulation and a glucocorticoid response is suspected, hyperaldosteronism serving to prevent retention of any lost cellular potassium.

Reduced or intermittent diuretic therapy may provoke less hyperaldosteronism but will not control symptoms satisfactorily in severe disease. The dried-out patient on 'the diuretic life' exchanges the discomfort and dangers of systemic and pulmonary oedema for the ill health of a low cardiac output state with cardiac cachexia and hyperaldosteronism. Medical treatment of the established situation is difficult, and my colleague Mr Gareth Rees suggests that if surgical treatment is feasible it should be considered before this degree of deterioration has occurred. We should regard the need for intensive diuretic therapy as an indication that surgical correction of the underlying heart disease should be considered.

Hyponatraemia in Congestive Heart Failure

Although in general retention of fluid in congestive heart failure is associated with Na retention, water being retained secondarily to maintain osmotic equilibrium, there have been suggestions that anti-diuretic hormone (ADH) might be involved. The cardinal feature of primary water retention from ADH is hyponatraemia, associated with a fall in plasma and tissue osmotic pressure due to dilution.

Hyponatraemia is not seen in the early stages of congestive heart failure but is a complication of prolonged failure usually with intensive treatment. However, there are hints that ADH may be involved and Lossnitzer and Bajusz (1974) found hyponatraemia at an early stage of failure in the spontaneous hereditary cardiomyopathy of the hamster; most authorities agree that ADH is not a major factor in the fluid retention of congestive heart failure (Laragh, 1962; Genest et al, 1968).

Possible causes of hyponatraemia in congestive heart failure are:

1. Inappropriate ADH activity, thought unlikely (see above),
2. the sick cell syndrome—cellular failure to maintain cellular osmolality transmitted to extracellular fluid,
3. renal mechanisms preventing the excretion of 'free water'.

The sick cell syndrome

In essence the suggestion is that interference with cellular metabolism may lead to a fall in intracellular osmolality leading to a secondary fall in extracellular fluid osmolality. Loss of anionic phosphate esters in congestive heart failure could have this effect (Flear, 1974) and could be associated with K loss. Leaf (1974) suggests that the loss of intracellular ions involved would be too great for hyponatraemia to arise in this way except as a transient event in agonal states with loss of renal function. In hyponatraemic congestive heart failure, Leaf (1974) concludes water is retained in excess of cations (Na and K) in the body.

Failure of 'free water' clearance

The renal disturbances of congestive heart failure provide a clear mechanism for excessive water retention in some severely affected patients (Bell, Schedl and Bartter, 1964). The excretion of free water, i.e. water absorbed or produced by the body without corresponding solute such as Na ions, relies on the arrival of a reasonable Na ion load at the distal tubules and collecting ducts. With excessive reabsorption of Na and water in the proximal tubules, less Na and water reaches the distal tubules and free water clearance is impaired. Dilutional hyponatraemia is generally met as a complication of phase c of congestive heart failure after a diuresis and while diuretic therapy is being used to maintain the dry weight or an optimal situation close to the dry weight.

Treatment is difficult and hyponatraemia generally heralds a terminal situation. In most patients with heart failure it is not necessary to restrict water intake as control of the Na balance is the primary problem. In dilutional hyponatraemia, water restriction may be helpful although it usually provokes intense thirst and it may be necessary to remove flower vases from the ward! The suggestion that plasma Na is reduced so some isotonic or even hypertonic saline should be given is erroneous, as total body Na is usually increased in these patients as the extracellular fluid although diluted remains expanded. Such treatment runs the risk of accentuating pulmonary oedema but is occasionally successful, presumably by increasing the Na load to the distal tubules. An osmotic diuretic such as intravenous mannitol may be helpful but must be used with caution because of the acute increase in blood volume provoked. Conventional diuretic therapy should continue to maintain the Na load, feeding the distal tubular water handling mechanism.

SOME ASPECTS OF DIGITALIS THERAPY

Mechanism of Digitalis Action

A unified theory of digitalis action (Langer, 1972; Langer and Serena, 1972) suggests that the action of digitalis glycosides relies on blockade of the myocardial cell membrane Na pump enzyme, a Na- and K-dependent adenosine triphosphatase (ATPase) responsible for the energy-dependent removal of Na ions from the cell in exchange for K ions, against the concentration gradients for these ions. The hypothesis further suggests that the consequent increase in intracellular Na with reduction in intracellular K concentration will disturb the membrane potential, leading to the production of ectopic arrhythmias, and that the inotropic actions of digitalis are due to a secondary effect of the increased intracellular Na on Ca ions either facilitating a membrane Na/Ca exchange process or by displacing Ca ions from intracellular stores, which may be in relation to the cell membrane (Naylor, 1975), with the net effect that Ca ion concentration is increased in the active region of the myofibrils augmenting the force and velocity of contraction which is dependent on Ca ions to release the actin and myosin interaction which produces myocardial contraction.

The work of Ogden, Selzer and Cohn (1969) shows that the effect of digitalis on AV conduction is independent of the inotropic action, the former being apparently related to changes in sympathetic activity (Mendez, Aceves and Mendez, 1961). Dissociation of the action on ectopic rhythms (via K ion) and the inotropic mechanism (via Ca ion) would not in itself upset the Langer theory, but the hypothesis in its simple form is rendered untenable by the observation of a dissociation between inhibition of the Na pump enzyme and the inotropic effect of digitalis glycosides (Okita, Richardson and Ruth-Schechter, 1973; Noble, 1975), although the pump enzyme is blocked by increasing concentrations. Although the unified theory may be rescued by adding secondary hypotheses and is still adequate to explain the arrhythmic action, it begins to look as though a different mechanism must be sought to explain the inotropic action of digitalis. Goldman et al (1975) indicate from their studies of the effect of hyperkalaemia on digoxin binding that the inotropic receptor must be closely linked to the Na- and K-dependent ATPase and Gervais et al (1975) suggest that changes in lipid Ca ion binding in relation to the enzyme may be responsible for the inotropic effect of ouabain. Lüllmann and Peters (1976) postulate a conformational change in the enzyme.

The Inotropic Effectiveness of Digitalis Treatment

Although an inotropic effect of digitalis has been accepted for many years (Mackenzie, 1911) and seems undoubted in experimental studies (Mason and Braunwald, 1963), sceptical physicians have long had doubts as to the long-term value of digitalis treatment used for an inotropic effect in patients in normal sinus rhythm (Scowen, 1965; Platt, 1975), the main clinical value of the drug being in the control of ventricular rate in atrial fibrillation by producing a suitable degree of AV block. Attempts to demonstrate a prolonged inotropic effect have been difficult, and using the velocity of the aortic ball valve as an index of left ventricular contraction, Davidson and Gibson (1973) showed only a slight but significant effect, one-third of the response produced by mild supine exercise, at 4 and 6 h after an oral dose, but not at 8 or 12 h. The inotropic action of digitalis is well known to be relatively weak compared to that of isoprenaline in animals (Ogden et al, 1969).

In a long-term cardiac catheterisation study, Cohn et al (1975) failed to show a sustained beneficial effect in eight patients with cardiomyopathy or ischaemic heart disease. When an improvement was noted, in three subjects, the peak effect was at 1 to $1\frac{1}{2}$ h after intravenous administration and was partially or totally lost at 2 to 4 h. A rise in arterial pressure was noticed if cardiac output increased, suggesting that arterial resistance did not fall. They suggest that the inotropic effect on myocardial contractility noted experimentally may not be translated effectively into an improved cardiac output in myocardial disease.

It seems possible that the inotropic effect of digitalis is obscured in clinical work by compensatory regulatory adjustment of other factors controlling myocardial performance, such as the Frank–Starling mechanism or the effect of stimulation by catecholamines (Davidson and Gibson, 1973; Cohn et al, 1975). It is suggested that therapeutic effects, such as diuresis or a fall in venous pressure, may be due to reflex effects, such as a reduction in sympathetic tone or an action elsewhere in the cardiovascular system, for instance venous dilatation (McMichael and Sharpey-Schafer, 1944).

If there is no descending limb of the Frank–Starling curve the advantage of a fall in venous pressure is difficult to judge, but such a response may help to relieve pulmonary congestion by dilating pulmonary veins or shifting fluid to a more compliant systemic venous system.

The pressor action may have an adverse effect and Katz (1973b) has questioned the value of driving the diseased myocardium by analogy with the situation in coronary artery disease, where inotropic interventions increasing myocardial oxygen consumption have been shown to accentuate ischaemia; a forced load on the abnormal myocardium in congestive heart failure may produce an adverse effect. If myocardial performance is limited, the compensatory mechanisms of the body may be obtaining an optimal response and adding the inotropic effect of digitalis may serve only to reduce the response through an existing mechanism. The response may be different in less diseased hearts; further work is clearly necessary to clarify the situation, particularly in paediatric practice where strong clinical suspicion exists of a response to digitalis as the sole therapy of heart failure.

Digitalis Dose

It is difficult to judge the correct dose when digitalis is used for its inotropic effect in sinus rhythm (Carruthers, Kelly and McDevitt, 1974; *British Medical Journal*, 1975a) as the gradual slowing of the ventricular rate which is such a useful feature of increasing dose in atrial fibrillation is not evident.

The concept of a 'full digitalising dose' conveying the impression of a progressive benefit up to toxic levels is also responsible for some excessive therapy (*British Medical Journal*, 1975a). The therapeutic margin is so narrow that it seems likely that many patients with sinus rhythm are being put at risk of toxic effects by digitalis therapy for an illusory advantage.

Effect of Potassium Depletion on Digitalis-induced Arrhythmias

An action of digitalis on the cell membrane Na pump suggests that digitalis glycosides produce ectopic arrhythmias by changing the ratio of intracellular

(K_i) to extracellular (K_o) potassium ion, so altering the membrane potential which is related to the ratio of $K_i:K_o$.

Potassium depletion may potentiate this effect in several ways. Intracellular potassium depletion replaced by Na to maintain osmotic balance might be expected to have such an effect, but must be gross to change the membrane potential seriously (see p. 410). A more likely mechanism is that reduction in plasma K concentration which will have relatively little effect on the K_o/K_i ratio potentiates the effect of digitalis on the Na pump. The Na- and K-dependent enzyme of the Na pump is orientated in the cell wall (Glynn, 1962; Naylor, 1975) to be driven by extracellular K and intracellular Na, and a reduction in extracellular K concentration might be expected to reduce the activity of the Na pump and potentiate the effects of digitalis. There is also competition between plasma potassium ion and digoxin for binding sites on the cell membrane (Goldman et al, 1975).

Binnion (1975) has challenged the conventional view that K depletion potentiates digitalis effect. He gives a preliminary report of animal work in which K depletion by various methods such as glucose–insulin infusion (low plasma K but no cellular depletion), thiazide treatment and a no K diet (most closely resembling the situation in congestive heart failure, with low plasma K probably associated with cellular K depletion) showed no sensitivity to digoxin infusion.

Although there has been little evidence to support the conventional view (Corbett, 1975), and a response to K treatment in digitalis toxicity may indicate only a therapeutic action of K ions rather than a preceding depletion, there is naturally caution in accepting these results as applicable to congestive heart failure in man.

A possible source of confusion is the likelihood that hypokalaemia from an increase in potent diuretic therapy will often be associated with reduced glomerular filtration rate, evident as a rising blood urea and falling creatinine clearance as renal blood flow falls further, and may potentiate digoxin effect as digoxin clearance will also be reduced. This situation should be distinguished by finding a plasma digoxin concentration in the toxic range (i.e. more than 2.0 ng/ml), whereas in digoxin toxicity potentiated by hypokalaemia the plasma digoxin is likely to be in the usual therapeutic range of 1 to 2 ng/ml.

Recently Shapiro and Taubert (1975) have produced some human data showing that hypokalaemia produces digoxin toxicity. In digoxin toxicity, normokalaemic patients (mean serum K 4.7 mEq/litre) had mean plasma digoxin concentrations over 3.7 ng/ml, but in hypokalaemic patients (mean serum K 3.0 mEq/litre) the mean digoxin was 1.1 ng/ml; the groups were comparable in other ways. There is thus good evidence to continue to avoid hypokalaemia in diuretic treatment of heart failure when patients are also being treated with digitalis glycosides.

(p. 404); the rationale is clear in stages 1 and 3 where the plasma aldosterone levels are raised, in stage 2 the phase of renin and aldosterone suppression antagonism of the low levels of aldosterone activity may still be important because of the large Na load reaching the distal tubule, increasing the quantitative importance of the aldosterone-controlled Na/K exchange system.

Spironolactone ('*Aldactone*') is an analogue of aldosterone which acts as a competitive antagonist and seems more likely to be effective in stages 1 and 2 of congestive heart failure (p. 404) than in stage 3 where the plasma aldosterone levels are very high. Spironolactone is moderately effective as a Na diuretic in addition to its action in retaining K ions and may be considered as a first line of diuretic treatment in moderately severe or mild congestive heart failure, where the rapid action of the 'loop diuretics' is not required. The more gradual effect of spironolactone avoids the rebound effect between doses seen with loop diuretics and thiazides.

Trimterene and amiloride have similar effect to spironolactone but are not specific competitors of aldosterone, acting to produce a contrary effect at the same level in the nephron. Their action is likely still to be evident in the face of very high plasma aldosterone levels. Amiloride (5 mg) with each dose of frusemide (40 mg) orally seems effective in preventing hypokalaemia and eliminates the need for K supplements in most patients.

Diet. Strict Na restriction is not generally necessary in association with modern potent diuretic treatment so long as excessive Na loading is avoided, and may have the disadvantage of provoking further hyperaldosteronism in congestive heart failure. Potassium supplements are not usually needed in patients on spironolactone or amiloride and may provoke dangerous hyperkalaemia in patients with impaired renal function.

Bed Rest

Excessive physical activity and the upright posture may direct blood flow from the kidneys (Wade and Bishop, 1962) accentuating the impairment of glomerular filtration rate and provoking further renin and aldosterone activity, so bed rest still has a useful part to play in treatment. There is an increased risk of venous thrombosis in association with the reduced peripheral blood flow in congestive heart failure and consideration should be given to long-term anticoagulant therapy if strict bed rest is recommended, as pulmonary embolism is a frequent and troublesome complication of congestive heart failure.

The recently reported response of patients with severe heart muscle disease to long-continued low-grade β-adrenergic blockade (Waagstein et al, 1975) could operate by interfering with renin release which is mediated by the sympathetic nervous system when provoked by dietary Na restriction in animals, and may operate via the renin angiotensin–aldosterone mechanism or within the kidney by local angiotensin formation to increase Na retention by a redistribution of renal blood flow (Warren and Ledingham, 1975), a possible 'third factor' (p. 407). This mechanism may operate in addition to any effect from the removal of inappropriate tachycardia as a result of sympathetic stimulation. This approach must be used with great caution as the myocardial effect of β-adrenergic blockade suddenly removing a major compensatory mechanism maintaining myocardial performance may produce disastrous acute failure.

REFERENCES

Asbury, M. J., Gatenbo, P. B. D., O'Sullivan, S. & Boarke, K. (1972) Bumetanide: potent new 'loop' diuretic. *British Medical Journal*, **1**, 211.

Bell, N. H., Schedl, H. P. & Bartter, F. C. (1964) An explanation for abnormal water retention and hypo-osmolality in congestive heart failure. *American Journal of Medicine*, **36**, 351.

Binnion, P. F. (1975) Hypokalaemia and digoxin-induced arrhythmias. *Lancet*, **1**, 343, 743.

British Medical Journal (1975a) Problems with digoxin. **1**, 49.

British Medical Journal (1975b) Picking a diuretic. **1**, 521.

Brod, J. (1972) Pathogenesis of cardiac oedema. *British Medical Journal*, **1**, 222.

Carruthers, S. G., Kelly, J. G. & McDevitt, P. G. (1974) Plasma digoxin correlations in patients on admission to hospital. *British Medical Journal*, **36**, 707.

Cohn, K., Selzer, A., Kersch, E. S., Karpman, L. S. & Goldschlager, N. (1975) Variability of haemodynamic responses to acute digitalisation in chronic cardiac failure due to cardio-myopathy and coronary artery disease. *American Journal of Cardiology*, **35**, 461.

Corbett, L. C. (1975) Hypokalaemia and digoxin induced arrhythmias. *Lancet*, **1**, 742.

Croxson, M. S., Neutze, J. M. & John, M. B. (1972) Exchangeable potassium in heart disease: long-term effect of potassium supplements and amiloride. *American Heart Journal*, **54**, 53.

Davidson, C., Burkinshaw, L., McLachlan, M. S. F. & Morgan, D. B. (1976) Effect of long-term diuretic treatment on body-potassium in heart-disease. *Lancet*, **2**, 1044.

Davidson, C. & Gibson, D. (1973) Clinical significance of positive inotropic action of digoxin in patients with left ventricular disease. *British Heart Journal*, **35**, 970.

Davidson, C. & Gillebrand, I. M. (1973) Use of amiloride as a potassium-conserving agent in severe cardiac disease. *British Heart Journal*, **35**, 456.

Davis, J. O. (1963) The role of the adrenal cortex and the kidney in the pathogenesis of cardiac oedema. *Yale Journal of Biology and Medicine*, **35**, 402.

Davis, J. O. (1974) The mechanisms of salt and water retention in cardiac failure. In *The Myocardium: Failure and Infarction*, ed. Braunwald, E., p. 50. New York: HP Publishing Co., Inc.

Edmonds, C. I. & Jasoni, B. M. (1972) Total body potassium changes in hypotensive patients during prolonged diuretic therapy. *Lancet* **2**, 8.

Edmondson, R. P. S., Thomas, R. D., Hilton, D. J., Patrick, J. & Jones, N. F. (1974) Leuco-cyte electrolytes in cardiac and non-cardiac patients receiving diuretics. *Lancet*, **1**, 12.

Edwards, R. H. T. (1975) Presented at the Joint Meeting of the British Cardiac Society and the Swedish Societies of Cardiology, Stockholm, 1st September 1975.

Flear, C. T. G. (1974) Hyponotraemia. *Lancet*, **1**, 164.

Genest, J., Granger, P., de Champlain, J. & Boucher, R. (1968) Endocrine factors in con-gestive cardiac failure. *American Journal of Cardiology*, **22**, 35.

Gervais, A., Lindenmayer, G., Entman, M. C., Pitts, B. I. R., Lane, L. K. & Schwartz, A. (1975) A mechanism for ouabain action involving calcium-Na^+, K^+-ATPase interaction. *Circulation*, **51/52**, Suppl. II, 25.

Gibson, D. G., Marshall, J. C. & Lockey, E. (1970) Assessment of proximal tubular sodium reabsorption during water diuresis in patients with heart disease. *British Heart Journal*, **32**, 399.

Glynn, I. M. (1962) Activation of adenosine triphosphatase activity in a cell by external potassium and internal sodium. *Journal of Physiology, London*, **160**, 18P.

Goldman, R. H., Coltart, P. J., Schweiger, E., Snidow, G. & Harrison, D. C. (1975) Dose response in vivo to digoxin in normo- and hyperkalaemia: associated biochemical changes. *Cardiovascular Research*, **9**, 515.

Guyton, A. C. (1963) *Cardiac Output and its Regulation*. Philadelphia: W. B. Saunders.

Hamer, J., Knight, R. K., Miall, D. A., Hawkins, L. A. & Dacombe, J. (1976) Plasma aldosterone levels in patients with severe, treated congestive heart failure. *British Heart Journal*, **38**, 534.

Hayward, G. W. (1955) Pulmonary oedema. *British Medical Journal*, **1**, 1361.

Johns, E. J. & Singer, B. (1974) Specificity and blockade of renal renin release by propranolol. *Clinical Science and Molecular Medicine*, **47**, 331.

Katz, A. M. (1973a) Effects of ischaemia on the contractile processes of heart muscle. *American Journal of Cardiology*, **32**, 456.

Katz, A. M. (1973b) Biochemical defect in the hypertrophied and failing heart. Deleterious or compensatory. *Circulation*, **47**, 1076.

Kilcoyne, N. M., Schmidt, D. H. & Cannon, P. J. (1971) Intrarenal blood flow in congestive heart failure. *Circulation*, **43/44**, Suppl. II, 65.

Langer, G. A. (1972) Effects of digitalis on myocardial ionic exchange. *Circulation*, **46**, 180.

Langer, G. A. & Serena, S. D. (1972) Effects of strophanthidin upon contraction and ionic exchange in rabbit ventricular myocardium: relation to control of active state. *Journal of Molecular and Cellular Cardiology*, **1**, 65.

Laragh, J. H. (1962) Hormones and the pathogenesis of congestive heart failure: vasopressin, aldosterone and angiotensin. II. Further evidence for renal-adrenal interaction from studies in hypertension and in cirrhosis. *Circulation*, **25**, 1015.

Lawson, R. H., Boddy, K., Gray, J. M. B., McHaffey, M. & Mills, E. (1976) Potassium supplements in patients receiving long-term diuretics for oedema. *Quarterly Journal of Medicine*, N.S. **45**, 469.

Leaf, A. (1974) Hyponatraemia. *Lancet*, **1**, 1119.

Linzbach, A. J. (1960) Heart failure from the point of view of quantitative anatomy. *American Journal of Cardiology*, **5**, 370.

Lockey, E., Longmore, D. B., Ross, D. N. & Sturridge, M. F. (1966) Potassium and open-heart surgery. *Lancet*, **1**, 671.

Lossnitzer, K. & Bajusz, E. (1976) Water and electrolyte alterations during the life course of the B.I.O. 14G. Syrian golden hamster. A disease model of hereditary cardiomyopathy. *Journal of Molecular and Cellular Cardiology*, **6**, 163.

Lüllmann, H. & Peters, Th. (1976) In *Proceedings of the 7th European Congress of Cardiology*, 325.

Mackenzie, J. (1911) Digitalis. *Heart*, **2**, 273.

Mason, D. T. (1973) Regulation of cardiac performances in clinical heart disease. Interactions between contractile state, mechanical abnormalities and ventricular compensatory mechanisms. *American Journal of Cardiology*, **33**, 437.

Mason, D. T. & Braunwald, E. (1963) Studies on digitalis. IX. Effects of ouabain on the non-failing human heart. *Journal of Clinical Investigation*, **42**, 1165.

McMichael, J. & Sharpey-Schafer, L. D. (1944) The action of intravenous digoxin in man. *Quarterly Journal of Medicine*, N.S. **13**, 123.

Mendez, C., Aceves, J. & Mendez, R. (1961) The anti-adrenergic action of digitalis on the refractory period of the AV transmission septum. *Journal of Pharmacology and Experimental Therapeutics*, **131**, 199.

Merrill, A. J. (1946) Oedema and decreased renal blood flow in patients with chronic congestive heart failure; evidence of 'forward failure' as the primary cause of oedema. *Journal of Clinical Investigation*, **23**, 389.

Nagent de Deuxchaisnes, C., Collet, R. A., Basset, R. & Mach, R. S. (1961) Exchangeable potassium in wasting amyolophy heart disease and cirrhosis of the liver. *Lancet*, **1**, 61.

Nagent de Deuxchaisnes, C. & Mach, R. S. (1974) Potassium depletion and potassium supplementation in cardiac failure. *Lancet*, **1**, 517.

Naylor, W. C. (1975) Ionic basis of contractility, relaxation and cardiac failure. *Modern Trends in Cardiology*, ed. Oliver, M. F., Vol. 3, p. 154. London: Butterworths.

Nicholls, M. G., Espiner, E. A., Donald, R. A. & Hughes, H. (1974) Aldosterone and its regulation during diuresis in patients with gross congestive heart failure. *Clinical Science and Molecular Medicine*, **47**, 301.

Noble, D. (1975) Action of cardiac glycosides. Presented to Cardiac Muscle Research Group, Oxford, 4th July 1975.

Ogden, P. C., Selzer, A. & Cohn, K. E. (1969) The relationship between the inotropic and dromotropic effects of digitalis. The modulation of these effects by autonomic influences. *American Heart Journal*, **77**, 628.

Okita, G. T., Richardson, F. & Ruth-Schechter, B. F. (1973) Dissociation of the positive inotropic action of digitalis from inhibition of sodium and potassium activated adenosive triphosphatase. *Journal of Pharmacology and Experimental Therapeutics*, **185**, 5.

Olesen, K. H. & Valentin, N. (1975) Total exchangeable potassium, sodium and chloride in patients with severe valvular heart disease. *Scandinavian Journal of Thoracic and Cardiovascular Surgery*, **7**, 37.

Platt, Lord (1975) Questionable dogma. How useful is digitalis? *World Medicine*, 7th May, p. 38.

Rutenberg, H. L. & Spann, J. F. (1973) Alterations of cardiac sympathetic neurotransmitter activity in congestive heart failure. *American Journal of Cardiology*, **33**, 472.

Sarnoff, S. J. & Mitchell, J. H. (1961) The regulation of the performance of the heart. *American Journal of Medicine*, **30**, 747.

Schimert, G., Hunt, O. R., Lillenstein, M. & Brennan, J. C. (1966) Sodium/potassium ratios in papillary muscle biopsic obtained during mitral valve replacement. *Journal of Thoracic and Cardiovascular Surgery*, **52**, 126.

Schrier, R. W. & de Wardener, H. E. (1971) Tubular reabsorption of sodium ion: influence of factors other than aldosterone and glomerular fibrillation rate. *New England Journal of Medicine*, **285**, 1231, 1292.

Schwartz, A., Sodahl, L. A., Entman, M. L., Allen, J. C., Reddy, T. S., Goldstein, M. A. & Wyburg, C. E. (1973) Abnormal biochemistry in myocardial failure. *American Journal of Cardiology*, **32**, 407.

Schwartz, A. B. & Swartz, C. D. (1974) Dosage of potassium to correct thiazide-induced hypokelemia. *Journal of American Medical Association*, **230**, 702.

Scowen, Sir E. F. (1965) Personal communication.

Scroop, G. C. & Whelan, R. F. (1966) Central vasomotor action of angiotensin in men. *Clinical Science*, **30**, 79.

Shapiro, W. & Taubert, K. (1975) Hypokalaemia and digoxin-induced arrhythmias. *Lancet*, **2**, 604.

Spann, J. F., Covell, J. W., Eckberg, D. C., Sonnenblick, E. K., Ross, T. & Braunwauld, E. (1967) Myocardial contractile state in hypertrophy and congestive failure: studies in the intact heart and the isolated muscle. *Circulation*, **36**, Suppl., 2, 241.

Spotnitz, H. M. & Sonnenblick, E. H. (1973) Structural conditions in the hypertrophied and failing heart. *American Journal of Cardiology*, **37**, 391.

Stampfer, M., Epstein, S. E., Beiser, G. D. & Braunwauld, E. (1968) Hemodynamic effects of diuresis at rest and during intense upright exercise in patients with impaired cardiac function. *Circulation*, **37**, 900.

Taylor, R. R., Covell, J. W. & Ross, J. (1965) Left ventricular function in experimental aorta-caval fistula with circulatory congestion and fluid retention. *Journal of Clinical Investigation*, **47**, 1333.

Urquhart, J., Davis, J. O. & Higgins, J. T. (1964) Simulation of spontaneous secondary hyperaldosteronism by intravenous infusion of angiotensin II in dogs with an arteriovenous fistula. *Journal of Clinical Investigation*, **43**, 1355.

Vander, A. J. (1967) Control of renin release. *Physiological Reviews*, **47**, 359.

Waagstein, F., Hjalmarson, A., Varnauskas, E. T Wallentin, I. (1975) Effect of chronic beta-adrenergic receptor blockade in congestive cardiomyopathy. *British Heart Journal*, **37**, 1022.

Wade, O. L. & Bishop, J. M. (1962) *Cardiac Output and Regional Blood Flow*. Oxford: Blackwell.

Warren, D. J. & Ledingham, J. G. G. (1975) Effects of beta-adrenergic receptor blockade on the renal vascular response to a low sodium diet in the rabbit. *Clinical Science and Molecular Medicine*, **48**, 533.

Watson, M. (1975) Picking a diuretic. *British Medical Journal*, **3**, 369.
White, R. J. (1970) Effect of potassium supplements on the exchangeable potassium in chronic heart disease. *British Medical Journal*, **3**, 141.
White, R. J., Chamberlain, D. A., Hamer, J., McAllister, J. & Hawkins, L. A. (1969) Potassium depletion in severe heart disease. *British Medical Journal*, **2**, 606.
Zelis, R., Longhurst, J., Capone, R. J. & Lee, G. (1973) Peripheral circulation central mechanism in congestive heart failure. *American Journal of Cardiology*, **32**, 481.

16
CLINICAL PHARMACOKINETICS
OF DIGITALIS

T. R. D. Shaw

In the last few years a new dimension was added to the study and use of digitalis when methods were introduced for assaying the cardiac glycosides in the body fluids. Unlike the early work with radioactive digoxin and digitoxin these assays could be used to study large numbers of cardiac patients in routine clinical situations and during use of standard digitalis preparations. They have been much used to study how the body handles the digitalis drugs (the pharmacokinetics) and how this handling is disturbed by disease or by interference from other drugs. The assays can be of considerable help in clinical situations. Failure to achieve a satisfactory effect from digitalisation is due either to insufficient glycoside reaching the tissues and receptors or to an abnormal type of response: assessment of the body stores of glycoside by measurement of the plasma glycoside level allows these two components of the problem to be separated. In addition, plasma levels can be a guide for the adjustment of dosage, and can help in deciding when digitalis toxicity is present, since this is more likely to occur when body glycoside levels are high.

In this chapter I shall try to outline the new knowledge gained about the processes which influence the body's handling of digitalis. An understanding of these processes is helpful in anticipating the effect of digitalisation and is needed for the full interpretation of plasma glycoside levels. The emphasis will be on digoxin since this is by far the commonest digitalis preparation used in the United Kingdom.

Use of Digitalis Assays: General Considerations

Assays

Considerable ingenuity produced several different techniques for assay of the cardiac glycosides during the 1960s. These were a double isotope dilution derivative assay, gas chromatography, two techniques using competitive binding (radioimmunoassay and radioreceptor assay), and two assays based on measurement of the inhibition by digitalis of the Na-K-dependent ATPase in cell membranes (using erythrocyte rubidium 86 uptake and ATP degradation by hog brain homogenates). Their characteristics have been compared by Butler (1972). The digoxin radioimmunoassay, using the principle of competition between the sample and a fixed amount of radioactive digoxin for binding sites on digoxin antibody, was based on the methodology developed for assay of peptide hormones. It became feasible when suitable antibodies to digoxin were raised in rabbits (Butler and Chen, 1967). Initially tritiated digoxin was used, requiring a beta counter. The radioimmunoassay subsequently developed for clinical use (Smith, Butler and Haber, 1969) has become by far the most widely used digoxin assay because of its advantages in speed, simplicity, sensitivity and accuracy. Radioimmunoassay kits are available commercially and are being increasingly used in clinical chemistry laboratories. Their use expanded further when kits were produced with iodine-isotopes which needed the simpler and more readily available gamma counter.

Pharmacokinetics

Recording at random the blood level of drugs would be of as little use as recording random blood glucose levels. The measurements have to be interpreted in the light of the physiological processes which are acting and of the setting in which the measurements were taken. Fortunately our understanding of the physiological principles which apply to the administration, absorption, distribution and excretion of drugs has become much more detailed during the last decade. Pharmacokinetics is the study of the drug concentration changes in the body resulting from these processes (Gibaldi, 1971; Notari, 1971). The use of drug assays is inseparable from pharmacokinetics. One of its most important concepts is that it is valid to consider the body simplified into one or more distinct, homogeneous, drug-containing compartments. In the commonly used 'two-compartment model' the body is conceived as consisting of a central compartment, corresponding to the blood and highly perfused tissues, and a larger peripheral compartment, corresponding to the tissues into and from which drugs diffuse more slowly. Absorption and excretion take place via the central compartment. The peripheral compartment is a larger pool in which the drug may be reversibly bound to the tissue proteins. When the very diverse tissues of the body are simplified into this anatomical model then the speed of absorption, diffusion between the tissues, and elimination can be considered as single rate constants. The practical use of this concept is that using measurement of drug concentration changes in readily accessible fluids such as blood and urine, conclusions can be made about the handling of the drug by the body as a whole, and processes such as elimination and tissue binding can be quantitated. In addition, simple equations based on such models are useful to predict how the body content of the drug will be affected by changes in excretion and absorption and how long it will take to reach a steady state of balance between absorption and excretion during repeated dosing.

The pharmacokinetic principles and equations are essential for quantitating absorption but are also very useful concepts in practical therapeutics, particularly for digitalis (Marcus, 1975). They are only now becoming more widely known by clinicians, although they were used in part in the initial studies with radioactive digoxin by Doherty and associates (1961, 1962) and in the pioneer attempts by Jelliffe (1967, 1968) to rationalise digitalis administration.

Bioavailability and biopharmaceutics

Two terms often associated with pharmacokinetics are 'bioavailability' and 'biopharmaceutics'. The term bioavailability or biological availability is awkward because it covers two aspects of drug absorption into the systemic circulation—how rapidly the drug is absorbed and how much is absorbed—and the two are sometimes unrelated. However it has the advantage of emphasising that the way a drug reaches the tissues depends both on the route of administration and on the formulation. The place of bioavailability in general therapeutics has been well summarised by Koch-Weser (1974). 'Biopharmaceutics' is the study of how the physical and chemical characteristics of tablets, elixirs, suspensions, etc., affect drug absorption (Wagner, 1971).

Bioavailability of Digoxin Tablets

Absorption characteristics

One of the most important advances produced by the use of the digitalis assays so far has been the demonstration that the absorption of digoxin is greatly influenced by its pharmaceutical formulation.

The first indication that there was a problem with the bioavailability of digoxin tablets came with reports of significant differences in plasma digoxin levels when patients were given different commercial brands of 0.25 mg tablets (Lindenbaum et al, 1971; Manninen, Melin and Härtel, 1971; Shaw, Howard and Hamer, 1972).

These observations led to more detailed studies of digoxin tablets and their absorption characteristics. Figure 16.1 is derived from a study by Johnson et al (1973a). They administered to fasting normal subjects two batches of tablets which contained exactly the same ingredients and varied only in the manufacturing technique. Batch A produced a peak plasma digoxin level which was higher and earlier than B. This indicates that absorption was more rapid with batch A, but differences in peak levels do not prove that the extent of absorption is different (Sorby and Tozer, 1973; Sanchez et al, 1973). In a single-dose study of this kind it is possible to compare the percentage absorption of the dose in two ways. The area under the plasma level–time curve is an index of the amount absorbed, providing the time axis extends to several times the elimination-half life of the drug (the elimination half-life of digoxin is approximately 36 h when renal function is normal). If the absorption curve is over only a few hours, there is bias in favour of the more rapidly absorbed drug. Using the 50 h curve, nearly 85 per cent more digoxin was absorbed from tablets A than from B. A second index of absorption is the amount of drug excreted in the urine. In this same study 46 per cent of the dose appeared in the urine within the first four days after A compared to 23 per cent after B.

Tablets B thus produced absorption which was both slower and less complete. Reports concerning digoxin bioavailability have sometimes been limited to absorption curves of short duration but impairment of absorption from several brands of digoxin tablet has been confirmed by single-dose studies of rigorous pharmacokinetic design (Huffman and Azarnoff, 1972; Wagner et al, 1973a; Greenblatt et al, 1973; Preibisz, Butler and Lindenbaum, 1974).

Absorption from different formulations can also be compared when each is administered on a regular daily basis and sufficient days have passed to reach a steady-state between absorption and excretion. This time to steady-state depends only on the half-life of drug elimination. After four half-lives 93.75 per cent of the change to the new steady state has been achieved so that with digoxin at least one week's treatment is needed, with longer periods if renal

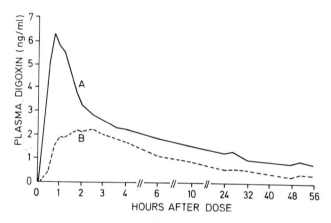

Figure 16.1   Absorption curves recorded in fasting normal volunteers after 1.5 mg digoxin doses of tablets A and tablets B. The tablets contained the same ingredients but differed in manufacturing technique. (Adapted from Johnson et al, 1973a.) 1 ng/ml = 1.3 mmol/l

function is impaired. With blood samples timed to avoid the 6 to 8 h after the dose during which absorption is taking place, the plasma level is an index of the amount of digoxin in the body. When the bioavailability of digoxin tablets was compared in this way, significant differences in the steady-state levels were found with different commercial brands (Lindenbaum et al, 1973; Shaw et al, 1973; Preibisz et al, 1974) and with experimental batches of the same brand (Johnson et al, 1973b). The impression that the magnitude of difference found in steady-state measurements was less than that calculated from single-dose studies was confirmed in the careful work by Preibisz and associates (1974) but the difference was still of considerable clinical importance.

Clinical effects

When brands of digoxin tablets available in the United Kingdom were administered for two-week periods to cardiac patients significant differences were found in the plasma digoxin levels and in the control of heart rate for patients with atrial fibrillation (Fig. 16.2).

In Scandinavia, Redfors et al (1973) found that when their patients were changed from a slowly absorbed to a rapidly absorbed digoxin preparation there was an increase of 28 per cent in the mean steady plasma digoxin level. Of their 91 patients, two developed ECG evidence of digoxin toxicity and four became nauseated and anorexic. The control of atrial fibrillation was significantly improved and 14 patients reported symptomatic improvement on the

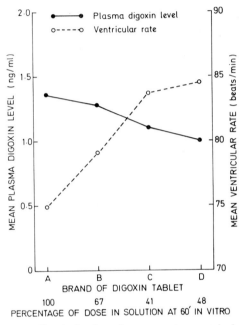

Figure 16.2   Mean plasma digoxin levels and mean resting ventricular rates in 13 patients with atrial fibrillation during use of four brands of digoxin tablets of different dissolution rate. (Adapted from Shaw et al, 1973)

new formulation, reflecting that many patients had been underdigitalised with the more poorly absorbed formulation.

It has been common for a patient to receive a variety of brands of tablets of the same drug. The traditional recommended doseses for digoxin were based on well-absorbed formulations, and underdigitalisation was common with poorly absorbed tablets. Digitalis toxicity is most likely to occur in patients stabilised with tablets of low bioavailability on a dosage that would normally be considered disproportionate to their size and renal function (Shaw, 1974).

Pharmaceutical standards

This variation between digoxin tablets was not detected by the pharmacopoeias disintegration test. This limits the time allowed to a tablet to break down into fragments under controlled conditions. However, the in vitro dissolution rate has been shown to correlate well with digoxin bioavailability (Lindenbaum et al, 1973; Johnson et al, 1973b; Shaw et al, 1973). This test measures the time taken for tablets to release the digoxin into solution. When applied to the two dozen brands of digoxin tablet available for dispensing in the United Kingdom it showed that there was a very wide spectrum of dissolution rates and that several makes varied markedly from batch to batch (Beckett and Cowan, 1973). The variation was from 19 to 92 per cent in solution after 30 min. Most of the inconsistency appears to have been due to the effects of different manufacturing methods on the particle size of the digoxin powder (Shaw and Carless, 1974), although changes in the crystalline structure may also play a part (Florence, Salole and Stenlake, 1974).

Changes in the production technique of the very widely used British Lanoxin brand had led to a change from high bioavailability to low bio-availability during the period of late 1969 to May 1972 (Johnson et al, 1973a; Shaw, Howard and Hamer, 1974a). As a result there was a period when this brand was dispensed in Britain only when it had been prescribed by its brand name (*Lancet*, 1972). It was subsequently shown that strict quality control of each Lanoxin batch by dissolution rate measurement ensured consistent high bioavailability (Johnson and Lader, 1974). Digoxin tablets made in different ways but all having a very rapid dissolution rate gave consistent digoxin levels and, very importantly, reduced the variance between individuals (Shaw, Raymond and Greenwood, 1974b; Johnson, Rye and Lader, 1974).

From 1st October 1975 all digoxin tablets dispensed in the United Kingdom must have a dissolution rate such that at least 75 per cent of the dose is in solution by 1 h. In the United States the FDA has stated that digoxin is to be regarded as a new drug and before it is marketed by any company certain information must be filed with them (Harter, 1975). Digoxin tablets with a dissolution rate under 55 per cent at 1 h cannot be marketed; those releasing between 55 and 95 per cent within 1 h are considered 'conventional' and can continue to be sold but the details of manufacturing and quality control must be approved. Formulations releasing more than 95 per cent in 1 h and more than 90 per cent within 15 min cannot be distributed until human studies have shown that, as seems likely, no adverse effects result from the rapid absorption. These are temporary measures and further change in the American regulations is likely.

Previous clinical and experimental experience with rapidly absorbed formulations has suggested that transient toxicity is not a significant problem. The response to digoxin is much delayed compared to the rise in plasma level during absorption. When single-loading doses of digoxin were given, producing very high plasma digoxin levels before distribution to the tissues, no evidence of toxicity was observed (Bertler, Bergdahl and Karlsson, 1974; Whiting and Sumner, 1974). It is my own impression that the occasional patient with digoxin intolerance producing nausea soon after each dose is commoner with rapidly dissolving tablets. If the nausea or vomiting persists when the tablets are taken after a meal, then changing to lanatoside C or digitoxin has been successful.

A separate problem of clinical importance was the finding that some brands showed wide fluctuation in the digoxin content of individual tablets, a few even ranging from 30 to 170 per cent of the stated 0.25 mg dose (van Oudtshoorn, 1972; Manninen and Korhonen, 1973). However, most pharmacopeias now specify that individual tablet content must be tested and remain within a relatively narrow range.

Bioavailability of Other Cardiac Glycosides

There is insufficient information at present about the bioavailability of most of the other glycosides. The lipid insolubility of ouabain prevents it from being adequately absorbed from the bowel even in liquid formulation. Methyl digoxin appears to be well absorbed, while lanatoside C has moderate absorption. Differences in the clinical response to commercial digitaline preparations were noted in the past (Evans, 1940; Dick, 1948) but Stoll et al (1973) did not find any significant difference in the total absorption from two American digitoxin preparations. However, neither of the brands they studied was very slowly dissolving and the bioavailability of digitoxin is still under review. Since digitalis leaf contains a mixture of glycosides its bioavailability would be hard to quantitate, but this preparation is well established. The patients I have seen using digitalis leaf have had their atrial fibrillation remarkably well controlled.

The new British standards ought to prevent inadequate digitalisation due to poor formulation but the possibility of a 'rogue' batch or a patient using very old tablets should perhaps be borne in mind. The present American standards do not eliminate some degree of variation between brands.

Gastrointestinal Absorption

When digoxin is taken by mouth as a solution or as quickly dissolving tablets, absorption is rapid when the patient has been fasting. Peak levels in the blood occur about 1 h after the dose. Only a short time is gained by giving the drug intravenously. If administration by mouth is not possible then intravenous infusion can be used. Intramuscular injection can be very painful, causes local muscle necrosis, and the digoxin reaches the circulation more slowly than with a rapidly absorbed oral formulation (Greenblatt et al, 1973).

Compliance to prescription

Clearly, if a tablet is not swallowed there will be no absorption. Compliance to the dosage instructions is better with digoxin than with many other drugs, but one-third of American patients admitted to being irregular in taking their tablets and these patients had lower steady-state digoxin levels than patients claiming not to have missed any doses (Weintraub, Au and Lasagna, 1973). Consistent with this was the finding that outpatients had a mean plasma digoxin level which was 72 per cent of that recorded in a similar group of hospitalised patients whose drug administration had been supervised (Sheiner et al, 1973). Fortunately, a patient's compliance appears to remain fairly consistent over a period of time. The usual reason given for failure to take the tablets was the very human one of absentmindedness, but suspected adverse reactions or a fear of addiction were also common and could be clarified by the physician. When digitalisation produces an unexpectedly poor response and there are low digoxin levels for the dose prescribed, then poor compliance with the dosage should be suspected. The patient and relatives should be questioned on this and a tablet count taken when possible.

Stomach

A recent meal prolongs absorption but does not change the extent of absorption (White et al, 1971; Sanchez et al, 1973). Absorption is not significantly affected by a previous partial gastrectomy (Beerman, Hellstrom and Rosen, 1973). Incubation of digoxin with gastric aspirates has been shown to produce cleavages at the three sugar groups to form active and inactive metabolites (Beerman, Hellstrom and Rosen, 1972). The extent to which this occurs depends on the pH and the duration of incubation. At pH of 1.4 to 1.9, incubation for 15 min hydrolysed 2 to 8 per cent of the digoxin. The importance of this effect in vivo is uncertain, but is probably small.

Intestine

Digoxin is absorbed mainly from the upper small intestine (Beerman et al, 1972). Even when administered as a solution, digoxin is not completely absorbed. It is hard to pinpoint the exact percentage of the dose which reaches the circulation since studies which have compared the urinary digoxin excretion after intravenous and oral doses vary somewhat in their estimates of the extent of absorption (Table 16.1). After an intravenous dose about 80 per cent of the digoxin can be found in the urine, with modest variation between individuals. When taken as an oral solution significantly less of the dose appears in the urine and the differences between individuals become much more marked. When intravenous digoxin was given daily for a two-week period, steady-state plasma levels and urinary excretion were higher than those recorded after the same doses of digoxin elixir; in the six normal subjects who were studied absorption from the elixir averaged 82 per cent (Huffman, Manion and Azarnoff, 1974). The absorption from any digoxin elixir, which contains alcohol and often propylene glycol, appears to be about three-quarters complete, with slightly less absorption when digoxin is dissolved in water alone or prepared as rapidly dissolving tablets.

The extent of the variation in digoxin absorption between and within individuals was shown in the study by Johnson, Bye and Lader (1974) when they administered rapidly absorbed formulations to eight normal volunteers on five different occasions. With each formulation there was a greater than twofold difference between subjects in the 10 day urinary digoxin recovery, but each individual subject tended to absorb a constant amount. There was a significant correlation between the individual's percentage absorption and his plasma digoxin level subsequently recorded during maintenance therapy (Johnson and Bye, 1975).

Table 16.1 Extent of digoxin absorption as assessed by cumulative urinary excretion in single dose studies using digoxin in solution

| Authors | Number of subjects | Mean cumulative urinary excretion (range) | | Estimate of percentage absorbed |
		Percentage of intravenous dose	Percentage of oral dose	
Doherty and Perkins (1962)	10	80.0 (72–97)	—	—
Doherty, Perkins and Mitchell (1961)	6		46 (31–58)	About 80
Huffman and Azarnoff (1972)	4	57 (not stated)	53 (not stated)	'Complete'
Greenblatt et al (1973)	8	76 (not stated)	49 (not stated)	65
Johnson, Bye and Lader (1974b)	8	71 (64–81)	54 (39–76)	75
Beerman, Hellstrom and Rosen (1972)	5	—	50 (43–62)	—
Hall and Doherty (1974)	13	—	47 (32–77)	—

Since absorption from oral formulations is incomplete, digoxin dosage should be reduced to at least three-quarters when it is given intravenously. The individual differences in absorption must contribute significantly to the variation seen in plasma levels and response.

Evidence conflicts about the effect of clinical malabsorption states. Heizer, Smith and Goldfinger (1971) found that steady-state digoxin levels were reduced to one-third in patients with sprue, intestinal resection or hyper-motility compared to a control group of cardiac patients, but the mean digoxin level in their controls was surprisingly high for the dosage used. Two patients with pancreatic insufficiency absorbed the drug normally. Hall and Doherty (1974) studied 12 patients with malabsorption syndromes and 13 subjects without overt intestinal disease. With malabsorption, cumulative urinary excretion of digoxin was reduced from 47 to 32 per cent of the administered dose but the excretion in stool rose by a smaller amount, 14 to 18 per cent. It seems probable that digoxin absorption can be reduced when there is intestinal disease, but there is no correlation with the degree of steatorrhoea.

The motility of the normal bowel has been shown to have a pronounced effect on plasma digoxin levels when very slowly dissolving tablets were taken on a maintenance dosage. Metoclopropramide (Maxolon), a drug which produces a shorter gastrointestinal transit time, decreased steady-state digoxin levels from 0.72 to 0.46 mg/ml, while propantheline, which slows gut motility, increased the level from 0.96 to 1.35 mg/ml (Manninen et al, 1973a). However, with rapidly dissolving tablets propantheline caused only a slight increase from 1.69 to 1.75 mg/ml (Manninen et al, 1973b). This suggests that the incomplete absorption of digoxin from solution is not due to the speed of transit through the bowel. On the other hand, when disease or diet produces very rapid transit times it may be that even well-formulated preparations have their absorption reduced.

Drug interaction in the bowel

Several drugs have been shown to inhibit the absorption of digoxin. Neomycin caused slowing of digoxin absorption and a reduction in steady-state levels to 69 per cent (Lindenbaum et al, 1972). Activated charcoal is a powerful binder of digoxin and reduces its diffusion from the bowel (Härtel, Manninen and Reissell, 1973): it is available in all biochemistry laboratories and would be useful to give in cases of deliberate overdose providing it can be given very soon after the tablets were taken. The binding resin cholestyramine also impairs digoxin absorption (Smith, 1973a). Kaopectate was found to cause low digoxin levels (Binnion and McDermott, 1972). A possibly more common interaction could be with antacids. Khalil (1974) noted that magnesium trisilicate was a very powerful binder of digoxin and quantities used clinically would inactivate a usual digoxin dose. Aluminium hydroxide and magnesium hydroxide had minimal effects.

Digitoxin absorption

To date digitoxin absorption has not been subjected to the same pharmacokinetic analysis as has digoxin. In clinical studies, the response after an oral dose was the same as after an intravenous one, suggesting 100 per cent absorption (Gold et al, 1953; Weissler et al, 1966). The same conclusion was made from a radioisotope study (Beerman, Hellstrom and Rosen, 1971) and when plasma digitoxin levels were measured by the rubidium 86 assays after i.v. and oral doses (Storstein, 1974b). This would be consistent with the greater lipid solubility of digitoxin, and in this particular respect digitoxin would have an advantage over digoxin.

Plasma Protein Binding

There are striking differences between digoxin and digitoxin in their degree of binding to plasma proteins: 23 per cent of digoxin in blood is bound compared to 97 per cent for digitoxin.

The low degree of binding of digoxin means that it is immune from interaction with other drugs competing for the binding sites on the albumin. The free digoxin level in the blood and tissues is insignificantly affected by changes in serum albumin concentration. The values recorded by radio-immunoassay are virtually unchanged by hypoalbuminaemia.

The more highly bound digitoxin can be displaced from the plasma protein binding sites by drugs such as warfarin and phenylbutazone but this does not occur to any significant extent with the doses of these drugs used clinically. Since the digitoxin in plasma is only a small fraction of the amount bound to tissue proteins, hypoproteinaemia has only a very slight effect on the free digitoxin in the body. The main consequence of a low albumin level is that the serum digitoxin level recorded by assay will be much reduced, although free digitoxin concentration and total body stores remain normal for the dosage used. Plasma protein concentration must be considered when interpreting a plasma digitoxin level. A reduction of serum albumin to 2 g/100 ml would approximately halve the digitoxin level recorded.

Distribution to the Tissues

After an intravenous dose the plasma digoxin level falls very rapidly and markedly since the drug is being distributed to the tissues as well as being excreted. Within 6 to 8 h the distribution process is almost complete and the plasma level and body stores then fall exponentially at the rate of elimination. After an oral dose, absorption and distribution take place simultaneously. Binding to tissue proteins is so extensive that only a small percentage of the digoxin or digitoxin dose remains in the blood after distribution has occurred. The degree of tissue binding can be estimated by calculating the 'apparent volume of distribution' (Fig. 16.3). The plasma levels recorded during the final elimination phase are extrapolated back to time zero to give the plasma level which would have existed if the dose had been instantaneously distributed. The volume of distribution is the volume of blood which would have been needed to dilute the dose to this concentration, i.e. dose divided by plasma level. This is of course a theoretical rather than an anatomical volume but as an index it combines the effects of body size and composition as well as the intensity of tissue binding.

Volume of distribution is an important determinant of the digoxin levels produced by a particular dosage. When no loading dose is given but the patient is started on a regular daily dose, the body digoxin content and, in equilibrium with this, the plasma digoxin level gradually rise until the steady-state is reached when the amount absorbed each day balances the amount excreted each day. This steady-state level is defined by the formula:

$$\text{steady-state digoxin level} = \frac{f}{V} \times \frac{D}{KE}$$

where D is the daily dose and f the fraction of the dose absorbed. The steady-state level has a direct inverse relationship to V, the volume of distribution, and KE the elimination rate constant. $KE = 0.693/T_{\frac{1}{2}}$, the digoxin elimination half-life in days. As was demonstrated by Marcus et al (1966) a loading dose is not essential for digitalisation but is an attempt to supply the digoxin

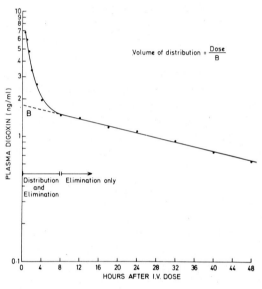

Figure 16.3 Method of calculation of apparent volume of distribution from plasma levels obtained after an intravenous dose

stores using one dose, given all at once or subdivided over a few hours. The final degree of digitalisation will depend on the daily doses which follow the loading dose. The same final result would be achieved by daily doses alone although several days then pass before digitalisation is completed. A loading dose therefore is needed only when digitalisation has to be rapid. The tissue levels obtained immediately after a loading dose will depend on the amount of digoxin given and on the volume of distribution and, unlike the maintenance doses, will be independent of elimination rate.

Body size is the most important variable for the volume of distribution. In a study of plasma digoxin levels before and after weight loss it appeared that lean body mass was the important element in the body size (Ewy et al, 1971). Changes in the patient's physiological status may also alter the distribution volume. Hyperkalaemia decreases tissue binding while hypokalaemia has the opposite effect. Goldman et al (1973) were able to show in dogs that infusions of potassium to produce serum K levels at between 5 and 7.5 mEq/litre reduced the myocardial concentration of digoxin by approximately 25 per cent and the microsomal-bound digoxin by one-third. This was associated with higher serum digoxin levels but a marked decrease in the inotropic response. Hyperthyroid patients have lower plasma digoxin levels than euthyroid patients given the same intravenous dose, with hypothyroidism giving the highest levels: alteration in tissue distribution appears to be one factor contributing to those differences (Doherty et al, 1973). Severe renal impairment alters the volume of distribution of digoxin. Reuning, Sams and Notari (1973) submitted to pharmacokinetic analysis some of the published data on plasma digoxin levels after intravenous administration. They found that the two-comparment model fitted closely to the recorded concentrations. The digoxin tissue levels they calculated corresponded to the extent and time course of pharmacologic effect. Patients with severe renal impairment had a volume of distribution reduced to two-thirds that of normal subjects, probably due to changes in the tissue protein binding. A similar effect in uraemia has been noted with other drugs (Gibaldi and Perrier, 1972). Thus in severe uraemia body size will overestimate the volume of distribution and both loading and maintenance doses should be appropriately reduced.

Excretion

The third characteristic of the patient which determines the body's digoxin levels is the rate of elimination. Digoxin is principally excreted in unchanged form into the urine. The rate of digoxin excretion depends on how much is cleared by glomerular filtration. There is a small contribution from tubular secretion and it has been suggested that this process can be blocked by spironolactone, which Steiness (1974) found to increase plasma digoxin levels by 25 per cent. Several workers have shown that there is a close correlation between digoxin clearance and creatinine clearance. The elimination rate of digoxin would therefore be expected to be dependent on the state of renal function and it has been shown that as renal function declines, so the digoxin half-life of elimination is increased.

Digoxin is also metabolised to a small but significant extent. In radioisotope studies which included measurement of polar molecules not extractable by chloroform it was found that about one-third of the digoxin dose was metabolised (Marcus et al, 1966; Beerman et al, 1972). Luchi and Gruber (1968) reported a patient who was able to tolerate very high doses of digoxin due to an abnormal degree of conversion to dihydrodigoxin. Other patients are now being recognised who show this phenomenon (Butler and Lindenbaum, 1975): since dihydrodigoxin is cardioinactive and is not detected by the radioimmunoassay such patients will have unexpectedly low plasma digoxin levels and a poor response.

Digitoxin is mainly eliminated by being metabolised in the liver. In very detailed studies using the rubidium-86 assay and chromatography, Storstein (1974a, b) discovered that although the urinary excretion of digitoxin is reduced in renal failure there are changes in the pattern of liver metabolism, with a result that there is no alteration in the overall digitalis effect in the plasma (as measured by inhibition of rubidium-86 uptake). The rate of decline of the digitalis effect remains the same as when renal function is normal. A similar state of balance is found in severe hepatic insufficiency, when changes in urinary excretion compensate for changes in metabolism (Lukas, 1973). The effect of hepatic insufficiency combined with renal failure has not been studied.

The liver metabolism of digitoxin can be altered by other drugs which induce increased activity of liver enzymes. Phenylbutazone and diphenyl-hydantoin markedly decreased plasma digitoxin levels and a 60 mg q.i.d. dosage of phenobarbitone reduced digitoxin levels by half (Solomon and Abrams, 1972).

Digitoxin has a half-life of approximately one week and when toxicity occurs it can persist for an uncomfortably long time after the dosage has been stopped or reduced. Oral cholestyramine, by binding the relatively large amounts of digitoxin undergoing enterohepatic recycling, has been shown to significantly reduce the persistence of digitoxin in human subjects (Caldwell, Bush and Greenberger, 1971). Giving 4 g cholestyramine four times a day should be a useful way of shortening the duration of digitoxin toxicity.

Radioimmunoassay studies have been carried out on the rapidly acting glycosides which can be used intravenously. Ouabain had an elimination half-life of 21 h (Selden and Smith, 1972) allowing relatively easy transfer to subsequent oral doses of digoxin, with its half-life of 36 h. Acetyl strophan-thidin, which is not available in this country for clinical use, had a half-life of 2.3 h consistent with its brief duration of effect (Selden, Klein and Smith, 1973).

Calculation of Digoxin Dosage

By the pharmacokinetic theory, the body stores and digoxin level will be determined by renal function and lean body mass, providing absorption is constant and other factors do not alter the volume of distribution or rate of elimination.

Jelliffe (1971) has tried to quantitate the maintenance dosage, using the relationship between digoxin elimination and creatinine clearance. He pointed out that in anephric patients 14 per cent of the body stores of digoxin are lost each day by non-renal routes, while, when creatinine clearance (CCr) is 100 ml/min, the daily loss is 34 per cent. Between these extremes of renal function the increase from 14 to 34 per cent will be directly related to creatinine clearance, i.e. an increase of 1 per cent per 5 ml/min of creatinine clearance. The daily digoxin loss can be calculated as (14 + CCr/5 per cent). Since creatinine clearance requires a 24 h collection of urine and with human error this collection is often incomplete, he suggested calculating the creatinine clearance from the serum creatinine (C) using the formulae CCr = [(100/serum creatinine) − 12] for men, and CCr = [(80/serum creatinine) − 7] for women. Rearrangement of these formulae (Smith, 1973b) gives:

$$\text{daily loss of digoxin body stores*} = 11.6 + \frac{20}{C} \text{ (men)}$$

$$= 12.6 + \frac{16}{C} \text{(women)}$$

If the body's digoxin content was known then the percentage daily loss would give the amount of digoxin needed as a maintenance dose to replace these daily losses. With Jelliffe's method one decides what would be the appropriate single loading dose for the particular patient under consideration, taking into account body size, etc. By deciding the appropriate loading dose the clinician has decided what he judges to be the required total body store for digitalisation. From this the maintenance dose can then be calculated: for a loading dose of 1.5 mg, a 30 per cent daily loss would correspond to a daily dose of 0.5 mg. It is not necessary to actually administer a loading dose, only to decide what loading dose would have been appropriate, and the method can be used for patients already on a maintenance regime.

Jelliffe suggested that for a 70 kg person the standard loading dose should be 0.75 mg of digoxin, which is lower than many physicians would consider usual. Single-dose pharmacokinetic studies tend to support the clinical impression that for a person of normal size and without factors predisposing to digitalis toxicity an oral loading dose of 1.5 mg would provide adequate body stores corresponding to a plasma digoxin level of 1.5 ng/ml. Any factor tending to reduce the volume of distribution, particularly a small body size, or to sensitise a patient to digitalis would indicate choosing a lower dosage. Since in the present day the available diuretics are so effective in the control of heart failure it is perhaps better in general to underestimate the required digoxin dose and so reduce the likelihood of digitalis toxicity.

Jelliffe and Brooker (1974) went on to construct a nomogram for the calculation of digoxin dose. The nomogram includes serum digoxin levels, based on those recorded with a Na-K-ATPase assay, which appear much higher than those found by some other investigators and the nomogram should perhaps be regarded with some reserve until it has been evaluated further. Jelliffe's

---

* Formulae are based on serum creatinine as mg/100 ml. To change serum creatinine from SI units (mmol/l) multiply by 11.3.

approach does, however, provide a simple technique for trying to take
account of individual patient differences in estimating digoxin dosage.

It would be pleasant to be able to say that such a pharmacokinetic approach
produced very precise digitalisation. Unfortunately it does not entirely solve
the problem. When such a regime of digitalisation was used by Christiansen
et al (1973) a wide range of plasma digoxin levels still existed (Fig. 16.4). A
computer program designed to take account of body size and renal function
also gave a wide scatter of steady-state serum digoxin values between different
individuals (Peck et al, 1973; Wagner et al, 1973b). The computer was only
very slightly better at predicting serum digoxin levels than physicians know-
ledgeable in digoxin pharmacokinetics. Both were similar to predictions based

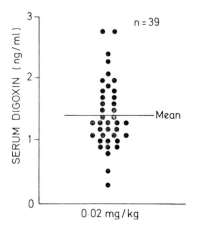

Figure 16.4 Steady-state plasma digoxin levels recorded in patients whose digoxin maintenance dosage had been calculated from a formula taking account of body weight and creatinine
clearance. An appropriate loading dosage was taken to be 0.02 mg digoxin per kilogram body
weight. (Adapted from Christiansen et al, 1973)

on dosage alone, disregarding body size and renal function. In addition to the
spectrum of size and renal function the variation between individuals appears
to depend considerably on factors such as compliance with the dosage regime,
percentage absorption, degree of metabolism and differences in volume of
distribution which cannot yet be easily quantified for individuals and are still
poorly understood.

Despite the disappointing results with dosage regimes adjusted for body
size and renal function such pharmacokinetic considerations are useful when
beginning digoxin treatment, particularly in patients with more severe renal
disease. After an educational programme of digoxin kinetics was introduced at
a Montreal hospital the incidences of digoxin toxicity and of digitalis-
associated deaths were markedly reduced (Ogilvie and Ruedy, 1972).

Once a steady-state has been reached on maintenance therapy clinical
judgement is still the best guide as to whether a satisfactory result with

digitalisation has been obtained. If the response is considered inadequate, measurement of the plasma digoxin level will help to decide if the suboptimal response is due to reduced delivery of digoxin to the body. This would call for a check on whether the patient is taking the tablets and if the tablets themselves are of suitable quality. Absorption could be estimated by a fasting absorption curve and by ensuring there is no drug interaction. Abnormalities in volume of distribution, elimination half-life, and metabolism would require more detailed studies.

Before a digoxin dose is increased on the basis of the plasma level recorded it would be wise to measure the level on more than one occasion if possible, since there is a moderate amount of variation in an individual from day to day even when on the same dosage. In a particular patient the steady-state plasma digoxin level should increase linearly with dose. Several studies have shown such a linear relationship but Huffman et al (1974) found that levels did not increase as much as expected at higher doses, and further work on this point would be useful. The value of monitoring digoxin dose by plasma level measurements was shown by the Boston Collaborative Drug Surveillance Program, during which the incidence of toxicity in patients on digoxin at the Massachusetts General Hospital fell from 14 to 6 per cent after the digoxin radioimmunoassay was introduced (Koch-Weser, Duhme and Greenblatt, 1974). As with any biochemical measurement, the clinician should discuss the quality control data with his clinical chemist before accepting that his local assay results will correspond with values quoted in the literature.

Plasma Digoxin Levels and Clinical Response

Smith (1975) has reviewed the use of plasma digoxin measurements when digoxin toxicity is suspected. All the surveys have shown that mean plasma levels are higher in toxic patients. Toxicity is relatively uncommon with levels below 2 ng/ml, becoming increasingly frequent with higher levels. There is, however, a lot of overlap in the levels recorded in non-toxic and toxic patients and clinical judgement and observations during adjustment of dosage must remain the final arbiters. Unfortunately, the symptoms and arrhythmias thought characteristic of digitalis toxicity are also very frequently found in non-toxic cardiac patients taking digitalis (Hillestad et al, 1973). A purely clinical decision can be difficult and inaccurate, particularly when made before the effect of an alteration in dose has been established. In this situation the finding of very high or very low levels can be useful.

Since plasma digoxin levels are related to dosage it would be surprising if they did not have some correlation with pharmacologic effect. Chamberlain and colleagues (1970) found that in patients with atrial fibrillation and known to be capable of achieving rapid ventricular rates the higher digoxin levels were associated with slower heart rates. Redfors (1973a, b) studied a group of patients with atrial fibrillation who were not taking diuretics. He progressively increased the digoxin dosage until there was any evidence of toxicity; there was a linear relationship between dosage and plasma digoxin level and as these increased there was a concomitant fall in the ventricular rate at rest and during exercise. There was a significant symptomatic improvement in these patients after digitalisation. His data does, however, emphasise the large individual differences in heart rate seen in patients with atrial fibrillation, due to natural variations in the properties of the atrioventricular node.

Conclusion

A course of treatment is a unique interaction between a drug and a patient. Our therapeutics improve as we learn more of each. The digitalis assays have helped to reveal how the body handles cardiac glycosides and have quantitated some of the processes involved. In this way they have clarified principles to be considered when digitalis treatment is practised. They have shown how much variation between individuals still remains unexplained. They are useful clinically in assessing how much delivery of the drug the dosage has achieved and by doing this have simplified the analysis of variations in response.

REFERENCES

Beckett, A. H. & Cowan, D. A. (1973) Differences in the dissolution rate of generic digoxin tablets. *Pharmaceutical Journal*, **211**, 111–112.

Beerman, B., Hellstrom, K. & Rosen, A. (1971) Fate of orally administered 3H-digitoxin in man with special reference to the absorption. *Circulation*, **43**, 852–861.

Beerman, B., Hellstrom, K. & Rosen, A. (1972) The absorption of orally administered 12α 3H digoxin in man. *Clinical Science*, **43**, 507–518.

Beerman, B., Hellstrom, K. & Rosen, A. (1973) The gastrointestinal absorption of digoxin in seven patients with gastric or small intestinal reconstructions. *Acta medica scandinavica*, **193**, 293–297.

Bertler, A., Bergdahl, B. & Karlsson, E. (1974) Plasma levels of digoxin after intravenous loading dose. *Lancet*, **2**, 958.

Binnion, P. F. & McDermott, M. (1972) Bioavailability of digoxin. *Lancet*, **2**, 592.

Butler, V. P. (1972) Assays of digitalis in the blood. *Progress in Cardiovascular Diseases*. **14**, 571–600.

Butler, V. P. & Chen, J. P. (1967) Digoxin-specific antibodies. *Proceedings of the National Academy of Sciences of the U.S.A.*, **57**, 71–78.

Butler, V. P. & Lindenbaum, J. (1975) Serum digitalis measurements in the assessment of digitalis resistance and sensitivity. *American Journal of Medicine*, **58**, 460–469.

Caldwell, J. H., Bush, C. A. & Greenberger, N. J. (1971) Interruption of the enterohepatic circulation of digitoxin by cholestyramine, II. Effect on metabolic disposition of tritium-labelled digitoxin and cardiac systolic intervals in man. *Journal of Clinical Investigation*, **50**, 2638–2644.

Chamberlain, D. A., White, R. J., Howard, M. R. & Smith, T. W. (1970) Plasma digoxin concentrations in patients with atrial fibrillation. *British Medical Journal*, **3**, 429–432.

Christiansen, N. J. B., Kolendorf, K., Siersback, K. & Molholm Hansen, J. (1973) Serum digoxin values following a dosage regimen based on body weight, sex, age and renal function. *Acta medica scandinavica*, **194**, 257–259.

Dick, P. (1948) The relative value of digitaline preparations in heart failure with auricular fibrillation. *British Heart Journal*, **10**, 122–124.

Doherty, J. E. & Perkins, W. H. (1962) Studies with tritiated digoxin in human subjects after intravenous administration. *American Heart Journal*, **63**, 528–536.

Doherty, J. E., Perkins, W. H. & Mitchell, G. K. (1961) Tritiated digoxin studies in human subjects. *Archives of Internal Medicine*, **108**, 531–539.

Doherty, J. E., Perkins, W. H., Gammill, J., Sherwood, J., Dodd, C. & Young, C. C. (1973) The influence of thyroid function on digoxin metabolism. In *Digitalis*, ed. Storstein, O., Nitter-Hauge, S. & Storstein, L., pp. 348–361. Oslo: Glydendal Norsk Forlag.

Evans, W. (1940) Relative value of certain digitalis preparations in heart failure with auricular fibrillation. *British Heart Journal*, **2**, 51–62.

Ewy, G. A., Groves, B. M., Ball, M. F., Nimmo, L., Jackson, B. & Marcus, F. I. (1971) Digoxin metabolism in obesity. *Circulation*, **44**, 810–814.

Florence, A. T., Salole, E. G. & Stenlake, J. B. (1974) The effect of particle size reduction on digoxin crystal properties. *Journal of Pharmacy and Pharmacology*, **26**, 479–480.

Gibaldi, M. (1971) *Introduction to Biopharmaceutics*. Philadelphia: Lea & Febiger.

Gibaldi, M. & Perrier, D. (1972) Drug distribution and renal failure. *Journal of Clinical Pharmacology*, **12**, 201–204.

Gold, H., Cattell, McK., Greiner, T., Hanlon, L. W., Kwit, N. T., Modell, W., Cotlove, E., Benton, J. & Otto, H. L. (1953) Clinical pharmacology of digoxin. *Journal of Pharmacology and Experimental Therapeutics*, **109**, 45–57.

Goldman, R. H., Coltart, D. J., Friedman, J. P., Nola, G. T., Berke, D. K., Schweizer, E. & Harrison, D. C. (1973) The inotropic effects of digoxin in hyperkalaemia: relation to Na–K ATPase inhibition in the intact animal. *Circulation*, **48**, 830–838.

Greenblatt, D. J., Duhme, D. W., Koch-Weser, J. & Smith, T. W. (1973) Evaluation of digoxin bioavailability in single dose studies. *New England Journal of Medicine*, **289**, 651–654.

Hall, W. H. & Doherty, J. E. (1974) Absorption and excretion in malabsorption syndromes. *American Journal of Medicine*, **56**, 437–442.

Härtel, G., Manninen, V. & Reissell, P. (1973) Treatment of digoxin intoxication. *Lancet*, **2**, 158.

Harter, J. G. (1975) Comments from the Food and Drug Administration. *American Journal of Medicine*, **58**, 477–478.

Heizer, W. D., Smith, T. W. & Goldfinger, S. E. (1971) Absorption of digoxin in patients with malabsorption syndromes. *New England Journal of Medicine*, **285**, 257–259.

Hillestad, L., Hansteen, V., Hatle, L., Storstein, L. & Storstein, O. (1973) Digitalis intoxication. In *Digitalis*, ed. Storstein, O., Nitter-Hauge, S. & Storstein, L., pp. 281–287. Oslo: Gyldendal Norsk Forlag.

Huffman, D. H. & Azarnoff, D. L. (1972) Absorption of orally given digoxin preparations. *Journal of the American Medical Association*, **222**, 957–960.

Huffman, D. H., Manion, C. V. & Azarnoff, D. L. (1974) Absorption of digoxin from different oral preparations in normal subjects during steady state. *Clinical Pharmacology and Therapeutics*, **16**, 310–317.

Jelliffe, R. W. (1967) A mathematical analysis of digitalis kinetics in patients with normal and reduced renal function. *Mathematical Biosciences*, **1**, 305–325.

Jelliffe, R. W. (1968) An improved method of digoxin therapy. *Annals of Internal Medicine*, **69**, 703–717.

Jelliffe, R. W. (1971) Factors to consider in planning digoxin therapy. *Journal of Chronic Diseases*, **24**, 407–416.

Jelliffe, R. W. & Brooker, G. (1974) A nomogram for digoxin therapy. *American Journal of Medicine*, **57**, 63–68.

Johnson, B. F. & Bye, C. (1975) Maximal intestinal absorption of digoxin, and its relation to steady-state plasma concentration. *British Heart Journal*, **37**, 203–208.

Johnson, B. F. & Lader, S. (1974) Bioavailability of digoxin from rapidly dissolving preparations. *British Journal of Clinical Pharmacology*, **1**, 329–333.

Johnson, B. F., Fowle, A. S. E., Lader, S., Fox, J. & Munroe-Faure, A. D. (1973a) Biological availability of digoxin from Lanoxin produced in the United Kingdom. *British Medical Journal*, **4**, 323–326.

Johnson, B. F., Greer, H., McCrerie, J., Bye, C. & Fowle, A. (1973b) Rate of dissolution of digoxin tablets as a predictor of absorption. *Lancet*, **1**, 1473–1475.

Johnson, B. F., Bye, C. & Lader, S. (1974) The bioavailability of other digoxin preparations compared with tablets. *Postgraduate Medical Journal*, **50**, Suppl. 6, 62–66.

Khalil, S. A. H. (1974) The uptake of digoxin and digitoxin by some antacids. *Journal of Pharmacy and Pharmacology*, **26**, 961–967.

Koch-Weser, J. (1974) Drug therapy: bioavailability of drugs. *New England Journal of Medicine*, **291**, 233–237, 503–506.

Koch-Weser, J., Duhme, D. W. & Greenblatt, D. J. (1974) Influence of serum digoxin conentration measurements on frequency of digitoxicity. *Clinical Pharmacology and Therapeutics*, **16**, 284–287.

Lancet (1972) The biolavailability of digoxin **2**, 311.

Lindenbaum, J., Mellow, M. H., Blackstone, M. O. & Butler, V. P. (1971) Variation in biologic availability of digoxin from four preparations. *New England Journal of Medicine*, **285**, 1344–1347.

Lindenbaum, J., Maulitz, R. M., Saha, J. R., Shea, N. & Butler, V. P. (1972) Impairment of digoxin absorption by neomycin. *Clinical Research*, **20**, 410.

Lindenbaum, J., Butler, V. P., Murphy, J. E. & Cresswell, R. M. (1973) Correlation of digoxin-tablet dissolution rate with biological availability. *Lancet*, **1**, 1215–1217.

Luchi, R. J. & Gruber, J. W. (1968) Unusually large digitalis requirements; a study of altered digoxin metabolism. *American Journal of Medicine*, **45**, 322–328.

Lukas, D. S. (1973) The role of the liver in the chemical transformation of digitoxin. In *Digitalis*, ed. Storstein, O., Nitter-Hauge, S. & Storstein, L., pp. 192–199. Oslo: Gyldendal Norsk Forlag.

Manninen, V. & Korhonen, A. (1973) Inequal digoxin tablets. *Lancet*, **2**, 1268.

Manninen, V., Melin, J. & Härtel, G. (1971) Serum digoxin concentrations during treatment with different preparations. *Lancet*, **2**, 934–935.

Manninen, V., Apajalahti, A., Melin, J. & Karesoja, M. (1973a) Altered absorption of digoxin in patients given propantheline and metoclopramide. *Lancet*, **1**, 398–400.

Manninen, V., Apajalahi, A., Simonen, H. & Reissell, P. (1973b) The effect of propantheline and metoclopramide on absorption of digoxin. *Lancet*, **1**, 1118–1119.

Marcus, F. I. (1975) Digitalis pharmacokinetics and metabolism. *American Journal of Medicine*, **58**, 452–459.

Marcus, F. I., Burkhalter, L., Cuccia, C., Pavlovich, J. & Kapadia, G. G. (1966) Administration of tritiated digoxin with and without a loading dose. *Circulation*, **34**, 865–874.

Notari, R. E. (1971) *Biopharmaceutics and Pharmacokinetics: an Introduction*. New York: Marcel Dekker.

Ogilvie, R. I. & Ruedy, J. (1972) An educational program in digitialis therapy. *Journal of the American Medical Association*, **222**, 50–55.

Van Oudtshoorn, M. C. B. (1972) Bioavailability of digoxin. *Lancet*, **2**, 1153.

Peck, C. C., Sheiner, L. B., Martin, C. M., Combs, D. T. & Melmon, K. L. (1973) Computer-assisted digoxin therapy. *New England Journal of Medicine*, **289**, 441–446.

Preibisz, J. J., Butler, V. P. & Lindenbaum, J. (1974) Digoxin tablet bioavailability: single-dose and steady-state assessment. *Annals of Internal Medicine*, **81**, 469–474.

Redfors, A. (1973a) The effect of different digoxin doses on subjective symptoms and physical working capacity in patients with atrial fibrillation. *Acta medica scandinavica*, **190**, 307–320.

Redfors, A. (1973b) Digoxin dosage and ventricular rate at rest and exercise in patients with atrial fibrillation. *Acta medica scandinavica*, **190**, 321–333.

Redfors, A., Bertler, A., Nilsen, R. & Wettre, S. (1973) Changing a population from one digoxin preparation to another. In *Digitalis*, ed. Storstein, O., Nitter-Hauge, S. & Storstein, L., pp. 390–395. Oslo: Gyldendal Norsk Forlag.

Reuning, R. H., Sams, R. A. & Notari, R. E. (1973) Role of pharmacokinetics in drug dosage adjustment. I. Pharmacologic effect, kinetics and apparent volume of distribution. *Journal of Clinical Pharmacology*, **13**, 127–141.

Sanchez, N., Sheiner, L. B., Halkin, H. & Melmon, K. L. (1973) Pharmacokinetics of digoxin: interpreting bioavailability. *British Medical Journal*, **4**, 132–134.

Selden, R. & Smith, T. W. (1972) Ouabain pharmacokinetics in dog and man: determination by radioimmunoassay. *Circulation*, **45**, 1176–1182.

Selden, R., Klein, M. D. & Smith, T. W. (1973) Plasma concentration and urinary excretion kinetics of acetyl strophanthidin. *Circulation*, **47**, 744–751.

Shaw, T. R. D. (1974) Non-equivalence of digoxin tablets in the UK and its clinical implications. *Postgraduate Medical Journal*, **50**, Suppl. 6, 24–29.

Shaw, T. R. D. & Carless, J. E. (1974) The effect of particle size on the absorption of digoxin. *European Journal of Clinical Pharmacology*, **7**, 269–273.

Shaw, T. R. D., Howard, M. R. & Hamer, J. (1972) Variation in the biological availability of digoxin. *Lancet*, **2**, 303–307.

Shaw, T. R. D., Raymond, K., Howard, M. R. & Hamer, J. (1973) Therapeutic non-equivalence of digoxin tablets in the United Kingdom: correlation with tablet dissolution rate. *British Medical Journal*, **4**, 763–766.

Shaw, T. R. D., Howard, M. R. & Hamer, J. (1974a) Recent changes in the biological availability of digoxin. Effect of an alteration in 'Lanoxin' tablets. *British Heart Journal*, **36**, 85–89.

Shaw, T. R. D., Raymond, K. & Greenwood, H. (1974b) The biological availability of very rapidly dissolving digoxin tablets. *Postgraduate Medical Journal*, **50**, Suppl. 6, 55–59.

Sheiner, L. B., Rosenberg, B., Marathe, V. V. & Peck, C. (1973) Differences in serum digoxin concentrations between out-patients and in-patients: an effect of compliance? *Clinical Pharmacology and Therapeutics*, **15**, 239–246.

Smith, T. W. (1973a) New approaches to the management of digitalis intoxication. In *Digitalis*, ed. Storstein, O., Nitter-Hauge, S. & Storstein, L., pp. 312–323. Oslo: Gyldendal Norsk Forlag.

Smith, T. W. (1973b) Digitalis glycosides. *New England Journal of Medicine*, **288**, 942–946.

Smith, T. W. (1975) Digitalis toxicity: epidemiology and clinical use of serum concentration measurements. *American Journal of Medicine*, **58**, 470–476.

Smith, T. W., Butler, V. P. & Haber, E. (1969) Determination of therapeutic and toxic serum digoxin concentrations by radioimmunoassay. *New England Journal of Medicine*, **281**, 1212–1216.

Solomon, H. M. & Abrams, W. B. (1972) Interactions between digitoxin and other drugs in man. *American Heart Journal*, **83**, 277–280.

Sorby, D. L. & Tozer, T. N. (1973) On the evaluation of biologic availability of digoxin from tablets. *Drug Intelligence and Clinical Pharmacy*, **7**, 79–83.

Steiness, E. (1974) Renal tubular secretion of digoxin. *Circulation*, **50**, 103–107.

Stoll, R. G., Christensen, M. S., Sakmar, E., Blair, D. & Wagner, J. G. (1973) Determination of bioavailability of digoxin using the radioimmunoassay procedure. *Journal of Pharmaceutical Sciences*, **62**, 1615–1620.

Storstein, L. (1974a) Studies on digitalis. I. Renal excretion of digitoxin and its cardioactive metabolites. *Clinical Pharmacology and Therapeutics*, **16**, 14–24.

Storstein, L. (1974b) Studies on digitalis. II. The influence of impaired renal function on the renal excretion of digitoxin and its cardioactive metabolites. *Clinical Pharmacology and Therapeutics*, **16**, 25–34.

Wagner, J. G. (1971) *Biopharmaceutics and Relevant Pharmacokinetics*. Hamilton: Drug Intelligence Publications.

Wagner, J. G., Christensen, M., Sakmar, E., Blair, D., Yates, J. D., Willis, P. W., Sedman, P. W. & Stoll, R. G. (1973a) Equivalence lack in digoxin plasma levels. *Journal of the American Medical Association*, **224**, 199–204.

Wagner, J. G., Yates, J. D., Willis, P. W., Sakmar, E. & Stoll, R. G. (1973b) Correlation of plasma levels of digoxin in cardiac patients with dose and measures of renal function. *Clinical Pharmacology and Therapeutics*, **15**, 291–301.

Weintraub, M., Au, W. Y. W. & Lasagna, L. (1973) Compliance as a determinant of a serum digoxin concentrations. *Journal of the American Medical Association*, **224**, 481–485.

Weissler, A. M., Snyder, J. R., Schoenfeld, C. D. & Cohen, S. (1966) Assay of digitalis glycosides in man. *American Journal of Cardiology*, **17**, 768–780.

White, R. J., Chamberlain, D. A., Howard, M. & Smith, T. W. (1971) Plasma concentrations of digoxin after oral administration in the fasting and postprandial state. *British Medical Journal*, **1**, 380–381.

Whiting, B. & Sumner, D. J. (1974) Oral digitalisation. *Lancet*, **2**, 1393.

447

17
INFECTIVE ENDOCARDITIS

John Hamer   Francis O'Grady

PATTERN OF THE DISEASE

The persisting problem of infective endocarditis is brought out by a review entitled 'The enigma of infective endocarditis' (Cole, 1975) which states 'It is a well-known and disturbing fact that the overall mortality (30 per cent) has not altered in the last 30 years'. The implication is that more effective antibiotic therapy ought to have reduced the mortality over this period and the persistence of a killing infectious disease to some extent reflects on the inadequacy of therapeutics. The enigma is further analysed by Cole (1975) as the *paradox of a changing disease*; a shift of peak age incidence to an older group without reduction in incidence since the introduction of penicillin (Weinstein, 1972), and the *paradox of persisting mortality* in spite of many factors tending to favour effective treatment including:

1. earlier diagnosis from a higher index of suspicion
2. improved microbiological techniques
3. more effective antibiotics
4. improved control of therapy by blood antibiotic level monitoring
5. widened indications for surgical intervention and improved surgical techniques.

Adverse factors such as:

1. delay in diagnosis in the elderly
2. inadequate therapy
3. mechanical factors, e.g. valve rupture

are held inadequate to account for the persisting high mortality and emphasis is placed on chronic immunological disturbances which may be unresponsive to antibiotic therapy.

The Changing Disease

Despite the general evidence of a changing incidence in disease towards an older age group with a different source of bacteraemia and a shift away from *Streptococcus viridans* of oral origin (Hayward, 1973), study of a restricted population of children only (Johnson, Rosenthal and Nadas, 1975) shows no real change in the type of infecting organisms although there has been a shift to older patients within the paediatric age group, as the dominant underlying disease shifts from rheumatic heart disease to treated congenital heart disease, and there has been increasing survival with a mortality of 24 per cent since the introduction of antibiotics (Table 17.1).

The *Streptococcus viridans* response is dramatic, and there is a hint that the *Staphylococcus aureus* mortality may have improved in the last decade.

The rarity of severe glomerulonephritis (one case) in this study may indicate that the immune response phenomena are mainly a problem of older age groups as suggested by Cole (1975).

Streptococcus viridans

Streptococcus viridans infection usually from a source in the mouth still remains the most frequent organism overall, but the incidence of infection with other streptococci, staphylococci, Gram-negative bacteria and various exotic organisms has been increasing in relation to the increase in average age of the patients.

Table 17.1 Changes in mortality rates from infective endocarditis (from Johnson et al, 1975)

| Period | Number | Mean age (years) | Total | Mortality rate, % | |
				S. viridans	Staph. aureus
1933–42	23	5.5	100	100	100
1943–52	18	7.9	28	30	33
1953–62	40	16.6	27	0	50
1963–72	68	12.7	19	7	26

Streptococcus 'viridans' defined on the basis of alpha haemolysis on blood agar is not a single species, but recognition of the group remains important therapeutically as these organisms are usually sensitive to penicillin. Various species of Streptococcus of the viridans group have been identified in the oral flora: *S. salivarius, S. sangius, S. mutans* and *S. mitior* (*Lancet*, 1974).

The production of endocarditis has been linked with the presence of a sticky surface polysaccharide, a dextran (corresponding to Group I serological type) (Elliott, 1973) in *S. sanguis*, the usual cause of endocarditis and less frequently in *S. mutans* and *S. bovis* (*Lancet*, 1974).

The other organisms reported with increasing frequency in recent years are in general less sensitive to penicillin and therefore present greater problems of management. In this connection it is important to distinguish the penicillin-resistant enterococcus (*Streptococcus faecalis*) from the closely similar but penicillin sensitive *Streptococcus mutans*.

Enterococci are normal commensals in the gut and genital tract, and a genitourinary disturbance is the usual source of infection. In a series of 38 such patients (Mardell et al, 1970) a genitourinary source such as urethral catheterisation was commonly found in the 22 men (average 59 years); the 16 women were younger (average age 37 years) and the infection usually occurred in relation to pregnancy, at normal delivery or abortion. Recently a patient was reported with bacterial endocarditis after the insertion of an intrauterine contraceptive device (de Swiet, Ramsey and Ross, 1975), so other forms of contraception may be preferable in susceptible patients.

An increase in the frequency of infection with anaerobic and micro-aerophilic streptococci was reported by Lerner and Weinstein (1960). This infection is important as the organism will not be isolated unless special culture techniques are used.

The distinction between acute and subacute bacterial endocarditis on the basis of survival for six weeks has become less relevant with the advent of effective antibiotic therapy. The usual causes of acute bacterial endocarditis were the pyogenic organisms *Streptococcus pyogenes* and *Staphylococcus aureus*, and these infections were characterised by a polymorph leucocytosis and purulent changes in the embolic lesions. Such changes are not seen with the blander infections producing subacute bacterial endocarditis. The classical association of particular species of bacteria with the acute form of bacterial endocarditis is not clear-cut, and in the elderly even *S. viridans* infection may run an acute course (Staffurth, 1970), as may also be seen in patients with a reduced resistance to infection from general disease. Bacterial endocarditis due to *Streptococcus pyogenes* has now almost completely disappeared (Finland and Barnes, 1970).

Staphylococcus aureus

Staphylococcus aureus is the commonest cause of acute endocarditis and an increase in the frequency of this infection was reported from Boston by Uwaydah and Weinberg (1965) and by Finland and Barnes (1970). The widespread use of penicillin in the United States seems to have encouraged the development of infections with resistant strains of this organism; fortunately the trend is much less evident in Europe, including Britain.

In spite of fears to the contrary the greater frequency of bacteraemia with Gram-negative bacilli in older people does not seem to have led to a serious increase in endocarditis due to these organisms (Uwaydah and Weinberg, 1965), although some increase was noted by Finland and Barnes (1970). In patients with Gram-negative bacteraemia the chance of developing endo-carditis is small in contrast to the situation in staphylococcal bacteraemia where persistent circulation of organisms more than 24 h after removal of all indwelling vascular catheters strongly suggests endocarditis even in the absence of clinical signs.

Clinical Features

The major features of the illness have not changed over the years, but a decreasing incidence of rheumatic heart disease as a basis, means that fewer patients give a history of previous rheumatic fever. It is now fortunately rare to see the classical syndrome of cachexia, enlarged spleen and anaemia with cafe-au-lait discoloration, as these changes are associated with prolonged uncontrolled infection which can generally be suppressed by antibiotic treatment even if a curative regime is not found.

The triad of fever (and other evidence of infection) with changing valve lesions and embolic phenomena has been modified by the evidence (Bacon, Davidson and Smith, 1974; Cole, 1975) that many of the lesions formerly attributed to microembolism are in fact immune complex phenomena. The transient suppression of fever by treatment with bacteriostatic antibiotics (e.g. tetracyclines) or inadequate doses of bactericidal agents often leads to delay in making the diagnosis and allows progression of the valve lesions and the auto-immune disturbances which are now the usual causes of death. Careless antibiotic therapy in a patient with heart disease and an undiagnosed fever is a cardinal sin of medical practice. Embolic manifestations are frequent and may continue to occur for a few weeks after effective treatment has begun. Infection of the right heart produces pulmonary emboli which may be mistaken for recurrent chest infection with dangerous delay in diagnosis and effective therapy.

Joint manifestations

Arthritis of a single major joint or a more general arthralgia are the usual findings (Doyle et al, 1967). High plasma gamma-globulin levels may produce positive latex-fixation tests giving rise to suspicion of rheumatoid disease (Messner et al, 1968; Bacon et al, 1974).

Neurological disturbances

Nearly one-third of patients show evidence of neurological involvement, which is often a major feature of the illness (Jones, Siebert and Gerias, 1969). Half these disturbances are strokes, with infarction four times as frequent as haemorrhage, and the major changes are sometimes preceded by transient ischaemic episodes. Subarachnoid haemorrhage may follow rupture of a mycotic aneurysm on a major cerebral artery.

Other features include confusional states, meningitis, headache, convulsions, visual impairment and mononeuritis. Diffuse cerebral vasculitis may account for the acute confusional states and diffuse organic cerebral changes (see below). The mortality in patients with neurological complications is considerably greater than usual.

Immune complex phenomena

Cole (1975) lists immune complex phenomena in infective endocarditis as:

Petechial rash
Osler's nodes
Roth's spots (retinal exudate with haemorrhage)

Janeway lesions (nodules on palms and soles)
Microscopic haematuria
Retinal haemorrhage
Cerebral vasculitis (presenting with psychiatric disturbance or diffuse neurological syndrome)
Arthralgia
Splinter haemorrhages and mycotic aneurysms.

In spite of the evidence that many of the symptoms and signs formerly attributed to microembolism are due to deposition of complexes of antibody, antigen and complement (Cordeiro, Costa and Leginha, 1965), it is difficult to exclude an embolic cause in the individual case. Focal lesions such as Osler's nodes, Roth's spots and Janeway lesions seem more likely to be embolic in origin and mycotic aneurysms may be due to embolism of vasa vasorum producing local damage to the arterial walls. However, evidence of a diffuse increase in vascular fragility, anaemia, changes in plasma proteins and diffuse glomerulonephritis are more likely to be related to the immune complex disturbance. The diffuse myocarditis evident histologically as the Bracht–Wächter bodies is a further candidate for a diffuse immune disturbance. Petechial haemorrhages are not infrequent and the common splinter haemorrhages in the nail beds may be a manifestation of increased capillary fragility as they resemble the lesions produced by trauma in normal subjects. In some cases major purpura is the dominant feature (Horwitz and Silber, 1967). The presence of splinter haemorrhages and diffuse renal disease in patients with lesions of the right side of the heart in which emboli are confined to the pulmonary vascular bed make an embolic cause of these systemic changes unlikely.

Evidence for the immunological basis of the diffuse changes is given by Cole (1975) as:

1. The clinical similarity to established autoimmune disease, e.g. disseminated lupus erythematosus, polyarteritis nodosa, rheumatoid arthritis.
2. The close relationship between the clinical course of the disease and the renal immune complex mediated complication.
3. The increase in serum gamma-globulins.
4. The occurrence of antiglobulins (rheumatoid factor) in approximately 50 per cent of cases.
5. The occurrence of specific antibodies to glomerular basement membrane, vascular endothelium and myocardium.
6. The deposition of immune complexes (seen by fluorescent labelling) on valvular endothelium and renal basement membrane.
7. The decreased serum complement.
8. The experimental demonstration of reaction of antiglobulins with specific opsonins.

Cole (1975) postulates that the abrupt fibrin deposition over the lesions found by Durack and Beeson (1972) in experimental endocarditis is evidence of an immune response with activation of clotting factors. The persistence of antigenic material from the infecting agent may produce a delayed hyper-sensitivity response producing further tissue damage as part of a process aimed at eliminating the antigen. High levels of antibody against the infecting organism and of immunoglobulin G are found (Phair, Klippel and Mackenzie, 1972).

The type of lesion produced by the immune responses varies with the ratio of antigen to antibody. Antigen excess leads to the production of increased capillary permeability, perhaps via release of vasoactive amines, which may allow immune complexes to accumulate by filtration through the vessel walls. Equivalence of antigen and antibody leads to granuloma formation (Spector and Heeson, 1969). The main antibodies involved in infective endocarditis are the IgG-opsonins (Laxdal et al, 1968). Beeson (1970) postulated a continued supply of antigen to the circulation as the basis of the immune response. The logical therapeutic step of adding drugs which suppress immune reactions to the treatment has seemed not yet to have been taken (Cole, 1975).

Many of the supposed autoimmune responses disappear with cure of the infection, e.g. acute confusional states recover and diffuse vascular damage will stop, but progression of the renal lesion may cause late death after elimination of the infection.

THE RENAL LESION OF INFECTIVE ENDOCARDITIS

The recognition of the importance of immune phenomena in infective endocarditis has led to the observation that the common diffuse renal disease responsible for the useful diagnostic finding of microscopic haematuria and often leading to renal failure is generally part of the immune response rather than a microembolic phenomenon, although frank major renal emboli also undoubtedly occur (Garrod, 1974). Gutman et al (1972) studied nine patients with glomerulonephritis in bacterial endocarditis and found the principal lesion to be a diffuse proliferative glomerulonephritis probably caused by circulating antigen/antibody deposits, but two patients had in addition local deposits of fibrin which might represent emboli. Immunofluorescence microscopy showed the presence of gamma-globulin and complement on the glomerular basement membranes in all four patients studied in this way.

Serological data showed a uniform pattern, the serum complement which may be low initially rose to normal levels during successful treatment. Rheumatoid factor and IgG titres rose at first and later fell. Two of these patients had staphylococcal infections, but in the other six blood cultures were negative, and in two patients the presumptive diagnosis was lupus erythema-tosus, emphasising the similarity of the immune response in the two conditions.

Wardle and Floyd (1973) demonstrated accelerated fibrinogen catabolism in three patients with bacterial endocarditis and renal failure and suggest that this is an important factor leading to proliferative glomerulonephritis.

Boulton-Jones et al (1974) studied five patients with glomerulonephritis complicating subacute infective endocarditis, but could demonstrate deposits of immunoglobulin and reduced serum complement in only three patients with segmental changes. The pathogenic mechanism could not be determined in the remaining two patients with diffuse proliferative glomerulonephritis.

They postulate that the site of deposition of immune complexes in the glomerulus depends on the size of the complex (Germuth, Senterfit and Drissman, 1972). Small complexes formed in antigen excess are subepithelial and may be associated with diffuse proliferation, but larger complexes formed in antibody excess deposit on the inside of the glomerular basement membrane and are accompanied by a focal nephritis, as in the three cases reported with segmental and focal proliferative glomerulonephritis. In keeping with this, Gutman et al (1972) found predominantly subepithelial deposits in their two patients with staphylococcal endocarditis, and subendothelial and intra-membranous deposits in their six patients with negative blood cultures.

That the immunoglomerulonephritis is not confined to patients with bacterial infection is shown by a report (Dathan and Heyworth, 1975) of a similar disturbance associated with *Coxiella burnetii* endocarditis which showed a particularly wide variety of circulating antibodies.

Bacterial endocarditis in addicts

Bacterial endocarditis in narcotic addicts is a special problem. The infection is due to the intravenous injection of grossly infected material and seems to be a frequent cause of death in these patients, although some over-reporting is suspected (Cherubin et al, 1968). Conway (1970) reviewed 60 patients. Perhaps because of the virulent nature of the organisms involved there is a strong tendency for normal valves to become infected, and preceding valve disease was known in only 16 of these patients; the usual incidence is 80 to 90 per cent. Although the aortic valve is usually involved, and mitral disease is next in frequency, there is a striking incidence of tricuspid valve involvement, and occasionally the lesion is on the pulmonary valve. There was tricuspid involvement in 24 of the 60 cases analysed by Conway (1970). The organism reported most often in the 1940s was Candida, but more recently *Staph. aureus* has been more frequent. Mixed infections may occur (Cherubin et al, 1968), as in an unusual case reported recently (Simberkoff et al, 1974), and may give rise to therapeutic problems (see later).

Aortic valve disease is often acute with rapid valve destruction and frequent emboli. In tricuspid valve disease, the pulmonary emboli may cavitate and form abscesses, but signs of tricuspid valve destruction are unusual and murmurs may be unimpressive or transient. All addicts with fever and evidence of pulmonary infection should have a blood culture, and if this is positive they should be treated as bacterial endocarditis, in spite of the difficulties of management in these patients. Recently successful complete surgical excision of the tricuspid valve in patients with resistant infection has been reported (Robin et al, 1975).

Candida endocarditis

Candida endocarditis is unusual as a spontaneous infection, but may complicate valve replacement surgery, presumably obtaining access from infected drip sites rather than as spores in imperfectly sterilised valves (Darrell, 1975). It is found in drug addicts, from grossly contaminated injections and as a superinfection during antibiotic therapy for bacterial endocarditis, presumably again from infected drip sites (Seelig et al, 1974). The infection is often silent without fever. The diagnosis may be made by marrow biopsy or from material removed at embolectomy. Large fungating vegetations are frequent and may embolise. Valve obstruction may occur if the masses are very large (Roberts et al, 1967) and is a particular problem of the infected prosthetic valve. Diagnosis by serological tests may be difficult (p. 457).

Experimental Model of Endocarditis

The experimental model utilised by Durack and Beeson (1972) has proved helpful in understanding the pathogenesis of bacterial endocarditis. Catheters placed in the right atrium or left ventricle of rabbits via the jugular vein or carotid artery lead to the formation of sterile vegetations on the valves on which they impinge. They have shown that these vegetations of non-infective thrombotic endocarditis have a high affinity for circulating *Streptococcus viridans* comparable to that of the liver or spleen in spite of the absence of special vascular arrangements or active cells in the vegetations, but not for L forms of *S. faecalis* or Coxsackie B_4 virus (Durack and Petersdorf, 1973). The bacteria grow rapidly after a lag phase of about $1\frac{1}{2}$ h. At about 20 h, a layer of fibrin appears over the endocardial lesion and its bacteria (Durack and Beeson, 1972): this fibrin roof may protect the bacterial colonies from phagocytic cells.

Non-bacterial thrombotic endocarditis

Sterile vegetations of platelets and fibrin are well known on heart valves in acute rheumatic fever. Similar changes in apparently normal valves have been known for many years as a terminal disturbance in severe disease, but MacDonald and Robbins (1957) reported that embolic complications from these vegetations may contribute to the death of the patient or may even be the first indication of systemic illness. Most cases are associated with extensive carcinoma, often a mucus-secreting adenocarcinoma (Rohner, Prior and Sipple, 1966; Ray Chauduri, 1971), and widespread venous thrombosis; a tendency to increased clotting has been postulated in these patients.

The experimental evidence referred to previously suggests that infection of a similar non-infective thrombotic endocarditis, forming on abnormal sites of blood flow in the circulation is the first step in the development of an infective endocarditis (Cole, 1975).

LABORATORY DIAGNOSIS

Blood Cultures

The bacteraemia is usually of low order (5–100 organisms/ml) but persistent so that blood cultures will ordinarily reveal the infecting organism and is of major importance in establishing diagnosis and determining management.

Technique

The common practice is to use blood culture bottles containing 50 ml nutrient broth with added anticoagulant (Liquoid; sodium polyanethyl sulphonate). This prevents the blood from clotting, and also neutralises the bactericidal activity of fresh blood, probably by inactivating components of complement.

The skin should be cleaned with 0.5 per cent chlorhexidine in 70 per cent ethanol and the vein entered with a single movement: blood obtained with difficulty is more likely to produce a contaminated culture.

Withdraw 10 ml of blood, and inject 5 ml into two blood culture bottles through the rubber seal.

It is important that the laboratory should know any antibiotic the patient is having or has had recently, and that the bottles be delivered directly to the laboratory for immediate incubation.

Number of cultures

Large numbers of cultures are not required. If two or three samples are negative, it is most unlikely that a later one will be positive. More than one sample should, however, be taken before treatment is started, because of the risk that contamination with skin bacteria may ruin a single sample.

When treatment is urgent, take two blood cultures (each in two bottles) separated by a few minutes. When treatment is less urgent, take three samples, an hour or so apart.

The time at which a blood culture is taken in relation to fever is not critical. Although showers of organisms may precede a febrile episode against a background of persistent bacteraemia (Weiss and Ottenburg, 1932), it is generally agreed that bacteraemia is constant and culture can be carried out at any time (Bennett and Beeson, 1954). In view of the urgency of the situation and the need for prompt diagnosis cultures should be taken without waiting for a febrile episode.

In the Laboratory

Practice varies greatly from one laboratory to another, but the principle is the same in all. The bottles are incubated, and inspected and subcultured after 24 and 48 h, and usually at further intervals for a week or more. In some hospitals 'pour plates' are made from the patient's blood, and special media may be inoculated at the bedside or from the blood culture bottles when they first reach the laboratory.

Most common pathogens will grow within 48 h. As soon as growth is obtained, the laboratory will report the likely identity of the organism and predict its probable antibiotic sensitivity. Confirmation of this preliminary information will take at least another 24 h. Aerobic and anaerobic cultures and cultures in 5 per cent CO_2 will reveal most of the possible infecting organisms.

Arterial sampling is said not to improve recovery (Bennett and Beeson, 1954) but the possibility of marrow culture should be kept in mind for the isolation of unusual organisms in view of the success reported with this technique in the recent Mexican epidemic of enteric fever (Gilman et al, 1975).

The Problem of Persistently Negative Blood Cultures

Persistently negative blood cultures are not infrequent even in expert hands (Shinebourne et al, 1969). Possible causes include:

1. Unusual organisms with specialised growth requirements; these seem to be becoming more frequent.
2. Previous inadequate antibiotic therapy.
3. Prolonged infection with signs mainly due to the immune response.
4. Non-bacterial thrombotic endocarditis (see above).
5. Infection with fungi (e.g. Candida) or rickettsia (e.g. *Coxiella burnetii*).
6. Another disease causing embolism and fever, such as left atrial myxoma.

Antibiotic therapy with bacteriostatic drugs or with bactericidal drugs at a dose inadequate to eradicate the infection may abolish the bacteraemia; repeated blood culture after several days may then be successful. Organisms may be visible in Gram-stained films of buffy coat although they cannot be identified; an inference from these films may be misleading in judging the most appropriate therapy. Cole (1975) envisages a bacteria-free phase of infective endocarditis when the immune response becomes dominant in the production of symptoms and the organisms are walled in by fibrin deposition. A similar situation with renal failure in patients with a very chronic illness in the preantibiotic era (Libman and Freiberg, 1968) is mentioned by Boulton-Jones et al (1974). Excess circulating antibody may account for the sterile blood cultures at this stage of the disease. However, in most patients with evidence of an immune response positive blood cultures can be obtained.

Rickettsial infections, i.e. *Q fever* endocarditis, are not uncommon (Dathan and Heyworth, 1975) and may be detected by antibody studies.

Candida endocarditis usually complicates valve replacement, drug addiction, or occurs as a superinfection during antibiotic treatment (e.g. from a drip site). Blood culture on Sabouraud's medium may be successful after ten days to three weeks, but may take even longer. Serological tests give more rapid results, but need expert interpretation (Remington, Gaines and Gilmer, 1972; Hellwege, Fischer and Blaker, 1972) as antibodies to Candida are frequent in bacterial endocarditis patients with no other evidence of Candida infection (Bacon et al, 1974).

Infective endocarditis may arise as part of an episode of *psittacosis* and is suspected when infective endocarditis with negative blood cultures is associated with pneumonitis and a cerebral disturbance. A history of bird contact and a high titre in the specific complement-fixation test will confirm the diagnosis. At necropsy prominent finger-like vegetations may be a feature (Levison et al, 1971).

Left atrial myxoma may cause confusion with infective endocarditis as it presents with murmurs suggesting mitral valve disease which may change from day to day, recurrent embolism, a low grade fever and a raised ESR. The diagnosis can usually be established by echocardiography showing a mass of echoes moving behind the anterior cusp of the mitral valve. Florid vegetations may produce similar echoes moving with the valve in infective endocarditis.

ANTIBIOTIC TREATMENT

The value of isolation of the infecting organism in planning treatment is so great that antibiotics should never be given before obtaining blood for culture. In most cases it is reasonable to delay treatment for a few days until the organism has been isolated and an initial impression of its sensitivity to antibiotics obtained, but occasionally the clinical situation demands speculative treatment before the results of blood culture are known.

The best speculative treatment, if the organism is not yet known, is penicillin with streptomycin (see below). If blood cultures are negative or the initial treatment is found to be inadequate, it is often necessary to stop all antibiotics for up to several weeks to obtain a satisfactory culture before a definitive antibiotic regime can be planned.

Cole (1975) points out the therapeutic paradox of the need for long periods (six to eight weeks) of high levels of bactericidal antibiotics to eliminate bacterial endocarditis (Cates and Christie, 1951; Kafer, Anderson and Hewitt, 1968) although the animal model data shows no evidence of failure of antibiotics to penetrate the vegetations. Although the original evidence as to the need for the six to eight weeks' therapy was not strong the dogma has stood the test of experience and shorter courses, although sometimes successful, seem to be associated with a greater incidence of relapse which may be difficult to manage.

Effective treatment requires a bactericidal antibiotic such as one of the penicillins, cephalosporins or aminoglycosides (for example, streptomycin). Bacteriostatic agents such as sulphonamides, tetracyclines or chloramphenicol will suppress the fever, but do not eradicate the infection and valve destruction may continue without clinical evidence of infection. It is necessary to test the isolated organism in culture to find the best bactericidal agent or combination of agents.

Assessment of Bactericidal Effect

The patient's organism is inoculated into tubes of appropriate medium containing serial dilutions of bactericidal antibiotics alone or in combination. After overnight incubation, the tubes that show no growth are subcultured to establish whether the organism has been killed or merely inhibited. From these results it can be judged which antibiotic, or antibiotic combination, will kill the organism in concentrations readily attainable in the patient's serum. The selection of the optimum bactericidal combination for unusual (or unusually resistant) organisms can involve the laboratory in a great deal of time-consuming work, but the combination of a beta-lactam antibiotic (penicillin or cephalosporin) together with an aminoglycoside (kanamycin, streptomycin or gentamicin) will prove bactericidal for the great majority of strains.

If the organisms survive in the presence of therapeutically attainable concentrations of such mixtures, it is likely that the planning and conduct of the patient's therapy will follow a stormy course. All other agents likely to be bactericidal for the bacterial species isolated (for example, in the case of staphylococci, sodium fusidate, lincomycin, erythromycin, vancomycin and rifamycins) must be additionally tested alone and in combination. It may be necessary to examine the possible benefit of adding a third agent such as erythromycin. In no circumstances should additional agents be introduced into the therapeutic regimen without laboratory evidence of benefit since the bactericidal effect of an already imperfect mixture may be further impaired by the speculative addition of another agent.

Coliform infections are particularly difficult to treat, but ampicillin and kanamycin (Hansing, Allen and Cherry, 1967) and a trimethoprim–sulphonamide combination (Fowle and Zorab, 1970) have been found effective. Some organisms cannot be eradicated by any known combination of antibiotics, and a policy of continuous suppression may be considered as an alternative to excision of an infected valve.

After treatment for 48 h the bactericidal action of a serum sample from the patient is tested at the time of minimal plasma level, when the next dose of antibiotic is due to see if the antibiotic regime is effective. A serum that is bactericidal at a dilution of 1 in 4 is considered satisfactory (Schlichter and MacLean, 1947; Jawetz, 1962).

There is naturally a tendency to err on the side of over-treatment in so dangerous a condition and it is conventional to continue high dose therapy for six to eight weeks (but see below).

In Q fever endocarditis, a policy of chronic suppression with tetracycline has generally been employed, but there is evidence that co-trimoxazole may be curative (Freeman and Hodson, 1972).

Penicillin, having high bactericidal activity and low toxicity, is almost the ideal antibiotic for the treatment of bacterial endocarditis, and is to be preferred if the infecting organism is sensitive. *S. viridans* is usually highly sensitive to penicillin, and will often respond to 1 megaunit four times a day, intramuscularly. Oral penicillins have been used in sensitive infections (Gray et al, 1964) with the assistance of probenecid to reduce renal excretion of the antibiotic, but such a regime is uncertain and needs close monitoring of the serum levels to ensure continued bactericidal effect. An additional problem is that if drug reactions, such as rashes or fever, occur; it may be uncertain whether the penicillin or the probenecid is responsible.

Gray (1975) has recently reinforced his suggestion for the use of oral therapy. He divides his patients with infective endocarditis into two groups, a 'naturally occurring' group sensitive to penicillin and usually responding to oral therapy and an 'extraneous' group, following soon after cardiac surgery or associated with narcotic abuse or haemodialysis and often needing intravenous antibiotics and combination therapy. He implies that ampicillin and amoxycillin may be useful antibiotics for oral use; presumably the more recently introduced ampicillins (Knudsen and Harding, 1975) must also be considered in this category. Many organisms need laboratory testing, particularly in view of the high incidence of pencillin-resistant infections in elderly patients with bedsores. He reports the remarkable treatment of 65 patients by oral therapy with only nine deaths (14 per cent), and only four patients needing to be changed to parenteral therapy or another antibiotic, but we would emphasise the importance of being certain that patients managed on such regimes are infected with fully penicillin-susceptible strains.

On the other hand, brief periods of therapy have been successful when more effective bactericidal mixtures have been employed. Penicillin kills the great majority of the staphylococcal or streptococcal populations but leaves a significant number of 'persisters'. These are indifferent to the action of penicillin and cannot be eradicated even by raising the penicillin to very high levels. Since all the killing that penicillin can achieve is completed after the first few doses it is arguable that nothing further is achieved by continuing very high dose therapy and that further treatment should aim to suppress the persisting minority long enough to allow clearance by the intrinsic defence mechanisms which in endocarditis seem to be peculiarly sluggish.

Streptomycin is not particularly active against streptococci because it cannot readily penetrate the cells. When the cell wall is damaged by a penicillin or a cephalosporin, however, the streptomycin enters readily and kills the great majority of the penicillin survivors. Hence the marked synergic effect between the two agents. This suggests that even sensitive *Streptococcus viridans* infection might be more effectively managed by a relatively brief period of treatment with a combination of penicillin and streptomycin followed by sufficient penicillin to suppress regrowth of the (hopefully very small number of) persisters. Such a regime has been successfully used by Tan et al (1971) who followed initial penicillin plus streptomycin therapy with oral phenoxymethyl penicillin. If oral penicillins are to be used in so dangerous a condition two warnings should be heeded. It should not be assumed that the oral penicillin will show the same activity against the infecting organism as benzylpenicillin and its activity should be tested in the laboratory. It is also essential to establish that effective plasma concentrations are attained, care must be taken that doses are not omitted, and the antibacterial effectiveness of the serum must be tested.

Mixed endocarditis, as often found in narcotic addicts, can produce therapeutic problems. An organism (such as *Enterobacter* species) producing a beta-lactamase can protect an otherwise sensitive organism (in this case *Staph. aureus*) against the action of penicillin or a cephalosporin (Simberkoff et al, 1974). Mixed infections may also be found in patients with leukaemia (Tattersall, Spiers and Darrell, 1972). Confusion may arise if a vigorous, easily demonstrable organism diverts attention from a more fastidious, slower-growing organism which may be more difficult to eradicate (Child et al, 1969).

More resistant organisms may need 2 to 8 megaunits of penicillin intramuscularly four times a day; if even larger doses are needed the possibility of giving the penicillin intravenously may be considered (see below).

Enterococci are relatively resistant to penicillin, but the synergistic effect of streptomycin with penicillin is very great, and this combination is usually effective. However, streptomycin must be used with care in these patients as there is often impairment of renal function as a result of the bacterial endocarditis; blood levels may be needed as a guide to dosage. Ampicillin is more active than penicillin against enterococci, but is usually inadequate alone. Mardell et al (1970) found that penicillin or ampicillin, with streptomycin in each case, were usually satisfactory, but other combinations may be required (Jawetz and Sonne, 1966).

Intravenous penicillin

When large doses of penicillin are needed, continuous intravenous therapy may be given. Comparatively larger doses are needed than for intramuscular injection as the renal loss is accentuated by the persistently high blood levels, and doses up to 100 megaunits a day can be used, although convulsions may be produced by extremely high blood levels if renal function is impaired. There is some risk of superimposed fresh infection, particularly with resistant staphylococci or Candida, from the indwelling catheter, and it has been suggested that the catheter should be changed every few days and replaced in a fresh site: however, in practice, with proper care at insertion of the catheter, the risk seems small. A further problem is the rapid inactivation of penicillin in alkaline sugar solutions; the usual 5 per cent glucose solution produces 75 per cent loss of activity in 6 h and 99 per cent loss in 24 h (Simberkoff et al, 1970) so penicillin solutions should be made up freshly for each infusion.

Hypersensitivity to penicillin

Penicillin hypersensitivity may be the cause of considerable difficulty in the management of bacterial endocarditis. If penicillin treatment is indicated and the evidence of sensitivity is not clear-cut a test dose should be given. Skin tests are not entirely reliable as reactions to a parenteral dose may still occur even if the test is negative. In most cases treatment can be continued while suppressing the sensitivity reaction with moderate doses of steroids (Raper and Kemp, 1965), although anaphylaxis may not be prevented and the additional precaution of gradually increasing the dose is suggested (Green, Peters and Geraci, 1967). Possible risks of this approach are the development of inadequate control of the sensitivity reaction. Another approach is to use an alternative antibiotic, but most other bactericidal agents are less effective against streptococci than penicillin. Cephaloridine, and the related drugs, cephalothin and cephazolin, are however suitable and good results were reported in 10 patients treated with cephalosporins by Rahal, Myers and Weinstein (1968). A minority of patients sensitive to penicillin are also sensitive to cephalosporins, no doubt because of the close chemical relationship between the two antibiotics (Assem and Vickers, 1974), but this is not a frequent problem (Apicella, Perkins and Saslaw, 1966).

Cephaloridine and, to a lesser extent, cephalothin, may produce renal tubular damage, particularly if renal function is impaired initially, or if potent diuretic drugs or aminoglycosides are given simultaneously.

Relapse may occur after an apparently successful course of treatment, and it has been suggested that bacterial variants (L-forms) with defective cell walls may be responsible (Beeson, 1970). These forms constitute at least part of the 'persister' fraction of the bacterial population remaining during treatment with penicillin which has its action in the cell wall (see page 459).

Treatment of Candida Endocarditis

Antibacterial agents are valueless in fungal endocarditis. The most widely used drug is amphotericin B which is fungistatic rather than fungicidal: it must be given by intravenous administration and may produce renal damage. An alternative treatment with 5-fluorocytosine has been suggested (Record et al, 1971): this can be given orally but is also fungistatic and may produce marrow or liver damage; the report shows little evidence of better results and resistant strains tend to be selected quickly. Darrell (1975) suggests that 5-fluorocytosine should be used only in association with amphotericin B which has some synergistic effect. Infected drip sites are often the source of infection and these should be replaced. Twice weekly flushing of drips with dilute amphotericin B has been suggested as a prophylactic (Brennan et al, 1972), but proper aseptic care is essential and generally effective.

For best results in *infected prosthetic valves*, the infected site must be removed before the infection can penetrate the myocardium. A mortality of only 20 per cent was found with removal of the infected valve within 48 h of diagnosis and with 15 min irrigation of the infected site with amphotericin B (1 g/litre in Ringer's solution) followed by amphotericin B 10 mg/day increasing up to 50 mg, if tolerated, three times a week up to a total of 2.5 g (Turnier et al, 1975). Similar principles apply to other fungal causes of endocarditis but only the yeasts and not the filamentous fungi respond to 5-fluorocytosine.

PROPHYLAXIS

It is generally believed on circumstantial evidence that a high circulating plasma level of a bactericidal antibiotic will prevent bacterial endocarditis in susceptible subjects with cardiac lesions having a transient bacteraemia, as after dental extraction, but there is no formal evidence to support this belief and current practice often fails to achieve the aim even when an attempt at prophylaxis is made (Durack, 1975). Evidence from experimental rabbit endocarditis indicates that highly bactericidal regimens are required (Durack and Petersdorf, 1973) and that bacteriostatic agents such as tetracycline and also many other antibiotics, including cephalexin and co-trimoxazole, are ineffective.

The frequency of bacteraemia is said to be related to the degree of gum disease and the amount of gum trauma (O'Kell and Elliot, 1934). The major risk is from dental extraction, and although bacterial endocarditis has been reported after filling or scaling the risk is so slight that routine cover for these procedures does not seem justified unless gingival bleeding is likely to be produced, as the frequency of bacteraemia is related to the degree of gum disease (Fleming, 1976). The suggestion that bacteraemia may be produced by chewing in some patients is probably erroneous (Cooke, 1970). Prophylaxis may not be necessary under the age of eight years (Fleming, 1976). The absence of any controlled trial, and the relative rarity of bacterial endocarditis in comparison with the frequency of dental extraction, has led some dentists to question the value of antibiotic cover. Hilson (1970) estimates the risk of bacterial endocarditis as 1 in 500 after extraction in a susceptible subject, and suggests that the risk of penicillin prophylaxis may outweigh the dangers of endocarditis. Such conclusions can only be based on a gross underestimate of the mortality and morbidity of bacterial endocarditis. Antibiotic cover for dental extraction should begin immediately before the procedure as the oral flora may become resistant to penicillin within two days (Garrod and Waterworth, 1962).

Evidence from experimental rabbit endocarditis (Durack and Petersdorf, 1973) indicates that highly bactericidal regimens are required and that bacteristatic agents such as tetracyclines and also many other antibiotics, including cephalexin and co-trimoxazole, are ineffective.

Regimens

The experimental work on rabbit endocarditis indicates that successful prophylaxis can be achieved in one of two ways: by giving a single dose of a 'totally bactericidal' antibiotic (or antibiotic combination), or, in the case of penicillin-sensitive organisms, by giving penicillin in such a way as to achieve a high initial plasma level followed by an inhibitory level that persists over two or three days. The first of these objectives can at present be achieved only by injection. Regimens that have been in use for some time and which appear to satisfy the experimental requirements are penicillin 1 megaunit plus strepto-mycin 0.5 g intramuscularly, or vancomycin 1 g intravenously. High initial levels of penicillin followed by relatively prolonged lower levels can be obtained from injections of one of the commercially available mixtures of benzyl-penicillin with procaine-, benethamine- or benzathine-penicillin.

There is obviously a demand for effective oral prophylaxis especially in children where the threat of prophylactic injections may increase the risk of endocarditis through refusal of necessary dental treatment (Hobson, 1975). More recent work on the rabbit model (Pelletier et al, 1975) suggests that phenoxymethyl penicillin 30 mg/kg followed by 7.5 mg/kg 6-hourly over 48 h should be effective against penicillin-sensitive streptococci. Unfortu-nately penicillin-resistant oral streptococci are now encountered relatively frequently especially in children and it has been suggested that preliminary antibiotic sensitivity testing is required (Dunbar and Elliott, 1975). It should be assumed that the oral streptococci will be penicillin resistant if the patient has received penicillin within the past six weeks. Penicillin-resistant strains are generally sensitive to parenteral cephalosporins but complete killing is likely to require the addition of streptomycin. Such strains are also likely to respond to vancomycin.

In seeking suitable oral therapy, consideration should be given to a three-day course of erythromycin. The drug is by no means completely protective when tested in the animal model but this may represent an unnaturally severe test of prophylactic agents and erythromycin provides substantial protection against the number of orgnaisms likely to be circulating in man. Prophylaxis for elderly patients for gynaecological and urological procedures raises difficult problems because the infecting organisms are often relatively resistant to antibiotics. The resistance patterns of such organisms and the comparative performance of prophylactic regimens against experimental infections with them has not yet been systematically studied and recommendations based on solid evidence cannot yet be made. General experience suggests that a penicillin plus an aminoglycoside is likely to be more effective than other agents that might be considered and the combination of ampicillin 1 g plus streptomycin 1 g has been employed. Some prefer the 'wider cover' offered by the potentially more toxic combination of gentamicin plus a cephalosporin. In normal delivery the risk is small and prophylaxis is unnecessary.

INDICATIONS FOR SURGICAL TREATMENT

The destructive process in the infected valves is a major problem in the management of these patients after the infection has been controlled. Infection of the aortic or mitral valves is most often found, and almost always leads to increasing incompetence. The only exception is the occasional production of obstruction by florid vegetations such as are found in Candida infections (see above). Damage to the aortic valve may be associated with fenestration or inversion of a cusp, or with the formation and rupture of mycotic aneurysms (Wise et al, 1971). Mitral valve lesions may be complicated by rupture of the chordae tendineae or perforation of the ventricular septum. The sudden appearance of gross aortic or mitral incompetence in an unprepared left ventricle quickly produces failure and urgent surgical treatment is often needed. There is no time for left ventricular hypertrophy to appear, and there is relatively little dilatation of the chamber. The left ventricle compensates to some extent by emptying to an unusually small end-diastolic volume. Characteristic clinical features are associated with the sudden onset of incompetence.

Sudden Aortic Incompetence

Acute aortic incompetence leads to a considerable fall in cardiac output with shock-like features which may obscure the usual changes in the arterial pulse. The left ventricular end-diastolic pressure rises steeply and may exceed the left atrial pressure (Wigle and Labrosse, 1966). Premature closure of the mitral valve in mid-diastole, which can be demonstrated by echocardiography, usually prevents any diastolic mitral incompetence, and a mitral closure sound may be heard in diastole. There may be a late diastolic outward thrust due to continued filling of the left ventricle from the aorta. The mitral first heart sound is absent, as the mitral valve has already closed, but there is often an early third sound or a mitral diastolic murmur due to the short period available for left ventricular filling. Wise and his colleagues (1971) stress the tachycardia and consequent abbreviation of diastole in these cases which may make auscultation difficult.

Echocardiography may show evidence of vegetations or high-frequency patterns associated with ruptured leaflets (Wray, 1975), and such florid changes may show the need for valve replacement (Sutton, Petch and Parker, 1976).

Sudden Mitral Incompetence

Acute mitral incompetence is usually due to ruptured chordae tendineae and also presents as severe pulmonary congestion with little cardiac enlargement. The left atrium is small unless there has been significant preceding mitral disease, and sinus rhythm is usually maintained. The systolic murmur often has a peak in mid-systole, and may well be heard in the neck, causing confusion with aortic stenosis. Cardiac catheterisation shows prominent 'v' waves as the large backflow occurs into the small left atrium.

Myocardial Damage

Myocardial disturbance may be an additional factor producing failure in bacterial endocarditis. There is some evidence of a worse prognosis in infections of a rheumatic valve than in a congenital abnormality, suggesting that rheumatic myocardial damage can have a deleterious effect, and pre-existing ischaemic heart disease may contribute to the development of failure in older patients (Shinebourne et al, 1969). Coronary emboli from the infected valves may produce frank infarction, and microemboli which are frequent at autopsy (Bracht–Wächter bodies) may be part of the immune response (see above), but the functional significance of these changes is uncertain. The possibility that myocardial disease is contributing to the development of heart failure suggests a conservative policy towards operation on the valve lesions in the acute stage of the disease. If improvement occurs with treatment it is best to defer operation until several weeks after the end of the antibiotic course, but the patient should be kept under close observation as there is a tendency for failure to return with increased activity in convalescence. More seriously affected patients, on the other hand, will not survive without immediate operation, and the risk of problems from myocardial damage must be accepted; relief of the load from the incompetent valve is usually enough to outweigh this effect and operation can reasonably be performed during antibiotic treatment if necessary (Stason et al, 1968; English and Ross, 1972).

Management

Unless the patient has had a long period of severe failure the operative risk is not unduly great in these patients (Wise et al, 1971) and it seems likely that prompt surgical treatment may reverse the changes and restore a reasonable long-term outlook as the ventricle has not suffered the effects of long-term hypertrophy and the dilatation found in established chronic aortic or mitral incompetence.

Early operation in patients with bacterial endocarditis presents some surgical difficulties. Failure of the sutures holding a valve replacement in the friable tissue of the ring of the infected valve may lead to a paravalvar leak

(Manhas et al, 1970) and there may be residual infection. However, cure of bacterial endocarditis may occur after successful operation on the underlying abnormality, as shown many years ago by Touroff (1943) and Tubbs (1944) following a ligation of a persistent ductus arteriosus, and a long course of antibiotic treatment is not usually needed after successful excision of an infected valve. In some cases excision may be the best way to deal with an infection which is resistant to antibiotic treatment.

Coliform infections have a particularly bad reputation in this respect (Simberkoff et al, 1974) but staphylococcal infection may present similar problems, as even the *Staphylococcus albus* may be resistant to many antibiotics; prompt treatment with rifampicin may be helpful (Peard et al, 1970) but it must be used in combination with another antibiotic, chosen on the basis of laboratory tests (see p. 458), to prevent the rapid emergence of resistance. A similar situation is seen in Q fever (*Coxiella burnetii*) endocarditis (Kristinsson and Bentall, 1967) where tetracycline has a suppressive effect but no effective agent killing the organism is known (see above).

Identification of the infected valve may be a problem if more than one valve is abnormal and echocardiography should be helpful. Replacement of the excised valve is the usual procedure, but the tricuspid valve may be excised without replacement (Robin et al, 1975), leaving a reasonable haemodynamic result and avoiding the problems of valve replacement in this position.

Infected prosthetic valves

Bacterial endocarditis involving the seating of a prosthetic valve is not unusual. English and Ross (1972) had six patients needing reoperation for endocarditis in their series. Infection may occur acutely following postoperative contamination, often by Candida from an infected drip site, or as a late complication. Profuse vegetations may obstruct the prosthesis or erosion alongside the ring may produce a paravalvar leak, but in either case reoperation may be needed on mechanical grounds. Removal of the infected valve seating is necessary to effect surgical cure of the infection of a prosthetic valve, and early operation with irrigation of the valve base is recommended in Candida infections (see above).

The incidence of infection of prosthetic valves at operation varies from 1 to 4 per cent; 70 per cent of these patients have staphylococcal infection, with about an equal proportion coagulase positive and negative. Many of the remainder are due to Candida infections, and in about half of these there is clear evidence of the use of antibiotics before operation which may favour the appearance of Candida infections, for instance, in drip sites, by eliminating competing organisms, and raises again the question of the value of the use of prophylactic antibiotics before operation. As the general reduction of septic complications is one of the factors allowing successful open heart surgery, it seems unlikely that a return to aseptic principles will be acceptable, but scrupulous attention to the aseptic insertion and management of drip sites is indicated, and prophylactic flushing with amphotericin B may be considered (see above).

Assessment after recovery

All patients recovering from bacterial endocarditis should be critically reviewed to assess the changes in the valve lesion. Although compensatory hypertrophy may allow a return to activities in spite of a greater degree of incompetence, early replacement may give a better outlook (Windsor and Shanahan, 1967). Further distortion of the valve may occur during healing, and lead to failure after an apparently successful recovery. If the aortic valve is involved an aortogram is useful to show any local mycotic disturbances such as sinus of Valsalva aneurysm that may require surgical treatment.

Patients who have recovered from bacterial endocarditis seem particularly liable to reinfection. Levison et al (1970) found 17 cases of reinfection in 251 patients, an incidence of 7 per cent. The recurrences were more frequent in younger patients, and were more often associated with congenital heart disease and *Streptococcus viridans* infection. The chance of cure did not seem unduly worse than usual in the second attack but in view of the risks of recurrent bacterial endocarditis, surgical treatment of minor congenital abnormalities such as ventricular septal defects that have been the site of infection should be considered.

MORTALITY

The persisting high mortality in spite of the advances in antibiotic therapy in recent years is due to:

1. Resistant infections not eradicable by current therapy.
2. Major embolism.
3. Acute heart failure due to severe sudden aortic or mitral valve rupture augmented by myocardial damage.
4. Severe immune-response glomerulonephritis, progressing to renal failure although the infection is overcome.
5. Late deaths due to worsening valve disease or mycotic aneurysm.
6. Delayed recognition allowing severe damage before treatment started.

REFERENCES

Apicella, M. A., Perkins, R. L. & Saslaw, S. (1966) Treatment of bacterial endocarditis with cephalosporin derivatives in penicillin-allergic patients. *New England Journal of Medicine*, **274**, 1002.

Assem, E. S. K. & Vickers, M. R. (1974) Penicillin allergy tests for in man. *Immunology*, **27**, 255.

Bacon, P. A., Davidson, C. & Smith, B. (1974) Antibodies to candida and autoantibodies in subacute bacterial endocarditis. *Quarterly Journal of Medicine*, N.S., **43**, 537.

Beeson, P. B. (1970) In *Bacterial Endocarditis*, ed. Beeson, P. B. & Ridley, M., p. 9. Beecham Research Laboratories.

Bennett, J. L. & Beeson, P. B. (1954) Bacteraemia. A consideration of some experimental and clinical facts. *Yale Journal of Biology and Medicine*, **26**, 241.

Boulton-Jones, J. M., Sissons, J. G. D., Evans, D. J. & Peters, D. K. (1974) Renal lesions of subacute infective endocarditis. *British Medical Journal*, **2**, 11.

Brennan, M. F., Goldman, M. H., O'Connell, R. C. & Kundsin, R. B. (1972) Prolonged parenteral alimentation: candida growth and prevention of candidaemia by amphotericin installation. *Annals of Surgery*, **176**, 265.

Cates, J. E. & Christie, R. V. (1951) Subacute bacterial endocarditis. *Quarterly Journal of Medicine, N.S.*, **26**, 93.

Cherubin, C. E., Baden, M., Kavaler, F., Lerner, S. & Cline, W. (1968) Infective endocarditis in narcotic addicts. *Annals of Internal Medicine*, **69**, 1091.

Child, J. A., Darrell, J. H., Rhys-Davies, N. & Davis-Dawson, L. (1969) Mixed infective endocarditis in a heroin addict. *Journal of Medical Microbiology*, **2**, 293.

Clinicopathological Conference (1968) *British Medical Journal*, **4**, 40.

Cole, P. (1975) The enigma of infective endocarditis. *Hospital Update*, p. 128.

Conway, N. (1970) Endocarditis in heroin addicts. *British Heart Journal*, **31**, 543.

Cooke, B. E. D. (1970) Relationship between oral disease and bacterial endocarditis. *Proceedings of the Royal Society of Medicine*, **63**, 263.

Cordeiro, A., Costa, H. & Leginha, F. (1965) Immunologic phase of subacute bacterial endocarditis. A new concept and general considerations. *American Journal of Cardiology*, **16**, 477.

Darrell, J. H. (1975) Candida endocarditis. *British Medical Journal*, **1**, 432.

Dathan, J. R. E. & Heyworth, M. F. (1975) Glomerulonephritis associated with *Coxiella burnetti* endocarditis. *British Medical Journal*, **1**, 376.

de Swiet, M., Ramsey, I. D. & Ross, G. M. (1975) Bacterial endocarditis after insertion of intrauterine contraceptive device. *British Medical Journal*, **3**, 76.

Doyle, E. F., Spanguolo, M., Taranta, A., Kuttner, A. G. & Markowitz, M. (1967) The risk of bacterial endocarditis during antirheumatic prophylaxis. *Journal of the American Medical Association*, **201**, 807.

Dunbar, J. M. & Elliott, R. H. (1975) The dentist and prevention of infective endocarditis. *British Dental Journal*, **139**, 125.

Durack, D. T. (1975) Current practice in prevention of bacterial endocarditis. *British Heart Journal*, **7**, 478.

Durack, D. T. & Beeson, P. B. (1972) Experimental bacterial endocarditis. I. Colonisation of a sterile vegetation. II. Survival of bacteria in endocardial vegetations. *British Journal of Experimental Pathology*, **53**, 44, 50.

Durack, D. T. & Petersdorf, R. G. (1973) Chemotherapy of experimental streptococcal endocarditis. I. Comparison of commonly recommended regimens. *Journal of Clinical Investigation*, **52**, 592.

Elliott, S. D. (1973) The incidence of group H streptococci in blood cultures (S.B.E.) *British Journal of Experimental Pathology*, **53**, 44.

English, T. A. H. & Ross, J. K. (1972) Surgical aspects of bacterial endocarditis. *British Medical Journal*, **4**, 598.

Finland, M. & Barnes, M. W. (1970) Changing etiology of bacterial endocarditis in the antibacterial era. Experiences at Boston City Hospital, 1933–1965. *Annals of Internal Medicine*, **72**, 341.

Fleming, H. A. (1976) Personal communication.

Fowle, A. S. E. & Zorab, P. A. (1970) *Esch. coli* endocarditis successfully treated with oral trimethoprin and sulphamethoxazole. *British Heart Journal*, **32**, 127.

Freeman, R. & Hodson, M. E. (1972) Q fever endocarditis treated with trimethoprim and sulphomethoxazole. *British Medical Journal*, **1**, 419.

Garrod, L. P. (1974) Letter: The kidney in infective endocarditis. *British Medical Journal*, **2**, 174.

Garrod, L. P. & Waterworth, P. M. (1962) The risks of dental extraction during penicillin treatment. *British Heart Journal*, **24**, 39.

Germuth, F. G., Senterfit, L. B. & Drissman, G. R. (1972) Immune complex disease. V. The nature of the circulating complexes associated with glomerular alteration in the chronic B.S.A. rabbit system. *Johns Hopkins Medical Journal*, **130**, 344.

Gilman, R. H., Terminal, M., Leverne, M. M., Herandez-Mendoya, P. & Hornick, R. B. (1975) Relative efficacy of blood, urine, rectal swab, bone-marrow and rose spot culture for recovery of *Salmonella typhi* in typhoid fever. *Lancet*, **1**, 1211.

Gray, I. R. (1975) The choice of antibiotic for treating infective endocarditis. *Quarterly Journal of Medicine, N.S.*, **44**, 419.

Gray, I. R., Tai, A. B., Wallace, J. G. & Calder, J. H. (1964) Oral treatment of bacterial endocarditis with penicillins. *Lancet*, **2**, 110.

Green, G. R., Peters, G. A. & Geraci, J. E. (1967) Treatment of bacterial endocarditis in patients with penicillin hypersensitivity. *Annals of Internal Medicine*, **67**, 235.

Gutman, R. A., Striber, G. E., Gilliland, B. C. & Cutler, R. E. (1972) The immune complex glomerulonephritis of bacterial endocarditis. *Medicine*, **51**, 1.

Hansing, C. E., Allen, V. D. & Cherry, J. D. (1967) *Escherichia coli* endocarditis. A review of the literature and a case study. *Archives of Internal Medicine*, **120**, 472.

Hayward, G. W. (1973) Infective endocarditis: a changing disease. *British Medical Journal*, **2**, 706, 763.

Hellwege, H. H., Fischer, K. & Blaker, F. (1972) Letter: Diagnostic value of *Candida precepitins*. *Lancet*, **2**, 386.

Hilson, G. F. R. (1970) Is chemoprophylaxis necessary? *Proceedings of the Royal Society of Medicine*, **63**, 267.

Hobson, P. (1975) The dentist and prevention of infective endocarditis. *British Dental Journal*, **139**, 87.

Horwitz, L. D. & Silber, R. (1967) Subacute bacterial endocarditis presenting as purpura. *Archives of Internal Medicine*, **120**, 483.

Jawetz, E. (1962) Assay of antibacterial activity in serum: useful guide for antimicrobial therapy. *American Journal for Diseases of Children*, **103**, 81.

Jawetz, E. & Sonne, M. (1966) Penicillin–streptomycin treatment of enterococcal endocarditis. A re-evaluation. *New England Journal of Medicine*, **274**, 710.

Johnson, D. H., Rosenthal, A. & Nadas, A. S. (1975) A forty-year review of bacterial endocarditis in infancy and childhood. *Circulation*, **51**, 581.

Jones, H. R., Siebert, R. G. & Gerais, J. E. (1969) Neurological manifestations of bacterial endocarditis. *Annals of Internal Medicine*, **71**, 21.

Kafer, C. S., Anderson, P. G. & Hewitt, W. L. (1968) End results in the treatment of bacterial endocarditis. *Transactions of the Association of American Physicians*, **61**, 112.

Knudsen, E. T. & Harding, J. W. (1975) A multicentre comparative trial of talampicillin and ampicillin in general practice. *British Journal of Clinical Practice*, **29**, 255.

Kristinsson, A. & Bentall, H. H. (1967) Medical and surgical treatment of Q-fever endocarditis. *Lancet*, **2**, 693.

Lancet (1974) Bacterial stickiness. **1**, 716.

Laxdal, T., Messner, R. P., Williams, R. C. & Quie, P. G. (1968) Opsonic agglutinating and complement-fixing antibodies in patients with subacute bacterial endocarditis. *Journal of Laboratory and Clinical Medicine*, **71**, 638.

Lerner, P. I. & Weinstein, L. (1960) Infective endocarditis in the antibiotic era. *New England Journal of Medicine*, **274**, 199, 323, 388.

Levison, D. A., Guthrie, W. W., Green, D. M. & Roberton, P. G. C. (1971) Infective endocarditis as part of psittacosis. *Lancet*, **2**, 844.

Levison, M. R., Kaye, D., Mandell, G. L. & Hook, E. W. (1970) Characteristics of patients with multiple episodes of bacterial endocarditis. *Journal of American Medical Association*, **211**, 1355.

Libman, E. & Freiberg, L. K. (1968) *Subacute bacterial endocarditis*, 2nd edn, p. 364. New York: Oxford Medical Publications.

MacDonald, R. A. & Robbins, S. L. (1957) The significance of non-bacterial thrombotic endocarditis; an autopsy and clinical study of 78 cases. *Annals of Internal Medicine*, **46**, 255.

Manhas, D. R., Hessel, E. A., Quie, P. G. & Williams, R. C. (1970) Open heart surgery in infective endocarditis. *Circulation*, **41**, 841.

Mardell, G. L., Kay, D., Levison, M. E. & Hook, E. W. (1970) Enterococcal endocarditis: an analysis of 38 patients observed at the New York Hospital–Cornell Medical Center.

Messner, R. R., Laxdal, T., Quie, P. G. & Williams, R. C. (1968) Rheumatoid factors in subacute bacterial endocarditis—bacterium, duration of disease or genetic predisposition? *Annals of Internal Medicine*, **68**, 746.

O'Kell, C. C. & Elliot, S. O. (1934) Bacteraemia and oral sepsis with special reference to the aetiology of subacute endocarditis. *Lancet*, **2**, 869.

Peard, M. C., Fleck, D. G., Garrod, L. P. & Waterworth, P. M. (1970) Combined rifampicin and erythromycin for bacterial endocarditis. *British Medical Journal*, **4**, 410.

Pelletier, L. L., Durack, D. T., Petersdorf, R. G. & Nielson, K. (1975) Chemotherapy of experimental streptococcal endocarditis. IV. Further observations on prophylaxis. *Journal of Clinical Investigation*, **56**, 319–330.

Phair, J. P., Klippel, T. & Mackenzie, M. R. (1972) Antiglobulins in endocarditis. *Infection and Immunity*, **5**, 24.

Rahal, J. J., Myers, B. R. & Weinstein, L. (1968) Treatment of bacterial endocarditis with cephalothin. *New England Journal of Medicine*, **279**, 1305.

Raper, A. J. & Kemp, V. E. (1965) Use of steroids in penicillin-sensitive patients with bacterial endocarditis. *New England Journal of Medicine*, **273**, 297.

Ray Chaudhuri, M. (1971) Non-bacterial thrombotic endocarditis in association with mucus-secreting adenocarcinomas. *British Journal of Diseases of the Chest*, **65**, 98.

Record, C. O., Skinner, J. M., Sleight, P. & Speller, D. C. E. (1971) Candida endocarditis treated with 5-fluorocytosine. *British Medical Journal*, **1**, 262.

Remington, J. S., Gaines, J. P. & Gilmer, M. A. (1972) Demonstration of *Candida precipitations* in human sera by immunoelectrophoresis. *Lancet*, **1**, 413.

Roberts, W. C., Ewy, G. A., Glancy, D. L. & Marcus, F. I. (1967) Valvular stenosis produced by active infective endocarditis. *Circulation*, **36**, 419.

Robin, E., Thoms, N. W., Arbulu, A., Ganguly, S. N. & Magnisalis, K. (1975) Haemodynamic consequences of total removal of the tricuspid valve without prosthetic replacement. *American Journal of Cardiology*, **35**, 481.

Rohner, R. F., Prior, J. T. & Sipple, J. H. (1966) Mucinous malignancies, venous thrombosis and terminal endocarditis with emboli. A syndrome. *Cancer (Philadelphia)*, **19**, 1805.

Schlichter, J. G. & MacLean, H. (1947) A method of determining the effective therapeutic level in the treatment of subacute bacterial endocarditis with penicillin. A preliminary report. *American Heart Journal*, **34**, 209.

Seelig, M. S., Speth, C. P., Kozinn, P. J., Taschdjian, C. L., Toni, E. F. & Goldberg, P. (1974) Patterns of *Candida* endocarditis following cardiac surgery: importance of early diagnosis and therapy (an analysis of 91 cases). *Progress in Cardiovascular Disease*, **17**, 125–180.

Shinebourne, E. A., Cripps, C. M., Hayward, G. W. & Shooter, R. A. (1969) Bacterial endocarditis 1956–1965: analysis of clinical features and treatment in relation to mortality. *British Heart Journal*, **31**, 536.

Simberkoff, M. S., Isom, W., Smithivos, T., Noriega, E. R. & Rahal, T. T. (1974) Two-stage tricuspid valve replacement for mixed bacterial endocarditis. *Archives of Internal Medicine*, **133**, 212.

Simberkoff, M. S., Thomas, L., McGregor, D., Shenkein, I. & Levine, B. B. (1970) Inactivation of penicillins by carbohydrate solutions at alkaline pH. *New England Journal of Medicine*, **283**, 116.

Spector, W. G. & Heeson, N. (1969) The production of granulomata by antigen–antibody complexes. *Journal of Pathology*, **98**, 31.

Staffurth, J. S. (1970) In *Bacterial Endocarditis*, ed. Beeson, P. B. & Ridley, M., p. 30. Beecham Research Laboratories.

Stason, W. B., de Sanctis, R. W., Weinberg, A. N. & Austen, W. G. (1968) Cardiac surgery in bacterial endocarditis. *Circulation*, **38**, 514.

Sutton, R., Petch, M. & Parker, T. (1976) Echocardiography in infective endocarditis (Abstract). *British Heart Journal*, **38**, 312P.

Tan, T. S., Terhune, C. A., Kaplan, S. & Hamburger, M. (1971) Successful two-week treatment schedule for penicillin-susceptible *Streptococcus viridans* endocarditis. *Lancet*, **2**, 1340.

Tattersall, M. N. H., Spiers, A. S. D. & Darrell, J. H. (1972) Initial therapy with combination of five antibiotics in febrile patients with leukaemia and neutropenia. *Lancet*, **1**, 162.

Touroff, A. S. W. (1943) The results of surgical treatment of patency of the ductus arteriosus complicated by subacute bacterial endocarditis. *American Heart Journal*, **25**, 187.

Tubbs, O. S. (1944) Effect of ligation on infection of the patent ductus arteriosus. *British Journal of Surgery*, **32**, 1.

Turnier, E., Kay, J. K., Bernstein, S., Mendez, A. M. & Zabiate, P. (1975) Surgical treatment of candida endocarditis. *Chest*, **67**, 262.

Uwaydah, M. M. & Weinberg, A. N. (1965) Bacterial endocarditis—a changing pattern. *New England Journal of Medicine*, **273**, 1231.

Wardle, E. N. & Floyd, M. (1973) Fibrinogen catabolism—study of three patients with bacterial endocarditis and renal disease. *British Medical Journal*, **3**, 255–257.

Weinstein, L. (1972) Endocarditis infective, past, present and future. *Journal of the Royal College of Physicians of London*, **6**, 161.

Weiss, H. & Ottenburg, R. (1932) Relation between bacteria and temperature in subacute bacterial endocarditis. *Journal of Infectious Diseases*, **50**, 61.

Wigle, E. D. & Labrosse, C. J. (1966) Sudden, severe aortic insufficiency. *Circulation*, **32**, 708.

Windsor, H. M. & Shanahan, M. X. (1967) Emergency valve replacement in bacterial endocarditis. *Thorax*, **22**, 25–33.

Wise, J. R., Bentall, H. H., Cleland, W. P., Goodwin, J. F., Hallidie-Smith, K. A. & Oakley, C. M. (1971) Urgent aortic valve replacement for acute aortic regurgitation due to infective endocarditis. *Lancet*, **2**, 115.

Wray, T. M. (1975) The variable echocardiographic features of aortic valve endocarditis. *Circulation*, **52**, 658.

16

18

SURGICAL TREATMENT

Gareth M. Rees

with a section on tachycardias by R. A. J. Spurrell

CARDIAC SURGERY IN INFANCY

Congenital heart disease occurs in six to eight of every thousand live births. Without treatment, approximately 50 per cent of these infants die within the first year. Considerable progress has been achieved in the investigation, management and surgical treatment of such infants and will be outlined in this section.

General Management

Sick infants with congenital heart disease generally have (1) severe forms of relatively simple abnormalities, (2) multiple complex defects, or (3) both. These babies should be managed in hospitals which can provide specialist care (Gersony and Hayes, 1972). Early transfer to such a hospital in a warmed oxygenated environment with a minimum of disturbance is advisable.

Accurate anatomical diagnosis can only be made by cardiac catheterisation and angiography. This should be performed as expeditiously as possible, without undue manipulation, heat or blood loss (Tatooles and Miller, 1973). In appropriate circumstances (e.g. simple transposition of the great arteries) this investigation is combined with therapeutic enlargement of an atrial septal defect by balloon septostomy which improves blood mixing and therefore the systemic oxygen saturation. No patient should be considered too ill to investigate, although the optimum time for this is a matter for skilled judgement.

In the cyanotic infant

The key to management lies in the amount of pulmonary blood flow (Rashkind, 1972). Decreased pulmonary blood flow due to an obstructive lesion resulting in shunting of blood from the right side of the heart to the left, produces a clinically 'hypoxic infant'. Intracardiac mixing may occur at atrial septal or ventricular septal level if distal obstruction allows sufficient pressure elevation in the appropriate chamber to facilitate shunting of blood from right to left. Thus, in cases with atrial septal defect (ASD), obstruction may occur at the tricuspid valve (e.g. tricuspid atresia), right ventricle (e.g. Ebstein's anomaly, where valvar dysfunction also occurs), pulmonary valve (e.g.

pulmonary stenosis with intact ventricular septum) or pulmonary artery (e.g. pulmonary atresia with intact ventricular septum). In cases where the communication occurs through the ventricular septum (VSD), obstruction may occur at infundibular or valvar level (e.g. Fallot's tetralogy), or in the pulmonary artery (e.g. pulmonary atresia). Obstruction due to narrowing of pulmonary arterioles causing a raised pulmonary vascular resistance is very rare in neonates, although it may later develop rapidly.

Cyanosis in infancy may also be due to extensive intracardiac mixing. Pulmonary blood flow is markedly increased due, in part, to the relatively lower pulmonary compared with systemic vascular resistance; additionally the pulmonary ventricle is more compliant than its systemic counterpart. Clinically, congestive cardiac failure results in hepatomegaly. Conditions where large communications are found between right and left sides include persistent truncus arteriosus, single ventricle and aortopulmonary window. They are also seen in association with partial or complete transposition of systemic arteries or veins and where obstructive left-sided lesions are associated with a left to right communication (e.g. left heart hypoplasia and preductal coarctation).

The non-cyanotic infant

Obstructive lesions causing left ventricular failure and pulmonary congestion include coarctation and aortic stenosis. Left to right shunts may also be of sufficient severity to precipitate cardiac failure, e.g. persistent ductus arteriosus, ventricular septal defect and total anomalous pulmonary venous drainage. Secundum atrial septal defects, however, unless associated with other complex lesions seldom cause difficulties at this stage.

Medical treatment should be commenced immediately. This is particularly relevant in patients with congestive failure where digitalis and diuretics may provide clinical improvement allowing surgery to be postponed. Attention to the baby's metabolic needs, e.g. fluid, acid/base balance, prevention and correction of hypothermia, and oxygenation, are all extremely important in addition to skilled specialist nursing care (Stark, 1972).

Surgical Treatment

This is now available for most of the common conditions causing serious disability in infancy. In relatively simple conditions, e.g. persistent ductus arteriosus and coarctation of the aorta, total correction may be readily performed. In more complex conditions an alternative surgical programme is available.

The established approach for babies requiring surgery has been to palliate initially and follow this when possible by a second totally corrective procedure when the child is bigger, ideally between five and ten years old. In some conditions there has been a trend towards early primary total correction. This is not yet practicable for all abnormalities, but Fallot's tetralogy provides an interesting example; when this condition does cause difficulties in the very young, hypoxia is the main problem, often as life-threatening cyanotic or anoxic 'spells'. The surgical alternatives lie between palliation with a systemic-pulmonary artery anastomosis or total correction of the defects. The advantages of the latter approach are impressive (Rees and Starr, 1973). Although the structures are small, a well-developed collateral circulation in infancy is usually absent so the operation is not attended by the occasionally severe haemorrhagic complications seen in older patients and the technical difficulties associated with shunt closure prior to total correction are absent.

Palliative shunt procedures, moreover, are often followed by progression of the tetralogy deformity with increasing infundibular hypertrophy and growth failure of the pulmonary valve and artery which may become atretic. Shunt procedures do not lower the risks of other complications such as cerebral thrombosis and sepsis in the form of subacute bacterial endocarditis and brain abscess. Physical development following total correction is marked, in contrast to the slow progress following palliative operations.

Starr's group (Starr, Bonchek and Sutherland, 1973) have reported total correction of 25 patients aged less than two years, 13 being under the age of one, with an operative mortality of 8 per cent. In 1971, Barrett-Boyes, Simpson and Neutze reported one operative death in a series of 12 infants undergoing total correction. Obviously such results cannot be extrapolated to all centres. The approach should be dictated by the available expertise. Nevertheless, the trend towards total correction will doubtless continue (*Lancet*, 1973).

Palliative Surgery

In conditions where cyanosis is due to pulmonary underperfusion, systemic-pulmonary artery anastomosis leads to palliation of symptoms with improvement in oxygenation. Three main alternatives are available.

Blalock–Taussig procedure: Anastomosis between subclavian and pulmonary arteries, preferably on the side of the innominate artery while satisfactory in older patients is difficult to perform below the age of six months and has a high incidence of occlusion, and is thus of limited value in young infants.

Potts' operation. Anastomosis between the pulmonary artery and descending thoracic aorta may be difficult to construct in the presence of a ductus: it is notoriously dangerous to close at a later total correction. It is now rarely performed.

Waterston's operation. Anastomosis of the ascending aorta and pulmonary artery is generally the procedure of choice in the very young. Certain technical considerations are critical. Too large an anastomosis over-perfuses the lungs and may lead to pulmonary oedema, often unilaterally; too small a shunt may spontaneously occlude. Failure to place the anastomosis directly behind the aorta may cause distortion of the pulmonary artery with stenosis and partial obstruction. Although closure at secondary total correction may be achieved by suture ligation through the lumen of the ascending aorta, a residual gradient may persist between proximal and distal pulmonary artery. This is particularly likely in cases of severe Fallot's tetralogy where the pulmonary arteries are either small or atretic. Such cases generally require more elaborate repair (Ross, 1973).

Prevention of closure of ductus. In some conditions, clinical deterioration is associated with spontaneous closure of a coexistent ductus arteriosus. Prevention or delaying closure by injecting therapeutic agents, e.g. prostaglandins or formalin solution, is a manoeuvre which may find an important clinical role (Olley, 1975).

Pulmonary artery banding. Excessive pulmonary blood flow in cyanotic or acyanotic patients leads to cardiac failure and damage to the intrapulmonary vessels with raised pulmonary vascular resistance. Constriction of the pulmonary artery with a non-reactive band, e.g. of Teflon or Dacron, decreases the flow (Muller and Dammann, 1952). Narrowing the pulmonary artery to roughly a third of its normal calibre generally reduces the distal pulmonary artery pressure to below 40 mmHg. The non-reactive band diminishes excessive fibrous reaction, facilitating later removal or patching. Conditions suitable for such measures include large left to right shunts, e.g. ventricular septal defect, single ventricle, common atrioventriclar canal defects and persistent truncus arteriosus.

Total Correction

The number of conditions in which a primary totally corrective procedure may be considered is gradually increasing. Such surgery is feasible following refinements in the management of infants in the perioperative period and particularly by developments in the technique of cardiopulmonary bypass.

Without cardiopulmonary bypass
Persistent ductus arteriosus. This is a common cause of refractory failure in infancy. Associated lesions are common and mainly account for the increased risks of surgical closure in infancy. Where persistence of the duct causes failure of clinical improvement, closure is indicated. This is best achieved by ligation with silk. Alternatively division with oversewing is advised and obviates the small risk of recannulation of the duct.

Coarctation of the aorta. Persistent cardiac failure and/or left ventricular hypertension provide the main indications for resection with primary end-to-end anastomosis. Graft replacement is not required; the anastomosis should in part at least be constructed with interrupted sutures to allow growth to occur. Restenosis may develop and is treated by reoperation (Stark, 1972).

With cardiopulmonary bypass

Cardiopulmonary bypass—technique. Two main alternatives are available in infancy.

(a) Deep hypothermia with circulatory arrest (Hikasa, Shirontani and Mori, 1967; Barratt-Boyes et al, 1971). Surface body cooling followed by further temperature reduction on bypass to 20 to 24°C allows complete circulatory arrest for periods up to 1 h.

The operative technique is then facilitated by a relaxed, bloodless field (Barratt-Boyes et al, 1972). Conditions suitable for correction under these circumstances are large ventricular septal defects, total anomalous pulmonary venous connection, partial atrioventricular canal defects, truncus arteriosus, pulmonary atresia with large ventricular septal defects, tetralogy of Fallot and transposition of the great arteries. Early results with total atrioventricular canal and complex transposition were disappointing. Postoperative pulmonary complications were remarkably absent.

The method has been criticised on two accounts. The operation time is prolonged by cooling, which is inevitably a slow procedure. Nevertheless the anaesthetic time seldom exceeded 4 h (Barratt-Boyes et al, 1972). Secondly there is a possibility that prolonged circulatory arrest produces cerebral damage. The difficulties of accurate neurological assessment in neonates has not allowed complete resolution of this doubt. The incidence of gross neurological defects thus far has been low, although the New Zealand workers stress the importance of carefully monitoring nasopharyngeal temperature as a guide to the duration of circulatory arrest. Long-term follow-up is essential and may provide further evidence to confirm or deny the safety of the technique.

Other modifications add little and have serious disadvantages. Deep hypothermia induced by bypass cooling followed by bypass rewarming increases the duration of perfusion and adds to metabolic complications, particularly acidosis. Surface cooling and surface rewarming, with an intervening period of circulatory arrest, is even more prolonged and requires a period of external cardiac massage when the cardiac output is particularly uncertain.

(b) Conventional cardiopulmonary bypass with miniaturisation of apparatus using normothermic or moderately hypothermic perfusate. This has considerable theoretical advantages having been carefully refined in adults and children (Gersony and Hayes, 1972). Psychological testing of patients with Fallot's tetralogy some years following total correction with moderate hypothermia showed normal to above-average intelligence quotients in all cases (Starr et al, 1973).

Ventricular septal defect (VSD). This is the commonest congenital cardiac malformation, and may occur as single or multiple defects. Most are in relation to the outflow tract of the right ventricle below the crista supraventricularis and are termed 'membranous defects'. Associated abnormalities are common. The high pulmonary vascular resistance of intrauterine life falls after birth and continues to do so for some months. The typical clinical features thus may take some time to develop. *Small* VSDs rarely cause difficulties in infancy and often close spontaneously; a conservative approach is advised. *Large* VSDs however may be attended by two serious complications; cardiac failure refractory to medical therapy and the development of a raised pulmonary vascular resistance. Surgical management is available either as palliative pulmonary artery banding or total correction. In many reported series (Henry et al, 1973), the combined mortality for a two-stage procedure (i.e. palliative surgery followed by total correction later) is 20 to 25 per cent and morbidity between operations is also considerable. Comparable or better figures have been obtained by one-stage total correction in infancy (Kirklin, 1971). Cardiac failure due to multiple VSDs is probably still best treated by palliation.

Total anomalous pulmonary venous drainage. Here, management depends on the exact anatomical features, in particular the size of an associated atrial septal defect (ASD) and on the presence of pulmonary venous obstruction. ASD is an almost invariable finding and allows oxygenated blood to return to the left side. If large, normal development occurs and surgery may be deferred. Small ASDs may be temporarily palliated by balloon septostomy. Pulmonary venous obstruction is commonest where the vein drains into the portal or hepatic veins or inferior vena cava (infracardiac type). It is less frequent where pulmonary venous drainage is to the left innominate or superior vena cava (supracardiac type) and rare where drainage is to the coronary sinus or right atrium (cardiac type). Pulmonary venous obstruction causes pulmonary oedema with associated clinical deterioration requiring urgent operative intervention. In infancy, total correction is best achieved under conditions of circulatory arrest under deep hypothermia. A commonly associated persistent ductus should be closed prior to anastomosis of the common venous trunk to the back of the left atrium in the supracardiac and infracardiac types. In the cardiac type, pulmonary venous return is redirected to the left atrium by repositioning the atrial septum or by use of a patch.

Fallot's tetralogy. This has been discussed elsewhere (p. 475). The prime anatomical consideration influencing whether palliation or total correction is advised in symptomatic infants is the size of the pulmonary artery. Recently it has been suggested that total correction should be undertaken in all: the pulmonary artery should be patched across the pulmonary annulus if hypoplastic, or if severely so, a homograft valve-bearing conduit is inserted from the right ventricle to distal pulmonary artery. The results after patching are satisfactory (Starr et al, 1973).

Transposition of the great arteries (TGA). Classical TGA is usually associated with normal anatomical relationships of atria and ventricles. Associated anomalies are common and include defects of atrial and ventricular septa, persistent ductus arteriosus and ventricular outflow tract obstruction. An accurate anatomical diagnosis is essential and determines management. Balloon septostomy should be performed within the first two months of life. This is followed by reassessment at six months or earlier if the clinical condition is unsatisfactory. In those with an intact ventricular septum, redirection of the venous flow by intra-atrial baffle should be undertaken between six and twelve months.

Associated defects increasing pulmonary blood flow (e.g. VSD or PDA) cause pulmonary vascular abnormalities with raised absolute pulmonary vascular resistance which when greater than 12 units provides a contra-indication to total correction. Thus a PDA should be closed at the time of balloon septostomy if there is evidence of heart failure or pulmonary hypertension. A small VSD requires no special management. If large, pulmonary artery banding is indicated in infants less than six months of age followed by total correction at one year. If the infant is older than six months, one-stage total correction should not be delayed. Transposition with VSD and localised left ventricular obstruction should be totally corrected at one year of age.

Below the age of six months, venous redirection by intra-atrial baffle (Mustard's operation) under deep hypothermia with circulatory arrest is the operation of choice. This may be performed using conventional bypass with moderate hypothermia in older patients. The baffle is tailored of autologous pericardium or Dacron and inserted to direct the systemic venous inflow to the mitral valve and thus to the pulmonary circulation. The pulmonary venous inflow goes to the tricuspid valve and systemic circulation. Special precautions are taken to avoid trauma to the region of the coronary sinus thus decreasing the incidence of postoperative dysrhythmias.

Tricuspid atresia. Systemic venous return to the left heart in this defect occurs through an ASD and in most a VSD allows some pulmonary flow. Associated transposition of the great arteries is common. Thus pulmonary blood flow may be greater or less than normal and palliative surgery is directed to modifying this. Balloon atrial septostomy may be necessary in early life if the septal defect is small. Aortopulmonary shunt improves poor lung perfusion while overperfusion associated with heart failure is decreased by banding the pulmonary artery. Superior vena cava to pulmonary artery anastomosis (Glenn procedure) is seldom indicated: the morbidity associated with high superior caval pressure is considerable; additionally, total correction at a later stage is rendered more difficult.

Pulmonary stenosis with intact ventricular septum. If severe this requires treatment in infancy either by closed or open valvotomy alone if the right ventricular cavity is of adequate size. If small and thick-walled a shunt procedure to improve pulmonary flow should be added. Where the pulmonary valve is atretic a shunt procedure is probably the best method of relief.

Aortic stenosis may cause cardiac failure in early infancy. Open valvotomy is the only procedure likely to prevent the development of a regurgitant valve and is thus advised when the obstruction is at valve level. Subvalvar stenosis may be resected while supravalvar stenosis may be patched.

Summary

Surgical correction of congenital cardiac defects in infancy has resulted in a markedly improved prognosis. This is due to advances in diagnostic technique and improvements in clinical management. Some children can therefore look forward to a normal life expectancy; in others, e.g. with transposition of the great arteries, the long-term results have yet to be determined, while in many conditions, e.g. congenital aortic stenosis, further surgery at a later date will almost certainly be required. At this time the aetiology of congenital heart disease is ill understood, and surgery provides the sole method whereby palliation and sometimes cure may be achieved.

ACQUIRED DYSFUNCTION OF THE TRICUSPID VALVE

The treatment of advanced tricuspid valve disease remains unsatisfactory. Problems encountered relate to effects of prolonged tricuspid valve dysfunction and the difficulties involved in restoring normal function in a high flow low-pressure situation where the attendant dangers of residual pressure gradients and risks of thromboembolic complications are high. Patients with severe tricuspid dysfunction are among the highest risk cases presenting for cardiac surgery. Severe metabolic derangements occur because of the associated pulmonary, hepatic and renal disturbances. Patients are often cachectic, cyanosed and mildly jaundiced. Electrolyte disturbances are complex: sodium and potassium levels may be modified by intensive diuretic therapy and coagulation factor abnormalities are common. Additional lesions of one or more of the other cardiac valves are almost invariable.

Less severe degrees of tricuspid valve dysfunction are difficult to evaluate, both preoperatively and at the time of surgery. Fluctuation of clinical signs with or without specific therapy is common. At operation cardiac output is additionally modified by the effects of anaesthesia and the open chest.

Tricuspid valve dysfunction is treated differently at various centres by techniques ranging from benign neglect to different varieties of repair or replacement of the valves. Evaluation of results requires understanding of the anatomy, the basic pathological abnormalities, methods for assessing the pathophysiology and finally the criteria for selection of patients for surgery.

Anatomy

The normal tricuspid valve orifice is oval and bears three cusps. The most constant leaflet, the anterior, is largest and is anchored anteriorly to papillary muscles and medially to the papillary muscles of the conus. The posterior leaflet is smaller and often divided into three portions: its chordae are derived mainly from the posterior and also the anterior papillary muscles. The septal leaflet is attached by short chordae directly to the septum, and to the posterior papillary muscles. The annulus fibrosus is generally poorly developed except at the anteroseptal commissure where it is reinforced by the fibrous trigone separating the tricuspid from the aortic valve. The bundle of His is located close to the atrial attachment of the septal leaflet, along a line extending 5 mm posterior to the anteroseptal commissure to the coronary sinus before descending along the lower border of the membranous septum to the ventricles. (Grondin et al, 1967; Carpentier et al, 1974).

Pathology

Rheumatic fever is the commonest cause of acquired tricuspid dysfunction, followed by infective and traumatic lesions. At necropsy, macroscopically abnormal tricuspid valves are seen in approximately one-third of patients with chronic rheumatic heart disease. Over 40 per cent of patients with advanced mitral valve disease also have right atrial pressure tracings which are diagnostic of tricuspid insufficiency (Sepulveda and Lukas, 1955). Intraoperative evidence of tricuspid valve dysfunction was found in one quarter of patients with mitral valve disease (Starr, Herr and Wood, 1966).

Fusion of the commissures, to a diaphragm with a central or eccentric orifice, and deformity of the subvalvar mechanism, is termed *organic* tricuspid valve disease, and is due to rheumatic involvement of the valve (Lillehei et al, 1966). Such valves almost always are both stenotic *and* incompetent. Calcification is unusual and rarely extensive.

The concept of *functional* tricuspid incompetence is the subject of controversy. Scarring and thickening of the leaflets with chordal shortening may well be due to trauma caused by the incompetent jet (Starr et al, 1966; Braunwald, Ross and Morrow, 1967). Functional changes, due to pulmonary hypertension following left heart (generally mitral valve) abnormalities, include right ventricular enlargement and dilation of the tricuspid annulus. Dysrhythmias, e.g. atrial fibrillation, are commonly associated and disrupt normal atrioventricular valve closure. Such tricuspid incompetence may improve with energetic antiheart-failure therapy and thereby influence intraoperative management.

Infective. Endocarditis of the tricuspid valve is commonly seen in drug abusers who inject bacteria-contaminated drugs intravenously: unusual bacterial forms are common (Child et al, 1969). Endocarditis may also complicate an infected VSD by a jet lesion (Kennedy et al, 1966).

Traumatic lesions. Tricuspid insufficiency following non-penetrating trauma to the chest wall is increasingly seen following road traffic accidents. Prolapse of the anterior leaflet generally occurs following either ruptured chordae or damage to or rupture of the anterior papillary muscles (Jahnke, Nelson and Aaby 1967; Tachovsky, Guiliani and Ellis, 1970). Additional dilatation of a persistent foramen ovale with right to left shunt has also been described (Shabetai, Adolph and Spencer, 1966).

Haemodynamic Assessment

No method is completely reliable; unfortunately, preoperative and intra-operative assessments are all made in a rapidly changing haemodynamic situation.

Tricuspid stenosis may be confirmed with a double lumen catheter simultaneously measuring pressures in the ventricle and atrium. Small gradients are particularly seen in early diastole and indicate organic valve disease (Braunwald et al, 1967). Systolic 'V' waves of tricuspid insufficiency are frequently but not invariably present (Cairns et al, 1968), while mean right atrial pressure is often elevated (Starr et al, 1966). Functional tricuspid insufficiency is most unlikely in the absence of elevation of pulmonary artery pressure and raised pulmonary vascular resistance. In these the lesion is almost certainly organic.

Digital assessment at surgery has been criticised as a method of assessing functional abnormalities (Carpentier et al, 1974). Most, however, would not support this view. There is no doubt that an accurate diagnosis of valve stenosis *can* be made in this way: additionally an easily palpable jet in a beating heart cannot be interpreted as anything but regurgitation, provided care is taken to avoid mechanical distortion. Digital palpation is likely to be most unreliable in the presence of factors depressing cardiac performance—here no abnormality may be detectable so erroneously excluding the presence of a malfunctioning valve.

Indications for Surgery

It is remarkable how well tricuspid insufficiency is tolerated in otherwise normal hearts (Shabetai et al, 1966). However, in chronic rheumatic heart disease, tricuspid dysfunction is a serious additional lesion, indicating the severity of the chronic rheumatic process, of the presence of pulmonary vascular disease with pulmonary hypertension, or both.

Organic lesions. Grossly stenotic valves with deformed cusps respond poorly to valvuloplasty (Lillehei et al, 1966). Most agree that in such situations valve replacement is indicated (Braunwald et al, 1967; Starr et al, 1966), although Carpentier and colleagues (1974) have claimed success with repair combined with narrowing the annulus with a cloth-covered metal ring. Traumatic and infected lesions may also respond best to replacement, although total excision of infected valves without replacement has been suggested.

Functional lesions. The fluctuant nature of tricuspid regurgitation is well recognised, and there is little doubt that in milder cases correction of other lesions (generally mitral valve disease) may be followed by complete regression of tricuspid insufficiency.

If medical treatment is instigated with success, such patients do not require surgery (Braunwald et al, 1967; Kirklin and Pacifico, 1973).

However, in more severe cases, a difficult decision has to be made during the operation. Having dealt with other valve lesions a choice is presented between operating on the tricuspid valve with undoubted resulting improvement in cardiac performance (Starr et al, 1966); alternatively the tricuspid valve lesion is accepted, thus avoiding the dangers associated with prolongation of both the bypass and total operation time. This decision is aided by inserting a finger into the right atrium before and again after bypass; persistent severe regurgitation should be corrected as it seldom resolves spontaneously.

Tricuspid Valve Replacement

Results. The combined results of tricuspid valve replacement carried out at several London Cardiothoracic Centres (Brompton Hospital, Hammersmith Hospital, National Heart Hospital and London Chest Hospital) were presented to the British Postgraduate Medical Federation Course in cardiac surgery in 1972 (G. M. Rees, personal communication): 124 patients were included, four required reoperation making a total of 128 tricuspid valve replacements: 94 patients were female and 30 male. The aetiology of tricuspid valve dysfunction was chronic rheumatic heart disease in 123, while one was due to infection. At operation the pathology was described as mainly organic in 90 and functional in 34. Prosthetic valves (mainly Starr–Edwards ball valves) were used on 79 occasions; 49 tissue valves were inserted (mostly homografts). Single tricuspid procedures were rare (four), and mostly re-operations. Double valve procedures, i.e. combined with replacement or repair of another valve (generally mitral valve) were carried out on 75 occasions. In a further 49, tricuspid valve replacement was part of a triple valve procedure (mostly triple valve replacement).

No operative deaths followed single tricuspid valve replacement. Where tricuspid replacement formed part of a double valve procedure the operative mortality (i.e. within 30 days of surgery) was 32 per cent. Where tricuspid replacement was part of a triple procedure the operative mortality was 55 per cent. Late mortality figures were difficult to evaluate, due to the variable duration of follow-up, etc. Early causes of death were primarily related to low cardiac output and associated dysrhythmias. Complete heart block was seen seven times (two recovered spontaneously). Thrombosis was a feature in patients receiving both mechanical prostheses (three occasions) and frame-mounted tissue valves (two occasions). Pulmonary embolic complications occurred three times. More than half the patients developed postoperative jaundice. Of 23 surviving homograft tricuspid valve replacements, 13 were satisfactory, 10 were either importantly stenotic or regurgitant and 3 required further replacement. There was no significant difference in early mortality rates between those considered to have primarily organic or functional pathological features, nor was the preoperatively pulmonary artery pressure a guide to survival.

These figures include patients operated on very early in the experience of these hospitals of open heart surgery: recently there has been a marked trend towards improvement in results. The results also reflect patient selection as many of the surgeons concerned undertook no therapy or simple annuloplasty for milder cases. Similarly, poor results following tricuspid valve replacement were obtained by Carpentier et al (1974). Their hospital mortality rate for replacement of mitral and tricuspid valves was 31 per cent while the rate for replacing mitral, aortic and tricuspid valves was 45 per cent. Starr's group have also experienced considerable problems with the use of a caged ball valve, where tissue ingrowth occurs from the small bellows-shaped right ventricular cavity with valve dysfunction and thrombosis (Van der Veer et al, 1971). Postoperative transprosthetic pressure gradients were common. Positive systolic venous pulses indicating persistent regurgitation possibly by interference with ball motion have been noted previously (Baragan et al, 1969). Replacement with a bulky intraventricular ball and cage valve can no longer be advised. Disc valves of the Starr low profile, or Björk–Shiley variety have theoretical advantages. However, information on their long-term function is sparse.

Surgical technique. Tricuspid valve replacement is generally preceded by procedures on the mitral and/or aortic valves. It can be conveniently undertaken on a beating perfused heart following closure of all left heart incisions. The right atrium is opened avoiding damage to the right atrial conducting tissue as far as possible. Careful inspection of the cusp and subvalvar anatomy is undertaken, and the position of the intracardiac conducting fibres are defined. For valve replacement, it is preferable to resect the leaflets and chordae rather than to leave them intact (Lillehei et al, 1966: Taguchi and Matsuura, 1968); this may help to prevent interference with the function of the prosthesis. The prosthesis may be sutured by either a continuous method or by an interrupted technique inserting sutures where the leaflets join the annulus; this is satisfactory, except near the conducting tissue where the annulus should be avoided to prevent the development of atrioventricular dissociation. Here a cuff of septal leaflet with attached chordae is left in situ. Recognition of this complication is facilitated by operating on a beating heart and may occasionally be corrected by removing the offending suture.

Special postoperative problems. Intensive postoperative care, with particular attention to maintaining a good cardiac output, is essential. Prolonged ventilation may be necessary. Heart block is a hazard and temporary pacemaker wires should be used (Starr et al, 1966; Carpentier et al, 1974). Permanent heart block requires long-term pacing. These patients are also susceptible to bradycardia, in the absence of complete heart block, and temporary or even permanent pacing may be required. Haemorrhage presents a particular problem—hepatic dysfunction, venous hypertension and division of adhesions in reoperations are all contributing factors: vitamin K should be given although the results are imperfect in the presence of hepatic dysfunction. Hepatic and renal failure are common.

Annuloplasty. Narrowing the tricuspid annulus to decrease tricuspid regurgitation is an attractive concept. Originally it was performed by placing sutures with Teflon buttresses in relation to the commissure between the anterior and posterior cusps. It is unlikely, however, that this approach solves a more generalised problem. The long-term failure rate is high due to tearing of the sutures. It may, however, tide patients over the early postoperative phase, is easy to perform and thus retains some devotees. Little reliable data are available about its efficacy.

Ring annuloplasty. A ring can be used to narrow the tricuspid valve annulus because pathological dilatation occurs mainly in relation to the anterior and posterior cusps: the annulus which is related to the septal cusp shows minimal enlargement (Deloche et al, 1973). The ring described by Carpentier has a rectlinear segment corresponding to the septal cusp, and a long curved segment corresponding to the anterior and posterior cusps. The ring size is chosen to match the septal cusp length which is facilitated by placing a suture at each end and fitting this to the marks on the most suitable size of ring. Sutures are then placed through the junction of the cusp and annulus, carefully avoiding conduction fibres.

Valve competence may be tested by the injection of saline through the orifice. Organic lesions may also be managed in this way by combination with triple commissurotomy if all cusps are reasonably well developed; if the posterior cusp is very shrunken it is divided at its middle. Ruptured chordae or perforated cusps may be treated by excision of a contiguous triangular section of the abnormal valve, reconstituting the defect with fine interrupted sutures. These procedures are then combined with placement of a ring as before.

Special postoperative measures are as detailed for tricuspid valve replacement: 150 patients with tricuspid valve disease were treated by this method in a four-year period (Carpentier et al, 1974). In those undergoing an additional mitral valve procedure (repair or replacement), the hospital mortality was 9.5 per cent. In those where mitral and aortic procedure were performed as well, the mortality rate was 14 per cent. Clinical and angiographic assessment showed considerable improvement sustained over a four to five year period. Conduction problems were rare and transient. Thromboembolic complications were virtually absent as were residual atrioventricular pressure gradients.

These results represent a considerable improvement on previous figures. There are some features which undoubtedly contribute to this. For example, all patients were operated on since the end of 1968 by which time patient management had become highly sophisticated. Many of the patients also had mild tricuspid valve disease. Nevertheless this new approach based on pathological anatomy is an important advance. Whether a rigid ring is necessary or whether a strip of non-absorbable flexible material would be equally effective to not known. Recently, placement of a running suture in relation to the anterior and posterior cusps only has been advised. Tension in this suture narrows the annulus to any desired size. The suture lies well away from conduction tissue.

Summary

Tricuspid valve dysfunction presents a continuing surgical challenge. A better understanding of the anatomy of the diseased valve has led to current efforts to repair rather than replace the valve and has produced a considerable improvement in results.

DIRECT MYOCARDIAL REVASCULARISATION

Since 1968 there has been a marked increase in the number of procedures undertaken to revascularise the myocardium. In the USA alone, it is estimated that in 1975 some 40 000 such operations were performed which, at an approximate cost of $10 000 per operation, gives a total cost of 400 million dollars. In the United Kingdom the number of operations is much less, although there is good evidence that the situation is changing rapidly. A procedure of such economic importance requires close evaluation as to its likely risks and benefits.

Historical Aspects

Cardiac surgeons have responded readily to the challenge of ischaemic heart disease. Earlier attempts to treat it were often reported with enthusiasm amounting to euphoria which waned as rapidly as the operations became discredited. *Cervical sympathectomy* to relieve pain; depression of metabolic activity by *total thyroidectomy*—both had their vogue. Increasing direct flow through the epicardial surface through apposed viscera or *by forming adhesions* also proved popular. Narrowing the *coronary sinus* or channelling arterial flow through the coronary sinus achieved success in Beck's hands. *Vineberg* developed an operation whereby a freely bleeding vessel was implanted into the myocardium to perfuse the sinusoids; postoperative studies confirmed myocardial perfusion, although the quantity was small. Coronary endarterectomy had a moderate success but was associated with a high mortality.

Direct *anastomosis* between the aorta and circumflex branch of the left coronary was accomplished in experimental animals using autogenous vein grafts by Julian et al (1957). The use of *autogenous vein grafts* in man was first reported by Favoloro (Effler, Favoloro and Groves, 1970) who excised segmental stenoses of the right coronary artery and bridged the gap with a venous autograft. Long saphenous ('jump') grafts placed end to side between the aorta and coronary artery beyond the stenosis were introduced in the late 1960s. This operation remains the current procedure of choice although it has undergone many subtle modifications, its basic concept remaining unchanged.

Saphenous Vein Grafts

Operative techniques

Successful surgery depends on the quality of preoperative coronary arteriograms combined with angiographic assessment of left ventricular performances discussed elsewhere in this book. The anatomical site and severity of stenoses are noted and either radiographs or a composite line diagram should be available for reference in the operating theatre. Most agree that stenoses exceeding 70 per cent give rise to significant obstruction: Green (1974) believes that stenoses exceeding 50 per cent provide an indication for bypass surgery.

The venous autograft. This may be obtained from the leg. However, when the saphenous vein is diseased or has previously been injected or removed, the cephalic vein provides a satisfactory alternative. The lower saphenous vein has advantages, often being of better quality and of a calibre similar to that of the coronary artery. Flow rates vary in inverse proportion to the internal diameter of the graft. Thus narrower vessels may be less likely to thrombose subsequently. The vein should be handled with care; damage due to excessive manipulation may cause late pathological changes of the vessel wall. On removal it is injected with heparinised blood to prevent thrombosis and marked to indicate the direction of blood flow. The graft should be placed to ensure antegrade flow as retrograde flow is prevented by venous valves.

Internal mammary implantation. The internal mammary artery may be used as an alternative to a venous autograft. It has the advantage of being pre-conditioned to systemic blood pressure. However, the operative technical problems are somewhat greater. Dissection from the back of the sternum is required and the artery may already have atherosclerotic changes or be of indifferent length or calibre. The internal mammary is mainly used for grafting the left coronary system: multiple anastomoses by this method is impossible and requires a combination of arterial and venous autografts. While flow rates measured at operation are somewhat less than for saphenous grafts, higher long-term patency rates have been claimed, although this may have been biased by careful patient selection.

The anastomoses. Although distal anastomoses have been constructed on a beating heart, it is unlikely that these can be constructed as well as when the heart is stationary. This requires cardiopulmonary bypass with cardiac standstill induced by ischaemic arrest or by induced ventricular fibrillation. A short period of ischaemic arrest or fibrillation required to construct the distal anastomosis is well tolerated in most patients. Moderate hypothermia affords additional myocardial protection and is probably advisable in more extensive procedures, e.g. multiple grafts or valve replacement or aneurysm resection. Fine suture material, e.g. Prolene, with a low coefficient of friction is essential. Interrupted or continuous suture technique or a combination of both is a matter of individual taste.

The proximal anastomosis is easily performed on the beating heart either

17

prior to or after discontinuation of bypass, thus reducing total bypass time. Each graft should have a separate aortic orifice. The temptation to join grafts which then have one proximal, but more distal anastomoses—'Y' grafts— should be resisted: these are notoriously susceptible to thrombosis, thus compromising at least two distal anastomoses.

The risks of surgery

Operative mortality rates are dependent on many factors, not least the criteria employed in selecting patients for surgery. Thus Tector and McNabb (1974) reported a series of over 190 patients operated upon in one year without mortality. From Houston, Cooley et al (1973) have recorded results in a series of 1492 patients operated upon between 1969 and 1972 with operative mortality rates for single grafts of 5.1 per cent, for double grafts of 7.1 per cent and for triple grafts of 8.8 per cent. The operative mortality for 397 triple coronary artery grafts performed at the Cleveland Clinic between 1970 and 1973 was 2.5 per cent (Cheanvechai et al, 1974). Most series reveal a progressive fall in the risks of surgery with increasing experience of the surgical team.

Deaths occurring in the perioperative period are mainly related to myocardial failure, often in association with myocardial infarction. Accurate figures on the frequency of myocardial infarction after coronary artery surgery are difficult to obtain. Electrocardiographic and enzyme changes are common postoperatively and mask the classical abnormalities associated with infarction. Cooley et al (1973) found that 14 per cent of patients developed infarcts after vein graft operations without additional procedures. Cheanvechai et al (1974) estimated the infarct incidence at 4 per cent although perhaps a more realistic estimate is 10 to 15 per cent. It should be noted that infarction is not necessarily related to graft occlusions but may follow progression of disease within the coronary arteries themselves.

Treatment of left ventricular aneurysm as well by resection or plication was associated with an operative mortality of 16 per cent (Cooley et al, 1973). Additional valve replacement also increased the risks of death following surgery to 24 per cent. Starr's experience with combined valve surgery and vein grafting is illuminating (Okies et al, 1974). The first three patients who were treated in this way died. Following modification of the surgical technique the next nine consecutive patients survived surgery. Emphasis is placed on a carefully organised approach with particular attention to myocardial protection. The mortality for combined valve replacement and coronary artery surgery was much higher for mitral replacement than for aortic replacement, due probably to impaired left ventricular performance.

Further analysis of Cooley's data identifies factors likely to increase the risks of surgery. These factors include evidence of left ventricular dysfunction (low left ventricular ejection fraction, high left ventricular end-diastolic pressure, clinical evidence of cardiac failure). Surprisingly, mortality rates did not correlate well with the number of grafts inserted; however, where significant stenoses were *not* bypassed, the risks were greater. The age of the patient did not increase the risks of surgery unduly.

Technical factors are clearly of prime importance, particularly the adequacy of the distal anastomosis and the 'run-off' into the distal coronary circulation.

The timing of surgery in relation to acute myocardial ischaemia is of considerable importance. Myocardial infarction within a month prior to surgery increases the dangers of surgery which is complicated by recurrent dysrhythmias.

'Unstable' or 'preinfarction' angina is difficult to define objectively. Most would include patients in whom angina is increasing in frequency and/or severity; where it occurs at rest, with or without transient ECG changes of ischaemic rather than infarction; where serum enzymes remain normal, or where pain persists in spite of therapy for 24 h. In clinical practice, however, many of these criteria are less well defined and categorisation of a particular patient may be impossible. The results of surgery in this group are very variable but in most surgeons' experience the risks are considerably increased; the incidence of intractable dysrhythmia or infarction are both raised.

Long-term effects
THE FATE OF THE GRAFT

Most reports of restudies within a few months of vein graft surgery indicate that patency rates range between 85 and 90 per cent (Walker et al, 1972). Factors biasing many of the quoted figures include a tendency to restudy patients where there is a failure to improve symptoms or who have recurrence of angina: refusal by the patient to have a repeat study may be interpreted variously. An additional 'late occlusion rate' between 13 and 22 per cent has also been recorded. A prospective follow-up of a group of patients studied at two weeks, one year and three years after surgery has produced important data (Grondin et al, 1974). Eleven per cent of grafts were found to be occluded two weeks after surgery; at one year the occlusion rate rose to 32 per cent. However, three years after operation only another 5 per cent had occluded. Most grafts showed angiographic evidence of luminal narrowing (mean 30 per cent reduction) although a quarter of all cases showed little change. Neither the initial calibre of the graft nor the run-off seemed to influence the development of narrowing. Severe diffuse or segmental reduction in diameter was associated with a poor run-off in the initial study and the graft showed a tendency to become occluded by the third study. Early occlusions are probably due to poor run-off, grafts with flow rates less than 40 ml/min are at particular risk (Grondin et al, 1971), or faulty surgical technique, particularly at the distal anastomosis. Late occlusion seems to be related to medial and intimal fibrous proliferation (Vlodaver and Edwards, 1971), the former being due to destruction of the vasa vasorum and the latter to high increased intraluminal pressure and/or high oxygen saturations. Fibrosis of grafts may also be due to the methods of dissection and handling the vein at the time of operation (Brody, Kosek and Angel, 1972). Grondin et al (1974) emaphsise the importance of stenosis of the aortic anastomosis which was associated with a high incidence of graft closure. Belief that the mural changes seen in the saphenous vein can be avoided by use of the internal mammary artery should be tempered by experimental evidence from dogs that when internal mammary artery anastomosis is associated with a poor run-off intimal changes may occur in the arterial wall (Yarborough et al, 1972). It is hoped that with increasing experience, the incidence of early occlusion may be reduced, thus leading to a higher late patency rate.

THE FATE OF THE ORIGINAL CORONARY CIRCULATION

The evidence here is somewhat conflicting. In a group of patients studied by Benchimol et al (1974), three to four months postoperatively there appeared to be no difference in the rate of progression of abnormalities in coronary arteries associated with patent or non-patent grafts. Their conclusion that progression of atherosclerosis within the native coronary circulation is rarely influenced by graft implantation, contradicts the earlier suggestions of Aldridge and Trimble (1971). In a group of 50 patients studied at the National Heart Hospital, London, the patency rate of grafts inserted into arteries with total proximal occlusion was significantly higher than those inserted into coronaries with a proximal stenosis (Rees, 1976). Rees suggests that when a graft is inserted into a narrowed coronary artery, a 'watershed' situation is created with competition between the graft and the original coronary artery to provide the main source of blood flow. Either the graft or the coronary artery is likely to occlude following relegation of the vessel to the role of minor provider of blood.

THE EFFECT OF VEIN GRAFTING ON LEFT VENTRICULAR PERFORMANCE

Quantitative analysis of left ventricular function before and after vein graft surgery had shown that where the graft is patent, improvement occurs while deterioration of function tends to accompany graft occlusion (Rees et al, 1971). The ability of the ventricle to empty is enhanced as measured by increase in ejection fraction and decrease in end-systolic volume. The rate of contraction at the ventricular equator increased after successful surgery. Improvement of dyskinetic regions of ventricular wall were also noted postoperatively in association with patent grafts. This significant improvement in ventricular wall motion and pump function following successful aorto-coronary bypass surgery was confirmed by Chatterjee et al (1973) even in the presence of old myocardial infarction. In both these reports it was emphasised that in these patients, end-diastolic volumes were normal before operation and that similar beneficial results would not necessarily follow in patients with cardiomegaly or evidence of heart failure.

Results

RELIEF OF SYMPTOMS

The paradox whereby an operation advised mainly to give relief from angina is difficult to assess by such results is in part related to the unpredictable course of the condition and also the complex nature of the symptoms themselves. The patient's emotional state following a dramatic procedure, complicated by bed rest, treatment with various medications, followed by prolonged convalescence, makes a symptom which many people find difficult to describe, almost impossible to assess. The interrelationship of patient and physician may further complicate the position. Reports of relief from pain should furthermore only be judged in the light of the known placebo response. Earlier procedures to treat angina were also associated with dramatic pain relief in many instances, although the improvement frequently was of short duration. Following vein bypass surgery, over 80 per cent are found to be either pain free or markedly improved; 10 to 20 per cent are unchanged while a very small group are worse. Most have found good correlation between graft patency and symptomatic improvement. Providing graft patency persists, symptomatic relief is generally sustained over a long period.

Stress testing by exercise or pacemaker-induced tachycardia provides increased objectivity in evaluating postoperative angina, particularly where preoperative data are also available. There is considerable evidence that angina may be abolished or decreased by successful surgery. Nevertheless, a small group with occluded grafts also experience relief. Some of these patients may experience perioperative myocardial infarction, converting painful ischaemic tissue into inert areas (Griffith et al, 1973).

LATE RESULTS

The natural history of patients with angina pectoris treated medically has been comprehensively reviewed by Reeves et al (1974). Earlier studies based on patients not investigated by coronary arteriography indicated the annual mortality was very variable but ranged between 3 and 9 per cent. Recent studies where the diagnosis was confirmed and the extent of the disease assessed by coronary angiography have indicated that the likelihood of early death is related to the number and severity of stenoses. Thus, where only one of either left anterior descending, circumflex or right coronary arteries is significantly stenosed, the annual mortality rate is 2 per cent. If two arteries are stenosed the rate is 7 per cent, while for triple vessel disease the annual mortality rate is 11 per cent. As noted by earlier workers, certain electrocardiographic features (mainly ST changes), hypertension, cardiac enlargement and congestive failure all influence the prognosis adversely. Left ventricular angiography also provides valuable prognostic evidence; local or generalised dysfunction are associated with a worse outlook. Conclusive evidence on whether surgery prolongs life awaits the results of prospective controlled trials with matched groups of patients randomly allocated surgical or medical treatment. At least two large multicentre studies are currently in progress (Veterans Administration Hospitals Cooperative Study for Surgery for Coronary Arterial Disease, and the European study (Hultgren et al, 1974)). The results of a small prospective randomised trial in patients with stable angina has been already reported at just over two years following entry to the trial (Mathur et al, 1975). Mortality of patients operated on was 9 per cent and those not operated on was 14 per cent; however, the difference was not statistically significant. The difficulties of such trials are great and will require many patients studied over a prolonged time before a definitive answer is provided.

SELECTED GROUPS

This aspect has been elaborated by McNeer et al (1974). In their series 89 base-line characteristics were recorded for each patient in an endeavour to identify subgroups where one form of therapy or another may prove to be superior. At two years 83 per cent of medical patients and 85 per cent of surgical patients were alive, although twice as many surgical patients (53 per cent) as medical (26 per cent) were pain free. Significantly more patients who have triple vessel disease, normal arterovenous oxygen difference and an abnormal left ventricular angiogram survive for two years if they are operated on than if they are treated medically. These patients may be those with localised muscle disease who are likely to infarct at an early stage and are prevented from so doing by surgery.

SPECIFIC CORONARY ARTERY LESIONS

A retrospective analysis of patients selected from a total of 3527 coronary angiograms performed at the Cleveland Clinic between 1960 and 1965 has been compared with the results of 1000 patients operated on between 1967 and 1970 (Sheldon et al, 1973). The patients selected for the first group were included on the basis of lesions now considered operable. They were carefully matched for age, sex and severity of disease with the surgical group. The surgical mortality was 4 per cent. The attrition rate for non-operated cases was 9.3 per cent per annum over the first four years of follow-up while that of surgical cases was 4.8 per cent. Patients with single vessel disease of the left anterior descending, double and triple vessel disease all fared better following surgery. While evey attempt was made to match the two groups, the effect of the temporal disparity is very difficult to evaluate and may bias the results. Cooley et al (1973) claim an overall attrition rate of 2.7 per cent per annum after the initial surgical mortality in a group of 1492 patients operated on between 1969 and 1972. The Duke University series of 490 operated patients has been compared with 611 non-operated patients (Rosati, 1975). Some baseline characteristic inequalities have however been noted: non-operated patients were older, had worse electrocardiographic and left ventricular angiographic characteristics with a high left ventricular end-diastolic pressure.

Survival at four years was remarkably similar in the two groups; 82 per cent of surgical patients and 78 per cent of medical patients were alive at this time.

Stenosis of the left main coronary artery is generally accepted as corresponding to two-vessel disease. The increased operative mortality of patients with this lesion has been demonstrated (Cooley et al, 1973). Nevertheless, the two-year survival figures are considerably better after surgery than in those treated medically; 40 per cent were dead with medical treatment compared with 21 per cent mortality if treated surgically. At 36 months the Veterans study indicated that 32 per cent of patients treated medically are dead compared with 20 per cent of those treated surgically (Hultgren, 1975).

UNSTABLE ANGINA

As indicated, this condition remains ill-defined, increasing the difficulty of interpreting the results. While Gazes et al (1972) indicate that the mortality following medical therapy in the first year is 43 per cent, Krauss, Hutter and DeSanctis (1972) emphasise that the early mortality (i.e. while in hospital) is low and that operation may be better deferred until the condition is more stable.

A prospective study where patients with acute coronary insufficiency were randomly allocated medical or surgical treatment has been carried out in 40 patients (Selden et al, 1975). At the end of four months the clinical course, changes in left ventricular function and response to exercise and pacemaker-induced tachycardia were compared in the two groups. One patient died in each group while the incidence of myocardial infarction was low in both (two in the medical group and three in the surgical group). Ejection fraction afterwards was similar in the two groups, but the surgical group fared better symptomatically either subjectively or on objective stress testing. The conclusion was that such patients should be treated medically in the first instance and operated on later if angina persists.

There have been successful reports of surgery during the acute phase of infarction (Cohn et al, 1972). The hazards of such surgery are likely to be great but so is the outlook without surgery, particularly where cardiogenic shock is present. Attempts to treat acute infarction by revascularisation remains an experimental procedure.

Summary

Aortocoronary bypass surgery has become an established treatment for coronary artery disease. In stable angina pectoris with reasonable left ventricular function, the operative mortality is low and most patients can anticipate an immediate marked improvement or total relief of symptoms. Return of symptoms occurs in some and is often associated with graft occlusion, a phenomenon that is more common early after surgery but less likely later. Its efficacy in patients with extensive myocardial damage either chronically or acutely, as in syndromes of preinfarction angina or definitive infarction, is not established. Prolongation of life similarly is not confirmed although in some groups suggestive evidence is accumulating. The operation at present finds its main indication in chronic, stable angina where it is at least a more effective and no more dangerous form of therapy than offered by conventional medical means.

THE SURGICAL TREATMENT OF TACHYCARDIAS
by R. A. J. Spurrell

In recent years an increasing interest has been shown in the surgical management of patients with intractable arrhythmias that cannot be controlled by drug or pacemaker therapy.

Mechanisms of Tachycardias

The surgical therapeutic approach to the management of tachycardias is dependent upon a proper understanding of the underlying mechanisms of the arrhythmia. Two main mechanisms are considered to underly most tachycardias. Firstly, there is the rapidly discharging ectopic focus either in the atria or atrioventricular (AV) junction to produce a supraventricular tachycardia or in the ventricle producing a ventricular tachycardia. Secondly, there is the re-entry or reciprocal mechanism which can occur either in the atria, AV junction or ventricles. For a re-entry mechanism to occur there have to be two connecting pathways present, one for antegrade conduction and the other for retrograde conduction. The activation impulse is conducted rapidly around these two pathways resulting in a tachycardia. Supraventricular tachycardias commonly result from the re-entry process occurring within the AV node (Goldreyer and Bigger, 1971) and under these circumstances both antegrade and retrograde pathways probably lie within the AV node.

The supraventricular tachycardia associated with the Wolff, Parkinson and White (1930) (WPW) syndrome is due to a re-entry mechanism in which antegrade conduction to the ventricles occurs by way of the AV node–His bundle pathway and retrograde conduction occurs by way of an accessory atrioventricular pathway which commonly occurs in either the right or left atrioventricular groove (Kent, 1893). In type A WPW the accessory pathway classically occurs in the left atrioventricular groove and in type B WPW it occurs in the right atrioventricular groove. With the advent of more sophisticated techniques for studying these arrhythmias it is now recognised that the anatomical site of accessory AV pathways is very varied and they may occur between the atrial septum and ventricular septum (Paladino fibres), between the atrial septum and His bundle, bypassing the AV node (pathways of this type have been described by James (1963)) and between the lower AV node or upper His bundle and the ventricular septum (Mahaim, 1947).

Patients who have accessory AV pathways present may suffer from re-entry or circus movement tachycardias as described above or they may suffer from paroxysmal atrial fibrillation or atrial flutter with a rapid ventricular response due to conduction over the accessory pathway.

Recently increasing interest has been shown in the underlying mechanism of ventricular tachycardia and Wellens et al (1972) have demonstrated using programmed stimulation techniques that in some patients with ventri-cular tachycardia a re-entry mechanism may be responsible. However, they were unable to identify the precise site of re-entry within the ventricles and they suggested that it could be either in the main bundle branches, the distal His–Purkinje system, in working myocardium or in combinations of these three tissues. Spurrell, Sowton and Deuchar (1973) using similar techniques presented evidence that in four patients with re-entry ventricular tachycardia the site of re-entry was the main intraventricular bundle branches.

Surgical Treatment of Supraventricular Tachycardias

Most patients with paroxysmal supraventricular tachycardias can be managed satisfactorily with antiarrhythmic agents. However, some patients develop attacks of paroxysmal atrial fibrillation, atrial flutter or supraventri-cular tachycardia due to re-entry involving the AV node, which are resistant to conventional drug therapy. These attacks may be sufficiently disabling for surgical intervention to be considered. Provided that there is no accessory atrioventricular pathway then the most satisfactory surgical approach to this problem is to interrupt the bundle of His. This is most satisfactorily done through a right atriotomy while on cardiopulmonary bypass, the His bundle is then interrupted just in front of the coronary sinus. Following interruption of the His bundle a junctional escape rhythm occurs which may have a satisfac-tory rate but a demand pacemaker should be implanted at the same procedure. In the author's experience this procedure has been found to be a highly satisfactory approach to the management of intractable supraventricular tachycardia.

WPW syndrome

The surgical management of the supraventricular tachycardias associated with the WPW syndrome is a totally different problem owing to the presence of an additional atrioventricular conduction pathway. In those patients who have a re-entry tachycardia involving the AV node–His pathway and the accessory pathway then interruption of the His bundle can certainly be effective in terminating tachycardias of this type. However, the accessory atrioventricular pathway remains which leaves the potential hazard of ventricular activation at high frequencies should atrial flutter or fibrillation occur. This potential hazard becomes more significant if the refractory period of the pathway is short. A more logical approach would be to interrupt the accessory pathway. This procedure was first carried out successfully by Cobb et al (1968), and since then similar procedures have been performed in many centres.

The technique used for identifying the site of insertion of the accessory pathway in the ventricle has been epicardial mapping. Following exposure of the heart at surgery the epicardial activation times during sinus rhythm or an atrially paced rhythm are obtained from about 50 preselected sites on each ventricle using a hand-held unipolar or bipolar electrode. Times of equal activation are joined together and an isochrone map of epicardial activation drawn for the ventricles. The earliest point of epicardial activation will classically be found in the right or left atrioventricular grooves in patients with anomalous activation of the ventricles due to the WPW syndrome. If the accessory pathway is in a rather more inaccessible site then mapping of the atrioventricular rings on the endocardial surface may be necessary to identify a site of insertion in the interventricular septum for instance. Once the site of insertion of the accessory pathway has been identified then surgical interruption is carried out. The technique for this varies but many authorities now believe that the most satisfactory approach is to detach the atrial wall along the AV ring in the region of the accessory pathway. Following the atrial incision and provided anomalous activation of the ventricles disappears on the surface ECG, the atrial incision is closed with sutures.

It has been found that interruption of accessory pathways in the right atrioventricular groove has been more successful than interruption of accessory pathways in the left atrioventricular groove and this has also been the author's experience.

The surgical management of patients with the WPW syndrome has recently been reviewed in detail by Gallagher et al (1975).

Surgery for Ventricular Tachycardias

Various approaches to the surgical management of refractory ventricular tachycardia have been made. Resection of a ventricular aneurysm is well recognised in the management of ventricular tachycardia (Thind, Blakemore and Zinsser (1971) and resection of an aneurysm or a hypokinetic area of left ventricular wall with additional aortocoronary bypass surgery has also been shown to be successful in the treatment of this arrhythmia (Graham et al, 1973). Spurrell et al (1973) have reported two patients with re-entry ventricular tachycardia who underwent surgical interruption of the anterior radiation of the left bundle branch in order to interrupt a re-entry mechanism involving the anterior radiation of the left bundle.

More recently Spurrell et al (1975) and Fontaine et al (1975) have reported the surgical interruption of a re-entry mechanism in patients with re-entry ventricular tachycardia following epicardial mapping. In this situation the heart is exposed at surgery and the ventricular tachycardia is initiated using correctly timed ventricular premature beats. Epicardial mapping, as described earlier, is then carried out during tachycardia to produce an isochrone map of epicardial activation. From this map the activation front during ventricular tachycardia is identified and then interrupted by a transmyocardial incision in the ventricle. This technique has proved successful in the management of patients with life threatening re-entry ventricular tachycardia.

Techniques of the sort described in this section have proved invaluable in the surgical management of patients with re-entry tachycardias. In patients with tachycardias which are due to a rapidly discharging ectopic focus, particularly in the ventricle, the problem is more difficult particularly in terms of identifying the site of the focus, and as yet no satisfactory techniques are available.

REFERENCES

CARDIAC SURGERY IN INFANCY

Barratt-Boyes, B. G., Simpson, M. & Neutze, J. M. (1971) Intracardiac surgery in neonates and infants using deep hypothermia with surface cooling and limited cardiopulmonary bypass. *Circulation*, **43**, Suppl. 1, 25–30.

Barratt-Boyes, B. G., Neutze, J. M., Seelye, E. R. & Simpson, M. (1972) Complete correction of cardiovascular malformation in the first year of life. *Progress in Cardiovascular Diseases*, **XV**, 229–253.

Gersony, W. M. & Hayes, C. J. (1972) Perioperative management of the infant with congenital heart disease. *Progress in Cardiovascular Diseases*, **XV**, 213–228.

Henry, J., Kaplan, S., Helmsworth, J. & Schreiber, T. (1973) Management of infants with large ventricular septal defects. *Annals of Thoracic Surgery*, **15**, 109–119.

Hikasa, Y., Shirontami, H. & Mori, C. (1967) Open heart surgery in infants with an aid of hypothermic anaesthesia. *Nippon Geka Hokan*, **36**, 495–508.

Kirklin, J. (1971) Pulmonary artery banding in babies with large ventricular septal defects. *Circulation*, **43**, 321–322.

Lancet (1973) Management of Fallot's tetralogy, *Lancet*. **2**, 305.

Muller, W. & Dammann, J. F. (1952) The treatment of certain congenital malformations of the heart by the creation of pulmonary stenosis to reduce pulmonary hypertension and excessive pulmonary flow. *Surgery, Gynecology and Obstetrics*, **95**, 215–219.

Olley, P. M. (1975) Non-surgical palliation of congenital heart malformations. *New England Journal of Medicine*, **292**, 1292–1294.

Rashkind, W. J. (1972) The cyanotic newborn: an approach to diagnosis and treatment. *Cardiovascular Clinics*, **4**, 275–280.

Rees, G. M. & Starr, A. (1973) Total correction of Fallot's tetralogy in patients aged less than one year. *British Heart Journal*, **35**, 898–901.

Ross, D. N. (1973) Personal communication.

Stark, J. (1972) Cardiac surgery in early infancy. *Postgraduate Medical Journal*, **48**, 478–485.

Starr, A., Bonchek, L. I. & Sutherland, C. (1973) Total correction of tetralogy of Fallot in infancy. *Journal of Thoracic and Cardiovascular Surgery*, **65**, 45–57.

Tatooles, C. J. & Miller, R. A. (1973) Palliative surgery in infants with congenital heart disease. *Progress in Cardiovascular Diseases*, **XV**, 331–340.

ACQUIRED DYSFUNCTION OF THE TRICUSPID VALVE

Baragan, J., Escher, J., Coblence, B., Mehrez, R. & Lenegre, J. (1969) Positive systolic venous pulses after replacement of the tricuspid valve by a Starr–Edwards ball valve prosthesis. *American Journal of Cardiology*, **23**, 785–791.

Bloomer, W., Emmanoulides, G. & Lipman, C. (1968) Prosthetic replacement of an insufficient tricuspid valve in a five-year-old child. *Annals of Thoracic Surgery*, **5**, 550 555.

Braunwald, N., Ross, J. & Morrow, A. G. (1967) Conservative management of tricuspid regurgitation in patients underoing mitral valve replacement. *Circulation*, Suppl. 1, 63–69.

Cairns, K. B., Kloster, F., Bristow, D., Lees, M. & Griswold, H. (1968) Problems in the haemodynamic diagnosis of tricuspid insufficiency. *American Heart Journal*, **75**, 173–179.

Carpentier, A., Blondeau, P., Laurens, B., Hay, A., Laurent, D. & Dubost, C. (1968) Mitral and tricuspid valve replacement with frame-mounted aortic homografts. *Journal of Thoracic Cardiovascular Surgery*, **56**, 388–394.

Carpentier, A., Deloche, A., Hanania, G., Forman, J., Sellier, P., Plivnica, A. & Dubost, C. (1974) Surgical management of acquired tricuspid valve disease. *Journal of Thoracic Cardiovascular Surgery*, **67**, 53–62.

Child, J., Darrell, J., Rhys Davies, N. & Davis-Dawson, L. (1969) Mixed infective endocarditis in a heroin addict. *Journal of Medical Microbiology*, **2**, 293–299.

Deloche, A., Guerinon, J., Fabiani, J.-N., Morillo, F., Caramanian, M., Carpentier, A., Maurice, P. & Dubost, Ch. (1973) Etude anatomique des valvulopathies rhumatismales tricuspidiennes. Application a l'étude des différentes valvuloplasties. *Annales de Chirurgie Thoracique et Cardio-vasculaire*, **4**, 32–40.

Grondin, P., Lepage, G., Castonguay, Y. & Meere, C. (1967) The tricuspid valve: a surgical challenge. *Journal of Thoracic and Cardiovascular Surgery*, **53**, 7–20.

Jahnke, E. J., Nelson, W. P. & Aaby, G. (1967) Tricuspid insufficiency: the result of non-penetrating cardiac trauma. *Archives of Surgery (Chicago)*, **95**, 880–887.

Kennedy, J., Sakga, G., Fisk, A. & Sancetta, S. (1966) Isolated tricuspid valve insufficiency due to subacute bacterial endocarditis. *Journal of Thoracic and Cardiovascular Surgery*, **51**, 498–506.

Kirklin, J. & Pacifico, A. (1973) Surgery for acquired valvar heart disease. *New England Journal of Medicine*, **288**, 194–9.

Lillehei, C. W., Gannon, P. G., Levy, M., Varco, R. & Wang, Y. (1966) Valve replacement for tricuspid stenosis or insufficiency associated with mitral valvar disease. *Circulation*, **33**, 34–42.

Sepulveda, G. & Lukas, D. S. (1955) The diagnosis of tricuspid insufficiency. *Circulation*, **11**, 552–560.

Shabetai, R., Adolph, R. & Spencer, F. (1966) Successful replacement of the tricuspid valve, ten years after traumatic incompetence. *American Journal of Cardiology*, **18**, 916–920.

Starr, A., Herr, R. H. & Wood, J. A. (1966) Tricuspid replacement for acquired valve disease. *Surgery, Gynecology and Obstetrics*, **122**, 1295–1310.

Tachovsky, R., Guiliani, E. & Ellis, F. (1970) Prosthetic valve replacement for tricuspid insufficiency. *American Journal of Cardiology*, **26**, 196–199.

Taguchi, K. & Matsuura, Y. (1968) Surgical treatment of tricuspid insufficiency. *Diseases of the Chest*, **53**, 599–604.

van der Veer, J., Rhyneer, G., Hodam, R. P. & Kloster, F. (1971) Obstruction of tricuspid ball valve prostheses. *Circulation*, **43**, Suppl. 1, 62–67.

DIRECT MYOCARDIAL REVASCULARISATION

Aldridge, H. E. & Trimble, A. S. (1971) Progression of proximal coronary artery lesions to total occlusion after aortocoronary saphenous vein bypass grafting. *Journal of Thoracic and Cardiovascular Surgery*, **62**, 7.

Benchimol, A., Harris, C. L., Fleming, H. & Desser, K. B. (1974) Progression of obstructive coronary artery disease after implantation of aortocoronary saphenous vein bypass grafts. *Journal of Thoracic and Cardiovascular Surgery*, **68**, 257–262.

Brody, W. R., Kosek, J. C. & Angel, W. W. (1972) Changes in vein grafts following aorto-coronary bypass induced by pressure and ischaemia. *Journal of Thoracic and Cardiovascular Surgery*, **64**, 847.

Chatterjee, K., Swan, H. J. C., Parmley, W. W., Sustaita, H., Marcus, H. S. & Matloff, J. (1973) Influence of direct myocardial revascularisation on left ventricular asynergy and function in patients with coronary heart disease. *Circulation*, **47**, 276–290.

Cheanvechai, C., Effler, D. B., Groves, L. K., Loop, F. D., Navia, J., Grinfield, R. & Sheldon, W. C. (1974) Triple bypass graft for the treatment of severe triple coronary vessel disease. *Annals of Thoracic Surgery*, **17**, 545–554.

Cohn, L. H., Gorlin, R., Herman, M. V. & Collins, J. J. (1972) Aortocoronary bypass for acute coronary occlusion. *Journal of Thoracic and Cardiovascular Surgery*, **64**, 503–509.

Cooley, D. A., Dawson, J. T., Hallman, G. L., Sandiford, F. M., Wukasch, D. C., Garcia, E. & Hall, R. J. (1973) Aorotocoronary saphenous vein bypass. *Annals of Thoracic Surgery*, **16**, 380–390.

Effler, D. B., Favoloro, R. G. & Groves, L. K. (1970) Coronary artery surgery utilising saphenous vein graft techniques. *Journal of Thoracic and Cardiovascular Surgery*, **59**, 147.

Gazes, P. C., Mobley, E. M., Faris, H. M., Duncan, R. C. & Humphries, B. (1972) Pre-infarction angina-prospective study. Ten-year follow-up (Abstract). *Circulation*, **46**, Suppl. II, 23.

Green, G. In discussion of Bruschke, A., Proudfit, W. L. & Sones, F. M. (1973) Progress study of 590 consecutive non-surgical cases of coronary disease followed five to nine years. *Circulation*, **47**, 1147.

Griffith, L. S. C., Achuff, S. C., Conti, C. R., Humphries, J. O'N., Brawley, R. K., Gott, V. L. & Ross, R. S. (1973) Changes in intrinsic coronary circulation and segmented ventricular motion after saphenous vein coronary bypass graft surgery. *New England Journal of Medicine*, **288**, 589–595.

Grondin, C., LaPage, G., Castonguay, Y., Meere, C. & Grondin, P. (1971) Aortocoronary bypass graft. Initial flow through the graft and early post-operative patency. *Circulation*, **44**, 815.

Grondin, C., Lesperance, J., Bourassa, M. G., Pasternac, A., Campeau, L. & Grondin, P. (1974) Serial angiographic evaluation in 60 consecutive patients with aortocoronary artery vein grafts, two weeks, one year and three years after operation. *Journal of Thoracic and Cardiovascular Surgery*, **67**, 1–6.

Hultgren, H. N., Takaro, T., Fowler, N. & Wright, E. C. (1974) Evaluation of surgery in angina pectoris. *American Journal of Medicine*, **56**, 1–3.

Hultgren, H. N. (1975) Coronary artery surgery: critical appraisal. Unpublished data presented at Royal Society of Medicine conference, 6th June.

Julian, O. C., Lopez-Belio, M., Moorhead, D. & Leba, A. (1957) Direct surgical procedures on the coronary arteries. *Journal of Thoracic Surgery*, **34**, 654.

Krauss, K. R., Hutter, A. M. & DeSanctis, R. W. (1972) Acute coronary insufficiency: course and follow-up. *Archives of Internal Medicine*, **129**, 808–813.

Mathur, V. S., Guinn, G. A., Anastassiades, L., Chahine, R. A., Korompai, F. L., Montero, A. C. & Luchi, R. J. (1975) Surgical treatment for stable angina pectoris. *New England Journal of Medicine*, **292**, 709–713.

McNeer, J. F., Starmer, C. F., Bartel, A. G., Behar, V. S., Kong, Y., Peter, R. H. & Rosati, R. A. (1974) The nature of treatment selection in coronary artery disease: experience with medical and surgical treatment of a chronic disease. *Circulation*, **49**, 606–614.

Okies, J. E., Phillips, S., Chartman, B. R. & Starr, A. (1974) Technical considerations in multiple valve and coronary artery surgery. *Journal of Thoracic and Cardiovascular Surgery*, **67**, 762–769.

Rees, G. M., Bristow, J. D., Kremkau, L., Green, G. S., Herr, R. H., Griswold, H. E. & Starr, A. (1971) Influence of aortocoronary bypass surgery on left ventricular performance. *New England Journal of Medicine*, **284**, 1116–1120.

Rees, R. S. O. (1976) The watershed: a factor in coronary vein graft occlusion. *British Heart Journal*, **38**, 197–200.

Reeves, T. J., Oberman, A., Jones, W. B. & Sheffield, L. T. (1974) Natural history of angina pectoris. *American Journal of Cardiology*, **33**, 423–430.

Rosati, R. A. (1975) Coronary artery surgery: critical appraisal. Unpublished data presented at Royal Society of Medicine conference, 6th June.

Selden, R., Neill, W. A., Ritzmann, L. W., Okies, J. E. & Anderson, R. P. (1975) Medical versus surgical therapy for acute coronary insufficiency. *New England Journal of Medicine*, **293**, 1329–1333.

Sheldon, W. C., Rincon, G., Effler, D. B., Proudfitt, W. L. & Sones, F. M. (1973) Vein graft surgery for coronary artery disease: survival and angiographic results in 1000 patients. *Circulation*, **48**, Suppl. III, 184–189.

Shlesinger, M. H. & Zoll, P. M. (1941) The incidence and localisation of coronary artery occlusions. *Archives of Pathology*, **32**, 178.

Tector, A. J. & McNabb, P. E. (1974) Direct coronary artery surgery for one year without an operative death. *Annals of Thoracic Surgery*, **17**, 345–350.

Vlodaver, Z. & Edwards, J. E. (1971) Pathologic changes in aortocoronary arterial saphenous vein grafts. *Circulation*, **44**, 719.

Walker, J. A., Friedberg, H. D., Flemma, R. J. & Johnson, W. D. (1972) Determinants of angiographic patency of aortocoronary vein bypass grafts. *Circulation*, **45**, Suppl. I, 86.

Yarborough, J. W., Roberts, W. C., Abel, R. M. & Reis, R. L. (1972) The cause of luminal narrowing in internal mammary arteries implanted into canine myocardium. *American Heart Journal*, **84**, 507.

SURGICAL TREATMENT OF TACHYCARDIAS

Cobb, F. R., Blumenschein, S. D., Sealy, W. C., Boineau, J. P., Wagner, G. S. & Wallace, A. G. (1968) Successful surgical interruption of the bundle of Kent in a patient with Wolff–Parkinson–White syndrome. *Circulation*, **38**, 1018.

Fontaine, G., Guiraudon, G., Frank, R., Gerbaux, A., Couteau, J. P., Barillou, A., Gay, J., Cabrol, C. & Facquet, J. (1975) La cartographie épicardique et le traitement chirurgical par simple ventriculotomie de certaines tachycardies ventriculaires rebelles par réentrée. *Archives des maladies du coeur et des vaisseaux*, **68**, 113.

Gallagher, J. J., Gilbert, M., Svenson, R. H., Sealy, W. C., Kassel, J. & Wallace, A. G. (1975) Wolff–Parkinson–White syndrome. The problem, evaluation and surgical correction. *Circulation*, **51**, 767.

Goldreyer, B. N. & Bigger, J. T. (1971) The site of re-entry in paroxysmal supraventricular tachycardia in man. *Circulation*, **43**, 15.

Graham, A. F., Craig Miller, D., Stinson, E. B., Daily, P. O., Fogarty, T. J. & Harrison, D. C. (1973) Surgical treatment of refractory life threatening ventricular tachycardia. *American Journal of Cardiology*, **32**, 909.

James, T. N. (1963) The connecting pathways between the sinus node and AV node and between the right and left atrium in the human heart. *American Heart Journal*, **66**, 498.

Kent, A. F. S. (1893) Researches on the structure and function of the mammalian heart. *Journal of Psychology*, **14**, 233.

Mahaim, I. (1947) Kent's fibres and paraspecific conduction through the upper connections of the bundle of His-Tawara. *American Heart Journal*, **33**, 651.

Spurrell, R. A. J., Sowton, E. & Deuchar, D. C. (1973) Ventricular tachycardia in four patents evaluated by programmed electrical stimulation of heart and treated in two patients by surgical division of anterior radiation of left bundle branch. *British Heart Journal*, **35**, 1014.

Spurrell, R. A. J., Yates, A. K., Thorburn, C. W., Sowton, G. E. & Deuchar, D. C. (1975) Surgical treatment of ventricular tachycardia after epicardial mapping studies. *British Heart Journal*, **37**, 115.

Thind, G. S., Blakemore, W. S. & Zinsser, H. F. (1971) Ventricular aneurysmectomy for the treatment of recurrent ventricular tachyarrhythmia. *American Journal of Cardiology*, **27**, 690.

Wellens, H. J. J., Schuilenburg, R. M. & Durrer, D. (1972) Electrical stimulation of the heart in patients with ventricular tachycardia. *Circulation*, **46**, 216.

Wolff, L., Parkinson, J. & White, P. D. (1930) Bundle branch block with short PR interval in healthy young people prone to paroxysmal tachycardia. *American Heart Journal*, **5**, 685.

INDEX

Note: Numbers in square brackets indicate the number of separate mentions on the page.

acebutolol
  elimination, 145, 146
  hypertension therapy, 250
acetyl strophanthidin, 438
actin, 267
adrenaline, inotropic effect, 272
α-adrenergic blocking drugs, 176, 192, 229, 388
  see also specific drugs
β-adrenergic blocking drugs, therapy with
  acute coronary insufficiency, 177
  angina pectoris, 171
    dosages, 175
    mechanism of action, 171
    side-effects, 174, 192
  arrhythmias, 163
  blood pressure control, 250
  cardiomyopathies, 184
  congestive heart failure, 184
  ectopic rhythms, 185
  Fallot's tetralogy, 184
  haemodynamic effects of, 245
  hypertension, 181, 229, 245–253
    along with other drugs, 250
    assessment, 253
    mode of action, 246
    selection of patients, 251
    side-effects, 252
  intermediate coronary syndrome, 71
  migraine, 193
  myocardial infarction, 66, 177
  phaeochromocytoma, 192
  psychiatric disturbances, 191
  side-effects of, 174, 192, 252
  subarachnoid haemorrhage, 185
  supraventricular tachycardias, 187
  surgery during, problems, 175
  thyrotoxicosis, 190
  see also specific drugs
adrenergic neurone inhibiting drugs (ANID)
  clinical use, 238
  haemodynamic effects, 236
  mode of action, 235
  side-effects, 238
  see also specific drugs

β-adrenoceptors, stimulation of, 377, 379
adrenocorticotrophic hormone-induced hypertension, 212
aerosols and arrhythmia, 137
airways resistance in heart failure, 377
ajmaline, 164
alcohol, 135, 185
alcoholism, propranolol therapy, 192
Aldactone see spironolactone
aldosterone, 200
  assay, 205
  in heart failure, 384, 403, 404
aldosterone antagonists, 418
alprenolol, 180, 247, 250
amiloride, 231, 233, 419
aminoglutethimide, 208
aminophylline, 418
amiodarone, 162
amitriptylene, 136
amoxycillin, 459
amphetamine inhibition of antihypertensives, 239
amphotericin B, 461, 462, 467
ampicillin, 458, 459, 460, 464
anaesthesia and arrhythmia, 135, 186
aneurysms, ventricular
  radiological diagnosis, 12, 32, 47, 48
  resection, 140, 496
angina
  with normal coronary arteries, 175
  myocardial oxygen consumption in, 171, 175, 309
  radiological investigation, 45, 48, 52
  treatment
    β-adrenergic blocking drugs, 171
    vein grafting, 59, 72, 486
angina, crescendo, 71
angina, Prinzmetal's variant, 71, 175, 176, 177
angina decubitus, 176
angiography, 31
  in diagnosing congenital heart disease, 11, 473
  of left ventricle, 47, 315, 330 [2]
    wall movements, 321, 322, 326, 329

angiography—*continued*
of saphenous vein grafts, 59
angiotensin, 200, 384, 404
annuloplasty, 485
Anrep effect, 302
Ansolysen *see* pentolinium tartrate
antacids and digoxin, 434
antazoline, 164
antibiotics, use in infective endocarditis, 457, 462
see also specific antibiotics
antidepressants, tricyclic, 135, 187, 236, 239
antidiuretic hormone (ADH) and hyponatraemia, 412
anxiety
ectopic rhythms in, 135, 185, 188
treatment of, 191
aorta
coarctation, surgical treatment, 1, 474, 476
malposition, 5, 19
stenosis
surgical treatment, 1, 4, 479
ultrasound investigation, 15
transposition, 5, 20, 473, 478
surgical treatment, 477, 479
aorta-left ventrical tunnel, 11
aortic valve
infection, 453, 464
replacement, 464, 484, 485, 488
aortocoronary bypass, 71, 486, 496
aortopulmonary window, 474
aprindine, 164
Arfonad *see* trimethapan
arrhythmias
contributory factors, 135
ECG features of, 81–130
early post-infarction, 64, 132
prevention, 178
ectopic, 135, 185, 415
see also bradycardia and tachycardia
arteries, great
malposition, 5, 19
transposition, 5, 20, 473, 478
surgical treatment, 477, 479
arthralgia in infective endocarditis, 450, 451
atenolol, 172
elimination, 146
in treatment of
angina, 173, 177
hypertension, 182, 247, 250
myocardial infarction, 180
atheroma and hypertension, 218
atria, physical properties, 293
atrial septal defect
effect of ventricular stiffness in, 291
management of, 473, 478
surgical, 1
myocardial biopsy in, 358
ultrasonic investigation, 14

atrioventricular block, ECG diagnosis, 92, 101
atrioventricular canal defects, surgery in, 476, 477
atrioventricular dissociation, 102
atropine therapy
postinfarction arrhythmias, 64, 178
sinoatrial block, 89
autonomic nervous system in cardiac control, 378, 381, 382

balloon pumping, intra-aortic (IABP), 69, 390
balloon septostomy, 473, 478 [2], 479
bendrofluazide, 232
benzothiadiazines, 230, 232
bethanidine
clinical use, 230, 238, 250
mode of action, 235
side-effects, 238
bioavailability, definition, 427
biopharmaceutics, definition, 427
biopsy, myocardial, 349–367
in assessing myocardial function, 361
bioptome, 351, 352, 358, 362
technique, 353
catheter, 350, 362
complications, 362
criteria for use, 349
damage artefact in, 358
diagnostic value, 355
drill, 350
enzymatic analysis in, 364
examination of specimen, 353
indications for, 352
needle, 349, 352, 358
reliability, 361
in studying effects of drugs, 361
bioptome, 351
see also biopsy, myocardial
Blalock–Taussig procedure, 6, 7, 475
blocks *see* specific types of block
Bowditch effect, 300
Bracht–Wächter bodies, 451, 465
bradycardia, 85
early post-infarction, 64
induced by β-adrenergic blockade, 171, 172, 174, 183
sinus, 85
breathlessness, 370, 371
bretylium tosylate, 163
bumetanide, 418

cachexia, cardiac, 408, 410, 411
caffeine, 135, 185, 301
calcium supply to heart, 266, 271, 272
in hypertrophy, 278
in ischaemia, 281
role in contraction, 300, 301

Candida endocarditis, 453, 454, 456, 466
  treatment, 460, 461
cannulation in infants, 2
carbenoxalone sodium, 212
carbonoic anhydrase inhibitors, 417
cardiac ballet, 123
cardiac cycle, 303
cardiomyopathy
  alcoholic, 307, 350, 361
  biopsy in, 349, 350, 356, 357, 361
  classification, 356
  congestive
    biopsy in, 357, 359, 361, 363
    ejection fraction, 339
    ventricular walls in, 334
  ejection fraction in, 338
  hypertrophic, 184
    β-adrenergic blocking drugs in, 184
    biopsy in, 357, 362, 364
    ejection fraction, 339
    ultrasound diagnosis, 16
    ventricular walls in, 333, 334
  myocardial changes in, 306
  obliterative, biopsy in, 357
  repolarisation, 184
cardiopulmonary bypass, 1, 2, 3, 477
catecholamines
  and arrhythmias, 135
  in heart failure, 377
  and hypertension, 216
  inotropic effect, 271, 301
central nervous system, effect of β-adrenergic
    blocking drugs on, 247
cephalexin, 462, 463
cephalic vein graft, 487
cephaloridine, 461
cephalosporins, use in infective endocarditis,
    458, 461, 463, 464
cephalothin, 461
cephazolin, 461
charcoal, activated, and digoxin, 434
chest radiography, use in heart failure, 373
children
  cardiology, 1–25
  heart failure in, 370
  surgery in, 473
  see also infants
chlordiazepoxide, 163
chloroform, 135, 186
chlorothalidone, 230, 233
chlorothiazide, 230
chlorpromazine inhibition of antihyper-
    tensives, 239
cholestyramine and digitalis, 434, 438
clonidine
  clinical use, 229, 243
  haemodynamic effects, 243
  mode of action, 242
  renal effects, 243

clonidine—continued
  side-effects, 244
coliform endocarditis, 458, 466
compliance, myocardial, 290
  left ventricle, 333
  measurement, 289
congenital heart disease
  and infective endocarditis, 448, 467
  investigation of, 10–21
  surgical treatment, 1–10, 473, 474
    corrective, 474, 476
    palliative, 475
contraceptives, oral, hypertension, 215
contractility see muscle, contractility
contraction see muscle, contraction and
    ventricle, left, contraction
cor triatriatum, 2, 19
Cordilox see verapamil
coronary arteries
  anatomy, 52
  calcification, 45
  disease
    development of collateral pathways, 56
    patterns of, 56
    vein grafting in, 59, 72, 73, 486
  dominance in, 54
  spasm of, 175, 176, 177
coronary arteriography, 39, 45
  complications, 51
  indications for, 52
  interpretation in, 57
  projections for, 51
  recording findings in, 59
  technical considerations, 50
coronary care
  prehospital, 63
  see also intermediate coronary syndrome
    and myocardial infarction
coronary insufficiency, acute, 71, 176
coronary syndrome, intermediate, 71, 176
corticosterone and hypertension, 211
co-trimaxazole, 459, 462, 463
counterpulsation, 69, 389
Coxiella burnetii, see Q fever
Coxsackie B4 virus, 454
Cushing's syndrome, ACTH-dependent, 211,
    213
cyanosis in infancy, 473
3′: 5′-cyclic adenosine monophosphate
    (cyclic AMP) in inotropic mecha-
    nisms, 272, 381
cyclopenthiazide, 232
cyclopropane, 186
cyclothiazide, 230

debrisoquine
  clinical use, 230, 239
  mode of action, 235

debrisoquine—*continued*
  side-effects, 238
defibrillation, electrical, 134, 138
dehydration, 417
dental surgery, infective endocarditis and, 462
deoxycorticosterone, role in hypertension, 209
dexamethasone, 210, 211
dextrocardia, 20
diabetes, anti-hypertensives and, 234, 253
diagnosis
  radioisotope, 27–43
  ultrasound, 13–21
diastole *see* myocardium, dilatation *and* ventricle, left, dilatation
diazepam, 163
diazoxide, 228
digitalis
  in angina therapy, 173, 174
  and arrhythmias, 108, 115, 117, 139, 186, 414
    effect of potassium depletion on, 415
  in atrial fibrillation therapy, 189
  clinical pharmacokinetics, 425–445
    use of assays in, 425
  in heart failure, 385, 413, 474
    dose, 415
  inotropic effectiveness, 414
  mechanism of action, 413
digitalis leaf, 431
digitoxin, 431
  bioavailability, 431, 434
  elimination, 145, 438
  plasma protein binding, 435
  toxicity, 438
digoxin
  absorption, 427
    gastrointestinal, 431
    inhibition of, 434
  distribution to tissues, 435
  dosage calculation, 438
  elimination, 145, 437
  plasma protein binding, 435
  radioimmunoassay, 425
  in stimulation of arrhythmias, 135
  toxicity, 416, 429, 441
  in treatment of tachyarrhythmias, 133, 134, 135
digoxin, methyl, 431
digoxin tablets
  bioavailability, variations in, 427
    clinical effects of, 428
  pharmaceutical standards, 429
dihydrallazine, 251
16α, 18-dihydroxy-deoxycorticosterone, 211
Dilantin *see* phenytoin
diphenylhydantoin and digitoxin, 438

disopyramide (Rythmodan, Norpace), 142
  pharmacokinetics, 146, 161
  therapy, 161
    side-effects, 162
diuretics
  and hypokalaemia, 233, 407, 416
  influence on aldosterone, 404
  and sodium retention, 418
  in treatment of
    heart failure, 404
      congestive, 417, 474
    hypertension, 230
      mechanism, 231
      side-effects, 233
    reninism, 201
dobutamine, 386, 388
dopamine, 217, 386
drip sites, infection from, 454, 456, 461, 466
drug addiction
  β-adrenergic blockade, 191
  infective endocarditis in, 453, 454, 456
drugs
  β-adrenergic blocking *see* β-adrenergic blocking drugs
  anti-arrhythmic
    bioavailability, 144
    classification, 140
    pharmacodynamics, 147
  anti-hypertensive, 67, 227–261
  diuretic, 417
  inotropic, 385
  vasodilator, 67, 387
  see also specific drugs and groups of drugs
ductus arteriosus
  prevention of closure, 476
  surgical treatment, 1, 474, 476
  ultrasound investigation, 15
dyskinesis, 48

Ebstein's anomaly, 19, 473
echocardiography *see* ultrasound
edrophonium, 133
Einsemenger syndrome, 4
ejection fraction, 338
electrical defibrillation *see* shock, d.c.
electrocardiography in arrhythmia diagnosis, 82
electrography, intracardiac, 83
  see also His bundle electrograms
endocardial cushion defect, 11, 12, 14
endocarditis, infective, 447–471
  assessment after recovery, 467
  clinical features, 449
  in drug addicts, 453, 454
    treatment, 459, 460
  experimental model, 454
  laboratory diagnosis, 455
    negative blood cultures in, 456

endocarditis, infective—*continued*
  mortality, 448, 467
  organisms causing
    bacterial, 448, 453, 454
      mixed, 460
    fungal, 453, 454, 456
    rickettsial, 453, 456
    viral, 457
      see also specific organisms
  prophylaxis, 462
  treatment
    antibiotic, 457
    surgical, 464
endocarditis, non-bacterial thrombotic, 454, 456
Epanutin *see* phenytoin
erythromycin, 463
ethacrynic acid, 231, 233, 418
excitation–contraction coupling, 265
  calcium in, 301
  in cardiac hypertrophy, 278, 402
  in ischaemia, 281
extrasystoles, 104

failure *see* heart failure
Fallot's tetralogy, 474
  β-adrenergic blockade in, 184
  surgical treatment, 1, 3, 475, 477, 478
    palliative, 476
    side-effects, 477
  ultrasound investigation, 15
fibrillation
  atrial, 115
    management, 133, 134, 189, 495
  ventricular, 116
    transient, 123
fluid depletion, 417
fluid retention, 399, 401, 402
fluorocarbons and arrhythmia, 137
5-fluorocytosine, 461, 462
Fluothane *see* halothane
flutter, atrial, 115
  management, 133, 134, 189, 495
Fontan operation, 4, 7, 8, 9
Framingham survey, 392
Frank–Starling mechanism, 288, 289, 292, 377, 378
frusemide, 231, 233, 405, 418, 419

gamma cameras, 30
gentamicin, 458, 464
Gerbode defect, 2, 19
Glenn operation, 6, 7, 8, 479
glomerular filtration rate in heart failure, 384, 403
  effect of diuretics, 418
glomerulonephritis in infective endocarditis, 452
glue sniffing, 137

glycosides, cardiac
  assay, 425, 438
  bioavailability, 431
  inotropic effect, 271
glycyrrhizic acid, 212
gout, 234
grafts *see* vein grafts
Gram-negative bacteria and endocarditis, 448
guancydine, 251
guanethidine
  clinical use, 229, 238
  mode of action, 235
  side-effects, 238
gum disease and endocarditis, 462

haemangiopericytoma, 201
haemodialysis, infective endocarditis and, 459
haemorrhage in infective endocarditis, 450, 451
halothane (Fluothane), 135, 186
heart
  growth, 273
  stroke output, 271
heart failure, 369–423
  β-adrenergic blocking drugs and, 252, 253
  clinical manifestations, 369
  congestive, 399
    fluid retention, 399, 402
    fundamental disturbances, 399
    hyponatraemia in, 412
    potassium depletion, 407
    therapy
      β-adrenergic blocking drugs, 184
      bed rest, 419
      digitalis, 413
      diuretics, 417
  contractility in, 336, 380
  dilatation of ventricle in, 310
  laboratory investigation, 373
    by chest radiography, 373
    by physiological measurements, 374
  myocardial changes in, 306, 308, 309, 379
  natural history, 391
  physiological basis of, 377
  salt retention, 383
  treatment, 385
    drugs, 385
    mechanical assistance, 389
    metabolic support, 391
  water retention, 383, 399
heart muscle
  changes in reflex control in heart failure, 378
  contractility, 271, 297
    effect of load changes, 302
    heart rate and, 300
    in hypertrophy, 278, 309
    inotropic mechanisms, 271
    role of calcium, 301

heart muscle—*continued*
  contraction of, 265, 285, 292
    atrial, 293
    calcium in, 300
    elastic elements in, 286
    oxygen consumption and, 304
  fibre shortening, 271, 287, 292
  radioisotope scanning, 34
  stretching of, 287, 293
  see also myocardium *and* ventricle, left
      and ventricular muscle disease
heart rate and contractility, 300
His bundle
  block, 98
  electrograms, 84, 85, 92
  surgical interruption, 495
homovanillic acid, 217
hydrallazine, 229, 251
hydrochlorothiazide, 232
hydromotive pressure, 298
16β-hydroxy-dehydroepiandrosterone, 212
18-hydroxy-11-deoxycorticosterone, 211
11β-hydroxylase deficiency syndrome, 204
17α-hydroxylase deficiency syndrome, 203,
      211
hyperaldosteronism, 205, 211, 411
hyperglycaemia, diuretics and, 234
hyperkalaemia, 417
hypertension
  ACTH-induced, 212
  aetiology, 199–226
  catecholamines and, 216
  classification, 199
  environment and, 218
  heredity and, 203, 218
  high renin, 199
  labile, 217
  low renin, 203
    congenital, 203
    essential, 207
      tests for, 209
  malignant, 202
  neurogenic, 217
  oral contraceptives and, 215
  in pregnancy, 213
  prostaglandins and, 215, 218
  renal, 200
    renin activity in, 202
  sensitivity factors, 219
  treatment, 227–261
    β-adrenergic blocking drugs in, 181, 245
    adrenergic neurone inhibiting drugs in,
        235
    clonidine in, 242
    diuretics in, 230
    in emergency situations, 227
    methyldopa in, 239
hypertensive pulmonary vascular disease, 4

hypertrophy, cardiac, 273
  biochemical defects in, 276
  myocardial changes in, 306
  in myocardial response, 401
  protein synthesis in, 275
    role of amino acids, 276
  ventricular walls in, 333, 334
hyperuricaemia in diuretic therapy, 234
hypoglycaemia, 253
hypokalaemia *see* potassium depletion
hyponatraemia in congestive heart failure,
      412, 417
hypoplasia, 4, 9, 16
  left heart, 474
hypotension
  in ANID therapy, 237, 238, 239
  in methyldopa therapy, 241
hypotensive therapy in myocardial infarction,
      67
hypothermia in treatment of congenital
      heart disease, 1[2], 477, 478, 479

IHSS *see* subaortic stenosis, idiopathic
      hypertrophic
immune complex phenomena in infective
      endocarditis, 450
impotence after myocardial infarction, 74
infants
  cyanosis in, 473
  surgery in, 2, 3, 473, 474
infarctectomy, 72
intra-aortic balloon pumping (IABP), 69, 390
intraventricular block, 99
ischaemia, 279
  fatty acid metabolism in, 280
  glycolysis in, 279
  mitochondrial function in, 280, 307
  myocardial changes in, 307, 308
  and oxygen supply and demand, 305
  radiological investigation, 34, 38
  revascularisation in, 486
  sarcoplasmic reticulum function in, 281
  ventricular wall movements in, 327, 330,
      331
isoprenaline, 125, 386
Isoptin *see* verapamil
isosorbide dinitrate, 388
isotopes, 28, 29

Janeway lesions, 451
joints in infective endocarditis, 450

kanamycin, 458 [2]
kaopectate and digoxin, 434
kidney disease
  hypertension in, 201
  in infective endocarditis, 452
kidneys
  in heart failure, 384, 402, 413

kidneys—*continued*
  role in hypertension, 199
    in pregnancy, 214

labetolol, 229, 250
laevocardia, 20
lanatoside C, 431 [2]
Lanoxin, 430
Laplace, law of, 295, 319
Liddle's syndrome, 205
lidocaine *see* lignocaine
lignocaine (lidocaine, Xylocaine), 149
  pharmacokinetics, 144, 145, 146, 150
  therapy, 64, 150, 178, 187
liquorice and hypertension, 212
liver in heart failure, 384
Lown–Ganong–Levine syndrome, 115

magnesium trisilicate and digoxin, 434
mammary artery, internal, graft of, 487, 490
mannitol, 413, 418
Maxolon, 434
metabolism, cardiac, 263–284
  in hypertrophy, 276
  in ischaemia, 279
methyclothiazide, 230
methyldigoxin, 431
methyldopa
  cardiovascular effects, 240
  clinical use, 229, 241, 250
  mode of action, 239
  side-effects, 241
metoclorpropamide, 434
metopolol, 172, 173, 180, 250
mexiletine
  pharmacokinetics, 146, 147, 164
  therapy, 164
migraine, β-adrenergic blockade, 193
mineralocorticoid excess in hypertension, 208, 209, 212
minoxidil, 251
mitral valve
  congenital abnormalities, 11
  infection, 453, 464, 465
  regurgitation, 46, 49
  surgery, 72, 483, 484, 485, 488
  tricuspid dysfunction and, 481
Möbitz blocks
  type I, 86, 87, 94
  type II, 86, 87, 95
Mustard procedure, 6, 7, 479
myocardial infarction
  management, 63–79, 132, 150, 152
    β-adrenergic blocking drugs, 177
    limiting infarct size in, 65, 179
    metabolic changes of ischaemia and, 281
    pre-hospital, 63
    surgical, 72
  radiological investigation, 34, 46

myocardial infarction—*continued*
    rehabilitation, 73
myocardial ischaemia *see* ischaemia
myocarditis, myocardial biopsy in, 358
myocardium
  biopsy *see* biopsy, myocardial
  blood flow, 38
  contractility, 271, 297
    assessment of, 336
    effect of load changes, 302
    heart rate and, 300
    in hypertrophy, 278, 309, 401
    role of calcium, 301
  contraction, 265, 285, 286, 292
    see also ventricle, left, contraction
  dilatation, 332
    see also ventricle, left, dilatation
    in failing heart, 380
  force-velocity relationships in, 294, 336
  Frank–Starling mechanism in, 292
  in infective endocarditis, 465
  jeopardised, 65
  mechanical performance, 285–314
    assessment in heart disease, 285, 375
    integration of, 303
  metabolism, 265
  oxygen consumption, 65
    angina and, 171, 175
    mechanics of contraction and, 304
  physical properties, 286
    changes in disease, 289
      hypertrophic, 306
      primary myocardial, 307
  radiological investigation, 35
  revascularisation, 486
  ultrastructure, 263
myofibrils, protein components, 267
myosin, 267
  in cardiac hypertrophy, 276, 277
  light chain subunits, 270
myosin ATP-ase
  control of, 268
  in hypertrophy, 277
myxoma, left atrial, 457

neomycin and digoxin, 434
nitroglycerin therapy, 67, 388
nitroprusside therapy, 228, 229, 388
noradrenaline
  cardiac stimulation, 379
  in treatment of heart failure, 386
Norpace *see* disopyramide

obesity and hypertension, 218
oestrogens and hypertension, 215
Osler's nodes, 450, 451
ostium primum defect, 2, 14
ouabain, 142, 414, 431, 438
oxprenolol, 172, 173, 174, 180, 250

oxygen
  consumption, myocardial, 65
    angina and, 171, 175, 309
    in heart failure, 310
    and mechanics of contraction, 304
  supply/demand, ischaemia and, 305

pacemakers
  in initiation of reciprocal tachycardia, 140
  after valve replacement, 484
pain, anginal, 370, 371
parasympathetic system *see* autonomic nervous system
parasystole, 109
Parkinson's disease, β-adrenergic blockade, 191
penicillin
  hypersensitivity to, 461
  use in infective endocarditis, 457 [2], 458, 459
    intravenous, 460, 463
pentolinium tartrate (Ansolysen), 229
perhexiline, 163
pericardial effusions, radioisotope diagnosis, 31
phaeochromocytoma
  effect of adrenergic neurone blockers in, 236
  and hypertension, 216, 228
  treatment, 192
Phenhydan, 157
phenobarbitone and digoxin, 438
phenothiazines and arrhythmia, 136
phenoxybenzamine, 192, 250
phentolamine, 68, 192, 388
phenylbutazone and digitoxin, 438
phenytoin (Epanutin, Dilantin)
  pharmacokinetics, 144, 145, 146, 158
  therapy, 157, 187
  side-effects, 160
phthalimidines, 230, 232
pindolol, 172
  therapy, 180, 247, 250
polythiazide, 230, 233
potassium depletion
  and arrhythmia, 137, 410, 415
  in congestive heart failure, 407
  and digoxin toxicity, 137, 416
  in diuretic therapy, 233, 407, 416
  treatment of, 233, 411, 418
potassium excess, 417
Pott's operation, 475
practolol, 172
  elimination, 145, 146
  haemodynamic effects, 245
  therapy
    angina, 172, 173 [2], 174
    anxiety, 191
    atrial fibrillation, 189

practolol therapy—*continued*
    cardiomyopathy, 184
    hypertension, 182, 245, 250
      mode of action, 247
    myocardial infarction, 66, 179, 180
    side-effects, 252, 253
prazosin hydrochloride, 251
preductal coarctation, 474
pre-eclamptic toxaemia, 213
pregnancy, hypertension in, 213
prenylamine, 163
Prinzmetal's variant angina, 71, 175, 176, 177
probenecid, 459
procainamide (Pronestyl), 149
  elimination, 145, 146
  metabolism, 144
  pharmacokinetics, 144, 145, 146, 152
  therapy, 151
    side-effects, 152, 153
procaine, 151
Pronestyl *see* procainamide
pronethanol, 245
propantheline, 434
propranolol, 142, 172, 182
  haemodynamic effects, 245, 246
  pharmacokinetics, 144, 145, 146
  therapy
    angina, 172, 173 [2], 174, 175 [2]
    hypertension, 183, 245
      along with other drugs, 250
      mode of action, 247 [2], 248 [3]
    intermediate coronary syndrome, 71, 177
    myocardial infarction, 66, 180
    psychiatric disturbances, 191, 192
    side-effects, 252
propranolol, dimethyl quaternary derivative of, 164
prostaglandins and hypertension, 218
  in pregnancy, 215
proteins, contractile, 267
  in cardiac hypertrophy, 275, 277
  synthesis, 274
psittacosis, infective endocarditis in, 457
pulmonary artery
  banding of, 476, 479
  malposition, 5, 19
  transposition, 5, 20, 473
    surgical treatment, 477
pulmonary atresia, 474
  blood supply in, 10
  surgical treatment, 9, 477
pulmonary emboli, radioisotope diagnosis, 31, 46
pulmonary stenosis
  surgical treatment, 1, 4, 479
  ultrasound investigation, 18
pulmonary valve
  infection of, 453
  obstruction at, 473

pulmonary venous connection, anomalous, 478
  surgical treatment, 1, 2, 477, 478
  ultrasound investigation, 20
pumps, 389

Q-fever (*Coxiella burnetii*) endocarditis, 453, 456, 458, 466
quinidine, 149
  pharmacokinetics, 144, 145, 146, 155, 156
  therapy, 154
    side-effects, 155

radioisotope diagnosis, 27–43
Rastelli operation, 4, 5
regurgitation, volume of, radiological investigation, 33, 46, 49
rehabilitation, 73
renal artery stenosis, hypertension in, 201
renin, release of
  in classification of hypertension, 199
  during oral contraception, 215
  effect of β-adrenergic blocking drugs on, 182, 183, 247
  in heart failure, 377, 384, 404
  in pregnancy, 214
renin-angiotensin system, 200
  inhibitors, 200, 203
reninism, 201
reserpine, 229
rheumatic heart disease
  endocarditis and, 448, 449
  tricuspid dysfunction and, 481, 482
rifampicin, 466
Roth's spots, 450, 451
Rythmodan *see* disopyramide

salbutamol, 388
salt
  dilution, in heart failure, 412
  intake, and hypertension, 218
  retention, in heart failure, 383, 402
    aldosterone and, 418
    diuretic therapy and, 417, 418
saphenous vein grafts, 59, 72, 487
  fate of, 489
Sapirstein principle, 38
saralasin, 200, 203
sarcolemma, 264, 307
sarcomere, 267
  in contraction, 271, 287, 292
    measurement, 288
  in diastole, 288, 293
  in hypertrophy, 308
sarcoplasmic reticulum, 264
  calcium uptake by, 172, 266, 300, 301
    in ischaemia, 281
scanners, radioisotope, 29

scanning
  cold spot, 34
  hot spot, 34, 35
schizophrenia, β-adrenergic blockade, 191
septum, defects of *see* atrial/ventricular septal defects
shock
  d.c., in treatment of arrhythmias, 134, 138
  post-infarction, treatment, 69
shunts, intracardiac, radiological diagnosis, 33
sickle cell syndrome and hyponatraemia, 412
sinoatrial block
  ECG diagnosis, 86–92
  management, 89
sodium *see* salt
sodium nitroprusside, 228, 229, 387
sotalol, 172, 178, 180, 247, 250
spironolactone (Aldactone) therapy
  effect on digoxin excretion, 437
  in heart failure, 405, 419
  in hypertension, 205, 210, 211, 212 [2], 231, 233
    side-effects, 234
staphylococcal endocarditis, 448, 449
  in drug addicts, 453
  post-operative, 466
  therapy, 459, 460 [2], 466
Staphylococcus albus, 466
Staphylococcus aureus, 448, 449, 453
streptococcal endocarditis, 448, 449
  prophylaxis, 463
  therapy, 459, 461
Streptococcus bovis, 448
Streptococcus faecalis, 448, 454
Streptococcus mitior, 448
Streptococcus mutans, 448
Streptococcus pyogenes, 449
Streptococcus salivarius, 448
Streptococcus sanguis, 448
Streptococcus viridans, 448, 454, 459 [2], 467
streptokinase therapy, 71
streptomycin, use in infective endocarditis
  prophylaxis, 463 [2], 464
  treatment, 457, 458, 459, 460
stress, estimation of, 319, 323, 333
subaortic stenosis, 15
  idiopathic hypertrophic (IHSS), 16
subarachnoid haemorrhage, β-adrenergic blockade in, 185
sulphonamides in infective endocarditis, 457, 458
supra-aortic stenosis, 16
surgery, 473–500
  bypass, 59, 72, 486, 496
  for congenital heart disease, 1–10, 473
  dental *see* dental surgery
  during β-adrenergic blockade, 175
  infective endocarditis following, 459

surgery—*continued*
  in infective endocarditis treatment, 464
    post-operative infection, 466
  in tachycardias, 494
  in tricuspid valve disease, 483
sympathetic nervous system
  cardiac stimulation by, 301, 379
    in heart failure, 377, 379
  and hypertension, 217
  stimulation of arrhythmia, 135, 185
systole *see* myocardium, contraction

tachycardia, 101
  contributory factors, 135
  diagnosis, 101, 131
    ECG analysis in, 101
  ectopic
    atrial, 113, 114
    paroxysmal, 103, 113, 114, 123
    supraventricular, treatment, 133
    treatment, 497
    ventricular, 113, 123
  idioventricular, 125
  management, 132
    drugs used in, 140
    early post-infarction, 64, 132
    surgical, 494
  mechanism, 494
  paroxysmal, 103, 113
    atrial, 82, 114, 133, 134
    supraventricular, 114, 188, 495
    treatment, 133, 495
    ventricular, 103, 122
      benign, 126
    see also fibrillation/flutter
  re-entry (reciprocal, reciprocating)
    paroxysmal, 103, 113, 123, 188
    supraventricular, 117, 495
    treatment, 133, 138, 187, 495
    ventricular, 123, 496
  sinus, treatment, 133, 190
tetracycline, use in infective endocarditis,
    458, 462, 463, 466
thrombolytic therapy in myocardial infarc-
    tion, 20
thymoxamine, 192
thyrotoxicosis, 190, 191
timolol, 250
tobacco, 135
tolamolol, 173
torsade de pointes, 123
transplantation, serial biopsies in, 360
tremor, treatment, 191
triamterene, 205, 231, 233
trichloroethylene (Trilene), 186
tricuspid pouch, 12
tricuspid valve
  acquired dysfunction, 480
    haemodynamic assessment, 482

tricuspid valve—*continued*
    pathology, 481
    surgical treatment, 483
      indication for, 482
  anatomy, 481
  Ebstein's anomaly of, 19
  infection, 453, 454, 481
  obstruction at (tricuspid atresia), 7, 473,
    479
  replacement, 483
    post-operative care, 484
    technique of, 484
trifascicular block, 99
Trilene *see* trichlorethylene
trimethaphan (Arfonad), 68, 229
trimethoprim, 458
triamterene, 419
tropomyosin (Tm), 267, 268, 270
troponin (Tn), 267, 268, 270
  components, 269
truncus arteriosus, persistent, 474
  surgical treatment, 4, 5, 477
    palliative, 476
  ultrasound investigation, 20
tumours
  myocardial biopsy, 358, 362
  ultrasound investigation, 21
tyrosine hydroxylase, 379, 381

ultrasound investigation
  B-scan techniques of, 21, 319
  in congenital heart disease, 13
  in infective endocarditis, 457, 464, 466
  left ventricle, 318, 322, 331
    wall movements, 327, 328, 329

Valsalva manoeuvre, 375
valves
  infection of, 453, 464
  regurgitation by, 33
  replacement, 1, 72, 464, 483, 488
    in children, 10
    infection following, 454, 456, 462, 466
  see also specific valves
valvotomy, 1
  aortic, 479
  pulmonary, 4, 479
vancomycin, 463 [2]
vasodilator drugs, 67, 387
vein grafts, to coronary artery, 59, 72, 486
  long term effects, 489
  results of, 491
  risks in, 488
ventricle, left
  aneurysms, radiological investigation, 47,
    48
  angiography, 47, 315, 322, 326, 328
  contractility, 336

ventricle, left—*continued*
  contraction pattern, 321
    disturbed contraction rates and, 328
    effect of abnormal architecture, 324
    effect of isovolumic shape changes, 330
    in heart failure, 375
    incoordinate, 326
  dilatation, 324, 332
  double outlet, surgical treatment, 6
  echocardiography, 318, 322, 327
  ejection fraction in, 338
  end-diastolic pressure in, 339
  filling pressure, and heart failure, 285, 374, 399
  function, clinical assessment, 315–347
    effect of vein graft on, 490, 493
    in heart failure, 374
  pressure-volume relations in, 333
  stress in walls of, 319, 323, 333
  volume of, 316
ventricle, right
  double outlet, 5, 19
  outflow tract, reconstruction, 4, 6
ventricle, single, 6, 9, 19, 474, 476
ventricles, distension of, 291, 293
ventricles, walls of
  abnormal movement, 48, 326, 329, 330

ventricles, walls of—*continued*
  estimation of stress, 319, 323, 333
  isovolumic movements, 330
  stiffness, 290, 333, 334, 399
ventricular muscle disease, 4, 9, 16
ventricular septal defect (VSD), 12, 474, 477
  radiological investigation, 46, 49
  surgical, treatment, 1, 2, 3, 72, 477, 478
    palliative, 476
  ultrasound investigation, 15
verapamil (Cordilox, Isoptin), 119, 139, 142, 160
videodensitometry, 317, 322

water retention in heart failure, 383, 402, 412
Waterston's operation, 475
Wedensky effect, 98
Wedensky facilitation, 98
Wedensky phenomena, 98
Wenckebach phenomenon, 86, 87, 94
Wolff–Parkinson–White syndrome, 114, 187, 494
  ECG features, 115, 118, 119
  management, 134, 139, 495

Xylocaine *see* lignocaine